Fundamentals of Immunohematology:
THEORY AND TECHNIQUE

Fundamentals of Immunohematology:
THEORY AND TECHNIQUE

MARY LOUISE TURGEON, Ed. D., MT(ASCP)

Assistant Director of Medical Education,
Robert Packer Hospital/Guthrie Medical Center
Sayre, Pennsylvania
Medical Educational Consultant
Mary L. Turgeon & Associates
Waverly, New York
Clinical Assistant Professor of Pathology
University of North Dakota, School of Medicine
Grand Forks, North Dakota

Lea & Febiger Philadelphia • London • 1989

Lea & Febiger
200 Chester Field Parkway
Malvern, Pennsylvania 19355-9725
U.S.A.
(215) 251-2230

**Cover art courtesy of
Ortho Diagnostic Systems, Inc.**

Library of Congress Cataloging-in-Publishing Data

Turgeon, Mary Louise.
    Fundamentals of immunohematology.

    Includes index.
    1. Blood banks. 2. Immunohematology. I. Title.
[DNLM: 1. Blood Grouping and Crossmatching—methods.
2. Blood Groups—immunology. 3. Blood Transfusion—
methods. WH 420 T936f]
RM172.T84 1989   615′.39   88-37253
ISBN 0-8121-1217-2

PRINTED IN THE UNITED STATES OF AMERICA
Print Number 3 2

*To my husband, parents, and family for their unwavering support
of my professional and personal goals*

Preface

Fundamentals of Immunohematology has been written to meet the needs of undergraduate clinical laboratory science students, educators, and blood bank personnel for a book that encompasses the concepts, clinical practices, and techniques associated with modern transfusion therapy. Students, educators, and practitioners in other allied health disciplines, nursing, and medicine can also use the book as a primary blood banking-transfusion therapy reference.

The purpose of this book is to integrate the basic foundations of blood banking with the technical aspects of the discipline and clinical real-world problems. Beginning with important safety and quality assurance information, the book progresses to theoretic concepts and technical issues of importance such as pretransfusion testing, blood components and synthetic blood substitutes, transfusion reactions, and blood-borne infectious diseases. It concludes with general and special procedural protocols that conform to the recommended format of the National Commission on Clinical Laboratory Standards (NCCLS) and a discussion of new directions in serologic testing. Basic genetic concepts are not reiterated in this book because molecular genetics and Mendelian principles are presented in general college biology courses and other clinical courses. Genetic applications, however, are given in appropriate chapters.

Specific chapter objectives are presented at the beginning of each chapter for the convenience of students who wish to use them to focus on the expected learning outcomes of the chapter. Topical outlines are placed at the beginning of each chapter to assist students in the organization of each chapter, may be of use to instructors in preparing lectures. Illustrations and diagrams are used to clarify conceptual themes. Tables are included to summarize complex content.

Thirty-one serologic case studies, each with a complete discussion, have been organized into a separate chapter for ease of use. These patient examples enhance the integration of theory and practice. Additional case studies and numerous examples are presented throughout the book. At the conclusion of each chapter, a chapter summary and licensure-type review questions, appropriate for preparation for the National Certifying Agency (NCA) or Board of Registry examinations, are provided. Because *Fundamentals of Immunohematology* is intended for medical laboratory technology/clinical laboratory techician (MLT/CLT) and medical technology/clinical laboratory science (MT/CLS) students and practitioners, some portions of the book may not be applicable to CLT students.

M. L. TURGEON
Waverly, N.Y.

Acknowledgments

My objective in writing *Fundamentals of Immunohematology* was to integrate the basic theory and current information in blood banking with real-world applications. This book has provided me with the opportunity to share my perspectives and experience as a practitioner and educator with others.

I would like to thank those at Lea & Febiger who have assisted me in this pursuit. Special thanks to Christian C. "Kit" Febiger Spahr, Jr. for his interest in my work and his continuing support of this project, and Jessica Martin for her editorial assistance. An additional thank you to Sam Rondinelli for his superb attention to every aspect of the production of this book, and to Terri Siegel for translating my book cover concepts into an outstanding cover design.

I also want to express gratitude to James A. Terzian, M. D., St. Joseph's Hospital, Elmira, New York; Zissis Vesoulis, M. D., Guthrie Medical Center/ Robert Packer Hospital, Sayre, Pennsylvania; and Jane Banzhaf, Ed.D., MT(ASCP) SBB, Rochester Regional Red Cross, Rochester, New York, who generously gave of their time to review portions of the manuscript. Thanks also to my friend, Patrick J. Steed, R. Ph., Waverly, New York, for his assistance with the substances that can cause a positive direct antiglobulin test; to Polly F. Kay, MT(ASCP) MHS and Marion Hursey, School of Medical Technology, Anderson Memorial Hospital, Anderson, South Carolina for their case studies; and to Mary Judith (Judy) Horvath, St. Joseph's Hospital, Elmira, New York for assisting me with the case studies. I would also like to acknowledge the technical information and photographs provided by David Gibbons, Olympus Corporation, and Thomas Williams, Dynatech Laboratories, Inc. In addition, I wish to thank Robert Kalt, Marketing Services Manager, Ortho Diagnostics Systems, Inc., Raritan, New Jersey, for his assistance in procuring the photograph that has been used on the front and back cover. I sincerely appreciate the interest and efforts of all at Ortho Diagnostic Systems and Johnson & Johnson who assisted me with the cover photograph.

Finally, special thanks to Don Turgeon for his patience and support, and for once again contributing to the artistic elements of this my second book.

Contents

Part ONE

Basic Foundations

1

Safety and Quality Assurance in Blood Banking

At the conclusion of this chapter, the reader will be able to:
- Describe the role of the medical technologist or medical technician in providing quality patient care.
- List at least four functions of the blood bank.
- Explain the purpose and contents of a safety manual.
- Define the term "universal precautions."
- Discuss the five protective techniques in the prevention of disease transmission.
- Describe four important safety practices.
- Name two types of hazardous waste and describe the appropriate management and control of these wastes.
- Name the essential components of a quality assurance program.
- Describe the major techniques for establishing quality in the blood bank.
- Identify the daily quality assurance practices in the blood bank.

Chapter Outline

An Overview of Immunohematology

Safety in the Blood Bank
  Universal Blood and Body Fluid Precautions
  Occupational Transmission of HBV and HIV
  Protective Techniques for Infection Control
    Selection and Use of Gloves
      Gloves as a Barrier Protection for Phlebotomy
      Gloves as a Barrier Protection During Testing
      Facial Barrier Protection and Occlusive Bandages
      Laboratory Coats or Gowns as Barrier Protection
  Important Safety Practices
    Hand Washing
    Decontamination of Work Surfaces, Equipment, and Spills
    Needle Precautions
    Other Safety Precautions
  Hazardous Waste Management and Control
    Infectious Waste
    Chemical Hazards
  Safety Documents
    Compliance with Universal Precautions
    Compliance with Chemical Hazard Precautions

Quality Assurance in the Blood Bank
  Qualified Personnel
    Evaluation of Competence

    Maintaining Competence
  Established Blood Bank Policies and Procedures
  Established Quality Assurance Techniques
    Daily Practices
    Peer Review
    External Quality Control Programs
    Accuracy in Communications and Records
    Recognition and Resolution of Problems

Daily Quality Assurance Practices
  Quality Control of Reagents
    Daily Quality Control of Antisera
    Daily Quality Control of Reagent Red Cells
    Daily Reagent Control Records
  Quality Control of Equipment
    Centrifuges
    Waterbaths and Heat Blocks
    Refrigerators and Freezers
    Rh Viewing Boxes

Chapter Summary

Review Questions and Answers

Bibliography

AN OVERVIEW OF IMMUNOHEMATOLOGY

Immunohematology is a specialized branch of medical science. Efforts to save human lives by transfusing blood have been

3

recorded for centuries. Although most of the blood initially used for transfusions was of animal origin, an unsuccessful attempt to intravenously transfuse Pope Innocent VII with blood from three human donors was recorded in 1492. Because of the many disastrous consequences resulting from blood transfusions, transfusions were forbidden from 1667 until 1829, when James Blundell successfully transfused human blood to English women suffering from postpartum hemorrhage.

Blood transfusions continued to produce unpredictable results and were used only as a last resort until Landsteiner's historic discovery of the ABO blood groups in 1900. This landmark event initiated the era of scientifically based transfusion therapy and was the foundation of immunohematology as a science. Since World War II, the modern age of blood banking and transfusion therapy has flourished.

Medical technologists (clinical laboratory scientists) and technicians (clinical laboratory technicians) in the blood bank render a major service to the patient. To provide excellence in patient care through accurate, efficient, and cost-effective testing, the blood bank technologist or technician must be familiar with the *theory* and *practice* of a wide variety of procedures.

The scope of functions in a modern blood bank can include the following:

1. Recruiting blood donors
2. Collecting and storing whole blood or components from volunteer or autologous donors
3. Typing, screening, and preparing patient and donor blood for transfusion
4. Detecting and identifying antibodies in potential blood recipients or pregnant women
5. Establishing a data base to support suspected or potential disorders
6. Processing and dispensing blood components
7. Performing paternity testing
8. Conducting tissue typing prior to organ transplantation and participating in the processing of human materials (e.g., bone banking)

SAFETY IN THE BLOOD BANK

In 1983, the Centers for Disease Control (CDC) recommended that blood and body fluid precautions be taken when a patient was known or suspected to be infected with blood-borne pathogens. The rapid increase in the number of patients identified with human immunodeficiency virus (HIV) was partially responsible for a change in this initial recommendation. In August, 1987, the CDC published the document, "Recommendations for Prevention of HIV Transmission in Health-Care Settings" (MMWR, Supp. 2S, 1987). Additional safety guidelines under the title "Protection of Laboratory Workers from Infectious Disease Transmitted by Blood and Tissue" were proposed by the National Committee for Clinical Laboratory Standards (NCCLS Document M29-P, 1987). In 1988, the CDC issued clarifications of the original guidelines (MMWR, *37* (24), June, 1988).

Universal Blood and Body Fluid Precautions

The 1987 CDC document introduced the concept of *universal blood and body fluid precautions* or *universal precautions* to prevent parenteral, mucous membrane, and nonintact skin exposures of health-care workers to blood-borne pathogens. Under universal precautions, blood and certain body fluids of *all* patients are treated as potentially infectious for HIV, hepatitis B virus (HBV), and other blood-borne pathogens.

Occupational Transmission of HBV and HIV

Blood bank personnel should be aware of the fact that HBV and HIV are different diseases caused by unrelated viruses. The most feared hazard of all, the transmission of HIV through occupational exposure, is among the least likely to occur if proper safety practices are followed. Exposure to HIV is uncommon, but cases of occupational transmission to health-care personnel with no other known high-risk factors have been documented. Although HIV is an unlikely work-related hazard, its danger cannot be underrated because it is the cause of the fatal disease acquired immunodeficiency syndrome (AIDS). The transmission of HBV, which can also be fatal, is more probable than that of HIV.

Blood is the single most important source of HIV, HBV, and other blood-borne pathogens in the occupational setting. HBV can be present in extraordinarily high concentrations in blood, but HIV is usually found in lower concentrations. HBV may be stable in dried blood and blood products at 25°C for up to 7 days. HIV retains infectivity for more than 3 days in dried specimens at room temperature and for more than a week in an aqueous environment at room temperature. The likelihood of infection after exposure to blood infected with HBV or HIV depends on a variety of factors, including:

1. The concentration of HBV or HIV virus. Viral concentration is higher for HBV than for HIV.
2. The duration of the contact.
3. The presence of skin lesions or abrasions on the hands or exposed skin of the health care worker.
4. The immune status of the health care worker for HBV.

Although HIV has been isolated from blood, semen, vaginal secretions, saliva, tears, breast milk, cerebrospinal fluid (CSF), amniotic fluid, and urine, only blood, semen, vaginal secretions, and possibly breast milk have been implicated in transmission of HIV to date. Evidence for the role of saliva in the transmission of virus is unclear; however, universal precautions do not apply to saliva uncontaminated with blood.

HBV and HIV may be *directly* transmitted by:

1. Percutaneous (parenteral) inoculation of blood, plasma, serum, or certain other body fluids due to accidental needle punctures, etc.
2. Contamination of the skin with blood or certain body fluids without overt puncture because of scratches, abra-

sions, burns, weeping, or exudative skin lesions.
3. Exposure of mucous membranes (oral, nasal, or conjunctiva) to blood or certain body fluids as a direct result of pipetting by mouth, splashes, or splattering.
4. Centrifuge accidents or improper removal of rubber stoppers from test tubes, which can produce droplets. If these aerosol products are infectious and come in direct contact with mucous membranes or nonintact skin, direct transmission of virus can potentially occur.

HBV and HIV may be *indirectly* transmitted. Viral transmission can result from contact with inanimate objects such as work surfaces or equipment contaminated with infected blood or certain body fluids. If the virus is transferred to broken skin or mucous membranes by hand contact, this contact can produce viral exposure.

Protective Techniques for Infection Control

Universal precautions are intended to supplement rather than replace recommendations for routine infection control, such as hand washing. Infection control efforts for HIV, HBV, and other blood-borne pathogens must focus on prevention of exposure to blood. It is possible to be vaccinated against HBV, and this is a wise preventive measure. The risk of nosocomial transmission of HBV, HIV, and other blood-borne pathogens can be minimized if blood bank personnel are aware of and adhere to essential safety guidelines.

SELECTION AND USE OF GLOVES

Gloves for medical use are either sterile surgical or nonsterile examination gloves made of vinyl or latex. There are no reported differences in barrier effectiveness between intact latex and intact vinyl gloves. Tactile differences have been observed between the two types of gloves, with latex gloves providing more tactile sensitivity; however, either type is usually satisfactory for phlebotomy and as a protective barrier when performing technical procedures. Rubber household gloves may be used for cleaning procedures.

The general guidelines related to the selection and general use of gloves include the following:

1. Use sterile gloves for procedures involving contact with normally sterile areas of the body, or during procedures where sterility has been established and must be maintained. Use nonsterile examination gloves for procedures that do not require the use of sterile gloves.
2. Wear gloves when processing blood specimens, reagents, or blood products. Gloves should be changed frequently and immediately if they become visibly contaminated with blood or certain body fluids, or if physical damage occurs.
3. Do not wash or disinfect latex or vinyl gloves for reuse. Washing with detergents may cause increased penetration of liquids through undetected holes in the gloves. Rubber gloves may be decontaminated and reused, but disinfectants may cause deterioration. Rubber gloves should be discarded if they have punctures, tears, or evidence of deterioration, or if they peel, crack, or become discolored.

GLOVES AS A BARRIER PROTECTION FOR PHLEBOTOMY

Properly fitting vinyl or latex gloves do not interfere with the proper collection of samples from patients (see Chapter 2) or donors. The use of gloves reduces the incidence of blood contamination of hands during phlebotomy, but cannot prevent skin punctures caused by accidental sticking with a needle or other sharp objects. The likelihood of hand contamination with HIV, HBV, or other blood-borne pathogens depends on many factors, including the following:

1. The skill, technique, and experience of the phlebotomist.

2. The number of phlebotomies performed: the cumulative risk of blood exposure increases for phlebotomists who perform more procedures.
3. The circumstances under which the specimen is obtained: in emergency situations contact may be more likely.
4. The prevalence of either HBV or HIV in the patient or donor population.

As a result of the CDC modifications published in June, 1988, some institutions have relaxed recommendations for using gloves for phlebotomy procedures by skilled phlebotomists in settings where the prevalence of blood-borne pathogens is known to be very low, for example, volunteer blood donation centers. Institutions or organizations that choose to modify the policy of requiring gloves for all phlebotomies must periodically re-evaluate their policy and must provide gloves to all personnel who wish to use them for phlebotomy. The guidelines for the use of gloves during phlebotomy procedures include the following:

1. Gloves must be used by phlebotomists who have cuts, scratches, or other breaks in their skin. The presence of skin lesions increases the likelihood of infection after skin exposure.
2. Gloves should be worn when the phlebotomist judges that hand contamination may occur, e.g., when he/she is performing phlebotomy on an uncooperative patient.
3. Gloves must be worn when performing finger and/or heel sticks on infants and children.
4. Gloves must be worn by personnel receiving phlebotomy training.
5. Gloves should be changed between all patient contacts.

GLOVES AS A BARRIER PROTECTION DURING TESTING

Gloves should be worn when:

1. Handling blood, serum, plasma, or certain body fluids.
2. Handling blood or potentially infectious blood products, e.g., antisera of

human origin and reagent red blood cells.

3. Testing serum, plasma, or red blood cells.

4. Using items potentially contaminated with blood or certain body fluids, e.g., specimen containers, laboratory instruments, counter tops, etc.

Care must be taken to avoid indirect contamination of work surfaces or objects in the work area. Gloves should be properly removed or covered with an uncontaminated glove or paper towel before answering the telephone, handling laboratory equipment, or touching doorknobs.

FACIAL BARRIER PROTECTION AND OCCLUSIVE BANDAGES

Facial protection should be used if there is a potential for splashing or spraying of blood or certain body fluids. Masks or other facial protection should be worn if mucous membrane contact with blood or certain body fluid is anticipated. All disruptions of exposed skin should be covered with a water-impermeable occlusive bandage. This includes defects on the arms, face, and neck. Blood should never be forced into an evacuated tube by exerting pressure on the syringe plunger. This practice may cause the rubber tube stopper to pop off and spray blood on nonintact skin.

LABORATORY COATS OR GOWNS AS BARRIER PROTECTION

A color-coded two-lab-coat system or equivalent system should be used whenever laboratory personnel are working with potentially infectious specimens. The garment worn in the lab must be changed or covered with an uncontaminated coat on leaving the immediate work area. Garments should be changed immediately if grossly contaminated with blood or body fluids to prevent seepage through to street clothes or skin. Contaminated coats or gowns should be placed in an appropriately designated biohazard bag for laundering. Disposable plastic aprons are recommended if there is a significant possibility that blood or certain body fluids may be splashed. Aprons

should be discarded into a biohazard container.

Important Safety Practices

HAND WASHING

Frequent hand washing is an important safety precaution. It should be performed after contact with patients and laboratory specimens. Hands should be washed with soap and water:

1. After completing lab work and before leaving the laboratory.
2. After removing gloves.
3. Before eating, drinking, applying makeup, changing contact lenses, and using the lavatory.
4. Before all activities that involve hand contact with mucous membranes or breaks in the skin.
5. Immediately after accidental skin contact with blood, body fluids, or tissues. If the contact occurs through breaks in gloves, the gloves should be removed immediately and the hands thoroughly washed. If accidental contamination occurs to an exposed area of the skin or because of a break in the gloves, wash first with a liquid soap, rinse well with water, and apply a 1:10 dilution of bleach or 50% isopropyl or ethyl alcohol. Leave the bleach or alcohol on the skin for at least one minute before final washing with liquid soap and water.

DECONTAMINATION OF WORK SURFACES, EQUIPMENT, AND SPILLS

All work surfaces should be cleaned and sanitized at the beginning and end of the shift with a 1:10 dilution of household bleach (Table 1-1). Instruments, such as scissors used to cut donor blood segments,

Table 1-1. Preparation of Diluted Household Bleach

Vol. of Bleach	Vol. of H_2O	Ratio	% Sodium Hypochlorite
1 mL	9 mL	1:10	0.5

or centrifuge carriages should be sanitized daily with a dilute solution of bleach. Diluted household bleach prepared *daily* inactivates HBV in 10 minutes and HIV in 2 minutes. Disposable materials contaminated with blood must be placed in containers marked *Biohazard* and properly discarded.

All blood spills should be treated as *potentially* hazardous. In the event of a blood spill, this procedure for cleaning up the spill should be used:

1. Wear gloves and a lab coat.
2. Absorb the blood with disposable towels. Bleach solutions are less effective in the presence of high concentrations of protein. Remove as much liquid blood or serum as possible before decontamination.
3. Using a diluted bleach solution, clean the spill site of all visible blood.
4. Wipe down the spill site with paper towels soaked with diluted bleach.
5. Place all disposable materials used for decontamination into a biohazard container.

NEEDLE PRECAUTIONS

To prevent needle-stick injuries, needles should *never* be recapped, separated from syringes, or otherwise manipulated by hand. Used needles should be placed intact into specifically designated orange or red, puncture-proof, biohazard containers. The same criteria should be applied to used scalpel blades and any other sharp devices that may be contaminated with blood. The container should be located as close as possible to the work area. Phlebotomists should carry puncture-resistant containers in their collection trays. Needles should not project from the top of the container. To discard the containers, close and place them into a biohazard waste container. An accidental needle stick must be reported to the blood bank supervisor or other designated individual.

OTHER SAFETY PRECAUTIONS

Several other safety practices should be followed to reduce the risk of inadvertent contamination with blood or certain body fluids. These include the following:

1. Food and drinks should not be consumed in work areas or stored in the same area as specimens. Containers, refrigerators, or freezers used for specimens should be marked as containing biohazards.
2. Specimens needing centrifugation should be capped and placed in a centrifuge with a sealed dome.
3. Personnel should slowly and carefully open rubber-stopped test tubes with a 2×2 gauze square placed over the stopper to minimize aerosol production (the introduction of substances into the air).
4. Use safety bulbs for pipetting. Pipetting *by mouth* of any clinical material must be strictly forbidden.

Hazardous Waste Management and Control

The control of infectious, chemical, and radioactive waste is regulated by various government agencies, including the Occupational Safety and Health Administration (OSHA) and the Food and Drug Administration (FDA). Legislation and regulations that affects laboratories include the Resource Recovery and Conservation Act (RCRA), the Toxic Substances Control Act (TOSCA), clean air and water laws, "right-to-know" laws, and hazardous communications (HAZCOM) regulations. Blood banks should implement applicable Federal, state, and local laws that pertain to hazardous material and waste management.

INFECTIOUS WASTE

Infectious waste, such as contaminated gauze squares and test tubes, must be discarded into proper biohazard containers. These containers should be:

1. Conspicuously marked **Biohazard** and bear the universal biohazard symbol.
2. Of the universal color, orange, or orange and black, or red.

3. Rigid, leakproof, and puncture-resistant. Cardboard boxes lined with a leakproof plastic bag are available.
4. Used for blood and certain body fluids* and disposable materials contaminated with them.

If the primary infectious waste containers are red plastic bags, they should be kept in secondary metal or plastic cans. Extreme care should be taken not to contaminate the exterior of these bags. If they do become contaminated on the outside, the entire bag must be placed into another red plastic bag. Secondary plastic or metal cans should be decontaminated regularly and immediately with an agent such as a 1:10 solution of household bleach after any grossly visible contamination.

Terminal disposal of infectious waste should be by incineration; an alternate method of terminal sterilization is autoclaving. If incineration is not done in the health-care facility or by an outside contractor, all contaminated disposables should be autoclaved before leaving the facility for disposal with routine waste.

CHEMICAL HAZARDS

OSHA recommends that all chemically hazardous material be properly labelled with the hazardous contents and severity of the material, and bear a hazard symbol. Excellent guidelines for chemical hazards can be found in the National Fire Prevention Association's document NFPA 704.

Recent government regulations require that all employees who handle hazardous material and waste be trained to use and handle these materials. Chemical hazard education sessions must be presented to new employees and conducted annually for *all* employees.

---

*Some local health codes currently permit blood and body fluids to be disposed of by pouring them down the sink into the sanitary sewerage system. If disposal by this method is used, care must be taken to prevent splashing. Water should not be running in the sink, and facial protection and a plastic apron should be worn in addition to gloves and a laboratory coat. Sinks used for hazardous waste disposal should not be used for hand washing.

Safety Documents

Each laboratory *must* have an up-to-date safety manual. This manual should contain a comprehensive listing of approved policies, acceptable practices, and precautions including universal blood and body fluid precautions. Specific regulations that conform to current state and Federal requirements such as OSHA regulations must be included in the manual. Other sources of mandatory and voluntary standards include the Joint Commission on Accreditation of Hospitals (JCAH), the College of American Pathologists (CAP), the Centers for Disease Control (CDC), and the American Association of Blood Banks (AABB) guidelines.

COMPLIANCE WITH UNIVERSAL PRECAUTIONS

In addition to a clear policy on the institutionally required universal precautions previously discussed, compliance with the enforcement of universal precautions also requires that categories of risk classifications for all routine and reasonably anticipated job-related tasks and personal protective equipment be included with the departmental procedures manual. Risk classification is divided into three categories:

Category I. Tasks that involve exposure to blood, body fluids, or tissues. All procedures of job-related tasks that involve an inherent potential for mucous membrane or skin contact with blood, body fluids, or tissues, or a potential for spills or splashes of them, are Category I tasks.

Category II. Tasks that involve no exposure to blood, body fluids, or tissues, but may require performing unplanned Category I tasks. Normal work responsibilities involve no exposure to blood, body fluids, or tissues, but exposure or potential exposure may be required as a condition of employment.

Category III. Tasks in which no exposure to blood, body fluids, or tissues is involved and Category I tasks are not a condition of employment. Normal work responsibilities involve no exposure to blood, body fluids, or tissues. A person in this category does not perform and is not expected to perform tasks that can lead to potential exposure. Activities such as answering the telephone or sharing bathroom facilities with workers in other categories is not considered a risk. For usual blood bank activities, personal protective equipment consists of gloves and a laboratory coat or gown. Other equipment such as masks is normally not needed.

COMPLIANCE WITH CHEMICAL HAZARD PRECAUTIONS

Legislation, such as state "right-to-know" laws, and OSHA document 29 CFR 1910, which sets the standards for chemical hazard communication (HAZCOM), determine the types of documents that must be on file in a laboratory. For example, a yearly physical inventory of all hazardous chemicals must be performed, and material safety data sheets (MSDs) should be available in each department of use. Each institution should also have at least one centralized area where all MSDs are stored.

QUALITY ASSURANCE IN THE BLOOD BANK

Quality assurance techniques are used in the blood bank to guarantee error-free performance in the delivery of the highest level of patient care. A systematic approach to quality ensures that patients will receive safe blood products and related transfusion services promptly and at a reasonable cost. Important factors in a comprehensive quality assurance program include the following:

1. Qualified personnel
2. Approved blood bank policies and procedures
3. Correct blood collection and storage
4. Established quality assurance techniques
5. Accuracy in communications and records
6. Recognition and resolution of problems

Qualified Personnel

One of the most important functions of a quality assurance program in the blood bank is the maintenance of high standards for personnel. The competence of personnel should be evaluated at the entry level and maintained by continuous evaluation and education.

EVALUATION OF COMPETENCE

Entry level examination of the competence of clinical laboratory technicians / medical technicians and clinical laboratory scientists / medical technologists in blood banking should be validated. Validation should be by both external certification and new employee orientation to the work environment.

At the beginning of employment and periodically throughout the year, an employee's written job description should be reviewed. This document is important to the employee because it describes the employer's expectations. A job description should include the duties and responsibilities of the position and measurable standards of performance for each task described, as well as position title, hours worked, major functions and responsibilities of the position, qualifications for the position, the employee's immediate supervisor, and the departments with which the employee frequently works and communicates. Staff members should be required to document the fact that they have read the required manuals that apply to their tasks.

The formal annual performance evaluation, as well as periodic informal sessions, should focus on the job description as a tool to open communication and professional growth. Action plans for the correction of deficiencies should be developed with specific activities and timelines noted. Evaluations should be maintained to document performance.

MAINTAINING COMPETENCE

Participation in continuing education activities is essential to maintaining competence. If an employee has a specific area that is weak on performance appraisal, continuing education should be used as a corrective action for the lack of competence.

For most personnel, continuing education should keep staff members abreast of new knowledge and practices in the field and maintain an employee's job interest and motivation. It is important for individuals to share information gained after attending continuing education activities. Forms of continuing education include antibody and journal clubs, self-instruction, professional meetings, writing for publication, and workshop presentations for peers. The job description should specify that continuing education is an expected professional activity. Participation in such education should be recognized and rewarded with positive comments on performance evaluations and appropriate merit pay increases.

Established Blood Bank Policies and Procedures

Laboratory policies should be included in a reference manual available to all hospital personnel. This manual should contain all approved policies, including safety rules. Transfusion practices, such as the length of time a unit of cross-matched blood will be reserved for a patient, should be *clearly* stated in this document. This manual should be reviewed periodically by all blood bank personnel and must be reviewed annually by the medical director.

The procedures manual should be a complete document of current techniques and approved policies that are available at all times in the immediate bench area of blood bank personnel. It is important for all blood bank personnel to review this manual at least annually. The manual should comply with the NCCLS format standards for a procedures manual. The manual should minimally include the name of the test method; the principle of the test and its clinical applications; specimen collection and storage; quality control; reagents, equipment, and supplies; the procedural protocol; expected or normal values; and sources of error. The procedural format found in Chapters 13 and 14 of this book follows these guidelines.

Established Quality Assurance Techniques

DAILY PRACTICES

Each procedure must have an established protocol to ensure the quality of the results. Documentation of results is essential to support a quality control program. Factors such as day-to-day variability, reagent variability, and differences between technologists need to be closely monitored. The daily testing of reagents and monitoring of refrigerators, freezers, and waterbaths (discussed in detail later in this chapter) guarantee the accuracy and safety of blood banking practice. If reagent control results are not acceptable, the accuracy of patient results cannot be guaranteed. In these cases, the source of error must be identified before results can be considered valid.

PEER REVIEW

Accreditation agencies require that peer review of the transfusion of blood and blood derivatives be conducted in each hospital. The hospital transfusion committee performs this peer review function. In addition to the medical director of the blood bank, all major medical departments that routinely order blood should be represented on the committee: surgery, anesthesiology, medicine, obstetrics, pediatrics, and high blood use subspecialties such as hemodialysis, oncology, hematology, and neonatology. Non-physician members should include a blood bank technologist, a hospital administrator, a nurse, and a medical records librarian. Although the blood bank medical director may make most of the day-to-day policy decisions, it is appropriate for the committee to review issues affecting the entire hospital staff, such as transfusion reactions, single units of blood administered, crossmatch:transfusion ratios, and blood use.

EXTERNAL QUALITY CONTROL PROGRAMS

Many voluntary or mandatory accrediting agencies, such as the AABB, JCAH, and state and Federal regulatory agencies, have requirements or laws designed to ensure the safety of blood transfusion and related activities. It is important not to simply satisfy various inspection and accreditation requirements, but to embrace the spirit as well as the letter of the law.

Participation in proficiency testing programs ensures maintenance of consistently high standards. Proficiency samples should not receive special handling by the blood bank. Testing should include weekend, evening, and night shift personnel.

ACCURACY IN COMMUNICATIONS AND RECORDS

Blood bank personnel have frequent contact with physicians, nurses, hospital support staff, and donors. In many cases, the events requiring verbal communication are situations of high stress. It is critical that excellent communication skills be developed for effective interaction with coworkers and others to deliver high-quality patient care.

It is equally important in reporting results to be alert to clerical errors, particularly in transcription. Clerical errors must be guarded against when:

1. Reporting results (grouping, typing, cross-matching)
2. Maintaining pre- and post-transfusion records
3. Releasing and transferring blood and blood components

RECOGNITION AND RESOLUTION OF PROBLEMS

A problem can be described as a "critical incident" or deviation from standard operating procedures. To resolve a critical incident, good communication and thorough analysis of the problem with identification of interconnected causes are necessary, and overlapping factors such as inadequate training or knowledge, substandard materials or reagents, or improper procedures, may need to be considered. The incident should be thoroughly documented (for example, loss of a thawed unit of fresh frozen plasma, a donor reaction, or clerical errors).

Ongoing assessment of the functioning of a blood bank requires objective appraisal of important aspects of patient care and correction of identified problems. No one wants to make a mistake, but in the day-to-day operation of a blood bank, errors, near-misses, and inefficient practices and problems develop. It is essential to detect and appropriately resolve problems.

Daily Quality Assurance Practices

To monitor and ensure the highest quality of patient care, some factors in the blood bank should be evaluated periodically, while others are an integral part of the daily operation of the blood bank. Reagents and equipment are critical components in the accuracy of daily testing.

Quality Control of Reagents

Commercial reagent antisera and reagent red cells are licensed for clinical use only after they meet minimum standards for specificity and potency. Manufacturer's directions must be followed exactly. To guard against the loss of potency or specificity, the following additional practices should be followed:

1. Store all antisera at 2 to 6° C when not in use.
2. Freeze all rare antisera for extended storage. It is best to divide antisera into aliquots to avoid repeated thawing and refreezing. Thaw at 37° C and mix thoroughly before use.

DAILY QUALITY CONTROL OF ANTISERA

The manufacturer's directions must be strictly followed. Because reagent antisera or cells may deteriorate or become contaminated with agents (such as other antisera, blood, or microorganisms) each blood bank must confirm that *each* reagent, on *each* day of use, is correctly reactive (see Daily Quality Control Procedures, Chapter 13).

Positive and negative controls must be used for each reagent tested. The cells selected as positive controls in the test system should be weakly reactive to provide the best indication of antisera potency. This is best accomplished by choosing reagent red blood cells that are heterozygous for the antigen being tested. The following antisera should be tested daily: anti-A, anti-B, anti-A,B, anti-Rh_o(D), Rh_o(D) control, and anti-human globulin (AHG).

For routine daily quality control testing of AHG reagent, it is sufficient to use Rh_o(D) positive red blood cells sensitized with anti-Rh_o(D). The anti-Rh_o(D) reagent should be diluted to coat, but not agglutinate, Rh_o(D) positive cells and produce no more than a 2+ reaction with AHG. Evaluation for anticomplementary activity is considered unnecessary because AHG reagent that has lost potency because of improper storage demonstrates comparable loss of both anti-IgG and anticomplement activity.

Antisera that are infrequently used should be tested in parallel with an actual test with simultaneous testing of both positive and negative control cells.

DAILY QUALITY CONTROL OF REAGENT RED CELLS

Reverse grouping cells (such as A_1, A_2, and B cells) and alloantibody detection screening cells should be tested on *each* day of use with both a positive and a negative control. The reverse grouping cells should be tested with anti-A and anti-B antisera. If a discrepancy is observed, the reagent cells and antisera should be tested independently with cells or antisera of known reactivity.

It is particularly important to visually inspect each vial of screening cells for hemolysis. If the supernatant fluid is hemoglobin-tinged and a single wash removes the color, the cells can be used as a freshly prepared saline suspension. Some prefer to use a saline suspension of washed reagent red blood cells, especially if there is a problem in antibody identification. Screening cells can be examined with a weak saline-reactive antibody and a weak AHG antibody. It is impractical to perform testing on each vial of antibody identification panel cells.

DAILY REAGENT CONTROL RECORDS

Records of daily quality control testing must be maintained. The form must include the reactions, the commercial source and lot identification numbers of the reagents tested, date of testing, and the initials of the person conducting the test (Fig. 1-1).

Quality Control of Equipment

All instruments and equipment used in the laboratory must be properly maintained and monitored to ensure accurate testing. Continual monitoring of the temperatures of waterbaths, refrigerators, and freezers is important to the maintenance of reagent quality and test performance.

Equipment such as centrifuges, automatic cell washers, Rh view boxes (if used), and equipment (such as refrigerators, freezers, and waterbaths) should be cleaned and checked for accuracy on a regularly scheduled basis. A preventive maintenance schedule should be followed on all pieces of equipment. Failure to monitor equipment regularly can produce inaccurate test results and lead to expensive repairs.

CENTRIFUGES

The purpose of centrifugation in serologic testing is to enhance in vitro red blood cell antigen-antibody reactions. Centrifugation should pack the red blood cells into a well-defined cell button; however, overly tight packing is undesirable because nonagglutinated red blood cells cannot be easily resuspended.

In the case of automated cell washers, the dual function of washing red blood cells and enhancing agglutination reactions is desired. In this situation, the supernatant fluid should be clear after centrifugation and produce a well-defined cell button. Some automated cell washing systems also add AHG reagent to each tube.

To ensure that a centrifuge is working efficiently, the operator's manual should describe initial quality control checks and calibration procedures following repairs and annually. With automated cell washers, a

REAGENT CONFIDENCE RECORD

+ = POSITIVE
N = NEGATIVE

Reagent - Antisera Control

CELLS	Anti A	Anti B	Anti A, B	Anti D	Rh-hr. control	AHG	Saline
A_1	1 +	4 N	7 +	10 N	12 N	13 N	
A_2	2 +	5 N	8 +				
B	3 N	6 +	9 +				
dilute ccc				11 +		14 +	15 N

	Searchcyte I				Seachcyte II			
	IS	37°	AHG	CCC	IS	37°	AHG	CCC
dilute Anti-D	16 N	N	+		18 N	N	+	
Saline	17 N	N	N	+	19 N	N	N	+

INTERPRETATION

REAGENT	LOT NO.	EXP.DATE	REAGENT	LOT NO.	EXP. DATE
Anti-A			Reverse Cyte		
Anti-B			Search Cyte		
Anti-A,B			Coombs Control Cells		
Anti-D			A_2 Cells		
Rh-hr. Control			Anti-human Serum		
Albumin					

EQUIPMENT CONTROL

	INCUBATOR TEMP (°C)				REFRIG. (°C)				
I.D.	37 ± 1 Bath	37 ± 1 Block	37 ± 1 Block	45–50 Rh Box	1 - 6 Top Shelf	1 - 6 Bottom Shelf	-20 to -35 Freezer	22 - 25 Rm.Tp.	56 ± 1
Temp.									

Date ______________________

Technician ______________________

Reagent - Antisera Control

CELLS	Anti A	Anti B	Anti A, B	Anti D	Rh-hr. control	AHG	Saline
A_1	1 +	4 N	7 +	10 N	12 N	13 N	
A_2	2 +	5 N	8 +				
B	3 N	6 +	9 +				
dilute ccc				11 +		14 +	15 N

	Searchcyte I				Seachcyte II			
	IS	37°	AHG	CCC	IS	37°	AHG	CCC
dilute Anti-D	16 N	N	+		18 N	N	+	
Saline	17 N	N	N	+	19 N	N	N	+

INTERPRETATION

REAGENT	LOT NO.	EXP. DATE	REAGENT	LOT NO.	EXP. DATE
Anti-A			Reverse Cyte		
Anti-B			Search Cyte		
Anti-A, B			Coombs Control Cells		
Anti-D			A_2 Cells		
Rh-hr. Control			Anti-human Serum		
Albumin					

EQUIPMENT CONTROL

	INCUBATOR TEMP (°C)				REFRIG. (°C)				
I.D.	37 ± 1 Bath	37 ± 1 Block	37 ± 1 Block	45 — 50 Rh Box	1 - 6 Top Shelf	1 - 6 Bottom Shelf	-20 to -35 Freezer	22 - 25 Rm.Tp.	56 ± 1
Temp.									

Date ______________________

Technician ______________________

Fig. 1–1. Reagent confidence record

number of factors must be checked. Procedures include the following:

1. Testing to ensure that an equal volume of saline is being dispensed into each tube.
2. Checking that the total volume of saline added to each tube is less than 80% of the total volume of the tube to eliminate the possibility of cross-contamination. Forceful overfilling of test tubes with saline can produce foaming of serum protein. Underfilling of test tubes produces inadequate washing and residual protein can neutralize AHG antisera.
3. Verification that the time and speed of centrifugation are correct.
4. Examination of red blood cell buttons to be sure that each is correctly resuspended between washings to allow them to be washed properly and packed properly on the final decant cycle.
5. Inspection to see that the addition of AHG is proper, if this step is part of the cell washer's function.

WATERBATHS AND HEAT BLOCKS

Waterbaths and/or heat blocks are usually maintained at 37.5° C in the blood bank for the detection of warm reactive antibodies and thawing blood components (such as fresh frozen plasma). The temperature of incubators should be monitored periodically by properly attaching a standard thermometer. The temperature of each piece of equipment needs to be checked and recorded on each day of use (Fig. 1-1).

In the case of a multi-well heat block, the temperature can vary in the different wells; but, it is impractical to check the temperature of each well with a thermometer. A quick method of observing the temperature is the use of cholesteric liquid crystals, which change color as the temperature changes (green at 37° C and blue at 37.5° C. A small amount of crystals can be permanently placed in a test tube in each well for 60 seconds and observed immediately.

REFRIGERATORS AND FREEZERS

Blood bank refrigerators and freezers must be equipped with an alarm system and a temperature recording device. Additional refrigerators and freezers must be connected to an emergency power system. Temperature checks must be performed and recorded daily. Alarms must be periodically tested.

RH VIEWING BOXES

When Rh testing is performed on a slide or plate, the purpose of a lighted viewing box is to facilitate reading of the test and to provide sufficient heat so that the temperature of the Rh_o (D) antisera and red blood cells is approximately 37° C. Therefore, the glass surface of the viewing box must remain between 40 and 50° C. A thermometer should be properly attached to the glass surface of the box and the temperature should be checked routinely before use. When a test is conducted, the slide should be placed in the middle part of the heated surface to avoid possible cold spots.

CHAPTER SUMMARY

The medical technicians and medical technologists working in the blood bank render a major service to patients. Personnel working in this area have diverse functions, which include collecting and processing donor blood, performing pretransfusion compatibility testing, and identifying alloantibodies that have been formed as the result of pregnancy or prior transfusion.

Safety in the Blood Bank

Implementing universal precautions eliminates the need for specific warning labels. All blood and certain body fluid specimens should be treated as infectious and capable of transmitting disease.

Safety issues for patients as well as employee protection are a major concern for blood banks. Blood bank personnel must comply with the latest safety practices.

Knowledge and use of the proper techniques to guard against infectious contamination and exposure to chemical hazards are mandatory.

Quality Assurance in the Blood Bank

Quality assurance is a method of ensuring error-free performance. Any system should encompass the categories of personnel, policies and procedures, and techniques. Techniques for accomplishing quality assurance include daily practices, peer review, external quality control programs, accuracy in communications and records, and recognition and resolution of problems.

Daily Quality Assurance Practices

Daily practices must include the monitoring of antisera and reagent red cells. Equipment (such as centrifuges and alarms) must be periodically tested for accuracy. Records of all of these procedures must be maintained.

REVIEW QUESTIONS

1. Which of the following is *not* a function of a blood bank?
   A. Recruiting and collecting homologous blood donors
   B. Typing, screening, and preparing blood for transfusion
   C. Directly administering blood or blood components to patients
   D. Detecting and identifying antibodies in potential recipients
   E. Conducting tissue typing or processing materials, (e.g., bone banking)
2. Universal blood and body fluid precautions mandate:
   A. Immunization against hepatitis B
   B. Immunization against tuberculosis
   C. Wearing gloves when handling specimens
   D. Wearing masks for routine testing
   E. Disposing of needles in plastic bags

3-7.
Match the following precautions (use an answer only once).

3. Food and drinks   A. Should be disinfected with diluted bleach
4. Needles   B. Should be disposed of in biohazard bags
5. Work surfaces   C. Should *not* be in the same area as specimens
6. Specimens   D. Should *not* be recapped
7. Contaminated gauze squares   E. Should be treated as potentially hazardous

8. The purpose of quality assurance in blood banking is:
   A. To regulate inventory management
   B. To guarantee error-free performance
   C. To regulate personnel standards
   D. To monitor hospital budget practices
   E. To establish pay scales for blood bank technologists.
9. Which activity is helpful in maintaining competency as a continuing education activity?
   A. Antibody and journal clubs
   B. Professional meetings
   C. Writing for publication
   D. Workshop attendance or presentation
   E. All of the above.
10. A daily practice or practices that constitute part of a quality assurance program is / are:
    A. Daily monitoring of reagents
    B. Daily monitoring of refrigerators
    C. Daily monitoring of freezers
    D. Daily monitoring of centrifuges
    E. All of the above, except D
11. Clerical errors must be guarded against when:
    A. Reporting results
    B. Maintaining pre- and post-transfusion records
    C. Releasing blood or components
    D. Transferring blood or components
    E. All of the above

12. Blood bank antisera should be stored at ___ ° C when not in use.
    A. −20 to −10
    B. −10 to 0
    C. 0 to 2
    D. 2 to 6
    E. 18 to 25
13. Reagent antisera and reagent erythrocytes should be tested one each day of use with:
    A. A positive control
    B. A negative control
    C. Either a positive or a negative control
    D. Patient's serum or erythrocytes
    E. Both A & B
14. Heat block or waterbaths should be maintained at ___ ° C.
    A. 2
    B. 15
    C. 25
    D. 37
    E. 98
15. The glass surface of an Rh viewbox should be ___ ° C.
    A. Between 0 and 15
    B. Between 16 and 25
    C. Between 26 and 39
    D. Between 40 and 50
    E. Between 50 and 75

ANSWERS TO REVIEW QUESTIONS

1. C	9. A
2. B	10. E
3. E	11. B
4. E	12. D
5. E	13. E
6. C	14. D
7. C	15. D
8. D	

BIBLIOGRAPHY

American Association of Blood Banks Government Affairs Update: CDC, AHA Issue Recommendations on Gloves, Health Worker Precautions, July 2, 1987.

Bauer, S. (Ed).: Protection of Laboratory Workers from Infectious Disease Transmitted by Blood and Tissue, NCCLS Document M29-P, 7-9. Villanova, Pa., National Committee for Clinical Laboratory Standards, November, 1987.

Federal Register, 52 (210): 4181-24, October 30, 1987.

Friedland, G.H., et al.: Lack of transmission of HTLV-III/LAV infection to household contacts of patients with AIDS or ARC with oral candidiasis. N. Engl. J. Med., 314:344-346, 1986.

Haber, S. L.: What every laboratorian should know about AIDS, Med. Lab. Obs., 20(12):55-59, 1985.

Hallam, K.: Protection against lab-acquired infection: A new safety manual. MLO, 21(1):59-60, 1988.

James, A. N.: Legal realities and practical applications in laboratory safety management. Lab. Med. 19(2):84-87, 1988.

Nielsen, K. and Gibbs, F. G.: Controlling quality in the blood bank. J. Med. Technol., 3(11):573-571, 1986.

Martin, L. S., et al.: Disinfection and inactivation of HTLV-III/LAV. J. Infect. Dis. 152:400-403, 1985.

Resnick, L., et al.: Stability and Inactivation of HTLV-III/LAV under clinical and laboratory environments. JAMA, 255(14):1887-1891, 1986.

Sher, Paul P. (Ed).: Recommendations for prevention of HIV transmission in health care settings. Lab. Med., 19(2):88-95, 1988.

Sher, Paul P. (Ed).: AIDS and the laboratory: A time for reason. Lab. Med., 19(2):77, 1988.

Tierno, M.: Preventing acquisition of human immunodeficiency virus in the laboratory: safe handling of AIDS specimens. Lab. Med., 17(11):696-698, 1986.

U.S. Dept. of Health and Human Services: Update: Universal precautions for prevention of transmission of human immunodeficiency virus, hepatitis B virus, and other bloodborne pathogens in health-care settings. MMWR 37(24), June, 1988.

U.S. Dept. of Health and Human Services: 1988 Agent summary statement for human immunodeficiency virus and report on laboratory-acquired infection with human immunodeficiency virus. MMWR 37(S-4), April 1, 1988.

U.S. Dept. of Health and Human Services: Recommendations for prevention of HIV transmission in health-care settings. MMWR, 36, Supp. 2S, 1987.

U.S. Dept. of Labor, Office of Health Compliance Assistance: Enforcement procedures for occupational exposure to hepatitis B virus (HBV), human immunodeficiency virus (HIV), and other bloodborne infectious agents in health care facilities. Correspondence, Jan. 19, 1988.

Warren, D. and Reid, M.: Rapid temperature check for heat blocks. Transfusion, 24(5):414, 1984.

Widmann, F. K.: Technical Manual (9th ed.). Arlington, VA, American Association of Blood Banks, 46-48, 369-376, 1985.

2

Blood Collection, Storage, Processing, and Issue

At the conclusion of this chapter, the reader will be able to:
- Discuss the proper procedure for collecting blood from patients.
- Name at least three types of problems that can be encountered in performing phlebotomy and describe the appropriate resolution of each of these problems.
- Describe the medical history and physical criteria that would exclude a homologous donor.
- Delineate the proper steps in the preparation of a donor venipuncture site and the collection of blood.
- Explain the possible donor reactions and the appropriate initial first aid procedure for each.
- Define the term "autologous donation."
- Compare the four forms of autologous donation-transfusion.
- State the only generally accepted criterion for autologous donation.
- Briefly explain the process and purposes of hemapheresis.

- List the types of donor reactions that may be encountered in hemapheresis donors.
- Name the commonly used anticoagulants for donated blood and the respective approved maximum storage time.
- State at least three changes that occur in stored, anticoagulated blood.
- Define the term "storage lesion."
- State the appropriate methods for the storage of blood and blood components.
- List the tests that must be conducted on a unit of homologous blood.
- Describe the relevant information that should be checked before a unit of blood is issued from the blood bank.
- State the proper conditions for the storage of a recipient sample and integral segment from a unit of blood.
- List the acceptable conditions for the reissue of blood.

Chapter Outline

The collection of blood from patients and donors is one of the important functions of a blood bank. In this chapter, the techniques for collecting pretransfusion venous blood specimens and information related to the processing, storage, and dispensing of blood are discussed.

PATIENT BLOOD SPECIMEN COLLECTION

A properly collected blood specimen is essential to the accuracy and safety of blood transfusion. Strict adherence to the rules of specimen collection is critical because identification errors involving either the patient or the specimen are *major* potential sources of error.

Blood Collection Equipment

Although disposable plastic syringes may be used in special cases, evacuated blood-collecting tubes are the most widely used system for collecting venous blood samples. This system (Fig. 2-1) consists of a collection needle, a holder, and an evacuated glass tube containing enough vacuum pressure to draw a specific amount of blood.

The collecting needle used routinely is a double-pointed needle. The longer end is inserted into the patient's vein and the shorter end pierces the rubber stopper of the collection tube. Sterile needles for use with a standard holder are used. Various needle sizes are available. In addition to length, needles are noted by gauge size. The higher the gauge number, the smaller the inner diameter or bore of the needle. Double-pointed needles are either single-sam-

ple or multiple-sample types. The multiple-sample type has a short rubber sleeve on its short end which punctures the rubber stopper. The rubber sleeve prevents blood from leaving the system when more than one evacuated tube is needed for testing. The specially designed needle-holder is used to secure the needle. This holder can be washed and reused.

Evacuated tubes are intended for one-time use only. With use of the evacuated tubes with the double-pointed collection needles, a closed sterile system for specimen collection is achieved. This not only preserves the quality of the specimen during transport prior to testing, but also protects the patient from potential infections.

Evacuated tubes come in various mL sizes, including pediatric sizes, with color-coded stoppers. The stopper color denotes the type of anticoagulant (for example, lavender indicates EDTA and red indicates no anticoagulant). Red-stoppered and lavender-stoppered tubes are used in routine blood banking. Because a red-stoppered tube contains no anticoagulant, venous blood clots normally and produces the straw-colored fluid, *serum.* A lavender-stoppered tube allows whole blood to be separated into *plasma,* a straw-colored fluid, and the cellular components: erythrocytes, leukocytes, and platelets. EDTA (K3 EDTA), tripotassium ethylenediamine tetra-acetate, removes ionized calcium (CA^{++}) through a process referred to as chelation. This process forms an insoluble form of calcium salt that prevents blood coagulation.

Blood Collection Techniques

GENERAL PROTOCOL

1. If the patient is awake and alert, medical personnel should pleasantly introduce themselves to him or her and briefly explain the phlebotomy procedure in easy-to-understand terms.
2. Patient identification is the *critical* first step in blood collection. Asking the patient his or her name and checking the hospital identification band,

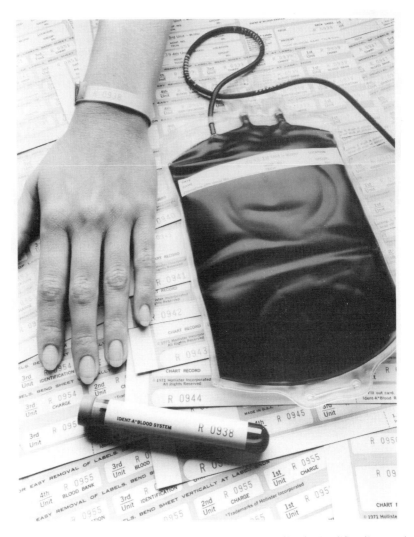

Figure 2-1. Blood bank identification system. A numbered patient identification system, such as the Ident-A-Blood Recipient System by Hollister Incorporated, Libertyville, IL, adds an additional safety precaution for correct identification of the patient, patient blood specimen, unit of blood, and related requisitions and reports. With this system, the patient receives a separate numbered bracelet at the time when the blood specimen is drawn. The number also appears on the blood specimen, any blood or blood components, the patient's chart, and related requisitions.

which *must* be physically attached to the patient, are necessary initial steps. In cases where a patient is unable to give his or her name or where identification is attached to the bed or missing, nursing personnel should be asked to physically identify the patient. Verbal identification of the patient should be noted on the test requisition. Many blood banks use a numbered blood-bank bracelet and requisition system to positively identify blood bank patients (Fig. 2-2). Positive identification is vitally important in emergency or other situations in which a patient lacks a hospital identification band.

3. Test requisitions should be checked and the appropriate equipment assembled. Requisitions must contain sufficient information for positive identification. First and last names and the identification numbers of patients are required. Optional information can

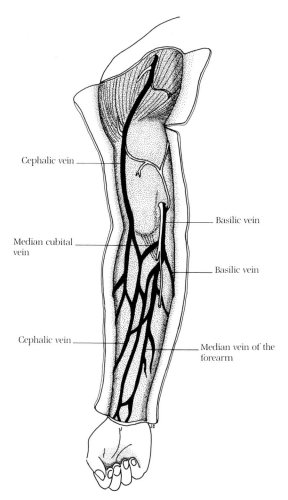

Cephalic vein

Median cubital vein

Cephalic vein

Basilic vein

Basilic vein

Median vein of the forearm

Figure 2-2. Veins of the arm. In the arm, the two most common veins used for venipuncture are the cephalic and median cubital. Illustration from Turgeon, M.L.: Clinical Hematology: Theory and Procedures. Boston, Little, Brown and Company, 1988. p. 9.

include sex, date of birth, clinical diagnosis, previous transfusion or pregnancy history, and attending physician's name. Incomplete or illegible forms are unacceptable.
4. All specimens must be properly labeled *immediately after* the specimen is drawn and *before* leaving the recipient's bedside. The label must state the recipient's first and last names, identification number, date, and name or initials of the phlebotomist. The specimen label and request form must agree.

VENOUS BLOOD COLLECTION (PHLEBOTOMY)

Supplies and Equipment. The following are necessary materials for venous blood collection:

1. Test requisition
2. Tourniquet
3. 70% alcohol and gauze square or alcohol wipes
4. Sterile disposable needles (vacutainer or syringe type)
5. Evacuated blood tubes and a needle holder or a syringe (in special cases)
6. Spirits of ammonia in breakable capsule (emergency use only)
7. Adhesive plastic strips or spots
8. Disposable gloves

Initiation of the Procedure

1. Identify the patient
2. Assemble all necessary equipment at the patient's bedside
3. Thoroughly wash your hands and put on disposable gloves.
4. If a needle and syringe are to be used, firmly secure the hub of the needle with the shield in place on the syringe. If an evacuated tube is to be used, screw the short end of the needle on the needle holder. The plastic shield is to remain on the needle until *immediately* before performing the venipuncture. The evacuated tube is placed into the holder and gently pushed until the top of the stopper reaches the guideline on the holder. Do not push the tube all the way into the holder or a loss of vacuum will result.

Selection of an Appropriate Site. Venous blood should not be drawn near an intravenous infusion IV site. It is preferable to draw the sample from the opposite arm if possible, or, if necessary, from below the infusion site. If possible, the IV should be shut off for 2 to 3 minutes before the sample is drawn. It should be noted on the test requisition if the sample was drawn from below an IV site, and the type of solution being administered should be recorded. Obtaining a blood specimen from an IV line should be avoided because it increases the risk of mixing the fluid with the blood sample.

1. Visually inspect both arms. Choose the arm that has not been repeatedly used for previous venipunctures and one that is free of bruises, abrasions, or sites of infection. In the arm, three veins can be used for venipuncture: the cephalic, basilic, and median cubital veins (Fig. 2-3).
2. Apply the tourniquet. Two general types of tourniquets are available. One type is a flat or rounded rubber tube, and the other has velcro ends for simple adjustment to the arm.
   A. If a rubber tourniquet is used, slide the tourniquet under the arm, a few inches above the expected venipuncture site. Evenly adjust both ends of the tourniquet (Fig. 2-3A).
   B. Grasp both ends of the tourniquet a few inches above the patient's arm. Pull up on the ends to create tension in the tourniquet. Cross the right side of the tourniquet over the left side. With the index finger of the right hand, create a small loop in the right side of the tourniquet while continuing to hold the tension in the tourniquet (Fig. 2-3B).
   C. Slip this small loop under the left side of the tourniquet. The resulting application allows easy removal of the tourniquet with one hand after the needle has been inserted into the vein (Fig. 2-3C).
3. Ask the patient to make a fist (sometimes a roll of gauze is placed in the patient's hand). This usually makes the veins more prominent. With the index finger, palpate (feel) for an appropriate vein (Fig. 2-3D). It is important to feel the vein, which has a resilient feeling compared to the surrounding tissues.

Large veins are not always a good choice because they have a tendency to roll as you attempt the venipuncture. Superficial and small veins should also be avoided. The ideal site is generally near or slightly below the bend in the arm (Fig. 2-3E). If no appropriate veins are found in one arm, examine the other arm by applying the tourniquet and palpating the arm. Do not leave the tourniquet on for more than 2 minutes. Veins in other areas such as the wrist, hands, or feet can be used as venipuncture sites, but only experienced phlebotomists should use these sites.

PREPARATION OF THE VENIPUNCTURE SITE

1. After an appropriate site has been chosen, release the tourniquet.
2. Using a cotton ball or an alcohol pad saturated with 70% alcohol, cleanse the skin in the area of the venipuncture site. Using a circular motion, clean the area from the center and move outward. Do not go back over an area once it has been cleansed.
3. Allow the site to dry.

PERFORMING THE VENIPUNCTURE

It is preferable to avoid touching the cleansed venipuncture site. In unusual situations, it may be allowable to touch the area with an alcohol-wiped finger to re-establish the location of the vein.

1. Reapply the tourniquet and have the patient make a fist if possible.
2. Use one hand to hold the evacuated tube or syringe. Use one or more fingers of the other hand to secure the skin area of the forearm below the intended venipuncture site. This tightens the skin and secures the vein. Position the patient's arm in a slightly downward position.
3. Hold the needle with the attached syringe or tube about 1 to 2 inches below, and in a straight line with, the intended venipuncture site. Position the blood-drawing unit at about a 20-degree angle. The bevel of the needle should be in an upward position.
4. Gently insert the needle through the skin and into the vein. This insertion motion should be smooth. If a vacuum tube is used, one hand should steady the needle holder unit while the other hand pushes the tube to the end of the plastic holder. It is important to hold

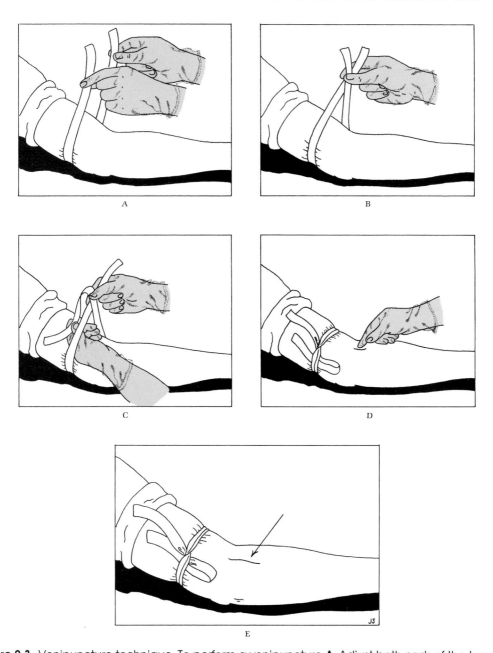

Figure 2-3. Venipuncture technique. To perform a venipuncture **A**, Adjust both ends of the tourniquet evenly. **B** and **C**, When applying the tourniquet place tension on the tourniquet, cross one side over the other, and slip a small loop under one side of the tourniquet. A properly applied tourniquet can be removed with one hand by simply pulling on one end of it. **D**, With the index finger, palpate the site for a suitable vein. **E**, The ideal site for venipuncture is usually near or slightly below the bend in the elbow. (Illustration from Turgeon, M.L.: Clinical Hematology: Theory and Procedures. Boston, Little, Brown and Company, 1988. p. 10.)

the needle still during the collection process to avoid interrupting the flow of blood. Multiple samples can be drawn by inserting each additional tube as soon as the tube attached to the needle holder has filled. If a syringe is used, one hand should steady the barrel of the syringe, while the other hand slowly pulls the plunger backward.

TERMINATION OF THE PROCEDURE

1. The tourniquet may be released as soon as the blood begins to flow into the evacuated tube or syringe, or immediately before the final amount of blood is drawn.
2. Ask the patient to open his/her hand.
3. After the desired amount of blood is drawn, place a gauze pad over the venipuncture site.
4. Withdraw the blood collecting unit with one hand and *immediately* press down on the gauze pad with the other hand.
5. If possible, have the patient elevate his/her entire arm and press on the gauze pad with the opposite hand. If the patient is unable to do this, apply pressure until bleeding ceases.
6. Place a nonallergenic adhesive spot or strip over the venipuncture site. Failure to apply sufficient pressure to the venipuncture site could result in a hematoma.
7. Mix tubes with anticoagulant by inverting the tubes several times. If a syringe was used, carefully remove the needle with an appropriate instrument *before* dispensing the blood into a test tube. Never manipulate a needle with your fingers! Discard the used needle in an appropriate biohazard container.
8. Label all tubes.
9. Clean up supplies from the work area. Remove gloves and wash hands before leaving the patient's room. Place gloves and other contaminated supplies in a biohazard bag. If a patient is an outpatient, have him/her wait for a few minutes after the venipuncture

is complete to be sure that he/she doesn't feel dizzy or nauseated.

PHLEBOTOMY PROBLEMS

Occasionally, a phlebotomist may experience an unsuccessful venipuncture. A venipuncture should not be attempted more than two times. If two attempts are unsuccessful, notify the blood bank supervisor or someone who can assist you. Problems encountered in phlebotomy can include the following:

1. Refusal by the patient to have blood drawn. The solution to this problem is to excuse yourself politely from the patient's room. Note the refusal on the requisition and notify the blood bank supervisor.
2. Difficulty in obtaining a specimen because the bore of the needle is against the wall of the vein. Slightly pulling back on the needle may solve this problem.
3. Movement of the vein. To guard against this problem, always have firm pressure on the arm below the intended venipuncture site. The needle can be moved around slightly to attempt to reach the vein, but *excessive* probing in the tissues must be avoided. Care must be exercised in moving the needle around because a hematoma can form if both sides of the vessel wall are pierced.
4. Sudden movement by the patient or phlebotomist that causes the needle to come out of the arm prematurely. Always anticipate the possibility of this situation. Quick action is needed! Immediately remove the tourniquet and place a gauze pad on the venipuncture site. Apply pressure until bleeding has stopped to prevent the formation of a hematoma. It is a good practice to have easy access to gauze pads whenever a venipuncture is being performed.
5. Blood clots may form in anticoagulated tubes. In the phlebotomy procedure, red top evacuated tubes should be drawn *first*. Promptly after terminating the venipuncture procedure, a tube containing EDTA anticoagulant should

be gently inverted at least six times to mix the specimen.

6. Fainting or illness after venipuncture. First-aid procedures should be practiced. It is important to be able to assist the patient immediately to prevent injury.

DONOR BLOOD COLLECTION

Although most donor blood is furnished by large regional collection agencies, many hospital blood banks maintain active donor facilities for the collection of blood from autologous or emergency donors, or for the collection of special products. In this section, information related to the collection and processing of homologous, hemapheresis, and autologous donors is presented.

Homologous Donors

The process of collecting blood from volunteer blood donors consists of three stages:

1. Registering and interviewing prospective donors to determine if they are appropriate candidates
2. Conducting a brief physical examination
3. Collecting a unit of blood or blood component

REGISTERING AND INTERVIEWING THE DONOR

Basic information from the donor includes the following:

1. Date of donation
2. Name: Last, first, and middle initial
3. Address: Residence and/or business
4. Telephone: Residence and/or business
5. Sex
6. Age and/or date of birth
   Acceptable donors can be between ages 17 through 65 years. Collection of blood from minors requires written consent obtained in accordance with applicable law. A person may donate after age 66; approval, however, is at

the discretion of the blood bank physician

7. Signed consent for the blood bank to take and use blood from the prospective donor

On the day of blood donation, the prospective donor's medical history must be confidentially evaluated to determine that donation will not be detrimental to either the donor or to the potential recipient. One of the important factors in ensuring a safe blood supply in the volunteer donor system is reliance on the donor's integrity and good intentions when answering the predonation medical history.

A form similar to Figure 2-4 is the basic guideline for the medical history interview. This record must be kept for at least 5 years or as required by local law, whichever is longer. Factors of importance include previous donations, previous deferral, surgery, past illnesses and weight loss, pregnancy, immunization, infectious diseases, hepatitis, and malaria.

Previous Donations. The donation interval should be at least 8 weeks, except for reasonable qualifying circumstances. Whole-blood donation must be deferred for at least 48 hours after hemapheresis.

Previous Deferral. It is important to determine if a donor has been previously rejected as a blood donor and the reason for the deferral. This information should be taken into consideration when evaluating the donor's current eligibility.

Donor deferral registries are an important supplement to screening procedures. These registries can alert blood banks to future donations from unacceptable donors, if the person returns to give blood, or if the original reason for rejection is no longer detectable. Records for permanent deferral as a donor must be maintained indefinitely.

Surgery. In cases of uncomplicated surgery, a donor is disqualified only until healing is complete and full activity has been resumed. If the donor has received blood or blood components, he/she should be deferred for 6 months (see the following discussion of Hepatitis).

Past Illnesses and Weight Loss. In some cases, potential donors with disorders such as diseases of the heart, liver, or lungs, a

DONOR REGISTRATION – BLOOD BANK

DONOR'S NAME	ADDRESS (Street, City, State & Zip Code)		HOME PHONE	DATE
DONOR'S BLOOD TYPE	SEX ☐ MALE ☐ FEMALE	I.D. INITIALS	DATE OF BIRTH	
DONOR'S EMPLOYER & ADDRESS			BUSINESS PHONE	

PLEASE ANSWER YES OR NO TO QUESTIONS BELOW

Ever had Yellow Jaundice, Liver Disease, Hepatitis or a Positive Blood Test for Hepatitis?	☐ YES ☐ NO	Ever Had Heart Disease, Chest Pain, or Shortness of Breath?	☐ YES ☐ NO
Ever Taken Self–Injected Drugs?	☐ YES ☐ NO	Ever Had Convulsions, Seizures, or Fainting Spells?	☐ YES ☐ NO
Received Blood Transfusions, Blood Injections, or Tattoos in Past Six Months?	☐ YES ☐ NO	Ever Had a Blood Disease or Cancer?	☐ YES ☐ NO
Been Exposed to Anyone With Yellow Jaundice, Hepatitis or a Kidney Machine in past Six Months?	☐ YES ☐ NO	Had any Vaccinations or Immunizations in the Past Year?	☐ YES ☐ NO
Ever Had Malaria?	☐ YES ☐ NO	Do You Have Any Acute Respiratory Disease or Trouble Breathing?	☐ YES ☐ NO
Ever Been Outside the U.S. in Past Three Years?	☐ YES ☐ NO	Had Any Dental Work in the Past Three Days?	☐ YES ☐ NO
Ever Had Any Serious Illness?	☐ YES ☐ NO	Been Exposed to Anyone With AIDS?	☐ YES ☐ NO
Been Hospitalized in Past Six Months?	☐ YES ☐ NO	Been to Haiti or Zaire?	☐ YES ☐ NO
Are You Feeling Well Today?	☐ YES ☐ NO	Pregnant in the Past Six Months?	☐ YES ☐ NO
Taken Any Medications in Past Month?	☐ YES ☐ NO	Had Sweats, Unexplained Fever or Weight Loss, Lumps in Neck, Arm Pits or Groin, Discolored Areas of Skin or Mouth, Persistent Cough, or Diarrhea?	☐ YES ☐ NO
Ever Been Deferred as a Blood Donor or Had Problems Donating Blood?	☐ YES ☐ NO		

The information I have given for this form is correct. I understand the information that has been given to me today about the spread of the AIDS virus through donated blood and plasma. If I am at risk for spreading the AIDS virus, I agree not to donate blood and plasma for transfusion to another person.

▶
DONOR'S SIGNATURE   DATE

FOR BLOOD BANK USE

PACK Q.C.	BLOOD DONATION WT.	LOT. No.	WHOLE BLOOD NO.	COMMENTS:
DONOR WEIGHT	TEMP.	B.P.	PULSE	
ARMS ☐ SATISFACTORY ☐ UNSATISFACTORY		SKIN DISEASE ☐ YES ☐ NO		
PHLEB ☐ SATISFACTORY ☐ UNSATISFACTORY		REACTION ☐ SLIGHT ☐ MODERATE ☐ SEVERE		
Hb ☐ SATISFACTORY ☐ UNSATISFACTORY		Hct.	TIME DONATION Completed	

Figure 2-4. Donor form.

history of cancer, or an abnormal bleeding tendency should be excluded, subject to evaluation by a physician. A previous history of tuberculosis which has been successfully treated and is no longer active does not disqualify a donor. Unexplained weight loss of 10% or more of previous weight should be investigated. Questionable conditions that might suggest that a potential donor is not in good health should be referred to a physician for further evaluation.

Pregnancy. If a woman knows that she is pregnant, she should be excluded from donating. Ordinarily, a prospective donor shall be excluded for 6 weeks, following delivery at term, or during the third trimester.

Medication. Most medications taken by a donor are not harmful to a recipient; therefore most donors taking medications, prescription, or nonprescription, are acceptable blood donors. Either a list of per-

Table 2-1. Drugs That May Be Permitted in a Prospective Blood Donor

1. Blood pressure medications, if the donor is free of side effects and cardiovascular symptoms
2. Bronchodilators and decongestants (nonprescription)
3. Hypnotics used at bedtime
4. Isoniazid, if no evidence of active tuberculosis exists
5. Oral hypoglycemic agents, if diabetes is well controlled without evidence of vascular complications
6. Tetracyclines and other antibiotics for acne. Isoretinoin disqualifies a donor
7. Topical steroid preparations applied to skin lesion not at the venipuncture site
8. Tranquilizers–a physician should evaluate the donor to exclude antipsychotic medications
9. Other medications–oral contraceptives, mild analgesics, vitamins, hormones or weight reduction pills. Marijuana may be permitted if the donor is not under the influence of the drug

mitted drugs (Table 2-1) or physician approval on an individual basis should be standard procedure. Ingestion of aspirin-containing medication within 3 days precludes use of a donor as the sole source of platelet preparations for an individual recipient.

Immunization. Persons recently immunized with toxoids and killed viral, bacterial, and rickettsial vaccines are acceptable if they are symptom-free and afebrile.

After smallpox vaccination, a donor is acceptable when the scab has fallen off or 2 weeks after an immune reaction.

If a donor has received an attenuated live virus vaccine (such as polio (oral), measles (rubeola), mumps, or yellow fever), the donor must be deferred for 2 weeks. In the case of German measles (rubella) vaccine, deferral is for 4 weeks. If rabies vaccination has been given following a bite by a rabid animal, the donor must be deferred for 1 year after the bite.

Prospective donors should be deferred for 12 months after receiving hepatitis B immunoglobulin (HBIG).

Infectious Diseases. A donor must be free from infectious diseases that are known to be transmitted through blood.

ACQUIRED IMMUNODEFICIENCY SYNDROME (AIDS). All donors must be given educational materials informing them of the high-risk behaviors associated with human immunodeficiency virus (HIV) infection and the resultant disease, acquired immune deficiency syndrome (AIDS). Persons at risk should refrain from donating blood for transfusion and should be provided with an opportunity to indicate in confidence that their blood, if collected, is not suitable for transfusion. A confidential self-administered questionnaire, which describes high risk behaviors and requires the donor to designate their blood for either laboratory purposes or for transfusions, is an effective way of implementing AIDS screening.

HEPATITIS. Recipients of blood or human blood components or derivatives known to be possible sources of hepatitis B are excluded for 6 months. Individuals who have been tattooed and those who have had close contact with an individual with viral hepatitis during the preceding 6 months must also be deferred for 6 months.

Reasons for permanent deferral include:

1. Viral hepatitis after age 11 years

2. Reactive test for hepatitis B surface antigen (HB$_s$Ag)
3. Donation of the only unit of blood or blood component transfused to a patient who developed transfusion-associated hepatitis within 6 months, who received no other blood component or derivative known to transmit viral hepatitis, and in whom there was no other probable source of hepatitis infection.

MALARIA. Permanent residents of nonendemic countries who have been in an area where malaria is endemic may be accepted 6 months after their return to a nonendemic area if they have been free of unexplained febrile illnesses and have not taken antimalarial drugs.

If a donor has a history of malaria or was previously a resident of an endemic area, he/she should be deferred for 3 years after becoming asymptomatic or leaving the endemic area, respectively. If a donor has had antimalarial prophylaxis and has been in an endemic area, deferral should be for 3 years after both cessation of therapy and departure from the area, if he/she remains asymptomatic in the interim. Donations for plasma, plasma components, or derivatives lacking intact red cells are exempted from the previous restrictions.

PHYSICAL EXAMINATION

The predonation physical examination should include the following:

1. Assessment of general appearance and health
2. Measurement of weight
3. Evaluation of temperature
4. Measurement of pulse and blood pressure
5. Quantitation of hemoglobin or microhematocrit (packed cell volume)

General Appearance. The prospective donor should appear to be in good health. Skin at the venipuncture site must be free of lesions. Evidence of repeated venipunctures narcotic use excludes a donor. Alcoholic intoxication also excludes a donor.

Measurement of Weight. Unexplained weight loss of a significant degree, such as more than 10 lbs. (4.54 kg), is a reason for exclusion. Donors who weigh 110 lbs. (50 kg) or more may donate 450 ± 45 mL of blood, in addition to any additional samples, which shall not exceed 30 mL. Donors weighing less than 110 lbs. (50 kg) may donate blood but shall donate proportionately less.

Anticoagulant restrictions. Packed red blood cells may be used for transfusion if 300 to 405 mL of blood have been collected into an anticoagulant volume calculated for 450 mL and the unit is identified as a "low volume unit." If less than 300 mL of blood is collected, it may be used for transfusion purposes if collected in a proportionately reduced volume of anticoagulant. The excess anticoagulant must be reduced proportionately by expressing the excess into an integrally attached satellite bag and sealing the tubing, and the volume of blood must be accurately measured. Other blood components shall not be made from low-volume units.

Example: Calculation of amount of anticoagulant to remove 63 mL:

$$\frac{\text{Donor's weight}}{50 \text{ kg (110 lbs.)}} \times 63 \text{ mL}$$

Example of amount of blood to draw:

$$\frac{\text{Donor's weight}}{50 \text{ kg (110 lbs.)}} \times 450 \text{ mL}$$

Evaluation of Temperature. A donor's temperature must not exceed 37.5°C. Care should be taken to remove the thermometer before obtaining a blood sample for hemoglobin/hematocrit testing.

Measurement of Pulse and Blood Pressure. Measurement of a donor's pulse must reveal no pathologic cardiac irregularities. The pulse should be between 50 and 100 beats per minute. If the prospective donor is an athlete with high exercise tolerance, a lower pulse rate may be acceptable.

In determination of blood pressure, the systolic pressure should be no higher than 180 mm Hg and the diastolic should be no higher than 100 mm Hg. Donors with values above these readings may be accepted only after evaluation by a qualified physician.

QUANTITATION OF HEMOGLOBIN OR MICROHEMATOCRIT (PACKED CELL VOLUME)

The donor's predonation hemoglobin should be no less than 12.5 g/dL (microhematocrit-packed cell volume 38%) for women and no less than 13.5 g/dL (microhematocrit-packed cell volume 41%) for men. If the specimen is from an earlobe puncture, the hemoglobin should be no less than 13.0 g/dL (microhematocrit-packed cell volume 39%) for women and 14.0 g/dL (microhematocrit-packed cell volume 42%) for men.

Capillary Blood Collection. Several types of micro-collection tubes are available for use in capillary blood collection. Normally, the micro-hematocrit type of capillary tube is the most frequently used. This small tube may be heparinized or plain. Capillary blood collection is performed using a sterile, disposable lancet. These lancets are individually wrapped and should be properly discarded in a puncture-proof container after a single use.

SUPPLIES AND EQUIPMENT. The following is a list of necessary materials:

1. Alcohol (70%) and gauze squares or alcohol wipes
2. Sterile small gauze squares
3. Sterile disposable blood lancets
4. Microhematocrit tubes
5. Disposable gloves

SELECTION OF AN APPROPRIATE SITE. The following steps must be taken in choosing a site:

1. The fingertip (usually of the third or fourth finger) is an appropriate site for the collection of small quantities of blood. The earlobe may also be used as a site of last resort in adults. *Do not puncture the skin through previous sites that may be infected.*
2. The site of blood collection must be warm to ensure free flow of blood; otherwise, the blood sample will not be truly representative of the blood in the vascular system. If necessary, massage the finger several times or place a warm cloth on the area for a few

minutes to increase blood circulation to the site.

PREPARATION OF THE SITE. The site is prepared as follows:

1. Hold the area to be punctured with the thumb and index finger of one hand, wearing a disposable glove.
2. Wipe the area with 70% alcohol and allow to air-dry.
3. Wipe the area with a dry gauze square or cotton ball. If the area is not dry, the blood will not form a rounded drop and will be difficult to collect.

PUNCTURING THE SKIN. The skin must be punctured according to the following procedure:

1. A disposable sterile lancet is used *once* and must be properly discarded in a puncture-proof container.
2. Securely hold the area. Puncture one time with a firm motion. The lancet should puncture across the creases of the fingerprint, not with the grooves. If the finger is the chosen site, the area to be punctured should be in the portion of the finger that is rich in capillaries—not the fleshy part (Fig. 2-5).
3. The first drop of blood should be wiped away because it is not a true sample. It is mixed with lymphatic fluid and possibly alcohol.
4. Subsequent drops are obtained by *gently* applying pressure to the area. A good capillary puncture should require *no* forcing or hard squeezing of the site. If the site is squeezed too hard, lymphatic fluid will mix with the blood and produce inaccurate test results.

Collecting the Sample. The sample is collected in the following way:

1. Filling of microhematocrit tubes is accomplished by allowing the tubes to fill with free-flowing blood by capillary action. The tubes must be held horizontally to avoid introducing air bubbles or breaks in the column of blood.

2. The site should be wiped frequently with a plain gauze square to prevent the accumulation of platelets, which slows down or stops the blood flow.

Termination of the Procedure. The procedure is terminated as follows:

1. Wipe the area with 70% alcohol on a gauze square or alcohol wipe.
2. Place a clean gauze square on the site and apply pressure. If the patient is unable to apply pressure to the site, hold the gauze square until the bleeding has stopped.
3. Label all specimens.
4. Place the used lancet into a puncture-proof container.

Alternate Method (Copper Sulfate Hemoglobin Determination). This method is based on specific gravity. Two solutions of copper sulfate are used. One solution with a specific gravity of 1.053, which is equivalent to 12.5 g/dL of hemoglobin, is used for women; and another solution with a specific gravity of 1.055, which is equivalent to 13.5 g/dL, is used for men. Twenty-five tests can be performed in a 30 mL container of solution before changing, or the solution should be changed daily.

After collecting a capillary blood sample in an anticoagulated tube, a drop of blood is allowed to fall gently from the tube at a height of about 1 cm above the surface of the solution. Observe the droplet. An acceptable specimen sinks within 15 seconds. Unacceptable specimens either remains suspended or sinks slightly and then rises to the top of the solution.

Although false-positive results are rare, false-negative results are common. In these cases, it is best to use a secondary method to verify the donor's ineligibility.

NOTIFICATION OF DONOR OF TEST RESULTS

The medical director of the facility collecting the blood is responsible for notifying donors of any clinically significant abnormalities detected during the predonation evaluation or during laboratory testing.

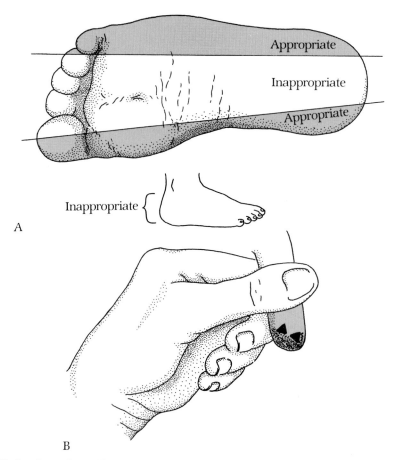

Figure 2-5. Collection of capillary blood. The heel is the preferred site for drawing capillary blood from the newborn. The puncture should be in either the heel or the toe areas designated in the drawing (A). The posterior curvature of the heel should never be used. The shaded areas of the fingertip (B) designated by arrows are the preferred sites for collection of capillary blood from the finger (B). Illustration from Turgeon, M.L.: Clinical Hematology: Theory and Procedures. Boston, Little, Brown and Company, 1988. p. 13.

COLLECTION OF BLOOD FROM THE DONOR

In the collection of a donor unit or of blood components, sterility must be maintained during processing by using aseptic methods and sterile pyrogen-free equipment and solutions. To maintain aseptic conditions, a sterile, closed system is used and a single venipuncture is performed. If more than one venipuncture is needed, another set and container must be used.

A numeric or alphanumeric system must be used that will make it possible to trace any unit of blood or component from the donor source to the final disposition. This system can be used to recheck records applying to the specific unit, including an investigation of any reported adverse reactions.

Supplies and Equipment. The following equipment is needed:

1. Anticoagulated collection bag or other specialized equipment
2. Phlebotomy site preparation solutions
   A. 15% aqueous soap or detergent solution
   B. 10% acetone in 70% isopropyl alcohol (1 part acetone and 9 parts isopropyl alcohol)
   C. Tincture of iodine (3 or 3½% in 70% ethyl alcohol)

or
   A. 0.7 % aqueous scrub solution of io-
      dophor compound, for example,
      PVP-iodine or poloxamer-iodine
      complex.
   B. Iodophor complex solution, for ex-
      ample, 10% PVP-iodine (This is
      available in pre-packaged form.)

3. Sterile applicator swabs (optional)
4. Sterile gauze squares and adhesive
   tape
5. A pair of hemostat clamps and a tube
   stripper
6. Disposable gloves
7. Metal clips and hand sealer, if heat
   sealer is not used
8. Emergency supplies, such as spirits of
   ammonia, emesis basin, etc.

Venipuncture Technique. PREPARATION
OF THE SITE. After selection of an appropriate vein (see selection of an appropriate
vein and venipuncture technique, discussed
previously), the area at least 1½ inches in
all directions from the intended venipuncture site needs to be prepared. Two methods of preparation are approved by the
AABB. The initial scrub and subsequent solutions should be applied at the intended
site, moving outward in a ring.

Method 1 involves the following steps:

1. Scrub vigorously with 15% aqueous
   soap or detergent solution for at least
   30 seconds to remove foreign substances, such as fats, oils, dead epithelial cells.
2. Remove soap and froth with 10% acetone in 70% isopropyl alcohol and allow to dry.
3. Apply tincture of iodine and allow to
   dry.
4. Remove the iodine with 10% acetone
   in 70% isopropyl alcohol and allow the
   solution to dry.
5. Cover the site with a dry sterile gauze
   if the venipuncture is not performed
   immediately.

The following procedure is used in
method 2:

1. Scrub area for 30 seconds with 0.7%
   aqueous scrub solution of iodophor

compound. Although excess foam
must be removed, the arm need not be
dry before the next step.
2. Apply iodophor complex solution and
   let stand for 30 seconds. This solution
   contains only 1% free iodine and need
   not be removed before completing the
   venipuncture. This solution has the advantage of having less odor and staining properties than tincture of iodine,
   and seldom causes skin reactions even
   in iodine-sensitive individuals.
3. Cover the area with dry sterile gauze
   if venipuncture is not done immediately.

THE PHLEBOTOMY PROCEDURE. This procedure involves the following steps:

1. Inspect the anticoagulant donor bag
   for leaks, cracks, or punctures. Be
   sure that the anticoagulant solution is
   clear.
2. Position the bag below the level of
   the donor arm balance system, making sure that the counterbalance is
   level and adjusted for the amount of
   blood to be drawn. A loose knot
   should be made in the tubing if metal
   clips and a hand sealer are not used.
   If a vacuum-assisted device is used,
   follow the manufacturer's instructions.
3. Reapply the tourniquet or blood pressure cuff (inflated to 40 to 60 mm Hg)
   and have the donor open and close
   the hand until the previously selected
   vein is again prominent.
4. Apply the hemostat clamp to the tubing, uncover the sterile needle, and
   perform the venipuncture immediately. A clean venipuncture guaran-
   tees a full, clot-free unit.
5. Open the hemostat and check to be
   sure that the blood flow is adequate.
   Carefully tape the tubing to hold the
   needle in place and cover the venipuncture site with a sterile gauze pad.
   Have the donor squeeze a rubber ball
   or other soft object every 10 to 12
   seconds during collection.
6. Keep the donor under observation
   throughout the phlebotomy. A person

should never be left unattended during or immediately after donation.

7. Mix the unit gently every 30 seconds. Rigid time limits for collecting a unit of blood are not fixed if the flow of blood is continuous. Units requiring more than 8 minutes may not be suitable for preparation of platelet concentrates, fresh frozen plasma, or cryoprecipitate. A unit containing 450 to 495 mL should weigh 425 to 520 g plus the weight of the container with its anticoagulant.

8. Additional samples may be obtained by disconnecting an in-line coupler or by tightening the preformed knot, hemostating the end toward the needle, and cutting the tubing on the needle side of the knot.

9. Deflate and remove the tourniquet. Lightly hold a sterile gauze square over the venipuncture site and remove the needle from the donor's arm. Apply pressure on the gauze. Have the donor raise his/her arm (elbow straight) and hold the gauze firmly over the phlebotomy site with the opposite hand.

10. Strip the donor tubing as completely as possible. Invert the donor unit and allow the line to refill; strip again. Seal the tubing attached to the bag into segments suitable for crossmatching with either a heat sealer or metal clips. It must be possible to separate segments from the container without breaking the sterility of the container. Reinspect the bag for defects.

POSTPHLEBOTOMY CARE. First, check the donor's arm and apply a bandage after bleeding has stopped.

Second, have the donor remain reclining for a few minutes under close observation by staff. When the donor appears to be in satisfactory condition, allow him/her to sit upright. Remain with donor as he/she assumes an upright position and walks to an observation area.

GENERAL TIPS. Have the donor take some nourishment such as orange juice before leaving the donor site and instruct him/her to increase fluids for the next few hours

and to refrain from smoking for 30 minutes. Instruct the donor to raise his/her arm and apply pressure if bleeding from the venipuncture site occurs. If the donor feels faint or dizzy, instruct him/her to lie or sit down with the head between the knees.

Instruct the donor to return to the blood bank or see a physician if symptoms persist. Symptomless donors may resume normal activities after 30 minutes. The bandage may be removed from the venipuncture site after a few hours.

Donor Reactions. All donor reactions must be noted on the donor form. The blood bank physician must provide written instructions for handling any donor reactions. These instructions must include a procedure for obtaining emergency medical help. In all cases, be sure that the donor feels stable before discharging him/her from the donor area.

GENERAL PROCEDURES. The following list gives the general procedures that should be followed in the event of a reaction.

1. Remove the tourniquet and immediately withdraw the needle at the first sign of a reaction.
2. If possible, move the donor to a private area.
3. Call the blood bank physician if necessary.

Donor reactions may include the following:

1. Fainting
2. Nausea and vomiting
3. Hyperventilation
4. Development of a hematoma

FAINTING. The symptoms of fainting include general weakness, sweating, dizziness, pallor, and loss of consciousness. The skin may feel cool and the blood pressure fall. In fainting, the pulse rate falls, as compared to cardiogenic or hypovolemic shock, in which the pulse rate rises. Convulsions with involuntary passage of feces or urine are rare.

First aid procedures for fainting include the following:

1. Place the donor on his/her back and raise the feet above the level of the head.
2. Loosen tight clothing.
3. Be sure that an adequate airway exists.
4. Apply cold compresses to the forehead or back of the neck.
5. Administer aromatic spirits of ammonia by inhalation. Lightly smell the broken capsule to test for strength. The donor should respond by coughing, which elevates the blood pressure.
6. Check the pulse, blood pressure, and respiration periodically.

NAUSEA AND VOMITING. If a patient feels nauseated:

1. Instruct him/her to breathe slowly and deeply.
2. Apply a cold compress to the forehead and turn the head to one side.
3. Provide an emesis basin and clean towels.
4. If the patient vomits, give him/her water and mouthwash to rinse the mouth.

HYPERVENTILATION. The early symptoms of hyperventilation may include twitching or muscular spasms. Nervousness may cause a donor to hyperventilate, which causes faint muscular twitching or tetanic spasms of the hands or face. In many cases, diverting the donor's attention with conversation can interrupt the hyperventilation pattern. If symptoms are apparent, have the donor breathe into a paper bag.

HEMATOMA. At the first sign of swelling in the venipuncture site, remove the tourniquet and the needle from the donor's arm. Place several sterile gauze pads over the hematoma and apply firm pressure for 7 to 10 minutes with the donor's arm held above heart level. Apply ice to the area for 5 minutes, if desired.

If an arterial puncture is suspected, immediately withdraw the needle and apply firm pressure for 10 minutes. Check for the presence of a radial pulse. If the pulse is not palpable, call the blood bank physician immediately.

Hemapheresis Donors

Hemapheresis is a unique form of blood donation. In this type of donation, whole blood is withdrawn from either a healthy donor or a patient. After removal, separation, and retention of the desired cellular elements or plasma, the remaining products are recombined and returned to the donor or patient. Plasmapheresis is an alternate term used to describe the removal of plasma with or without replacement of the lost fluid with a physiologic solution such as normal saline. The process of hemapheresis may be performed with an intermittent flow instrument that requires only a single venipuncture or with continuous-flow equipment that usually requires two venipunctures, one for removal of whole blood and the other for the return of the undesired components. With automated equipment, citrate solution is added in a measured quantity to the whole blood as it enters the primary tubing. All personnel involved in performing hemapheresis procedures should be thoroughly familiar with current regulations and qualified by training or experience to perform the procedure.

The harvested components (see Chapter 9) of hemapheresis from healthy donors are valuable to a wide variety of patients, particularly those who require multiple transfusions of platelets. Therapeutic hemapheresis is directly beneficial to patients with specific disorders, such as Waldenstrom's macroglobulinemia, myasthenia gravis, Goodpasture's syndrome, and Guillain-Barré syndrome. In therapeutic circumstances, hemapheresis is directed at removing a plasma component or excessive numbers of platelets or leukocytes (therapeutic cytapheresis).

In the early 1960s, Judson, an engineer employed by International Business Machines (IBM), spearheaded the initial efforts to design an automated instrument to selectively remove cells from the extracorporeal circulation. Judson was interested in cytodepletion because he wished to help his son, who was suffering from acute leukemia, to avoid the toxic side effects of chemotherapy. It was hoped that maintenance of a low circulating leukocyte count would avert organ damage. In 1964, it was demonstrated that lowering the leukocyte count of leukemia patients would not reduce organ damage. Although depletion of leukocytes through cytopheresis was not found advantageous to leukemia patients, components provided by hemapheresis therapy have proven beneficial to patients suffering from the toxic side effects of chemotherapy as well as to other neutropenic and thrombocytopenic patients.

DONOR GUIDELINES

If the frequency of donation does not exceed one donation every eight weeks, donors of components prepared by hemapheresis must meet the same previously described requirements as donors of whole blood. If the frequency of repeated mechanical plasma-and-cytopheresis donations is more often than once every 8 weeks, the rate should be guided by the following recommendations.

Additional general criteria include the following:

1. At least 48 hours should elapse between successive donations.
2. Incidental red blood cell loss should be no more than 25 mL per week.
3. The loss of plasma, exclusive of anticoagulant, should be less than 1000 mL per week for donors weighing less than 175 lbs. (89 Kg) and less than 1200 mL for heavier donors.
4. To avoid severe lymphocytopenia, individuals should not be permitted to donate if the predonation lymphocyte count is less than 1.2×10^9/L.

ASSESSMENT OF DONORS

Hemapheresis donors must have a routine measurement of hemoglobin and/or hematocrit before donation. In addition, it is desirable to evaluate the platelet count, the leukocyte count, and a leukocyte differential.

A donor with a platelet count below 150 $\times 10^9$ should be deferred from donating platelets (platelet pheresis). In addition, donors who have taken aspirin or aspirin-containing medications within 3 days of donation must be deferred.

If a donor is providing granulocytes, the absolute granulocyte value should be greater than 4×10^9/L. Granulocytapheresis donors who will receive predonation steroid stimulation to increase granulocyte yields should be carefully questioned about hypertension, diabetes, and any history of ulcers or symptoms of ulcers. A signed informed consent must include specific permission for the administration of steroids or hydroxyethyl starch, which enhances granulocyte harvest and minimizes red blood cell contamination of the granulocytes.

Coagulation studies are indicated only if the donor's medical history suggests a congenital or acquired bleeding tendency. A serum protein electrophoresis or quantitative determination of immunoglobulin must be determined once every 4 months for donors undergoing frequent plasmapheresis. The donor's serum protein level must be above 6.0 g/dL and the quantity of IgG and IgM must be normal.

Donors who do not meet these requirements may donate if the component will be of special value to the intended recipient, such as an HLA-matched platelet donor. If a donor does not meet the established guidelines, a physician must certify in writing that the donor's health permits the donation and that the donor's condition will not produce a risk to the recipient. The recipient's physician should also be notified.

DONOR REACTIONS TO HEMAPHERESIS

Although infrequent, unusual reactions may be observed in hemapheresis donors. The negative consequences of component donation can include procedural reactions, vascular complications, or reactions specific to the type of component, such as leukapheresis. Procedural reactions can include a reaction to the citrate anticoagulant, hypovolemia, hypervolemia, hemolysis, chilling, and allergic or anaphylactic reactions. Vascular complications can involve development of sclerosis or thrombosis. Reactions subsequent to leukapheresis can encompass a state of hypervolemia, edema, skin manifestations, or reactions to steroids. Immediate hypersensitivity reactions have been observed occasionally in healthy platelet pheresis donors. This type of anaphylactic reaction due to basophil histamine release during an automated platelet pheresis procedure is believed to be caused by sensitization to the ethylene oxide gas used to sterilize the disposable plastic equipment used in the procedure.

If a donor reaction occurs, first aid procedures should be instituted, with the approval of the medical director of the blood bank. If symptoms such as shortness of breath or other severe reactions occur, the pheresis procedure should be stopped and the blood bank physician should be notified. Examples of donor reactions and the immediate steps that should be taken include the following:

1. Chills should be treated by covering the donor with a blanket and connecting a blood warmer to the blood return channel.
2. Bleeding from the infusion site may occur in heparinized donors. If this occurs, the needle should be removed and light pressure applied. If applying pressure does not control the bleeding, both cold and pressure should be applied.
3. Paresthesia and muscle cramping related to the binding of calcium by citrate anticoagulant should be treated by slowly reinfusing the donor's blood and delaying the next centrifugation cycle until symptoms disappear.
4. Heparin or protamine sensitivity may produce epistaxis or unusual bleeding, chills, urticaria, or symptoms of anaphylactic shock. The infusion should be disconnected immediately and emergency treatment, such as administration of steroids or epinephrine, instituted.
5. Chest pain, shortness of breath, shock, pallor, sweating, and syncope can be symptoms of an air embolism. Immediately place the donor on his/her left side, administer oxygen, and obtain emergency care.

IMMEDIATE AND CHRONIC EFFECTS OF HEMAPHERESIS

The immediate effects of hemapheresis donation may demonstrate changes in the donor's hemoglobin and hematocrit, platelet count, or leukocyte count, depending on the harvested components and the type of equipment. Postdonation changes are generally considered acceptable with approved equipment. The platelet count in thrombocytapheresis donors decreases about 30% after donation and may require up to 72 hours to return to normal. Immediate slight to moderate decreases in the blood lymphocyte count and plasma immunoglobin concentrations are without known adverse effects.

Automated hemapheresis has made it possible to selectively remove large quantities of cellular elements or plasma proteins. As a result, the concentration of these substances in the donor's circulation can fall below normal. Platelet pheresis may remove 2.0×10^9 to 3.0×10^9 leukocytes per procedure from the circulation of a normal donor. This represents a loss of approximately four times more mononuclear cells than from a typical single unit donation; during leukopheresis approximately eight times the number of mononuclear cells is lost. Mononuclear cell depletion produces significant decreases in both the absolute number and percentage of T4+ lymphocytes and the absolute number of both T8+ and Leu-7+ lymphocytes. The normal ratio of T4:T8 cells is also altered.

The quantities of components, such as lymphocytes and immunoglobulins, that can be removed without causing significant immediate or long-term consequence is unknown, but frequent and sustained non-lymphocyte-sparing platelet pheresis is associated with changes in laboratory findings related to the immune system. Body defense mechanisms can become defective when plasma IgG levels are less than 200 mg/dL or when the circulating lymphocyte count is less than 1.0×10^9/L.

The chronic effects of hemapheresis donation have been studied less extensively than the immediate effects. Frequent donors have been found to exhibit a small but statistically significant decrease in their absolute lymphocyte count and percent of T lymphocytes, and IgM levels compared to controls. Current Food and Drug Administration (FDA) standards for whole blood donation allow an estimated loss of 6 to 8 $\times 10^9$ mononuclear cells per year. Intensive lymphocytapheresis for the treatment of rheumatoid arthritis demonstrates that lymphocyte depletion and immunosuppression are feasible with current technology. A concern exists that depletion of lymphocytes during routine cytopheresis may lead to immunosuppressive and associated infections, malignancy, or autoimmune disease.

HEMAPHERESIS DONOR RECORDS

In addition to the records required for all blood donors, such as medical history, physical examination, duration of the procedure, and occurrence and treatment of any reaction, the records for hemapheresis donors must include the type and amount of anticoagulants given, the quantity and name of any drugs administered, and the volumes of each product collected. The average red blood cell loss for each type of procedure should be calculated and recorded on the donor record. Repeat hemapheresis donors must have all their laboratory findings and collection data reviewed by physician at least once every 4 months.

Autologous Donors

Autologous donation or self-donation has gained in popularity since preoperative patients and their physicians have become more concerned about the risk of transmission of blood-borne infectious diseases in homologous blood. The two major categories of autologous donation are predeposit and autotransfusion.

PREDEPOSIT

Predeposit refers to the removal and storage of blood or blood components from the donor-patient. One or more units of blood are collected before an elective surgical procedure for reinfusion during or after the procedure. This form of autologous trans-

fusion is important in blood banking and is discussed in more detail later in this section.

AUTOTRANSFUSION

Autotransfusion can be divided into the following categories:

1. Intraoperative autotransfusion
2. Hemodilution
3. Postoperative autotransfusion

In *intraoperative autotransfusion,* whole blood is collected from a body cavity or wound, processed, and returned to the patient.

In hemodilution, whole blood is collected before a surgical procedure and simultaneously replaced with a comparable volume of crystalloid or colloid solution. Hemodilution was developed by cardiac surgeons, with the primary function being a decrease in blood viscosity. The decrease in viscosity reduces stress on the heart and increases the microcirculation. Blood collected during hemodilution can be saved and retransfused as fresh whole blood. Beneficial results from hemodilution have been achieved in cardiovascular surgery, vascular surgery, spinal surgery for scoliosis, and total hip replacements.

Postoperative autotransfusion utilizes shed mediastinal blood, blood from the chest, or blood from other sterile operative sites. This sterile blood is defibrinogenated to prevent clotting. Collection and processing of the blood is with the same devices as are used in intraoperative autotransfusion. The blood is retransfused following open heart surgery and traumatic hemothorax.

HISTORY OF AUTOLOGOUS TRANSFUSION

Autologous blood transfusion is not a new procedure. The first recorded use of autologous transfusion dates to 1818, when Dr. John Blundell used salvaged blood and returned it to ten patients with severe postpartum hemorrhage. Despite Dr. Blundell's innovative therapy and reasonable rate of success (half of the 10 treated patients survived), little serious attention was given to autotransfusion. Sporadic reports do appear in the medical literature throughout the remainder of the 19th century.

The direction of autotransfusion changed dramatically in 1915 with the development of the first sodium citrate blood anticoagulant. This made it possible to store blood in vitro. In 1921, Grant performed the first documented autologous predeposit collection. Autologous transfusion became standard practice in the 1920s and early 1930s. However, with the introduction of an organized blood bank in 1937 at Cook County Hospital in Chicago, Illinois, and the onset of World War II, homologous donation and transfusion emerged as the standard of practice and interest in autologous transfusion diminished.

The modern period of autologous transfusion began in the 1960s. Renewed interest in autologous transfusion in the form of intraoperative salvage gained momentum as post-transfusion hepatitis B became an issue of concern. The phenomenal growth in autologous predeposit programs has been fueled by anxiety about transfusion-associated HIV. Although it is well out of proportion to the actual risk, this concern has spurred public demand for a safe supply of blood, and it is widely accepted that autologous blood is the safest blood available.

ADVANTAGES AND DISADVANTAGES OF PREDEPOSIT AUTOLOGOUS DONATION AND TRANSFUSION

The autologous predeposit of blood has many benefits (Table 2-2), including individual benefits such as elimination of sensitization to cellular blood components and allergic reactions, as well as exposure to infectious agents, such as hepatitis virus and HIV. Societal benefits of autologous transfusion include reduction of the demand for homologous blood and the potential reduction of costs associated with compatibility testing.

Some of the disadvantages of autologous predeposit (Table 2-3) include the fact that it is not possible for medically-indicated transfusion, nor does it meet unanticipated needs. The most common adverse effects of predeposit autologous blood donation are anemia and hypovolemia. This situation

Table 2-2. Potential Benefits of Autologous Donation

1. Potentially extends the homologous blood supply by either not using available homologous blood or by adding to the blood supply, when the autologous donation is not used by the donor and meets acceptable standards
2. Often decreases overall health care costs if only minimal pretransfusion testing is performed
3. Provides peace of mind to surgical candidates with anxiety about contracting infectious diseases such as AIDS
4. Has no risk of alloimmunization to erythrocyte, leukocyte, platelet, or plasma protein antigens
5. Causes no transfusion-related reactions such as hemolytic, febrile, allergic, or graft-verus-host reactions
6. Supplies compatible blood for persons with rare red blood cell antibodies or blood types when compatible blood is not available
7. Is acceptable in the form of intraoperative autotransfusion and cell salvage to some Jehovah's Witnesses who would otherwise refuse blood transfusion for major surgery or trauma
8. Stimulates erythropoiesis

can be minimized by the administration of an oral iron supplement in advance of the planned donations and by following a recommended phlebotomy schedule. Other adverse reactions are not unlike those seen in homologous donors.

CRITERIA FOR PREDEPOSIT AUTOLOGOUS DONATION

The predeposit of autologous blood requires a written order from the patient's physician as well as the donor's informed consent (Fig. 2-6). Suitable guidelines need to be established by the blood bank medical director and must be retained in the blood

Table 2-3. Potential Problems of Predeposit Autologous Transfusion

1. Presurgical anemia
2. Presurgical volemia
3. Clerical identification errors
4. Outdating of liquid stored blood
5. Homologous blood transfused instead of autologous
6. Patient/donor unable to donate (e.g., poor veins or a preexisting medical condition that precludes donation)
7. Inadequate length of time to collect a suitable number of units

---

Blood Bank and Transfusion Service
Statement of Consent for Autologous Donation and Transfusion

I consent to the withdrawal of my own blood by authorized members of the staff of the Blood Bank for autologous transfusion purposes. The purpose, nature, and advantages of autologous transfusion, the risks involved, and the possibility of complications have been explained to me by _____, M.D. I understand that:

1. The procedure for donating my own blood is identical to routine blood donation. Each unit (approximately one pint) is collected by placing a needle into a vein in my arm; blood flows into a sterile plastic bag containing an anticoagulant. After the procedure, the needle is removed, and pressure and a bandage are applied to my arm to prevent bleeding. Each unit is labeled and stored for my own use during my subsequent hospitalization.

2. I will be asked to take oral iron supplements to replenish the iron lost with each donated unit.

3. A mild anemia or decrease in my blood volume may be a temporary result after frequent blood donation for autologous transfusion. Symptoms of anemia may include feeling faint, lightheaded, or weak. Because of these possible symptoms, I understand I should refrain from strenuous athletic events or hazardous occupation during the period of time I am donating blood.

4. While every effort will be made to transfuse me with only my own units of blood, there may be occasional situations where additional blood products are required, or where my own blood is no longer available. I will accept homologous (other donors') blood if my physician deems it necessary.

I further consent to such additional procedures related to autologous transfusion as may be necessary or desirable.

Should I not require transfusion of the blood withdrawn from me, I consent to the use or disposal of my blood in any manner deemed appropriate by the Blood Bank Medical Director.

Donor Signature _____   Date_____

Hospital Unit Number _____   or S.S. #_____

Witness _____   Date_____

Figure 2-6. Autologous donor's consent form.

bank procedures manual. Individual deviations from these guidelines require approval by the blood bank physician, usually in consultation with the donor-patient's physician. Diseases and conditions such as localized infections that usually preclude blood donation do not necessarily exclude autologous blood donation. If a patient's status is stable enough to allow elective surgery, he / she can usually donate several units of blood. Pregnant women may donate safely, especially during the second trimester. In some cases, patients with a cardiac history must be approved as donors by a cardiologist. Pre-existing medical conditions, such as active asthma or chronic obstructive pulmonary disease, and the presence of bacteremia, exclude the person as a donor. Donors with a history of seizures should also be excluded.

No age limits have been established for autologous donation. Children between ages 8 and 18 years have successfully predeposited autologous blood. Younger children have also been autologous donors. However, the volume collected must comply with the donor's weight and the ratio of anticoagulant guidelines.

Hemoglobin levels should be no less than 11 g/dL (or microhematocrit-packed cell volume no less than 34%). The interval between donations is usually 1 week with the final unit not to be drawn within 72 hours of the anticipated operation or transfusion. Usually two, but up to a total of five units of whole blood may be collected, providing that the patient's hemoglobin/hematocrit remains above 34%. Oral iron supplementation (ferrous sulfate, 300 mg, t.i.d.) should be prescribed.

Directed Donation

Some patients, anticipating the need for transfusion, have turned to family and friends as a means of protecting themselves against transfusion-associated AIDS. In most cases, this is futile. Directed donations have been found to be no safer than transfusions from random homologous donations. The incidence of regular donors testing positive for diseases transmitted by blood is comparable in voluntary and directed donors.

Some of the advantages of directed donation include a reduction in the anxiety a patient or his/her family may have about the safety and availability of blood and an increase in donor participation, which extends the general availability of blood and components to all patients.

A disadvantage of directed donations is that donors are under pressure to donate, which might motivate them to conceal information about exposure to high-risk behaviors. Another disadvantage is that directed donors often do not realize that they forego donor confidentiality and may be legally liable if the recipient experiences an adverse reaction such as contracting an infectious disease.

STORAGE AND PROCESSING OF DONOR BLOOD

Types of Anticoagulants

The storage of blood has evolved since the initial preservation of whole blood in glass bottles containing a sufficient concentration of acid-citrate-dextrose (ACD) to bind the ionized calcium of a unit of whole blood with excess citrate remaining available to complex with calcium in the recipient. A variety of anticoagulants and anticoagulant-preservative media is now available and plastic collection bags have replaced glass bottles.

Anticoagulants and/or anticoagulant-preservatives for whole blood and red cell concentrate storage include:

1. ACD (Acid-citrate-dextrose)
2. CPD (Citrate-phosphate-dextrose)
3. Heparin
4. CPD-A1 and CPD-A2 (citrate-phosphate-dextrose-adenine)
5. Adsol (AS-1)

The composition of two anticoagulant-preservative solutions in general use today are presented in Table 2-4.

Approved Storage Times

Because different media produce distinct effects on stored blood at 4° C, the approved length of storage differs. Whole blood or red blood cells collected and stored in CPD or ACD have an expiration date not exceeding 21 days after phlebotomy. Whole blood or red blood cells collected and

Table 2-4. Two Anticoagulant-Preservative Solutions in General Use*

	CPD†	CPDA-1‡
Na$_3$ citrate	26.3 g	26.3 g
Citric acid	3.27 g	3.27 g
Dextrose	25.2 g	31.9 g
NaH$_2$PO$_4$. H$_2$O	2.22 g	2.22 g
Adenine	—	0.275 g
Water	1000 mL	1000 mL
Volume per 100 mL	14 mL	14 mL
Storage Limit	21 days	35 days

* By permission from Perkins, A.: Strategies for massive transfusion, *In:* Clinical Practice of Blood Transfusion (Edited by L. D. Petz and S. N. Swisher). New York, Churchill Livingstone, 1981. pp. 485-499.
† CPD = Citrate-Phosphate-dextrose solution
‡ CPDA-1 = Citrate-phosphate-dextrose-adenine solution

stored in CPD-A1 have an expiration date not exceeding 35 days after phlebotomy. Whole blood or red blood cells collected and stored in heparin solution have an expiration date not exceeding 48 hours after phlebotomy.

Red blood cells that are separated and frozen have an approved storage time of 7 years and other components have variable storage times (see Chapter 9). Studies of the use of rejuvenation solutions for red blood cells have demonstrated that red blood cells in PIPA AS-1 can be satisfactorily rejuvenated. However, anticoagulant-preservative additive solutions, such as Adsol (AS-1) or Nutricel (AS-3), are not presently licensed for use with rejuvenation solutions.

The Effects of Anticoagulants on Stored Blood

Although the use of plastic bags improved red blood cell respiration and viability compared to glass bottles and research on the effects of anticoagulants on red cell metabolism has led to improved anticoagulant-preservatives, whole blood or red blood cells exhibit changes (Table 2-5) when stored at 4° C. The critical changes include decreased red blood cell viability, diminished 2,3-diphosphoglycerate (2,3-DPG) levels, and an increase in toxic materials such as plasma potassium.

When one of the anticoagulant-preservative solutions, such as CPD or CPDA-1, is used in a normal blood donation, 63 mL of anticoagulant-preservative are mixed with 450 mL of donor whole blood. This solution dilutes the whole blood constituents to 88% of their original concentration. These solutions also add 18 meq of sodium and 3 meq of phosphorus to each unit and alter the pH of freshly collected blood to between 7.0 and 7.2. When anticoagulants designed for long-term storage are used, a certain amount of hemolysis occurs whenever red blood cells are stored for 35 days or more. However, additives protect red blood cells membranes against hypotonic shock and reduce the degree of hemolysis during storage.

Red Cell Viability

When blood is collected in a plastic bag with a standard anticoagulant-preservative solution and stored at 4° C, the red blood cells slowly undergo metabolic changes in vivo that lead to a loss of red blood cell function, primarily the capacity to offload oxygen normally. To decrease metabolic demands, red blood cells are stored at 4° C. This temperature slows down enzyme activity, which partially protects hemoglobin or the red blood cell membrane. The proportion of viable, transfused red blood cells remaining in the circulation of the recipient 24 hours after transfusion is referred to as *post-transfusion viability.*

Factors leading to the loss of post-transfusion viability and contributing to extravascular catabolism include the following:

1. A decrease of surface-area-to-volume ratio. This may be caused by a loss of surface area or a volume increase, which leads to entrapment because of the inability of the red blood cells to

Table 2-5. Changes in Bank Blood on Storage at 4°C*

I. Decrease of Essential Components	II. Increase in Toxic Materials	III. Formation of Microaggregates
Red cell viability	Plasma potassium	
Red cell 2,3(DPG)diphosphoglycerate	Free hemoglobin	
Platelet viability	Plasma lactate	
Granulocyte viability	Plasma ammonium	
Coagulation factors, (factor V and factor VII)	Plasticizers	

* Modified by permission from Perkins, H. A.: Strategies for massive transfusion. *In:* Clinical Practice of Blood Transfusion. (Edited by Lawrence D. Petz and Scott N. Swisher). New York: Churchill Livingstone, 1981. pp. 485-499.

pass through the microcirculation of the mononuclear phagocyte system.

2. Changes in membrane deformability, either from intrinsic conditions such as sickled hemoglobin, or extrinsic factors such as low pH or changes in membrane surface properties.
3. Decreases in pH to between 4.5 and 5.5 induce an immediate decrease in the deformability of intact red blood cells, and cessation of ATP generation occurs.

FDA regulations require that at least 70% of the red blood cells in a donor unit remain viable in the anticoagulant-preservative solution at the end of the approved storage period; for example, viability of red blood cells in CPD solution after 21 days of storage averages 80 to 85% and red blood cells in AS-1 solution demonstrate a mean post-transfusion recovery of 83% after 42 days of storage. Increased survival of red cells in liquid storage can be achieved by rejuvenation of adenosine triphosphate (ATP) levels with adenosine, which produces an improvement in membrane-related functions.

There is considerable variability in the percentage of viable red blood cells because of the characteristics of the anticoagulant-preservatives, such as the initial osmolarity, the pH of the solution, and the ability of the solution to support ATP levels. The characteristics of the red blood cells of individual donors can also effect viability. Women donors often have been found to have better red blood cell survival rates. It has been suggested that this may be related to higher concentrations of steroid hormones that may act as red blood cell-membrane-stabilizing agents during storage.

When red blood cells are allowed to settle during the storage of whole blood without agitation, poorer post-transfusion survival has been observed. Storage of packed red blood cells with a hematocrit greater than 75% limits the availability of substrate around each cell and leads to shortened survival, even with high concentrations of glucose or the presence of purine nucleotides.

Storage Lesion

Viability, or post-transfusion survival, is believed to be related to the structural and metabolic status of the red blood cell membrane, for example the ATP level, the red blood cell shape, and the red blood cell deformability. The ATP-independent, irreversible loss of surface area of the red cell is referred to as *storage lesion.* The disruption of normal membrane architecture or membrane lesion can lead to recognition and destruction of transfused red blood cells (extravascular catabolism) by the mononuclear phagocyte system.

Red Blood Cell Membrane Changes and Adenosine Triphosphate Depletion

Red blood cells undergo changes in shape and membrane structure during metabolic depletion. These changes include

Early Stage: Shape changes, cellular swelling
Middle Stage: Oxidation of hemoglobin
Middle-Late Stage: Binding of cytoplasmic proteins to the membrane, increased intracellular Ca^{++}, loss of K^+ and H_2O
Late Stage: Irreversible membrane protein crosslinking, loss of lipid vesicles, echinocyte-sphero-echinocyte shape change.

The basic red blood cell membrane structure includes the lipid bilayer, the proteins spanning it (integral membrane proteins), and a filamentous meshwork of proteins along the cytoplasmic surface (peripheral membrane proteins) that form a membrane skeleton. Membrane changes are involved in red blood cell destruction. These changes include the following:

1. Loss of phospholipid asymmetry promotes the adherence of red blood cells to endothelial surfaces and may stimulate recognition and phagocytosis by monocytes.
2. Modification of cell surface antigens, including glycoproteins, glycolipids, and proteolipids, or rearrangement of antigen topography can alter red blood

cell survival. An antibody in the plasma appears to be directed against antigens that only reveal themselves in aged red blood cells in vivo or during in vitro storage.

When ATP levels in a red blood cell fall below 10 to 15% of normal, the cell begins to develop spicules and the shape changes. A change in shape is reversible, following up to 20 hours of ATP depletion, by incubation with glucose and purine nucleotides. This treatment returns ATP levels to normal or supernormal. After 28 hours of ATP depletion; however, the formation of irreversible spheroechinocytes with reduced surface area to volume ratio occurs.

The mechanism by which ATP depletion produces permanent surface area loss has not been completely described, but it is known that it directly or indirectly promotes the loss of lipid-rich vesicles. This loss of lipid from the membrane begins immediately with the onset of storage, and represents the major lethal injury, irreversible deformability of the membrane, to the red blood cell.

Storage of Blood

Immediately after collection, blood must be stored at 1 to 6° C, unless it is to be used as a source of platelets. For harvesting platelets, blood should be placed in storage at a temperature of 20 to 24° C for no longer than 6 hours.

When a unit of blood is collected, the integral donor tubing should be filled with anticoagulated blood and sealed into segments to be available for testing and compatibility examination. These segments can be separated from the collection bag without breaking the sterility of the unit. If the sterility of the collection bag is broken during processing or pooling, the blood or blood components must be stored at 1 to 6° C and transfused within 24 hours. If the sterility of components stored at 20 to 24° C is compromised, the unit must be transfused as soon as possible, or within a maximum of 6 hours.

Processing of Blood

In-House Donor Blood

Donor blood must be tested for ABO, Rh_o (D), and D^u antigens. These blood group systems are discussed in Chapters 4 and 5. If both the Rh_o (D) and D^u tests are negative, the donor unit is Rh negative. If either the Rh_o (D) or D^u test is positive, the donor is Rh positive.

Additional testing should include serum or plasma testing of previously transfused persons or pregnant women for clinically significant antibodies (discussed in Chapter 6). If antibodies are detected, the blood should be processed into components which contain only minimal amounts of plasma. Tests for HB_sAg and anti-HIV are also required. Because of the absence of specific tests for non-A, non-B (NANB) hepatitis at the present time, surrogate testing should be performed as an interim measure to reduce the risk of disease transmission. Surrogate tests for NANB are the anti-hepatitis B core (anti-HBc) screening test and the alanine aminotransferase (ALT) assay.

Donor Blood from Outside Sources

The hospital blood bank must be assured that the collection agency from which the blood was obtained has vigorously applied all appropriate standards of practice to the collection of blood.

Autologous Blood

The processing of blood for autologous transfusion must include ABO and Rh determination by the collecting facility. Other testing may be considered optional—depending upon the specific protocol used.

Proper identification of autologous units is of critical importance. The label must contain the patient's name and an identifying number, for example, Social Security number or birthdate, as well as ABO and Rh type, and the expiration date of the unit (Fig. 2-7A). This unit must also have a label stating "For Autologous Use Only" (Fig. 2-7B). Autologous units must be segregated and used *solely* for this purpose unless the

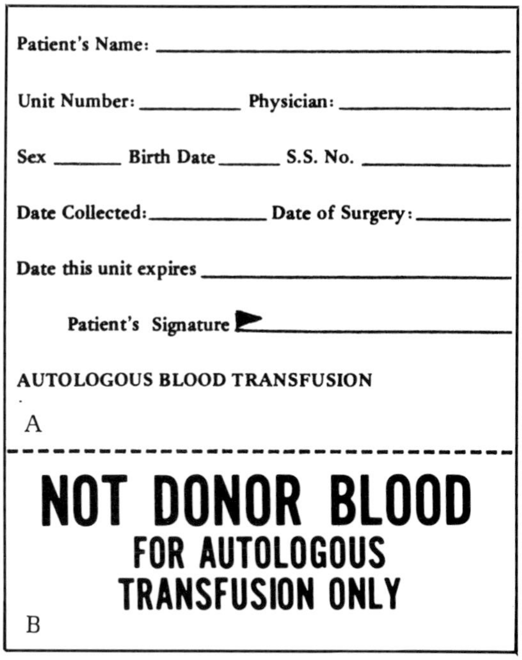

Patient's Name: _____

Unit Number: _____ Physician: _____

Sex _____ Birth Date _____ S.S. No. _____

Date Collected: _____ Date of Surgery: _____

Date this unit expires _____

    Patient's Signature ▶ _____

AUTOLOGOUS BLOOD TRANSFUSION

A

- -

NOT DONOR BLOOD
FOR AUTOLOGOUS
TRANSFUSION ONLY

B

Figure 2-7. A, Autologous donor label. B, Autologous donor sticker.

donor-patient and the donated blood meet all the requirements of a normal donation.

BLOOD COMPONENTS

Processing of blood components must follow the protocol described above for either in-house donor collection or units imported from other sources.

ISSUING BLOOD FOR TRANSFUSION

Blood must be inspected for abnormalities in appearance, such as hemolysis, immediately before issue from the blood bank. If any abnormality is observed, the unit cannot be used.

A transfusion requisition similar to the form shown in Figure 2-8 must be completed for each unit requested blood product. This form must minimally indicate the following:

1. Intended recipient's name, identification number, and ABO and Rh types
2. Donor unit or pool identification number and donor ABO and Rh types
3. Compatibility results, if performed

A copy of the transfusion form must be attached to the recipient's chart. A label or tag with the recipient's first and last names, identification number, unit number assigned by transfusing or collecting facility, and interpretation of compatibility tests, if performed, must be attached securely to the blood container before its release for transfusion.

Both the blood bank technologist and the nurse obtaining the blood must check the patient's identifying information, the blood types of the patient and donor unit, and the expiration date of the unit. Both individuals must sign the appropriate forms or the blood bank ledger book.

Retention of Blood Samples

A segment of the integral tubing from each donor unit and a stoppered sample of the recipient's blood must be stored at 1 to 6° C for at least 7 days *after* transfusion. Some facilities prefer to save these samples for up to 2 weeks.

Reissue of Blood

If returned, blood cannot be reissued unless:

1. The container closure has not been disturbed.
2. The unit has not been allowed to warm above 10° C or cool below 1° C during storage or transportation. If the temperature of off-site storage, for example an operating room refrigerator, cannot be documented, the blood should not be away from the blood bank for more than 20 minutes.
3. The records indicate that the blood has been reissued.
4. The blood is inspected prior to reissue.

CHAPTER SUMMARY

Patient Blood Specimen Collection

A properly collected blood specimen is essential to the accuracy and safety of

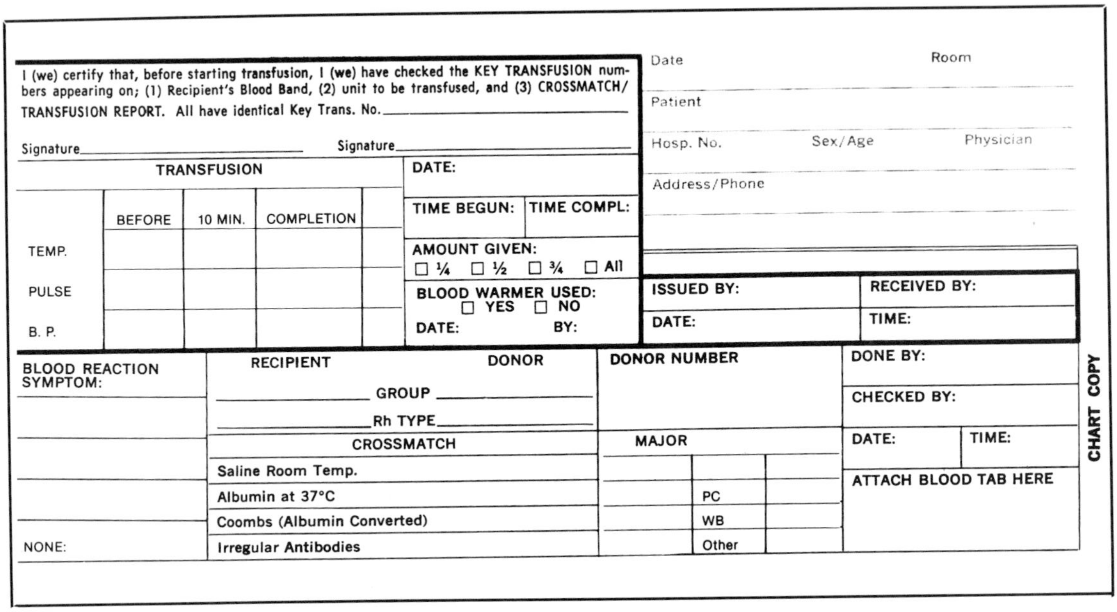

I (we) certify that, before starting transfusion, I (we) have checked the KEY TRANSFUSION numbers appearing on; (1) Recipient's Blood Band, (2) unit to be transfused, and (3) CROSSMATCH/ TRANSFUSION REPORT. All have identical Key Trans. No._____					Date Room
Signature_____ Signature_____					Patient

TRANSFUSION				DATE:	Hosp. No. Sex/Age Physician
	BEFORE	10 MIN.	COMPLETION	TIME BEGUN:	TIME COMPL:	Address/Phone
TEMP.				AMOUNT GIVEN: ☐ ¼ ☐ ½ ☐ ¾ ☐ All	
PULSE				BLOOD WARMER USED: ☐ YES ☐ NO	ISSUED BY: RECEIVED BY:
B. P.				DATE: BY:	DATE: TIME:

BLOOD REACTION SYMPTOM:	RECIPIENT DONOR		DONOR NUMBER	DONE BY:
	_____ GROUP _____			CHECKED BY:
	_____Rh TYPE_____			
	CROSSMATCH		MAJOR	DATE: TIME:
	Saline Room Temp.			ATTACH BLOOD TAB HERE
	Albumin at 37°C	PC		
	Coombs (Albumin Converted)	WB		
NONE:	Irregular Antibodies	Other		

CHART COPY

Figure 2-8. Transfusion requisition.

blood transfusion. Strict adherence to the rules of specimen collection is critical because identification errors involving either the patient or the specimen are *major* potential sources of error.

Collection of blood must follow a carefully prescribed protocol. After pleasantly introducing himself / herself to a patient, the phlebotomist should briefly explain the phlebotomy procedure in easy-to-understand terms. Patient identification is the *critical* first step in blood collection. The other steps in properly collecting a specimen include checking the test requisitions, assembling the appropriate equipment, and washing the hands before putting on a pair of disposable vinyl or latex gloves. After selecting an appropriate site and performing the venipuncture, all specimens should be properly labelled *immediately after* the specimen is drawn and *before* leaving the patient's bedside. The label must state the recipient's first and last names, identification number, date, and name or initials of the phlebotomist. The specimen label and request form must agree. Any contaminated disposable supplies and the used needle should be immediately placed in appropriate biohazard containers.

Occasionally, problems are encountered in obtaining a blood specimen. If two at-

tempts are unsuccessful, notify the appropriate supervisor. Other types of problems may be encountered in phlebotomy. These can include refusal by the patient to have blood drawn, difficulty in obtaining a specimen because the bore of the needle is against the wall of the vein, movement of the vein, sudden movement by the patient or phlebotomist that causes the needle to come out of the arm prematurely, or fainting or illness subsequent to venipuncture.

Donor Blood Collection

Although many hospitals receive donor blood from large regional collection agencies, many hospital blood banks also maintain active donor facilities for specialized purposes such as autologous predeposit of blood, emergency donors, or hemapheresis. Standard procedures must be followed in the processing of donors before blood collection. A thorough medical history and physical examination of donors are essential to the donor's safety as well as the safety of potential recipients. If the medical director approves, persons who deviate from the state criteria may be accepted as donors. The medical director is additionally responsible for notifying donors of any clinically significant abnormalities detected during the predonation evaluation or during laboratory testing.

Sterility must be maintained while collecting donor blood intended for recipient transfusion. To maintain aseptic conditions, a sterile, closed system is used and a single venipuncture is performed. After selection of an appropriate vein, the intended venipuncture site must be properly prepared and the phlebotomy procedure correctly performed. If more than one venipuncture is needed, another set and container must be used. Each unit collected must be labelled with a numeric or alphanumeric system to trace any unit of blood or component from the donor source to the final disposition. Postphlebotomy care is essential to the blood donation process. The blood bank physician must provide written instructions for handling donor reactions. This must include a procedure for obtaining emergency medical help.

Hemapheresis is a unique type of blood donation. In this process, whole blood from either a healthy donor or a patient is separated. Desired cellular elements or plasma are retained and the remaining products are recombined and returned to the donor or patient. Plasmapheresis is an alternate term used to describe the removal of plasma with or without replacement of the lost fluid with a physiologic solution. The process of hemapheresis may be performed using intermittent-flow or continuous-flow equipment. All personnel involved in performing hemapheresis procedures should be thoroughly familiar with current regulations and qualified by training or experience to perform the procedure. The products of hemapheresis from healthy donors are valuable to a wide variety of patients; therapeutic hemapheresis is directly beneficial to patients with specific disorders. Donors of components prepared by hemapheresis must meet the same requirements as donors of whole blood. If donation is more often than once every 8 weeks, the frequency should comply with the accepted guidelines. The immediate postdonation changes are generally considered to be acceptable with approved equipment; however, the chronic effects have been studied less extensively.

Autologous donation or self-donation may take the form of predeposit or autotransfusion. Although autologous donation is not a new procedure, public concern about the transmission of infectious diseases through blood transfusion has expanded interest in autologous donation because autologous blood is the safest blood available. Predeposit of autologous blood has many benefits, including the elimination of sensitization to cellular blood components and allergic reactions as well as blood-borne exposure to infectious diseases. Some of the disadvantages of autologous predeposit include the fact that it is not a feasible alternative in medically indicated transfusions, nor can it satisfy unanticipated needs. The most common adverse effects of autologous blood donation are anemia and hypovolemia. The predeposit of autologous blood requires the consent of the patient's physician and the blood bank physician. Autologous donors do not have to meet the same requirements as homologous donors, but suitable guidelines should be established by the blood bank medical director; individual deviations from the guidelines require approval by the blood bank physician, usually in consultation with the donor-patient's physician.

Some patients, anticipating the need for transfusion, have turned to directed donations from relatives and friends as a means of protecting themselves against blood-borne infectious disease. Although having blood donated by persons known to the patient may alleviate anxiety about the safety and availability of blood, directed donations are no safer than screened blood from homologous donors.

Storage and Processing of Donor Blood

Blood was initially preserved in glass bottles containing a sufficient concentration of acid-citrate-dextrose (ACD) to bind the ionized calcium and thus prevent coagulation. Plastic bags have replaced glass bottles and several types of anticoagulants or anticoagulant-preservative media are now used. The approved length of storage at 4° C depends on the anticoagulant or anticoagulant-preservative solution. Red blood cells that are separated and frozen can be stored for a considerably longer period than blood in the liquid state.

Red blood cells exhibit changes when stored at 4° C. Critical changes include a decrease of red blood cell viability and 2,3 diphosphoglycerate (2,3 DPG) levels, and an increase in constituents such as plasma potassium. At least 70% of the red blood cells must remain viable at the end of the permitted storage period. Red blood cell viability or post-transfusion survival is believed to be related to characteristics such as the level of adenosine triphosphate and red cell shape and deformability. The ATP-independent, irreversible loss of surface area of the red cell is referred to as *storage lesion.*

Immediately after collection, blood must be refrigerated at 1 to 6° C. If platelets are to be harvested, the unit of blood should be stored at 20 to 24° C and the platelets must be separated from the unit within 6 hours. If the sterility of a donor unit is compromised, the unit must be transfused promptly.

Homologous donor blood must be tested for ABO, Rh_o (D), D^u, HB_sAg and, anti-HIV and surrogate tests for non-A, non-B hepatitis should be performed. The surrogate tests are the anti-hepatitis B core (anti-HB_c) screening test and the alanine aminotransferase (ALT) assay. Additional testing should include serum or plasma testing of previously transfused persons or pregnant women for clinically significant antibodies. Modifications in the processing of blood are appropriate for autologous donors and blood received from other donor collection sources.

Issuing Blood for Transfusion

Blood must be inspected for abnormalities in appearance immediately before issue from the blood bank. All relevant patient and donor information must be checked. This information includes the recipient's name, identification number, and ABO and Rh types, as well as the donor unit or pool identification number and the donor ABO and Rh types. Compatibility results, if per-

formed, must also be checked. A label or tag with this information must be attached securely to the blood bag before release for transfusion.

An integral segment from the blood bag and a sealed sample of the recipient's blood must be stored at 1 to 6° C for at least 7 days after transfusion. If a unit of blood is returned to the blood bank, it cannot be reissued unless certain requirements have been met.

REVIEW QUESTIONS

1. The characteristics of EDTA include:
   A. Chelates Ca^{++}, which occur in plasma in a test tube
   B. Chelates Ca^{++}, which occur in serum in a test tube
   C. Forms an insoluble calcium salt that prevents blood coagulation
   D. Reduces the level of complement in a blood sample
   E. All of the above, except B

2–6. Organize the following steps in blood procurement in the proper order.
   A. Label the specimen tubes
   B. Palpate venipuncture site
   C. Identify the patient
   D. Put on disposable gloves
   E. Check the test requisition and assemble the appropriate equipment

2. ____
3. ____
4. ____
5. ____
6. ____

7–10. Match the phlebotomy with its respective correct solution.
7. Movement of the vein
8. Sudden movement that causes the needle to come out of the patient's arm
9. Refusal by patient to have blood drawn
10. Prevention of a hematoma
   A. Immediately remove the tourniquet and place gauze pad on the venipuncture site
   B. Move the needle around until the vein is located
   C. Politely excuse yourself and note refusal on requisition
   D. Avoid piercing both sides of a blood vessel and apply pressure to an oozing venipuncture site

E. Always place firm pressure on the arm below the intended venipuncture site

11–13. Arrange the steps in the process of collecting blood from donors.
A. Conduct a brief physical examination
B. Interview the prospective donor
C. Collect the unit of blood

11. ____
12. ____
13. ____

14. The usual acceptable age for homologous blood donation is:
A. 15 through 65
B. 17 through 65
C. 18 through 70
D. 21 through 75
E. Any age over 16 years

15. The acceptable interval between homologous whole blood donation is:
A. 4 weeks
B. 6 weeks
C. 8 weeks
D. 10 weeks
E. 12 weeks

16. Fill in the blank. If a prospective homologous donor has received blood or blood components known to be sources of hepatitis because of conditions such as surgery, the donor should be deferred from donating for ____ after the transfusion.
A. 6 weeks
B. 2 months
C. 3 months
D. 6 months
E. 1 year

17. If a prospective donor is taking a prescription or nonprescription medication, he/she should be:
A. Deferred until 10 days after stopping the medication
B. Accepted without reservation
C. Accepted if the drug is on the list of permitted drugs
D. Accepted on an individual basis by a physician
E. Either C or D

18. A reason or reasons for permanent donor deferral include(s):
A. A reactive test for hepatitis B surface antigen (HB$_s$Ag)

B. A person involved in a high-risk behavior associated with acquired immunodeficiency syndrome (AIDS).
C. A history of malaria
D. Vaccination with rabies vaccine
E. Both A and B

19. If a donor weighs 105 lbs., how much blood can safely be drawn?
A. 450 mL
B. 440 mL
C. 432 mL
D. 427 mL
E. 420 mL

20. The acceptable pulse rate for a homologous donor is ____ beats per minute.
A. 20–40
B. 50–75
C. 50–100
D. 100–180
E. Over 180

21. The lowest acceptable fingertip hematocrit from a woman donor is:
A. 32
B. 34
C. 36
D. 38
E. 40

22. In the copper sulfate hemoglobin method, the correct specific gravity of the solution for a male donor is:
A. 1.051
B. 1.053
C. 1.055
D. 1.057
E. 1.059

23. All the following are acceptable solutions for one of the two methods of donor arm preparation except:
A. 70% ethyl alcohol
B. 15% aqueous soap
C. 10 acetone in 70% isopropyl alcohol
D. 3% tincture of iodine
E. 10% PVP-iodine

24. The appropriate method of applying solutions to a donor's arm in preparation for venipuncture is:
A. Liberally apply all solutions
B. Allow all solutions to remain in contact with the skin for 20 seconds
C. Apply solutions at the intended venipuncture site and move the applicator outward in a ring

D. Apply solutions about 1 inch from the intended venipuncture site and move the applicator toward the site

E. Apply gauze pads saturated with various solutions to the intended venipuncture site

25–29. Arrange the following steps in the phlebotomy procedure of a blood donor in the correct sequence.

A. Apply a tourniquet or blood pressure cuff to the donor's arm

B. Strip the donor tubing

C. Perform the venipuncture

D. Have the donor drink fluids

E. Inspect the anticoagulant bag for leaks and cloudiness

25. ____

26. ____

27. ____

28. ____

29. ____

30–33. Match the following possible donor reactions with the appropriate initial first aid procedure.

30. Fainting

31. Nausea and vomiting

32. Hyperventilation

33. Hematoma

A. Divert the donor's attention with conversation

B. Place the donor on his / her back and raise the feet above the level of the head

C. Remove the tourniquet and needle from the donor's arm

D. Instruct the donor to breathe slowly and deeply

34–37. Match the following terms with their respective definitions.

34. Predeposit autologous donation

35. Intraoperative autotransfusion

36. Hemodilution

37. Postoperative autotransfusion

A. The collection of blood from a body cavity or wound, processing, and return to the donor-patient

B. The removal and storage of blood or blood components from a donor-patient

C. Collection of blood and retransfusion following open heart and traumatic hemothorax

D. Collection of blood with replacement using a crystalloid or colloid solution

38. Which of the following is *not* a benefit of autologous donation?

A. Complete elimination of homologous transfusion

B. Decrease in health care costs

C. No risk of alloimmunization

D. Stimulation of erythropoiesis

E. No transfusion-related reactions

39. The only generally accepted criterion for autologous donation is:

A. Patient over 18 years of age

B. Absence of all medications

C. Blood pressure not above 180 / 100

40–42. Match the anticoagulant with the respective approved maximum storage time.

40. CPD or ACD   A. 35 days

41. CPD-A1   B. 21 days

42. Heparin   C. 48 hours

43. FDA regulations require that at least ____% of erythrocytes remain viable in an anticoagulant-preservative solution at the end of the permitted storage period.

A. 35

B. 50

C. 65

D. 70

E. 95

44. All of the listed factors, except ____, lead to the loss of posttransfusion viability.

A. Increased pH

B. Decreased pH

C. Changes in membrane surface properties

D. A decrease of surface area to volume ratio

E. Changes in membrane deformability

45. The proper storage temperature for whole blood is ____° C.

A. −20 to −10

B. 0 to 4

C. 1 to 6

D. 2 to 10

E. 12 to 18

46. Homologous donor blood collected and processed from outside sources must have the following tests repeated by the hospital blood bank:

1. ABO

2. Rh
3. HB$_s$Ag
4. HIV
5. Alloantibodies
A. 1 and 2
B. 1, 2, and 5
C. 3 and 4
D. 3, 4, and 5
E. All of the above

47. Autologous blood donor units must be tested for the following:
1. ABO
2. Rh
3. HB$_s$Ag
4. HIV
5. Alloantibodies
A. 1 and 2
B. 1, 2, and 5
C. 3 and 4
D. 3, 4, and 5
E. All of the above

48. Samples of recipient's blood and donor units must be stored for __ days after transfusion.
A. 1
B. 3
C. 5
D. 7
E. 10

49. Which of the following is the exception? If a unit of blood is returned to the blood bank after issue, it cannot be reissued unless:
A. The closure has not been opened
B. The records indicate that it has been reissued
C. The blood is inspected prior to reissue
D. The blood is away from the blood bank for less than 20 minutes (unmonitored)
E. Administered to the same patient

ANSWERS

1. E	9. C
2. C	10. D
3. E	11. B
4. B	12. A
5. D	13. C
6. A	14. B
7. E	15. C
8. A	16. D

17. E	34. B
18. E	35. A
19. C	36. D
20. C	37. C
21. D	38. A
22. C	39. D
23. A	40. B
24. C	41. A
25. E	42. C
26. A	43. D
27. C	44. A
28. B	45. C
29. D	46. A
30. B	47. A
31. D	48. D
32. A	49. E
33. C	

BIBLIOGRAPHY

Bello, K.: Managing an autologous blood program. Med. Lab. Obs., 19(2):63-66, 1987.

Braine, H.G., Elfenbein, G.J., and Mellits, D.E.: Peripheral blood lymphocyte proliferative responses in vitro, and serum immunoglobulins in regular hemapheresis Donors, J. Clin. Apheresis, 2:213-218, 1985.

Brecher, M.E., Borchers, B., Rosen, N.R., and Lord, M.: Directed donations: An underutilized blood donor resource, Lab. Med., 19(2):103-105, 1988.

Brzica, S., Alvaro, A.P., and Taswell, H.F.: To each his own, QRB, 3(12):3-6, 1977.

Button, L., Kruskall, M.S., Scanlan, A., and Kevy, S.: Rejuvenation of red cells drawn in adsol to extend autologous red cell storage. Transfusion, 26(6):558, 1986.

Cable, R.G.: Implementation of a predonation system. International Anesthesiology Clinics. Boston: Little, Brown and Company, 12:59-76, 1984.

Council on Scientific Affairs. Autologous Blood Transfusions, JAMA, 256(17):2378-2380, 1986.

Cowell, H.R.: Prior deposit of autologous blood for transfusion. J. Bone Joint Surg., 69A(3):319, 1987.

Dodds, T.A., Sullivan, R.G., and Beck, J.R.: Cost-effectiveness of screening donor blood for non-A, non-B hepatitis using alanine aminotransferase and anti-hepatitis B core antibody. Transfusion, 26(6):597, 1986.

Fenwal Product Brochure, Fenwal Laboratories, Deerfield, Ill.,1986.

Finch, C.A.: Adenine-supplemented blood. Vox Sang., 48:319-322, 1985.

Greenwalt, T.J.: Autologous and aged blood donors. JAMA, 257(9):1220-1221, 1987.

Haber, S.L.: What every laboratorian should know about AIDS. Med. Lab. Observer, 20(12):55-59, 1985.

Holland, P.V., and Schmidt, P.J. (eds.): Standards for Blood Bank and Transfusion Services. 12th Ed.

Arlington, Va., American Association of Blood Banks, 1987.

Huestis, D.W., Bove, J.R., and Case, J.: Blood donation. *In* Practical Blood Transfusion, 4th ed., Boston: Little, Brown and Co., 1988, pp. 1-54.

Kruskall, M.S., et al.: Utilization and effectiveness of a hospital autologous preoperative blood donor program. Transfusion, 26(4):335-340, 1986.

Kumar, B.: The haemonetic cell saver, Anaesthesia, 41(7):774-775, 1986.

Leitman, S.F., et al. Allergic Reactions in healthy plateletpheresis donors caused by sensitization to ethylene oxide gas, Transfusion, 26(6):580, 1986.

Mallory, T.H., and Kennedy, M.: The use of banked autologous blood in total hip replacement surgery. Clin. Orthop. Rel. Res., (117):254-257, 1976.

Matsui, Y., et al.: Effects of frequent and sustained plateletapheresis on peripheral blood mononuclear cell populations and lymphocyte functions of normal volunteer donors, Transfusion, 26(5)446-452, 1986.

Nusbacher, J., et al.: Evaluation of a confidential method of excluding blood donors exposed to human immunodeficiency virus. Transfusion, 26(6):539, 1986.

Meryman, H.T., Hornblower, M.L-S. and Syring, R.L.: Prolonged storage of red cells at 4°C. Transfusion, 26(6):500-505, 1986.

Myhre, B.A., Demaniew, S., and Nelson, E.J.,: Preservation of red cell antigens during storage of blood with different anticoagulants. Transfusion, 24(6):499-501, 1984.

Oberman, H.A.: Surgical blood ordering, blood shortage situations, and emergency transfusion. *In* Clinical Practice of Blood Transfusion. Edited by L.D. Petz, and S.N. Swisher. New York, Churchill Livingstone, 1981. pp. 393-404.

Perkins, H.A.: Strategies for massive transfusion. *In* Clinical Practice of Blood Transfusion. Edited by L.D. Petz, and S.N. Swisher. New York, Churchill Livingstone, 1981, pp. 485-499.

Popovsky, M.A.: Autologous patients with localized infections, AABB News Briefs, 11(6):9-10, 1988.

Sandler, S.G. (Ed.): Autologous Transfusion. Arlington, Va., American Association of Blood Banks, 1983.

Schmidt, P.J.: Autologous blood transfusion, JAMA, 257(7):928-929, 1987.

Schoenleber, D.G.: Everybody wins with this autologous donor program. Med. Lab. Observer, 18:39-42, 1987.

Silvergleid, A.J.: Safety and effectiveness of pre-deposit autologous transfusions in pre-teenage and adolescent children. Transfusion, 26(6):580, 1986.

Silvergleid, A.J.: Autologous transfusions, JAMA, 241(25):2724-2725, 1979.

Strauss, R.G. Apheresis donor safety—Changes in humoral and cellular immunity, J. Clin. Apheresis 2:68-80, 1984.

Toy, P.T.C.Y., et al.: Predeposited autologous blood for elective surgery. N. Engl. J. Med., Vol. 316(9):517-520, 1987.

Turgeon, M.L.: Clinical Hematology: Theory and Procedures. Boston, Little, Brown and Co., 1988. pp. 6-14.

Wasman, J. and Goodnough, L.T.: Autologous Blood Donation for Elective Surgery, JAMA, 258(21):3135-3137, 1987.

Widmann, F.K. (Ed.): Technical Manual of the American Association of Blood Banks (9th Ed.). Arlington, Va., American Association of Blood Banks, 1985, pp. 19-33, 359-367.

Wolfe, L.C.: The membrane and the lesions of storage in preserved red cells. Transfusion, 25(3):185-201, 1985.

Yomtovian, R.A.: Autologous blood transfusion: Past Performance and current concerns. Minn. Med., 69:353-356, 1986.

Yomtovian, R.A.: Predeposit autologous blood transfusion: An analysis of donor attitudes and attributes. QRB, 13(2):45-50, 1987.

3

Principles of Antigens and Antibodies

At the conclusion of this chapter, the reader will be able to:
- Define the term "immunity."
- Describe the functions of the immune system.
- Outline the organization of the immune system.
- List cell types and effector mechanisms triggered by or involved in immune reactions.
- Describe the structure of the organs that house immunologic cells.
- Explain the general characteristics of the specific immune response.
- Compare and contrast humoral immunity to cell-mediated immunity.
- Discuss the formation of cell products of the specific immune response.
- Explain the role of the thymus in self-recognition.
- Describe the chemical composition of an antigen.
- Define the terms "isotype," "allotype," and "idiotype."
- Describe the chemical composition of an antibody.
- List the classes of immunoglobulins.
- Explain the physical and chemical properties of IgM antibodies.
- Explain the physical and chemical properties of IgG antibodies.
- Compare the characteristics of IgM, IgG, IgA, IgD, and IgE.
- Contrast the characteristics of a primary and secondary (anamnestic) response.
- Describe the production of monoclonal antibodies.
- Name the four types of noncovalent bonds formed in antigen-antibody reactions.
- State the most commonly used technique to detect and measure the consequences of antigen-antibody interaction.
- Define the term and process of agglutination.
- Name the four major methods commonly used in routine blood banking to enhance the agglutination of erythrocytes.
- Describe the purpose of the AHG test.
- Explain the method of grading the strength of agglutination reactions.
- State the reason for pseudoagglutination.
- Describe the results of the prozone phenomenon.

Chapter Outline

An *antigen* can be defined as a foreign substance that is able to elicit an *antibody* response. Not all foreign substances are capable of stimulating an antibody response, however, and the production of antibodies in response to antigenic stimulation depends on two major factors:

1. A person's immunologic ability both to recognize an antigen as foreign or non-self and to respond to this foreignness.
2. The physical and chemical nature of the antigen.

THE IMMUNE SYSTEM

The ability of the body to recognize the foreignness of a substance and produce an-

tibodies in response depends on several body cells, including several kinds of lymphocyte-type leukocytes, plasma cells, and macrophages. Lymphocytes recognize foreign antigens and/or produce antibodies, whereas plasma cells only produce antibodies. Macrophages, which are phagocytic cells, are important in the processing of antigens.

Development and Differentiation of Lymphocytes

During embryonic development, lymphocytes arise from pluripotent, precursor stem cells of the yolk sac and liver. Later, in fetal development and throughout the life cycle, the bone marrow becomes the sole provider of undifferentiated stem cells, which can further develop into lymphocyte precursors. Continued cellular development of these precursors and their subsequent proliferation occurs as the cells travel to specific sites, with the majority of cells differentiating into the two major categories of lymphocytes, *T lymphocytes* (T cells) or *B lymphocytes* (B cells).

PRIMARY LYMPHOID TISSUES

In humans, both the *bone marrow* and *thymus* are classified as primary or central lymphoid tissues (Fig. 3-1). Stem cells that migrate to the thymus proliferate and differentiate under the influence of the humoral factor thymosin. These cells acquire thymus-dependent characteristics to become *immunocompetent* (able to function in the immune response) T lymphocytes. It is believed that the bone marrow functions as the bursal equivalent in humans. It is from the term *bursa* that the B lymphocytes derive their name. Most of the cells produced in the primary sites die before leaving, with only a small percentage migrating to the secondary tissues.

SECONDARY LYMPHOID TISSUES

The secondary lymphoid tissues include the *lymph nodes, spleen,* and *Peyer's patches* in the intestine (Fig. 3-1). Proliferation of the T and B cells in the secondary

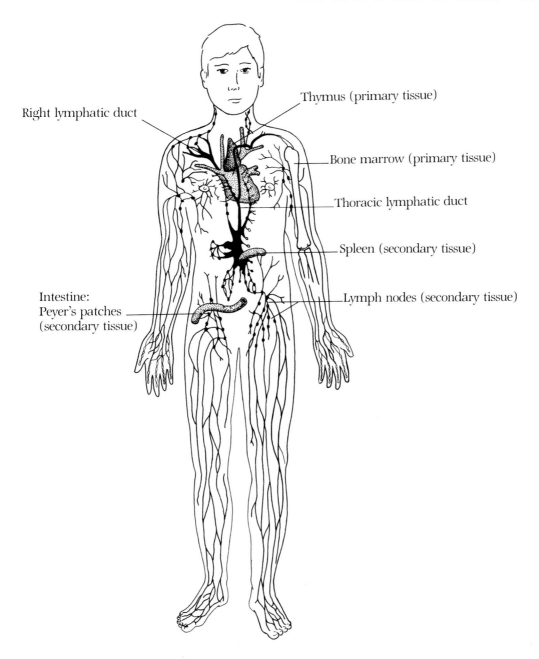

Figure 3-1 The primary and secondary lymphoid tissues. The primary lymphoid tissues are the bone marrow and the thymus. The secondary tissues consist of the spleen, lymph nodes, and Peyer's patches of the small intestine. (Illustration from Turgeon, M.L.: *Clinical Hematology: Theory and Procedures.* Boston; Little, Brown and Company, 1988. p. 98.)

or peripheral lymphoid tissues depends primarily on antigenic stimulation. The T cells (Fig. 3-2) populate the perifollicular and paracortical regions of the lymph node, the medullary cords of the lymph nodes, the periarteriolar regions of the spleen, and the thoracic duct of the circulatory system. The B cells (Fig. 3-2) multiply and populate the follicular and medullary (germinal centers) of the lymph nodes, the primary follicles

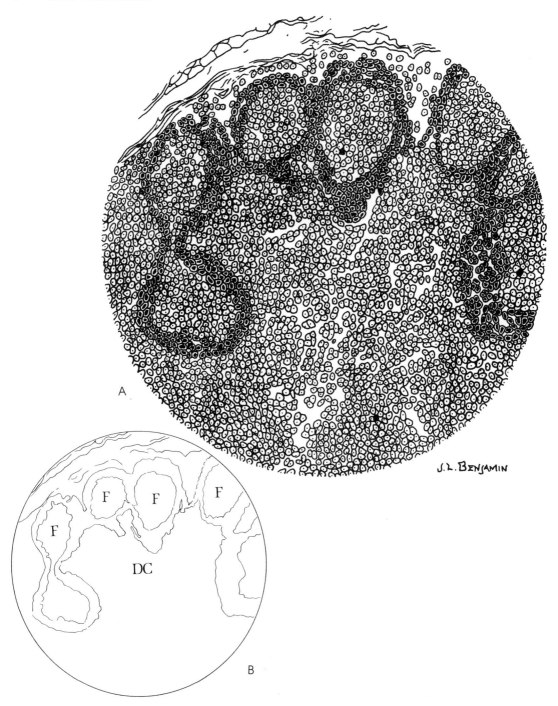

Figure 3-2 A, B. Lymph node. T and B cell areas are found in the lymph node. The lymphocytes of the outer cortex are mainly arranged in lymphoid follicles (F), which are the major sites of B lymphocyte localization and proliferation. The deep cortical zone (DC), or paracortex, is composed mainly of T lymphocytes that are never arranged in follicles. The number of cortical follicles and the depth of the deep cortical zone vary, both according to the immunologic state of each lymph node and in each individual. (Illustration from Turgeon, M.L.: *Clinical Hematology: Theory and Procedures.* Boston; Little, Brown and Company, 1988. p. 99)

and red pulp of the spleen, the follicular regions of gut-associated lymphoid tissue (GALT), and the medullary cords of the lymph nodes.

Cellular Activities of the Immune System

MACROPHAGES

Macrophages exist as either "fixed" or "wandering" cells. Fixed macrophages line the endothelium of the capillaries and the sinuses of organs such as the bone marrow, spleen, and lymph nodes. These cells, along with the network of reticular cells of the spleen, thymus, and other lymphoid tissues, comprise the *mononuclear phagocytic system* (Fig. 3-3). Macrophages and their known precursors, the monocytes, migrate freely into the tissues from the blood to replenish and reinforce the macrophage population.

The immunologic functions of the macrophage cells are to phagocytize, process, and present antigens to T cells. Enzymes released by the macrophages degrade engulfed antigens, but the antigenic determinants seem to be preserved. T cells receive RNA or other messages from macrophages and extracts from macrophages containing an RNA-antigen determinant-linked complex that can be used to stimulate IgG synthesis by lymphocytes. Antigen modification may not be required of all antigens. Low molecular weight antigens may activate T and B cells directly.

LYMPHOCYTES

Several major categories of lymphocytes are recognized as functionally active. These categories are the *T cells, B cells,* and the *natural killer (NK)* and *K-type* lymphocytes.

T Cells. T cells are responsible for foreign antigen recognition or cellular immune responses, which include chronic rejection in organ transplantation, the regulation of antibody reactions by either helping or suppressing the activation of B lymphocytes, and the secretion of soluble mediators.

T cells are divided into two subsets, the *helper/inducer* subset and the *suppressor/*

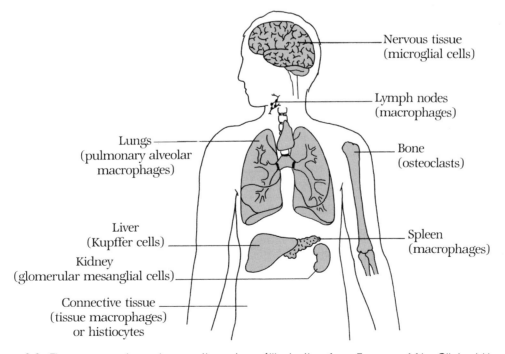

Figure 3-3. The mononuclear phagocytic system. (Illustration from Turgeon, M.L.: *Clinical Hematology: Theory and Procedures.* Boston; Little, Brown and Company, 1988. p. 75.)

cytotoxic subset. Functionally, the helper/
inducer subset signals B cells to generate
antibodies, to control production and
switching of types of antibodies that are
formed, and to activate suppressor cells.
The suppressor-cytotoxic lymphocytes control and inhibit antibody production by
either suppressing helper cells or turning off
B-cell differentiation.

T cells are also associated with the production of soluble mediators, *lymphokines,*
which provide the language for cell-to-cell
communication. Important lymphokines include those listed below:

1 *Migration inhibition factor (MIF)*—Affects macrophage migration during delayed hypersensitivity reactions.
2. *Interleukin 2 (T cell growth factor)*—
   Major factor stimulating T cell proliferation.
3. *Chemotactic factor*—Attracts granulocytes to affected areas in phagocytosis.
4. *Interleukin 1*—Released by macrophages; activates T-helper cells.

B Cells. B cells serve as the primary
source of cells responsible for humoral (antibody) responses. Participation of B cells
in the humoral immune response is accomplished by their maturation into plasma
cells, which subsequently synthesize and
secrete immune antibodies (immunoglobulins). Stimulation of B cells to produce antibodies is a complex process, usually
requiring interactions between *macrophages, T cells,* and *B cells.* The condition
of hyperacute rejection of transplanted organs is mediated by the B cell.

Natural Killer and K-type Lymphocytes.
These cells, which lack the recognizable
surface markers of mature T or B lymphocytes, include the *natural killer (NK)* and
K-type. The NK and K cells destroy target
cells through an extracellular nonphagocytic mechanism referred to as a cytotoxic
reaction.

NK-cells have the ability to nonspecifically attack certain types of tumor cells and
cells infected with a number of different
viruses. NK-cells are classified as a population of effector lymphocytes that produce
such mediators as *interferon* and *interleu-*

kin 2. These cells have long been classified
as *null* cells, but monoclonal antibodies
have revealed several membrane markers
that affirm their T-cell nature. They cannot
be absolutely classified as T cells, however,
because they have an unmistakably prim-
itive lineage.

K-type cells exhibit a different kind of
cytotoxic mechanism from NK cells. The
target cell must be coated with low concentrations of IgG antibody (to be discussed later in this chapter.) This is referred
to as an *antibody-dependent, cell-mediated,
cytotoxicity (ADCC)* reaction. An ADCC reaction may be exhibited by both K cells and
phagocytic and nonphagocytic myelogen-
ous-type leukocytes. K cells are capable of
lysing tumor cells. The precise lineage of
the K cell is uncertain.

Plasma Cells. The development of
plasma cells may follow two pathways;
they develop either directly from plasma
cell precursors or from stimulated B lymphocytes by way of intermediate cells. The
pathway from the B lymphocyte to the an-
tibody-synthesizing plasma cell (Fig. 3-4)
occurs when the B cell is antigenically stimulated and undergoes *blast transformation.*
The immune antibody response begins
when B lymphocytes encounter antigens
that bind to their specific immunoglobulin
surface receptors. After receiving an appropriate "second signal" provided by interaction with helper T cells, these antigen-
bound B lymphocyte cells undergo blast cell
transformation and proliferation to generate a clone of mature plasma cells, which
secrete a specific type of antibody.

ANTIGEN CHARACTERISTICS

Foreign substances, such as erythrocytes,
can be *immunogenic* or *antigenic* (capable
of provoking an immune response) if their
membrane contains a number of areas recognized as foreign. These areas are called
antigenic determinants or *epitopes.* Not all
surface areas act as antigenic determinants.
Only prominent determinants on the surface of a protein are normally recognized
by the immune system, and some of these
are much more immunogenic than others.
An immune response is directed against

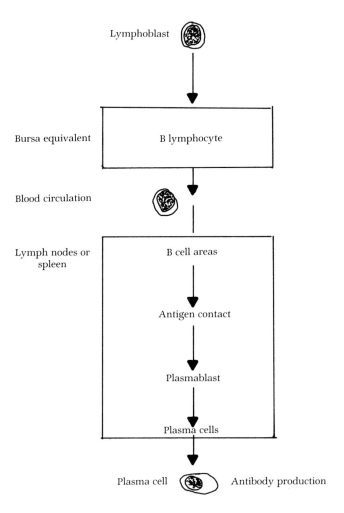

Figure 3-4. Plasma cell development from B lymphocytes. (Illustration from Turgeon, M.L.: *Clinical Hematology: Theory and Procedures.* Boston; Little, Brown and Company, 1988. p. 116.)

specific determinants and resultant antibodies bind to them, with much of the remainder of the molecule being non-immunogenic. Functionally, immunogenic determinants are said to be *immunodominant.*

Cell Surface Antigens

The cellular membrane of all mammalian cells consists of proteins, phospholipids, cholesterol, and traces of polysaccharide. The most popular hypothesis to explain the arrangement of these molecular components is the *fluid mosaic model.* According to this model, the cell membrane is a dy-namic fluid structure with globular proteins floating in lipids. The lipids, as phospholipids, are arranged in two layers. The polar (charged) phosphate ends of the phospholipids are oriented toward the inner and outer surfaces, whereas the nonpolar (fatty acid) ends point toward each other in the interior of the membrane. Protein molecules may be either intrinsic (incorporated into the lipid bilayer) or extrinsic (associated with either the outer or the inner surface of the membrane). Polysaccharides (carbohydrates) in the form of either glycoproteins or glycolipids can be found attached to the lipid and protein molecules of the membrane. Most of these proteins are immunogenic when injected into an individual of another species or even into a different individual of the same species.

Cellular antigens of importance to immunohematologists are blood group antigens, histocompatibility (HLA) antigens, and autoantigens.

BLOOD GROUP ANTIGENS

Blood group substances are widely distributed throughout the tissues, blood cells, and body fluids. The literature does not agree on the presence of the major blood group antigen systems on certain cells, particularly leukocytes. Recent studies (Table 3-1) have documented the fact that many erythrocyte antigens are not as widely distributed as previously thought. Some blood group antigens are restricted to specific types of cells. For example, Kell blood group antigens, with one exception, are found only on erythrocytes.

Certain antigens, especially those of the Rh system, are integral structural components of the erythrocyte membrane. If these antigens are missing, the erythrocyte membrane is defective and causes hemolytic anemia. When antigens do not form part of the essential membrane structure such as A, B and H (ABH), the absence of antigen has no effect on membrane integrity. The Lewis antigens are passively absorbed by selective uptake onto erythrocytes from the plasma.

HISTOCOMPATIBILITY ANTIGENS (HLA)

General Characteristics. The histocompatibility complex that encodes cell surface antigens was first discovered in graft rejection experiments with mice. When the antigens were matched between donor and recipient, the ability of a graft to survive was remarkably improved. These antigens are of primary importance, second only to the A and B antigens in influencing the survival or graft rejection of transplanted organs. The term *histocompatibility antigens* was coined for these antigens.

A comparable genetic system of alloantigens was later identified in humans. The presence of histocompatibility antigens was first recognized when multiply transfused patients experienced transfusion reactions despite proper crossmatching. It was discovered that these reactions resulted from leukocyte antibodies rather than antibodies directed against erythrocyte antigens. These same antibodies were subsequently discovered in the sera of multiparous women.

In humans, the major histocompatibility complex is referred to as human leukocyte antigen (HLA). It is the most complex immunogenetic system presently known in humans and is controlled by a major histocompatibility complex, or supergene, which includes several loci closely linked on the short arm of chromosome 6. Each of these loci involves numerous alleles, having at least 10 to 40 alleles per locus that control the production of their corresponding antigens. The antigens are found on body cells such as leukocytes, platelets, and other tissue cells as well as on some non-nucleated cells, and in body fluids. Some groups of these antigens exhibit cross-reacting characteristics that further increase the complexity of the system.

Although HLA was originally identified by its role in transplant rejection, it is now recognized that proteins encoded in this

Table 3-1. Erythrocyte Antigen Incidence on Leukocytes

Investigator(s)	Date	Occurrence of Major RBC Antigens on Leukocytes
Gaidulis et al.	1985	Not detectable on human granulocytes: A, B, D, U, Gerbich, Jk^a, Jk^b (Jk3), and Cartwright (Yt^a)
Kelton and Bebenek	1985	Granulocytes do not have surface A or B antigens
Dunstan	1986	Lymphocytes express A, B, Le^a and Le^b depending on the secretor status
		ABH and Lewis antigens are not detectable on monocytes and segmented neutrophils (PMNs) regardless of secretor (Se) status
		Lymphocytes, monocytes, and PMNs do not express D, E, e, C, c, Fy^a, Fy^b, Fy^5, Jk^a, Jk^b, K, k, M, m, S, s, U, Vel, Co^a, Lan, Jk^3, Yt^a, Di^b, Ge, Sc:1 or Lu^b antigens
		Lymphocytes, monocytes, and PMNs all express I, i, P and P$_1$ antigens

region are involved in many aspects of immunologic recognition, including interaction between different lymphoid cells and between lymphocytes and antigen-presenting cells.

The products of HLA genes play a crucial role in our immune system. The HLA genes encode for three classes of molecules: class I, class II, and class III. The class I major transplantation antigens are serologically defined. This class includes the main HLA-A, B, and C antigens. The three principal loci are termed A, B, and C, and their respective antigens are numbered 1, 2, 3, etc. The class II immune response gene region antigens are encoded in the HLA-D region and can be subdivided into three families, called HLA-DR, -DC (DQ), and -SB (DP). Class I and class II molecules are surface membrane proteins. Class I molecules are transmembrane glycoproteins, but the class II dimer molecule differs from class I in that both dimers span the cell membrane. Class I and class II gene products are biochemically distinct, although they appear to be distantly related through evolution. Both class I and class II antigens function as targets of T lymphocytes that regulate the immune response. The presence of self-class I antigens is a requisite for cytotoxic T lymphocytes to recognize and lyse virus-infected cells. Another function of class II molecules is to restrict the activity or regulatory T cells (T helper, suppressor, and amplifier subsets). Class II molecules are normally expressed by only a few types of cells such as B lymphocytes and macrophages; they may also appear under certain circumstances on activated T lymphocytes and epithelial cells. Many of the genes in both class I and class II gene families have no known functions. Class III molecules bear no clear relation to class I and II molecules aside from their genetic linkage. Class III molecules are involved in immunologic phenomena because they represent components of the complement pathways.

Class I antigens are determined by several techniques; the most popular and reproducible is the lymphocyte microcytotoxicity method. With this technique, a living lymphocyte suspension from peripheral blood or lymphatic tissue is mixed with antisera and complement. In the presence of the corresponding antigen, complement is fixed and the cells are killed. Cell death is determined by staining. A stain such as trypan blue penetrates dead cells but not living ones. Unaffected cells remain brilliantly refractile when observed microscopically. Other methods of analysis include leukocyte agglutination and complement fixation on platelets in suspension.

HLA Applications. HLA matching is of value in organ transplantation as well as in the transplantation of bone marrow. HLA-matched platelets are useful to patients who are refractile to random donor platelets. In paternity testing, HLA typing, along with the determination of ABO, Rh, MNSs, Kell, Duffy, and Kidd erythrocyte antigen, is used. In the past, most laboratories involved in testing individuals in disputed parentage cases used only the ABO, Rh, and MNSs systems. The chance of identifying a falsely accused man with these tests was 58%. Additional testing for Kell, Duffy, and Kidd erythrocyte antigens, and HLA typing offers an exclusion rate estimated at 92%. HLA typing is also useful in forensic medicine, anthropology, and basic research in immunology.

HLA testing is being used increasingly as a diagnostic and genetic counseling tool. An intriguing peculiarity of certain HLA alleles is that they appear to be genetically linked to the predisposition to various diseases, mainly of an autoimmune nature.

AUTOANTIGENS

In some situations (not always abnormal), antibodies may be produced in response to normal self-antigens. This failure to recognize self-antigens can result in autoantibodies directed at hormones, such as thyroglobulin, and cell-membrane antigens, such as the Ii blood group system. Antibodies of this type are discussed in detail in Chapter Five.

The Chemical Nature of Antigens

Antigens or *immunogens* are usually large organic molecules that are either proteins or large polysaccharides, and rarely (if ever) lipids. Antigens, especially cell surface or membrane-bound antigens, can be composed of combinations of the biochemical classes, for example, glycoproteins or glycolipids. For example, HLA antigens are glycoprotein in nature and are found on the surface membranes of nucleated body cells comprising both solid tissue and most circulating blood cells. The Lewis antigens are glycolipids, ceramide pentasaccharides (Le^a), or hexasaccharides (Le^b), which are absorbed from the plasma where they circulate on lipoproteins.

Proteins are excellent antigens because of their high molecular weight and structural complexity; lipids are considered inferior antigens because of their relative simplicity and lack of structural stability. When lipids are linked to proteins or polysaccharides, they may function as antigens. Nucleic acids are poor antigens because of their relative simplicity, molecular flexibility, and rapid degradation. Antinucleic acid antibodies can be produced by artificially stabilizing these acids and linking them to an immunogenic carrier. Carbohydrates (polysaccharides) by themselves are considered too small to function as antigens. However, in the case of erythrocyte blood group antigens, protein or lipid carriers may contribute to the necessary size and the polysaccharides present in the form of side chains, confer the immunologic specificity (immunodominant carbohydrate) and are considered the *antigenic determinant* groups or combining sites with which antibodies react.

The Physical Nature of Antigens

For antigens to function effectively, the following factors are important: foreignness, degradability, molecular weight, structural stability, and complexity.

FOREIGNNESS

The more foreign the antigenic determinant or the greater the degree to which it is recognized as non-self by an individual's immune system, the more antigenic it is. The immunogenicity of a molecule depends greatly on its degree of foreignness. Nor-

mally, an individual's immune system does not respond to self-antigens.

DEGRADABILITY

For an antigen to be recognized as foreign by an individual's immune system, a sufficient amount of antigen must be present to stimulate an immune response. Foreign molecules, which are rapidly destroyed, will not be present for enough time to provide the necessary antigenic exposure.

MOLECULAR WEIGHT

The higher the molecular weight, the better the molecule functions as an antigen. The number of antigenic determinants on a molecule is directly related to its size. Although large foreign molecules (molecular weight greater than 10,000) are better antigens; *haptens,* which are very small molecules, can bind to a larger carrier molecule and behave as antigens. If a hapten is chemically linked to a large molecule, a new surface structure is formed on the large molecule, which may function as an antigenic determinant.

STRUCTURAL STABILITY

If a molecule is to function as an effective antigen, structural stability is an essential characteristic. Molecules such as gelatin are poor antigens because of their structural instability. Totally inert molecules are also poor antigens.

COMPLEXITY

The more complex an antigen is, the more effective it will be. Complex proteins are better antigens than large repeating polymers such as lipids, carbohydrates, and nucleic acids, which are relatively poor antigens.

ANTIBODY CHARACTERISTICS

Antibodies, chemically classified as globulins, can be found in blood plasma and many body fluids such as tears, saliva, and breast milk. These specific glycoproteins are referred to as *immunoglobulins,* abbreviated Ig. Five distinct classes of immunoglobulin molecules are recognized in most higher mammals: IgM, IgG, IgA, IgD, and IgE.

The immunoglobulin classes differ from each other in characteristics such as molecular weight, sedimentation coefficient, and carbohydrate content (Table 3-2). In addition to the differences between classes, the immunoglobulins also vary within each class.

Antibody Response to Antigen

Production of antibodies is induced when the host's immune system comes into contact with a foreign antigenic substance and reacts to this antigenic stimulation. When an antigen is initially encountered, the cells of the immune system recognize the antigen as non-self and either elicit an immune response or become tolerant to it, depending on the circumstances. An immune reaction can take the form of cell-mediated immunity (immunity dependent on T cells and macrophages) or involve the production of antibodies directed against the antigen. Whether a cell-mediated response or an antibody response takes place depends on the way in which the antigen is presented to the lymphocytes; many immune reactions display both kinds of responses. The antigenicity of a foreign substance is also related to the route of entry. Intravenous and intraperitoneal routes are stronger stimuli than subcutaneous and intramuscular routes. Subsequent exposure to the same antigen produces a memory response, also known as a secondary or *anamnestic response,* and reflects the outcome of the initial challenge. In the case of antibody production, both the quantity and class of immunoglobulins produced varies.

THE PRIMARY ANTIBODY RESPONSE

Following a foreign antigen challenge, the primary IgM antibody-producing response proceeds in four phases (Fig. 3-5) but the

Table 3-2. Comparison of Characteristics of the Five Immunoglobulin Classes

Characteristic	IgM	IgG	IgA	IgE	IgD
Molecular weight	900,000	160,000	360,000	200,000	160,000
Sedimentation coefficient	19S	7S	11S	8S	7S
Percent carbohydrate	12	3	7	12	12
Subclasses	None	IgG1–4	alpha 1, 2	None	None
Serum concentration, mg/100 mL	50 to 200	800 to 1600	150 to 400	0.002 to 0.05	1.5 to 40
Half-life days	5	21	6	2	3

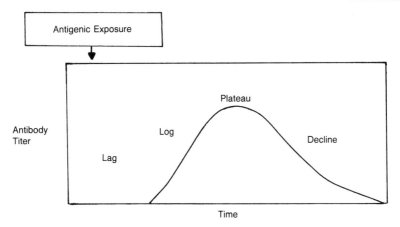

Figure 3-5. The four phases of an antibody response. Following an antigenic challenge, the antibody response in an immunocompetent proceeds in four phases: lag, log, plateau, and decline.

actual time period and levels of antibody (titer) depend on the characteristics of the antigen and the individual. The four phases are the following:

1. A *lag* phase, when no antibody is detectable
2. A *log* phase, in which the antibody titer rises logarithmically
3. A *plateau* phase, during which the antibody titer stabilizes
4. A *decline* phase, in which the antibody is catabolized

THE SECONDARY ANTIBODY (ANAMNESTIC) RESPONSE

Subsequent exposure to the same antigenic stimulus produces an antibody response that exhibits the same pattern as a primary response. Repeated exposure to an antigen can take place many years after the initial exposure, but clones of the T memory cells will be stimulated to proliferate, with subsequent production of antibody by the individual. Thus an anamnestic response, differs from a primary response in several important aspects (Fig. 3-6). The major dif-

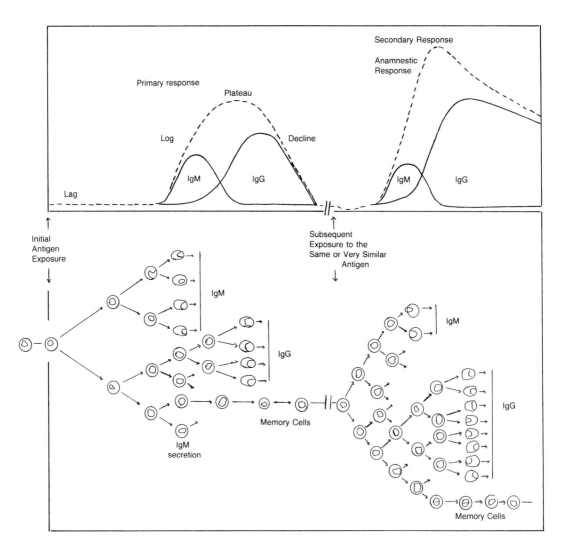

Figure 3-6. The primary and secondary (anamnestic) response. The differences between a primary and secondary response include the length of the lag phase, the type of antibody produced, and the antibody titer.

ferences between a primary and secondary response include the following:

Time. A secondary response has a shorter lag phase, a longer plateau, and a more gradual decline.

Type of Antibody. IgM-type antibodies are the principal class formed in the primary response. Although some IgM antibodies are formed in a secondary response, IgG antibodies are the predominant type of antibody formed.

Antibody Titer. In a secondary response, antibody levels attain a higher titer. The plateau levels in a secondary response are typically ten-fold more, or greater, than the plateau levels in the primary response.

Antibody Structure

Antibodies exhibit diversity among the different classes, which suggests that they perform different functions in addition to their primary function of antigen binding. Essentially, each immunoglobulin molecule is bifunctional. One region of the molecule is concerned with binding to an antigen, whereas a different region mediates binding of the immunoglobulin to host tissues, including cells of the immune system and the first component (C1q) of the classical complement system.

The primary structure of a protein is based on the sequence of amino acid residues linked together by peptide bonds. All antibodies have a common, basic polypeptide structure that has a three-dimensional configuration. The polypeptide chains are linked together by covalent and noncovalent bonds, which produce a unit composed of a four-chain structure based on pairs of identical heavy and light chains. The immunoglobulins IgG, IgD, and IgE occur only as monomers of the four-chain unit. IgA occurs in both monomeric and polymeric forms; IgM occurs as a pentamer with five four-chain subunits linked together.

A TYPICAL IMMUNOGLOBULIN MOLECULE

A classic model of antibody structure is displayed by the IgG molecule. Using electron microscopy, it can be seen to be Y-shaped (Figure 3-7). If the molecule is treated with a compound, such as 2-mercaptoethanol, which breaks interchain disulfide bonds, the molecule separates into four separate polypeptide chains. The basic molecule consists of two identical light polypeptide chains and two identical heavy polypeptide chains linked together by disulfide bonds. The light chains are found in the N-terminal half of the molecule. Light chains are small chains (MW 25,000) and are common to all classes of immunoglobulins. The light chains are of two subtypes termed kappa (κ) and lambda (λ), which have very different amino acid sequences and are antigenically different. In humans, about 65% of immunoglobulin molecules have kappa chains, while 35% have lambda. The larger, heavy chains (MW, 50,000-77,000) extend the full length of the molecule.

A general feature of the immunoglobulin chains is their amino acid sequence. The first 110 to 120 amino acids of both the light

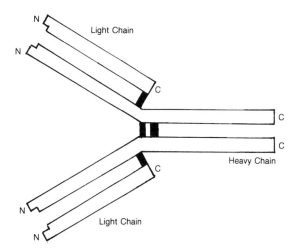

Figure 3-7. Basic immunoglobulin molecule configuration. The basic structure of an immunoglobulin molecule consists of two identical light polypeptide chains and two identical heavy polypeptide chains linked together by disulfide bond (heavy dark bars). At one end of the molecule, the amino (N) terminal ends are located; the opposite end has carboxy (C) terminals.

and heavy chains have a variable sequence and form the variable (V) region; the remainder of the light chains represent a constant (C) region with an amino acid sequence that is similar for each type and subtype. The remaining portion of the heavy chain is also constant for each type and has a hinge region. The class and subclass of an immunoglobulin molecule are determined by its heavy chain type (Fig. 3-8).

THE FAB, FC, AND HINGE MOLECULAR COMPONENTS

A typical monomeric IgG molecule consists of three globular regions (two Fab regions and an Fc portion) linked by a flexible hinge region. If the molecule is digested with a proteolytic enzyme (Fig. 3-9) such as papain, it splits into three approximately equal-sized fragments. Two of these fragments retain the ability to bind antigen and are referred to as *antigen-binding (Fab) fragments.* The third fragment, which is sometimes crystallizable, is referred to as the *Fc portion.* If IgG is treated with another proteolytic enzyme, pepsin, the molecule separates in a somewhat different manner. The Fc portion is split into very small peptides and completely destroyed. The two Fab fragments remain joined together to produce a structure called F(ab)'2. This structure has two antigen-binding sites. If F(ab)'2 is treated to reduce its disulfide bonds, it breaks into two Fab fragments with only one antigen binding site each. Further disruption of the interchain disulfide bonds in the two Fab fragments demonstrates that each contains a light chain and half of a heavy chain, the *Fd portion.*

Immunoglobulin Classes and Subclasses

Five major immunoglobulin classes exist. Each is unique and possesses its own characteristic antigenic determinants.

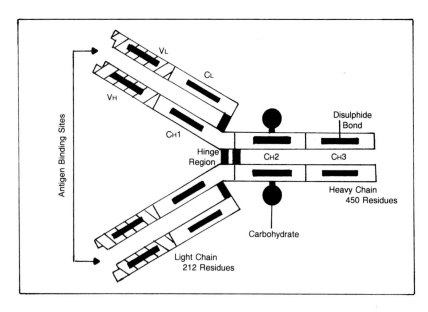

Figure 3-8. The basic structure of IgG. In the IgG molecule, the amino terminal end is characterized by sequence variability (V) in both the light (L) and heavy (H) chains. These are referred to as the VL and VH regions. The sites where antibody binds to antigen are located in these variable regions. The remainder of the molecule has a relatively constant (C) structure. The constant region of the light chain is the CL region; the constant region of the heavy chain is CH. The CH regions are divided into three distinct regions: CH1, CH2, and CH3. These sections are stabilized by intrachain disulfide bonds. The hinge region is a segment of heavy chain between the CH1 and CH2 domains. The flexibility of the hinge region permits variation in the distance between the two antigen-binding sites; therefore, they can react independently.

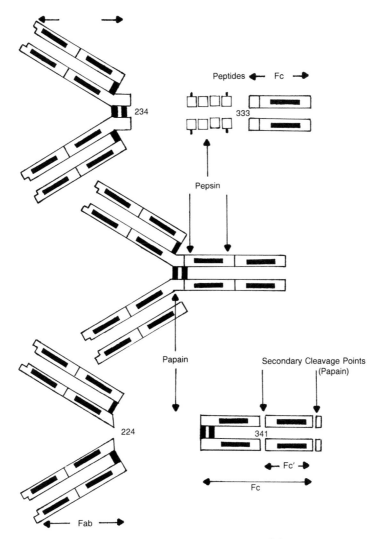

Figure 3-9. Enzymatic cleavage of human IgG1.

IgG

The most prominent immunoglobulin in normal serum is IgG. It is a 7S molecule with a molecular weight of approximately 150,000. IgG accounts for 70 to 75% of the total immunoglobulin pool. One of the subclasses, IgG_3, is slightly larger (MW 170,000) than the other subclasses.

Subclasses of IgG. Within the major immunoglobulin classes are variants known as subclasses and subtypes. These subclasses differ in their heavy chain composition (Fig. 3-10) and in some of their characteristics such as biologic activities (see Table 3-3). Four IgG subclasses (IgG_1, IgG_2, IgG_3, IgG_4) exist. The subclasses occur in the approximate proportions of 66, 23, 7, and 4%, respectively, in humans.

IgM

IgM accounts for about 10% of the immunoglobulin pool. It is largely confined to the intravascular pool, and is the predominant antibody produced in a primary immune response. In humans, it is found in smaller concentrations than IgG or IgA. The pentamer configuration of the molecule has

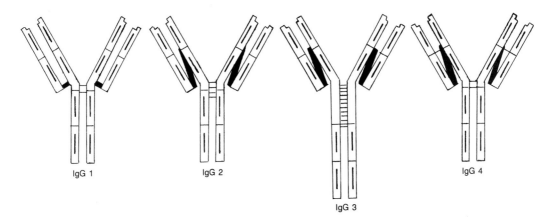

Figure 3-10. The molecular structures of the polypeptide chains of the four human IgG subclasses. The subclasses have different numbers and arrangements of the interchain disulfide bonds. In IgG1, the disulfide bond linking the light and heavy chains goes to the hinge region. In IgG2, IgG3, and IgG4, the bond goes to the junction between the variable and constant regions.

individual heavy chains with an MW of 65,000; the whole molecule has an MW of 970,000 and a sedimentation coefficient of 19S.

The IgM molecule is structurally composed of five basic subunits. Each basic subunit consists of two kappa or two lambda light chains and two mu heavy chains. The individual monomers of IgM are linked together by disulfide bonds in a circular fashion (Fig. 3-11). A small cystein-rich polypeptide called the J chain must be considered an integral part of the molecule. IgM has carbohydrate residues attached to the C_{H3} and C_{H4} domains. The site for complement activation by IgM is located on this C_{H4} region. IgM is more efficient than IgG in activities, such as the activation of complement cascade and agglutination.

IgA

IgA represents 15 to 20% of the total circulatory immunoglobulin pool. It is the predominant immunoglobulin in secretions, such as tears, saliva, colostrum, breast milk, and intestinal secretions. IgA is synthesized largely by plasma cells located on body surfaces. If the IgA is produced by cells in the intestinal wall, it may pass directly into the intestinal lumen or diffuse into the blood circulation. As IgA is transported through intestinal epithelial cells or hepatocytes, it binds to a glycoprotein called the secretory piece. This secretory piece protects IgA from digestion by gastrointestinal proteolytic enzymes and forms a complex molecule named secretory IgA (SIgA). Secretory IgA is of critical importance in protecting body surfaces against invading microorganisms.

In humans, more than 80% of IgA occurs as a typical four-chain structure consisting of paired kappa or lambda chains and two heavy chains. The basic four-chain monomer has an MW of 160,000. However, in most mammals plasma IgA occurs mostly as a dimer. In dimeric IgA, the molecules are joined by a J-chain linked to the Fc regions. Secretory IgA exists mainly in the

Table 3-3. Variations in Subclasses of IgG

Characteristic	IgG₁	IgG₂	IgG₃	IgG₄
% of total IgG in serum	65	24	7	4
Complement fixation	4+	2+	4+	(+)
Half-life in days	23	23	8	23
Placental passage	+	?	+	+

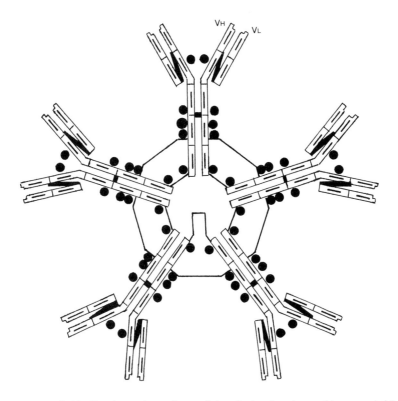

Figure 3-11. Pentameric polypeptide chain structure of human IgM.

11S, dimeric form and has an MW of 385,000. In humans, variations in the heavy chains account for the subclasses IgA_1 and IgA_2.

IgD

IgD, found in very low concentrations in plasma, accounts for less than 1% of the total immunoglobulin pool and is susceptible to proteolysis. This is primarily a cell membrane immunoglobulin found on the surface of B lymphocytes in association with IgM. The molecule has an MW of 184,000 and consists of two kappa or lambda light chains and two delta heavy chains. It has no interchain disulfide bonds between its heavy chains and it has a very exposed hinge region.

IgE

IgE is a trace plasma protein in the blood plasma of nonparasitized individuals. It has an MW of 188,000. IgE is of major importance because it mediates some types of allergic reactions, allergies, and anaphylaxis, and is generally responsible for an individual's immunity to invading parasites.

The IgE molecule is composed of paired kappa or lambda light chains and two epsilon heavy chains. It is unique in that its Fc region binds strongly to a receptor on mast cells and basophils and, together with antigen, mediates the release of histamines and heparin from these cells.

Other Immunoglobulin Variants

An antigenic determinant is the specific chemical determinant group or molecular configuration against which the immune response is directed. Immunoglobulins can function as effective antigens when used to immunize mammals of a different species because they are proteins. When the re-

Table 3-4. Principal Categories of Antigenic Determinants

Variant	Distribution	Variant	Location	Examples
Isotypic	All variants in normal persons	Classes, subclasses, types	C_H, C_H, C_L	IgM, IgE, IgA$_1$, IgA$_2$, kappa, lambda
Allotypic	Genetically controlled alternate forms—not present in all persons	Allotypes	Mainly C_H/C_L, sometimes V_H/V_L	Gm groups in humans
Idiotypic	Individually specific to each immunoglobulin molecule	Idiotypes	Variable regions	Probably one or more hypervariable regions forming the antigen-combining site

Modified from Roitt, Ivan M.: *Essential Immunology,* Fifth edition. Oxford, England, Blackwell Scientific Publications, 1984. p. 42.

sulting anti-immunoglobulins or antiglobulin antibodies are analyzed, three principal categories of antigenic determinants (Table 3-4) can be recognized: isotype, allotype, and idiotype determinants (Fig. 3-12).

ISOTYPIC DETERMINANTS

This class of antigenic determinant is the dominant type found on the immunoglobulins of all animals of a species. The heavy-chain, constant-region structures associated with the different classes and subclasses are termed *isotypic variants.* Genes for isotypic variants are present in all healthy members of a species. Determinants included in this category include those that are specific for each immuno-globulin class, such as gamma for IgG, mu for IgM, and alpha for IgA, as well as the subclass-specific determinants, kappa and lambda.

ALLOTYPIC DETERMINANTS

The second principal group of determinants is found on the immunoglobulins of some, but not all, animals of a species. Antibodies to these allotypes (*alloantibodies*) may be produced by injecting the immunoglobulins of one animal into another member of the same species. The allotypic determinants are genetically determined variations representing the presence of allelic genes at a single locus within a species. Typical allotypes in humans are the Gm

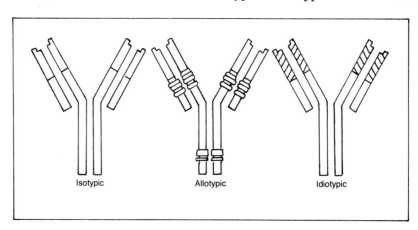

Figure 3-12. Variants of antibodies. Isotypic variation refers to the different heavy and light chain classes and subclasses. These variants are present in all healthy members of a species. Allotypic variations are not all present in all healthy members of a species. This type of variation occurs mostly in the constant region of the molecule. Idiotypic variations are specific to each antibody molecule. These variations occur only in the variable region of the molecule.

specificities on IgG (Gm = marker on IgG). In humans, the following five sets of allotypic markers have been found: Gm, Km, Mm, Am, and Hv.

IDIOTYPIC DETERMINANTS

Idiotypes exist as a result of the unique structures on light and heavy chains. These individual determinants characteristic of each antibody are termed the *idiotypes.* The idiotypic determinants are located in the variable part of the antibody associated with the hypervariable regions that form the antigen-combining site.

The Functions of Antibodies

The principal function of an antibody is to bind antigen. Antibodies, however, may exhibit secondary effector functions, as well as behaving as antigens. The significant secondary effector functions of antibodies (Table 3-5) are complement fixation and placental transfer. The activation of complement (discussed in detail later in this chapter) is one of the most important effector mechanisms of IgG_1 and IgG_3 molecules. IgG_2 seems to be less effective in activating complement; IgG_4, IgA, IgD, and IgE are ineffective in terms of complement activation. In man, most of the IgG subclass molecules are capable of crossing the placental barrier. It is not universally agreed whether or not IgG_2 crosses the placenta. Passage of antibodies across the placental barrier is an important mechanism in hemolytic disease of the newborn (HDN, discussed in Chapter 10) and in conferring passive immunity to the newborn during the first few months of life.

Antibody Avidity

Each four-polypeptide-chain antibody unit has two antigen binding sites that allow the unit to be potentially multivalent in its reaction with an antigen. The strength with which a multivalent antibody binds a multivalent antigen is termed *avidity;* this term contrasts with *affinity,* which is the bond between a single antigenic determinant and an individual combining site. When a multivalent antigen combines with more than one of an antibody's combining sites, the strength of the bonding is significantly increased. For the antigen and antibody to dissociate, all of the antigen-antibody bonds must be broken simultaneously.

Decreased avidity can result from the fact that an antigen has only one antigenic determinant (monovalent). Additionally, a hapten is monovalent and therefore can react only with one antigen combining site.

Antibody Specificity and Cross-Reactivity

Antigen-antibody reactions can show a high level of *specificity.* Specificity refers to the fact that the binding sites of antibodies directed against determinants of one antigen are not complementary to determinants of another dissimilar antigen. When some of the determinants of an antigen are shared by similar antigenic determinants on the surface of apparently unrelated molecules, a proportion of the antibodies directed against one kind of antigen will also react with the other kind of antigen. This is called *cross-reactivity.* Antibodies directed against a protein in one species may also react in a detectable manner with the homologous protein in another species, which is also an example of cross-reactivity.

Examples of cross-reactivity also occur between bacteria that possess cell-wall polysaccharides in common with mammalian

Table 3-5. Properties of Immunoglobulins

	IgG_1	IgG_2	IgG_3	IgG_4	IgM	IgA	IgD	IgE
Complement fixation	2+	1+	3+	0	3+	0	0	0
Placental transfer	1+	+/−	+	1+	0	0	0	0

erythrocytes. Intestinal bacteria and other substances found in the environment possess A- or B-like antigens similar to the A and B erythrocyte antigens. If A or B antigens are foreign to an individual, production of anti-A or anti-B occurs even though the person has never been exposed to these erythrocyte antigens. Cross-reacting antibodies of this type are *heterophile antibodies.*

Monoclonal Antibodies

Monoclonal antibodies are purified antibodies that are cloned from a single cell and engineered to bind to a single specific antigen. Monoclonal antibodies to cell surface antigens now provide a method for classifying and identifying specific cellular membrane characteristics, such as in the typing of erythrocyte and leukocyte antigens, and as a reagent in the detection of coating of erythrocyte antigens in the antihuman globulin (AHG) test.

DISCOVERY OF THE TECHNIQUE

In 1975, George Kohler, a postdoctoral student at Cambridge University, was examining cell hybrids developed from different lines of cultured myeloma cells (plasma cells derived from malignant tumor strains) by using Sendai virus to induce the cells to fuse together. (Sendai virus is an influenza virus that characteristically causes cell fusion.)

Initially, he immunized donors with sheep erythrocytes to provide a marker for the normal cells. After making the hybrids, he tested them to see if they still produced antibodies against the sheep erythrocytes and discovered that some of the hybrids were manufacturing large quantities of specific antisheep erythrocyte antibodies.

This technique is referred to as *somatic cell hybridization.* The resulting hybrid cells secrete the antibody characteristic of the parent cell, antisheep erythrocyte antibodies. The multiplying hybrid cell culture is called a *hybridoma.* Hybridoma cells can be cloned (the process in which single cells are selected and grown). The immunoglob-

ulins derived from a single clone of cells are named *monoclonal antibodies.*

MONOCLONAL ANTIBODY PRODUCTION

Modern methods for producing monoclonal antibodies (Fig. 3-13) are refinements of the original technique developed by Kohler. Basically, hybridoma technique enables scientists to inoculate crude antigen mixtures into mice and then select clones producing specific antibodies, each directed against a single cell surface antigen. The process of producing monoclonal antibodies takes from 3 to 6 months to complete.

To initiate the production of monoclonal antibodies, mice are immunized with a specific antigen. Several doses of the antigen are given to ensure a vigorous immune response. From 2 to 4 days later, spleen cells are then mixed with cultured mouse myeloma cells. Myeloma parent cells, which lack the enzyme hypoxanthine phosphoribosyl transferase, are selected because these cells cannot use hypoxanthine derived from the culture medium to manufacture purines and pyrimidines, and if unfused, will not survive in the culture medium. Additionally, the mouse myeloma cell lines usually do not secrete immunoglobulins, which simplifies the purification process.

Polyethylene glycol rather than Sendai virus is added to the cell mixture to promote cell-membrane fusion. Only 1 in every 200,000 spleen cells actually forms a viable hybrid with a myeloma cell. Normal spleen cells do not survive in culture. The fused-cell mixture is placed in a medium containing hypoxanthine, aminopterin, and thymidine (HAT medium). Aminopterin is a drug that prevents myeloma cells from making their own purines and pyrimidines, and because they cannot use hypoxanthine from the medium, the cells die.

Hybrids resulting from the fusion of spleen cells and myeloma cells contain transferase provided by the normal spleen cells. Consequently, the hybridoma cells are able to use the hypoxanthine and thymidine in the culture medium and survive. They divide rapidly in HAT medium, doubling their numbers every 24 to 48 hours.

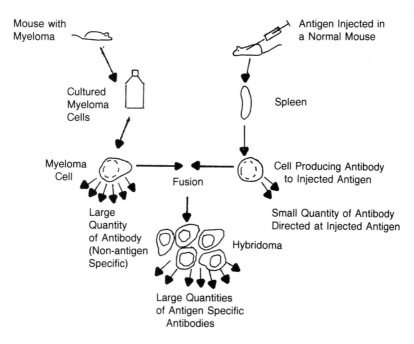

Figure 3-13 Monoclonal antibody production. Monoclonal antibodies are produced from hybridoma cells. The cells result from the fusion of neoplastic myeloma cells and specific antibody-producing cells.

About 300 to 500 different hybrids can be generated from the cells of a single mouse spleen, although not all make the desired antibodies. After the hybridomas have been growing for 2 to 4 weeks, the supernatant is tested for specific antibody, using methods such as the enzyme-linked immunoabsorbent assay (ELISA) or radioimmunoassay (RIA). Clones that produce the desired antibody are grown in mass culture and recloned to eliminate nonantibody-producing cells.

Antibody-producing clones lose their ability after being cultured for several months. It is usual to freeze and store hybridoma cells in small aliquots. They may then be grown in mass culture or injected intraperitoneally into mice. Because hybridomas are tumor cells, they grow rapidly and induce the effusion of large quantities of fluid into the peritoneal cavity. This ascites fluid is rich in monoclonal antibody and can be easily harvested.

In the case of the production of Anti-Human Globulin Murine Monoclonal BioClone (by Ortho Diagnostic Systems, Inc.), the reagent is prepared from a pool of mouse monoclonal anti-C3b and anti-C3d. The mouse anti-C3b and anti-C3d portions are obtained by intraperitoneally injecting a group of mice with an anti-C3b-secreting hybridoma and another group of mice with an anti-C3d-secreting hybridoma. After a suitable time, the mouse ascitic fluid is harvested from each of the groups, pooled, and manufactured into the specific anti-C3b,-C3d anti-human globulin (AHG) reagent.

APPLICATIONS OF MONOCLONAL ANTIBODIES IN BLOOD BANKING

The greatest impact of monoclonal antibodies in blood banking has been on the analysis of cell-membrane antigens. Because monoclonal antibodies have a single specificity compared to the range of antibody molecules present in the serum, they are useful in erythrocyte typing, leukocyte typing (lymphocyte subsets), and tissue typing.

The use of monoclonal antibodies can potentially reduce the overall cost of erythrocyte antigen determinations. Monoclonal antibodies produced by individual murine hybridomas to human blood group A cells can be used to detect A antigens as well as weak subgroups of A. Although not all anti-D monoclonal antibodies may be sensitive enough to detect weak D^u reactions, the use of monoclonal anti-D can eliminate the need for supplemental D^u testing.

Occasional instances of incorrect ABO typing have been observed because of inappropriate monoclonal antibody sensitivity. In these reported cases, inaccurate reactivity with some group B specimens has been noted with anti-A reagent.

THE MOLECULAR BASIS OF ANTIGEN-ANTIBODY REACTIONS

The basic Y-shaped immunoglobulin molecule is a bifunctional structure. The V domains are primarily concerned with antigen binding. When an antigenic determinant and its specific antibody combine, they interact through the chemical groups found on the surface of the antigenic determinant and on the surface of the *hypervariable* regions of the immunoglobulin molecule. Although the C domains do not form the antigen binding sites, the arrangement of the C domains and hinge region give the molecule segmental flexibility, which allows it to combine with separated antigenic determinants.

Types of Bonding

The bonding of an antigen to an antibody takes place because of the formation of multiple reversible intermolecular attractions between an antigen and amino acids of the binding site. These forces require close proximity of the interacting groups. The optimum distance separating the interacting groups varies for different types of bonds. Bonds form across short distances and weaken very rapidly as the distance increases (Fig. 3-14).

The bonding of antigens to antibodies is exclusively *noncovalent*. The attractive force of noncovalent bonds is weak when compared to covalent bonds; however, the formation of multiple noncovalent bonds produces considerable total binding energy.

The strength of a single antigen-antibody bond is termed the *antibody affinity* and is produced by the summation of the attractive and repulsive forces. The types of noncovalent bonds involved in antigen-antibody reactions are the following:

1. Hydrophobic bonds
2. Hydrogen bonding
3. Van der Waals forces
4. Electrostatic forces

HYDROPHOBIC BONDS

The major bonds formed between antigens and antibodies are hydrophobic. Many of the nonpolar side chains of proteins are hydrophobic. When antigen and antibody molecules come together, these side chains interact and exclude water molecules from the area of the interaction. The exclusion of water eliminates some of the constraints imposed by the proteins, which results in a gain in energy and forms an energetically stable complex.

HYDROGEN BONDING

Hydrogen bonding results from the formation of hydrogen bridges between appropriate atoms. Common hydrogen bonds in antigen-antibody interactions are O-H-O, N-H-N, and O-H-N.

VAN DER WAALS FORCES

Van der Waals forces are nonspecific attractive forces that are generated by the interaction between electron clouds and hydrophobic bonds. These bonds occur as a result of a minor asymmetry in the charge of an atom because of the position of its electrons. Van der Waals forces rely on the association of nonpolar, hydrophobic groups so that contact with water molecules is minimized. Although these forces are very weak, they may become collectively important in an antigen-antibody reaction.

ELECTROSTATIC FORCES

Electrostatic forces develop because of the attraction of oppositely charged amino acids located on two protein side chains.

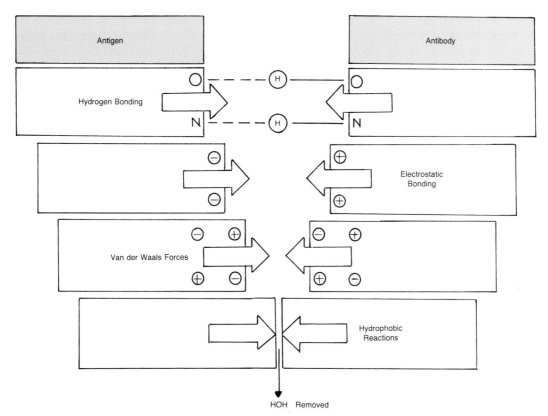

Figure 3-14. The types of bonds or forces that can bind antibodies and antigens. Various bonds or forces can be formed when the interacting groups of antigens and antibodies closely approach each other. The distance between interacting groups of molecules that produces optimum binding varies for different bond types.

The relative importance of electrostatic bonds is unclear.

Goodness of Fit

The strongest bonding develops when antigens and antibodies are in close proximity to each other and when the shapes of both the antigenic determinants and the antigen-binding site conform to each other. The complementary matching of determinants and binding sites is referred to as "goodness of fit."

A good fit creates ample opportunities for the simultaneous formation of several noncovalent bonds and few opportunities for disruption of the bond. If a poor fit exists, repulsive forces can dominate any small forces of attraction. Variations from the ideal complementary shape produce a de-crease in the total binding energy because of increased repulsive forces and decreased attractive forces. Therefore, "goodness of fit" is important in determining the binding of an antibody molecule to a particular antigen.

IN VITRO DETECTION OF ANTIGEN-ANTIBODY REACTIONS

Laboratory Tests

In vitro tests detect the combination of antigens and antibodies. Tests such as the RIA and ELISA measure immune complexes formed in an in vitro system. Tests such as agglutination tests are the most widely used to detect and measure the consequences of antigen-antibody interaction. Other test types include precipitation reactions, hemolysis testing, and inhibition of agglutination. Because of the widespread use of agglutination testing in blood banking procedures, such as blood grouping and compatibility testing, agglutination reactions are presented in detail in the following section. The reader should consult an immunology text for detailed descriptions of the other types of serologic procedures that have applications to transfusion therapy, such as hepatitis testing.

The Mechanism of Agglutination

Agglutination is the clumping of those particles with antigens on their surface, such as erythrocytes, by antibody molecules that form bridges between the antigenic determinants. This is the endpoint for most tests involving erythrocyte antigens and blood group antibodies. Agglutination, which is influenced by a number of factors, is believed to occur in two stages: *sensitization* and *lattice formation.*

SENSITIZATION

The first phase of agglutination, *sensitization,* represents the physical attachment of antibody molecules to antigens on the erythrocytic membrane. In this initial reversible interaction, antibodies combine rapidly with antigenic particles. The amount of antibody that will react is affected by the equilibrium constant, or affinity constant, of the antibody. In most cases, the higher the equilibrium constant, the higher the rate of association and the slower the rate of dissociation of antibody molecules. The degree of association of antigen with antibody is affected by a variety of factors and can be altered in some cases in vitro by altering some of these factors. The factors influencing antigen-antibody association include the following:

1. The antigen-antibody ratio or the number of antibody molecules in relation to the number of antigen sites per cell.
2. Physical conditions such as pH, temperature, and length of time of incubation, ionic strength, and steric hindrance.

Antigen-antibody Ratio. Under conditions of antibody excess, a surplus of molecular antigen-combining sites which are not bound to antigenic determinants exists. The outcome of excessive antibody concentration is known as the *prozone phenomenon,* which can produce false-negative reactions. This phenomenon can be overcome by serially diluting the antibody-containing serum until optimum amounts of antigen and antibody are present in the test system.

pH. Although the optimum pH for all reactions has not been determined, a pH of 7.0 is used for routine laboratory testing. It is known that some antibodies such as anti-M and anti-D react best at a lower pH. For example, anti-D reacts best at a pH between 6.5 and 7.0.

Temperature and Length of Incubation. The optimum temperature for reaching equilibrium in an antibody-antigen reaction differs for different antibodies. IgM (19S) type antibodies are cold-reacting (thermal range 4 to 22°C) and IgG (7S) antibodies are warm reacting with an optimum temperature of reaction of 37°C. The length of time of incubation required to achieve maximum results depends upon the rate of association and dissociation of each specific antibody. In laboratory testing, incubation times range from 15 to 60 minutes. The optimum time of incubation varies according to the class of immunoglobulin and how tightly an antibody attaches to its specific antigen.

Ionic Strength. The concentration of salt in the reaction medium has an effect on antibody uptake by the membrane-bound erythrocyte antigens. Sodium (Na^+) and chloride (Cl^-) ions in a solution have a shielding effect. These ions cluster around and partially neutralize the opposite charges on antigen and antibody molecules, which hinders the association of antibody with antigen. Reducing or lowering the ionic strength of a reaction medium with agents such as low ionic strength saline (LISS) or polybrene enhances antibody uptake.

Steric Hindrance. Steric hindrance is an important physiochemical effect that influences antibody uptake by cell surface antigens. If dissimilar antibodies with approximately the same binding constant are directed against antigenic determinants located in close proximity to each other, they will compete for space in reaching their specific receptor sites. The effect of this competition can be mutual blocking or *steric hindrance,* and neither antibody type will be bound to its respective antigenic determinant. Steric hindrance can occur whenever a conformational change in the relationship of an antigenic receptor site to the outside surface occurs. In addition to antibody competition, competition with bound complement, other protein molecules, or the action of agents that interfere with the structural integrity of the cell surface can produce steric hindrance.

Knowledge of the physical conditions on the uptake of antibody is important to the blood bank technologist. Because the combination of antigen and antibody is a reversible chemical reaction, altering the physical conditions can cause the release of antibody from the antigen-binding site. When physical conditions are purposely manipulated to break the antigen-antibody complex with subsequent release of the antibody into the surrounding medium, the procedure is referred to as an *elution procedure* (see Chapter 14). The product of this procedure, antibody suspended in a medium, is called an *eluate.* This procedure is of practical application in the investigation of positive direct anti-human globulin (DAT) tests and in alloantibody investigation.

LATTICE FORMATION

Lattice formation, or the establishment of crosslinks between sensitized particles such as erythrocytes and antibodies resulting in aggregation (clumping), is a much slower process than the sensitization phase. The formation of chemical bonds and resultant lattice formation depend on the ability of a cell with attached antibody on its surface to come close enough to another cell to permit the antibody molecules to bridge the gap and combine with the antigen receptor site on the second cell. Crosslinking is influenced by factors such as the *zeta potential.*

Zeta Potential. In the blood circulation, erythrocytes have a net negative surface charge (Fig. 3-15). Because like charges repel one another, erythrocytes in suspension remain separated from each other. The actual distance of separation is governed by the effective net surface charge density. When erythrocytes are suspended in electrolyte solutions such as sodium chloride, the ions in a suspending solution arrange themselves about the surface of the cell and become more diffuse as the distance from the cell surface increases. As an erythrocyte floats in an electrolyte solution, some ions remain with it. The diffuse double layer surrounding the cell is called the *ionic cloud* and the outer edge of this layer is referred to as the *surface of shear.*

A difference in electrostatic potential exists between the net charge at the cell membrane and the charge at the surface of shear. This electrostatic potential is referred to as the *zeta potential.* Zeta potential is believed to depend on the actual net surface charge density at the surface of the cell membrane and the *dielectric constant* of the surrounding medium (dielectric constant is a measure of the electrical conductivity of a suspending medium). The zeta potential as well as the distance between adjacent cells can be manipulated by altering the net surface charge density of the cells or the dielectric constant of the medium.

The Influence of Antibody Types on Agglutination. Immunoglobulins are relatively positively charged, and following sensitization or coating by particles, they reduce the zeta potential. Antibodies can bridge charged particles by extending beyond the effective range of the zeta potential, which results in the erythrocytes closely approaching each other, binding together, and agglutinating.

Antibodies differ in their ability to agglutinate. IgM antibodies, sometimes referred to as *complete antibodies,* are considerably more efficient than IgG or IgA antibodies in exhibiting in vitro agglutination when the antigen-bearing erythrocytes are suspended in physiologic (0.85%) sodium chloride (saline). Antibodies that do not exhibit visible agglutination of saline-suspended erythrocytes even when bound to the cell's surface membrane are considered nonagglutinating antibodies and may be called *incomplete antibodies.* Incomplete antibod-

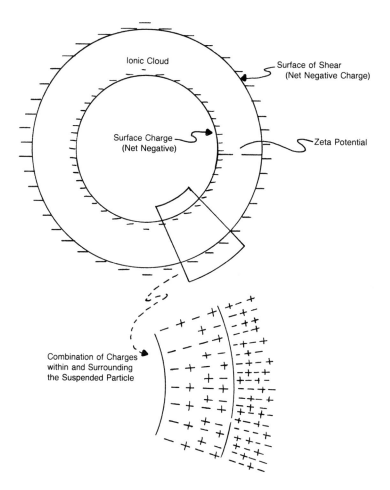

Figure 3-15. Zeta potential. Particles, such as erythrocytes, in suspension have a net negative surface charge. The zeta potential is the difference in electrostatic potential between the net charge at the cell membrane and the charge at the surface of shear.

ies may fail to exhibit agglutination because the antigenic determinants are located deep within the surface membrane or may demonstrate restricted movement in their hinge region, causing them to be functionally *monovalent.*

The Effect of Antigen Dosage. The term "double dose" is sometimes used to depict the homozygous genotypic expression of an antigen (such as "cc"), in comparison to the heterozygous genotypic expression of an antigen (such as "Cc"), which is referred to as a single dose. In some blood group systems, the presence of a homozygous genotype expresses itself with more antigen than the heterozygous genotype. The consequence of possessing a double dose of some blood group antigens (such as "c"),

is that a greater proportion of erythrocytes is agglutinated. This variation in strength of agglutination is referred to as the *dosage effect.*

Methods of Enhancing Agglutination. Several methods are commonly used in routine blood banking to enhance agglutination. These techniques include centrifugation, treatment with proteolytic enzymes, use of colloids, and addition of anti-human globulin (AHG) reagent.

CENTRIFUGATION. Centrifugation at high speed is a common technique incorporated into the protocol of many blood banking methods. Centrifugation attempts to overcome the problem of distance by subjecting sensitized cells to a high gravitational force, which counteracts the repulsive effect and physically forces the cells together.

ENZYME TREATMENT. Alteration of the zeta potential to enhance the chances of demonstrable agglutination is commonly used in the blood bank. Treatment with a weak proteolytic enzyme can strip off some of the negative charges on the cell membrane by removing surface sialic acid (cleaving sialoglycoproteins from the cell surface) residues; thereby reducing the surface charge on the cells, lowering the zeta potential, and permitting the cells to come closer together for chemical linking by specific antibody molecules. The risk of enzyme treatment is that it destroys some blood group antigens such as M, N, and Duffy.

COLLOIDAL MEDIA. In 1945, Cameron and Diamond established that certain anti-D (anti-Rh$_o$) sera would agglutinate Rh positive erythrocytes suspended in a colloid, bovine albumin. In 1964, Pollack first investigated the mechanism of action of bovine albumin. He concluded that agglutination of sensitized erythrocytes depended on factors such as the characteristics of the reaction medium. Therefore, some IgG antibodies, especially those with Rh-hr specificity, agglutinate if the zeta potential is carefully adjusted by the addition of colloids and salts. Although colloids can enhance agglutination, the effectiveness of the medium depends on the chemical properties and composition of the specific type of colloidal medium. The most frequently used colloidal reagent is bovine albumin solution. This product is manufactured from raw bovine serum. Processing results in a solution with a 22% protein concentration and a pH of 7.2, specifically designed for laboratory use. The solution additionally contains 0.1% sodium azide as a preservative.

OTHER ENHANCEMENT MEDIA. Additional enhancement media can be used to detect low-titered antibodies in routine alloantibody screening or compatibility testing. These media include low ionic strength saline (LISS), polybrene, and polyethylene glycol (PEG).

The principle of LISS is that the rate of antibody association increases as the ionic strength of the medium decreases. The use of LISS not only increases the sensitivity of antibody detection compared to bovine albumin, but also allows a shortened period of incubation. The most frequent disadvantage of a LISS technique is the increased number of nonspecific or false positive reactions observed. A more serious problem is the difficulty in detecting some examples of anti-Kell using low ionic strength solutions.

Enhancement of erythrocyte agglutination can also be achieved by using a low ionic strength medium with added positively charged macromolecules, such as polybrene or protamine. Although this technique was originally used in automated antibody detection systems, it has been adapted to manual procedures. With this technique, serum and erythrocytes are incubated in a low ionic strength medium, followed by aggregation of the cells with polybrene. The principle of this technique is that the addition of the macromolecule brings the red cells closer together to facilitate strong crosslinking by cell-bound antibodies. The use of enhancement media, such as polybrene, displays ABO incompatibility as effectively as a room temperature cross match and offers the added benefit of detecting most other clinically significant blood group alloantibodies reported to have been missed by saline-albumin screening techniques.

The addition of polyethylene glycol to serum-cell test mixtures has been reported to be more effective in detecting weak antibodies than LISS and manual polybrene. In general, polyethylene glycol does not produce nonspecific reactions.

CHEMICALLY MODIFIED ANTISERA. Chemical modification of antisera involves the conversion of some "incomplete" IgG antibodies, which are not capable of causing direct agglutination of saline-suspended erythrocytes, into saline agglutinins. This modification is achieved by reducing the disulfide bond near the hinge region of the IgG molecule with dithiothreitol, followed by an alkylation step to make the change permanent. Reduction of the disulfide bond enables the two IgG Fab structures to span a greater distance. The modified molecules can bridge the space separating erythrocyte suspended in saline and agglutinate them. Chemically modified antisera are available for detection of D and Kell antigens. Chemically modified anti-D sera are also suitable for the D^u test.

The Anti-Human Globulin (AHG) Test

In some cases, antigens may be so deeply imbedded in the membrane surface that the previously described techniques will not bring the antigens and antibodies close enough to crosslink. The anti-human globulin test is frequently incorporated into the protocol of many laboratory techniques to facilitate agglutination.

REAGENT PREPARATION

Because immunoglobulins are proteins, they function as effective antigens when injected into mammals of a different species. For example, human immunoglobulins promote a strong antibody response when injected into a rabbit. In the traditional preparation of anti-human globulin reagent, one colony of rabbits is injected with purified human gamma globulin and a second colony of rabbits is injected with purified components of human beta globulin. After a suitable time, plasma is harvested from the whole blood of the rabbits as the raw material. It is pooled and manufactured into a specific reagent for use in detecting human gamma globulin or components of complement. The product is buffered with bovine albumin and 0.1% sodium azide is added as a preservative. If color is added, such as in Ortho Anti-Human Globulin (green), FD&C Blue No. 1 and FD&C Yellow No. 5 dye are added.

Reagents, such as AHG, can be produced through genetic engineering. The synthesis of antibodies through biotechnology is discussed in detail in the section on monoclonal antibodies.

Using either the classic method or biotechnology, the resulting anti-immunoglobulin is useful in demonstrating that erythrocytes have been sensitized but fail to produce visible agglutination. The sensitizing globulins may be gamma globulin (antibody) and/or beta globulin (components of complement).

PRINCIPLES OF THE PROCEDURE

The principle of the AHG technique was rediscovered by Coombs in 1945; therefore the procedure was called *Coombs' test* for many years. The AHG method is routinely applied in direct and indirect testing (Table 3-6). The direct antiglobulin test (DAT) is used to detect in vivo sensitization or coating. If it is necessary to test for the presence of incomplete antibodies or complement on the surface of erythrocytes as in cases of suspected hemolytic anemia the DAT is used. A patient's washed erythrocytes are mixed with AHG, and if incomplete antibodies are present, agglutination occurs. To test for the presence of incomplete antibodies in a serum, an indirect antiglobulin test (IAT) is used. In the indirect technique, the serum containing antibodies is initially incubated with erythrocytes containing antigens that adsorb the incomplete antibodies. After washing with saline to remove unbound antibodies, the coated erythrocytes are mixed with AHG. On reacting with bound antibody, the AHG crosslinks and produces agglutination.

TYPES OF ANTI-HUMAN GLOBULIN (AHG) REAGENT

Two types of anti-human globulin reagent can be used in laboratory testing procedures (Tables 3-7 and 3-8): broad-spectrum (*polyspecific*) sera and *monospecific* sera.

Polyspecific serum is the basic type of reagent used in routine blood banking procedures, such as compatibility testing or antibody screening. A polyspecific serum is defined as one that must contain anti-IgG and anti-C3d (anticomplement component). The reagent may contain antibodies of other specificities, such as anti-IgM, anti-IgA, anti-C3b, or anti-C4. If the test is positive with polyspecific sera, a monospecific sera may used for follow-up testing.

Monospecific sera such as anti-IgG and anticomplement containing C3b + C3d (previously called anti-non-gamma) are the most commonly used types of monospecific sera. Anti-IgG can detect most clinically significant antibodies. This type of reagent is useful in differentiating agglutination produced by IgG antibodies rather than agglu-

Table 3-6. A Comparison of the Direct and Indirect Anti-Human Globulin Procedures

Type of Test	Patient's Erythrocytes	Patient's Serum
Direct anti-human globulin test (DAT)	Tested for *in vivo* coating of erythrocytes	—
Indirect anti-human globulin test (IAT)	—	Tested for the presence of alloantibodies

Table 3-7. Indications for Use and Limitations of AHG Reagents with Direct Antiglobulin Test (DAT)

Disorder	Polyspecific	Anti-IgG (Rabbit)	Indications for Use Anti-C3b, C3d (Murine Monoclonal BioClone)	Anti-C3d (Murine Monoclonal BioClone)
Hemolytic disease of the newborn (HDN)	Yes	Yes		
Transfusion reactions	Yes	Yes*	Yes*	Yes*
Drug-induced RBC sensitization	Yes	Yes*	Yes*	Yes*
Autoimmune hemolytic anemia	Yes	Yes*	Yes*	Yes*
Differentiation of immunoglobulin from complement coating of RBCs		Yes	Yes†	
Specific identification of coating substance		Yes		Yes

* This reagent should not be used as the sole antiglobulin reagent. To avoid false negative results, both IgG and C3d need to be included in the testing protocol.

† Except for C4.

Modified from Anti-Human Globulin (Rabbit and Murine Monoclonal BioClone® Product Brochure, June, 1986. Ortho Diagnostic Systems, Inc., Raritan, New Jersey.

Table 3-8. Indications for Use and Limitations of AHG Reagents with Indirect Antiglobulin Tests (IAT)

Disorder	Polyspecific	Anti-IgG (Rabbit)	Anti-C3b, C3d (Murine Monoclonal BioClone)
Pretransfusion compatibility testing (X-match)	Yes	Yes*	
Alloantibody screening	Yes	Yes*	
Antigen detection	Yes	Yes	
Serum antibody identification	Yes	Yes	Yes
Identification of antibody in an elution	Yes	Yes	

* The results of some studies indicate that anti-IgG may occasionally fail to detect antibodies, which are demonstrable only with polyspecific AHG reagent. Therefore, anti-IgG should not be used exclusively for the detection of clinically significant antibodies in antibody screening or pretransfusion compatibility testing. Anti-IgG should be used in conjunction with a polyspecific type of AHG.

Modified from Anti-Human Globulin (Rabbit and Murine Monoclonal BioClone® Product Brochure, June, 1986. Ortho Diagnostic Systems, Inc., Raritan, New Jersey.

tination due to complement fixation produced by cold agglutinins. Although various components of complement can sensitize erythrocytes, the C3d component is associated with immune hemolysis; therefore, it is important that this component be included in anticomplement reagents to facilitate the investigation of immune hemolytic anemias. Monospecific sera containing anti-IgM or anti-IgA are not routinely used in clinical laboratories because the need for them is rare, but they are used by reference and research immunohematology laboratories.

Grading Agglutination Reactions

In the blood bank, it is important to observe the strength of agglutination when it occurs. The combining of antigens (also referred to as *agglutinogens*) on the surface of erythrocytes and their corresponding antibodies (also referred to as *agglutinins*) should result in agglutination (synonymously referred to as hemagglutination if the cells are erythrocytes).

Observation of agglutination is initially made by gently shaking the test tube containing the serum and cells and viewing the lower portion, *the button,* as it is dispersed with a magnifying glass. Because agglutination is a reversible reaction, the test tube must be treated delicately and hard shaking must be avoided; however, all the cells in the button must be resuspended before an accurate observation can be determined. Observations are made both *macroscopically* (using a magnifying lens) and *microscopically* (using a microscope). Attention should also be given to observing whether or not discoloration of the fluid above the cells, *the supernatant,* is present. If the erythrocytes have been *hemolyzed,* this is as important a finding as agglutination.

The strength of agglutination, called *grading,* uses a scale of 0 or negative (meaning no agglutination) to 4+ (meaning all the erythrocytes are clumped). A standardized system has been developed by the American Association of Blood Banks for the grading of macroscopic agglutination reactions (Table 3-9).

Pseudoagglutination, or false appearance of clumping, may occur because of the presence of *rouleaux formation.* Rouleaux formation can be encountered in patients with high or abnormal types of globulins in their blood, such as in multiple myeloma or after receiving dextran as a plasma expander. If this condition is present, the erythrocytes microscopically resemble rolls of stacked coins. To disperse pseudoagglutination, a few drops of physiologic sodium chloride can be added to the reaction tube, remixed, and re-examined. This procedure, *saline replacement,* should be performed carefully if pseudoagglutination is suspected. It should never be done before the initial testing protocol is followed because the dilutional effect of the saline may produce a false negative result.

THE COMPLEMENT SYSTEM

Complement is a complex series of proteins, many of which are enzymes, proteinases. Collectively, these proteins are a major fraction of the beta 1 and beta 2 globulins. In the laboratory, it is often desirable to inactivate complement for certain tests. To inactivate serum, it must be heated for 30 minutes at 56° C. The sequential activation of the complement enzymes and products formed during the reaction chain, referred to as the complement cascade, has a variety of physiologic and cellular consequences. The physiologic consequences include blood vessel dilation and increased vascular permeability. The cellular effects of complement activation include the following:

1. Cell activation.
2. Cytolysis or hemolysis, if the cells are erythrocytes. The most important biologic role of complement in blood group serology is the production of cell membrane lysis of antibody-coated targets.
3. Opsonization, which renders cells vulnerable to phagocytosis.

The complement system is composed of two interrelated enzyme cascades, the *classical* and *alternative pathways* (Fig. 3-16). The classical pathway is initiated by the complexing of antigen to its specific antibody, either IgG or IgM, and is the primary amplifier of the biologic effects of humoral immunity. The alternative pathway is activated by contact with a foreign surface, such as the polysaccharide coating of a microorganism, and amplifies nonimmune defense against microbial infection and other biologic alterations. It is probable that under normal physiologic conditions, activation of one pathway also leads to acti-

Table 3-9. Grading Agglutination Reactions

Grade	Description
Negative	No aggregates.
Mixed field (MF)	Few isolated aggregates, mostly free floating cells, supernatant, appears red
Weak $(+/-)$	Tiny aggregates that are barely visible macroscopically, many free erythrocytes, turbid and reddish supernatant
1+	A few small aggregates just visible macroscopically, many free erythrocytes, turbid and reddish supernatant
2+	Medium-sized aggregates, some free erythrocytes, clear supernatant
3+	Several large aggregates, some free erythrocytes, clear supernatant
4+	All the erythrocytes are combined into one solid aggregate, clear supernatant

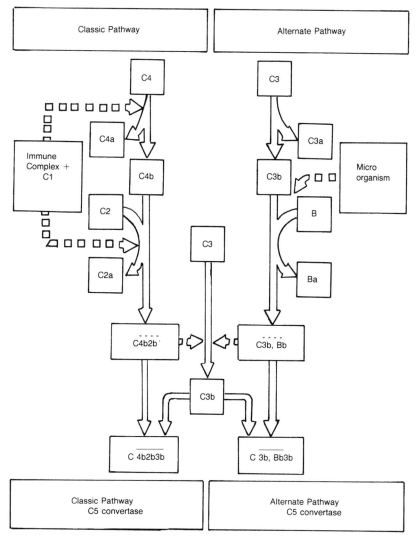

Figure 3-16. The complement cascade.

vation of the other. Either of the two routes leads to a common final pathway. Both pathways convert C3 to C3b, the central event of the common final pathway, which in turn leads to the activation of the lytic complement sequence, C5-C9, and cell destruction. A third set of plasma proteins, which function as the membrane attack complexes, become assembled into the structures responsible for lytic lesions in the lipid bilayer of the cell membrane and disrupt membrane integrity.

Once complement is initially activated, each enzyme precursor is activated by the previous complement component or complex, which is a highly specialized proteinase. This converts the enzyme precursor to its catalytically active form by limited proteolysis. During this activation process, a small peptide fragment is cleaved, a membrane-binding site is exposed, and the major fragment binds. As a consequence, the next active enzyme of the sequence is formed. It is important to note that because each enzyme can activate many enzyme precursors, each step up to C3 is amplified; therefore, the system forms an *amplifying cascade*.

The Classical Pathway

The principal components of the pathway are numbered C1 through C9. The sequence of component activation does not follow the expected numeric order. The sequence is C1, C4, C2, C3, C5, C6, C7, C8, and C9.

C3 is present in the plasma in the largest quantities and fixation of C3 is the major quantitative reaction of the complement cascade. Although the principal source of synthesis of complement in vivo is debatable, the majority of the plasma complement components are synthesized in hepatic parenchymal cells, except for C1, which is primarily manufactured in the epithelium of the gastrointestinal and urogenital tracts.

The classical pathway is composed of the following 3 stages:

1. Recognition
2. Enzymatic activation

3. Membrane attack leading to cellular destruction

FIXATION OF THE C1 COMPLEX

The recognition unit of the complement system is the C1 complex: C1q, C1r, and C1s, an interlocking enzyme system. The C1 complex is a unique feature of the classical pathway leading to C3 conversion. C1 fixation occurs when the C1q subcomponent binds directly to an immunoglobulin molecule. The other two subcomponents, C1r and C1s, do not bind to the immunoglobulin but are involved in subsequent activation of the classical pathway. Whether or not C1 fixation occurs depends on a number of factors. These conditions include the following:

1. Subclass of immunoglobulin. Only certain subclasses of immunoglobulin, such as IgM, and most of the IgG subclasses, can fix C1 even under optimal conditions.
2. Spatial or configurational constraints.

A single IgM molecule is potentially able to fix C1, but at least a pair of IgG molecules is required for this purpose. The amount of C1 fixed is directly proportional to the concentration of IgM antibodies; however, this is not true for IgG molecules.

The C1q molecule is potentially multivalent for attachment to the complement fixation sites of immunoglobulin. The structures of C1q peptide chains are formed into 3 subunits of 6 chains each. Each subunit consists of a Y-shaped pair of triple helices joined at the stem and ending in a globular head. The globular ends are assumed to be the sites for multivalent attachment to the complement-fixing sites in immune-complexed immunoglobulin. The sites on the IgG molecule are on the C_{H2} domains and probably the C_{H4} domain of IgM. The complement-fixing site may become exposed following complexing of the immunoglobulin, or the sites may always be available but need multiple attachments by C1q with critical geometry to achieve the necessary avidity.

C1r and C1s are chemically similar, but C1r forms dimers whereas C1s binds monovalently to C1r. C1r and C1s form a tetrad complex that binds to C1q in the presence of Ca^{++} ion. The binding mechanism of C1r by C1q is unknown because C1q is not known to have enzymatic activity. However, it is known that C1r and C1s activate in sequence while attached to C1q, and that both proteins become typical serine-histidine esterases on activation. C1s is the only substrate for C1r. C1s activates C4 and C2, the next components in the classical complement sequence, but C1r does not.

Fixation and Activation of C4 by the C1qrs Complex

C1s splits a peptide C4a from the N-terminal part of the alpha chain of the C4 component, leaving a large fragment, C4b. This reaction occurs in the fluid phase of the plasma around the C1s catalytic site and a reactive internal thioester bond is revealed on C4b. The stable binding of C4b molecules to membranes is less than 10% efficient. Binding occurs in close proximity to the site of activation, to either the C1qrs complex or the adjacent erythrocyte membrane. C4b molecules, which fail to bind, become inactive and decay.

C1s is weakly proteolytic for free intact C2 but highly active against C2, which has complexed with C4b molecules in the presence of Mg^{++} ions. This reaction will occur only if the C4b, C2 complex forms close to the C1s. The resultant C2b fragment joins with C4b to form the new C4b2b enzyme, the classical pathway C3 convertase. The catalytic site of the C4b2b complex is probably in the C2b peptide. A smaller, C2a fragment from the C2 component is lost to the surrounding environment. The C4b2b enzyme is unstable and decays with a half-life of 5 minutes at 37°C because of the release and decay of C2b.

There are two chief constraints on the activities of C1s on C4 and C2, and on the stable formation of the C4b2b complex:

1. The action of the proteinase inhibitor, C1 esterase
2. The effect of C3b inactivator

C1 esterase inhibitor binds to C1s and C1r. This activity may not be important in restraining the action of C1s at a local membrane site, but is extremely important in preventing the excessive action of free C1 on C4 and C2 in the fluid phase.

C3b-inactivator has the ability to disintegrate membrane-bound C4b. This action destroys the acceptor site for C2, which prevents the formation of C4b2b convertase.

The Action of C4b2b Complex on C3

The complement cascade reaches its full amplitude at the C3 stage, which represents the heart of the system. The C4b2b complex, referred to as the classical pathway C3 convertase, activates C3 molecules by splitting a peptide, the C3 anaphylatoxin, from the N-terminal end of the peptide of C3. This exposes a reactive binding site on the larger fragment, C3b. Consequently, clusters of C3b molecules are activated and bound near the C4b2b complex. Each catalytic site can bind several hundred C3b molecules, although the reaction is very inefficient. Only one C3b molecule combines with C4b2b to form the final proteolytic complex of the complement cascade.

Action of C3b on C5

C3b splits C5a from the alpha chain of C5 to initiate C5b fixation and the beginning of the membrane attack complex. No further proteinases are generated in the classical complement sequence. Other bound C3b molecules not involved in the C4b2b3b complex form an opsonic macromolecular coat on the erythrocyte or other target cell, which renders it susceptible to immune adherence by C3b receptors on phagocytic cells.

The C5-9 Membrane Complex

The fixation of C5b to biologic membranes is followed by the sequential addition of C6, C7, C8, and C9. When fully assembled in the correct proportions, they form the membrane attack complex. The C5b-C6 complex is hydrophilic, but with the addition of C7 to the C567 complex, the complex has additional detergent and phospholipid binding properties as well. This occurrence of both hydrophobic and hydrophilic groups within the same complex may account for its tendency to polymerize and form small protein micelles (a packet of chain molecules in a parallel arrangement). In free solution, uncombined C567 has a half-life of about 0.1 seconds. It can attach to any lipid bilayer within its effective diffusion radius, which produces the phenomenon of *"reactive lysis"* on innocent bystander cells. Once membrane-bound, C567 is relatively stable and can interact with C8 and C9.

C5-8 polymerizes C9 to form a tubule, known as the membrane attack complex, which bridges the membrane. This is a hollow cylinder (15 nm in length and 10 nm in diameter), which is inserted at one end into the lipid bilayer with the other end projecting from the membrane. Although the micellar arrangement of the membrane insertion region has not been positively established, a structure of this form can be assumed to disturb the lipid bilayer sufficiently to allow the free exchange of ions as well as water molecules across the membrane. The consequence in a living cell is that the influx of Na^+ and H_2O leads to disruption of osmotic balance, which produces cell lysis.

The Alternate (Properdin) Pathway

The alternate pathway shows points of similarity with the classical sequence and both pathways generate a C3 convertase, which activates C3 to provide the pivotal event in the final common pathway of both systems. However, in contrast to the classic pathway which is initiated by the formation of antigen-antibody reactions, the alternate complement pathway is predominantly a nonantibody-initiated pathway.

A key feature of the alternate pathway is that the first three proteins of the classic activation pathway, C1, C4, and C2, do *not* participate in the cascade sequence. The C3a component is considered the counterpart of C2a in the classic pathway, and C2 of the classic pathway structurally resembles factor B of the alternate pathway. The omission of C1, C4, and C2 is possible because activators of the alternate pathway catalyze the conversion of another series of normal serum proteins, which lead to the activation of C3. It was previously believed that *properdin,* a normal protein of human serum, was the first protein to function in the alternate pathway; thus, the pathway was originally named after this protein.

Activators of the alternative pathway are now known usually to be polysaccharides or carbohydrate-containing molecules such as lipopolysaccharides or glycoproteins. Known activators of the alternative pathway include zymosan, a polysaccharide complex from the surface of yeast cells, bacterial endotoxin, and aggregated IgA or IgE. In paroxysmal noctural hemoglobinuria (PNH), the patient's erythrocytes act as an activator, and the result is excessive lysis of the patient's erythrocytes.

The uptake of factor B onto C3b occurs when C3b is bound to an activator surface. However, C3b in the fluid phase or attached to a nonactivator surface preferentially binds to factor H and so prevents C3b,B formation. C3b and factor B combine to form C3b,B, which is converted into an active C3 convertase, C3b,Bb. This occurs because of the loss of a small fragment, Ba (a glycine-rich alpha$_2$ globulin which is believed to be physiologically inert) through the action of the enzyme, factor D. The C3b,Bb complex is able to convert more C3 to C3b, which binds more factor B and so the feedback cycle continues.

The major controlling event of this pathway is factor H, which prevents the association between C3b and factor B. Factor H blocks the formation of C3b,Bb, the catalytically active C3 convertase of the feedback loop. Factor H (previously Beta$_1$H) competes with factor B for its combining site on C3b, eventually leading to C3 inactivation. Factors B and H apparently occupy a common site on C3b. The factor that is preferentially bound to C3b depends on the nature of the surface to which C3b is attached. Polysaccharides are called activator surfaces and favor the uptake of factor B on the chain of C3b with the corresponding displacement of factor H. In this situation, binding of factor H is inhibited and consequently factor B replaces H at the common binding site. When factor H is excluded, C3b is thought to be formed continuously in small amounts. Another controlling point in the amplification loop depends on the stability of the C3b, Bb convertase. Ordinarily, C3b,Bb decays because of the loss of Bb with a half-life of approximately 5 minutes. However, if properdin (P) binds to C3b,Bb, forming C3b,BbP, the half-life is extended to 30 minutes.

The association on the surface of an aggregate of protein or the surface of a microorganism of numerous C3b units, factor Bb, and properdin has potent activity as a C5 convertase. With the cleavage of C5, the remainder of complement cascade continues as in the classical pathway.

CHAPTER SUMMARY

The Immune System

An antigen can be defined as a foreign substance that can elicit an antibody response. Production of antibodies in response to antigenic stimulation depends on a person's immunologic ability to recognize an antigen as foreign and on the physical and chemical nature of the antigen. Recognition of foreign antigens and production of antibodies depend on several T and B lymphocytes, plasma cells, and macrophages.

Antigen Characteristics

Foreign substances such as erythrocytes can be immunogenic if the membrane contains a number of antigenic determinants or epitopes. An immune response is directed against these determinants, and resultant antibodies bind to them. The cellular membrane of all mammalian cells chemically consists of proteins, phospholipids, cholesterol, and traces of polysaccharide. Most of the proteins are immunogenic. Cellular antigens of importance to immunohematologists are the blood group antigens, histocompatibility (HLA) antigens, and auto-antigens. Nucleated cells, such as leukocytes, possess many cell-surface-protein antigens, which readily provoke an immune response if transferred into a genetically different individual of the same species. Some of these antigens are much more potent than others in provoking an immune response and are called the major histocompatibility (HLA) antigens. In some situations (not always abnormal), antibodies may be produced in response to normal self-antigens. This failure to recognize self-antigens can result in autoantibodies directed at hormones, such as thyroglobulin, and cell-membrane antigens, such as the Ii blood group system.

Antigens are usually large organic molecules that are either proteins or large polysaccharides and rarely, if ever, lipids. Proteins are excellent antigens because of their high molecular weight and structural complexity. Polysaccharides by themselves are considered too small to function as antigens. In the case of erythrocyte antigens, protein or lipid carriers may contribute to the necessary size and the polysaccharides present in the form of side chains, confer the immunologic specificity and function as the combining sites with which antibodies react. For antigens to function effectively, several factors are important: foreignness, degradability, molecular weight, structural stability, and complexity.

Antibody Characteristics

Antibodies can be found in blood plasma and many body fluids such as tears, saliva, and breast milk. These specific glycoproteins are referred to as immunoglobulins, abbreviated Ig. Five distinct classes of immunoglobulin molecules are recognized in most higher mammals: IgM, IgG, IgA, IgD and IgE. These immunoglobulin classes differ from each other in characteristics such as molecular weight, sedimentation coefficient, and carbohydrate content.

After a foreign antigen challenge, an IgM antibody response proceeds in four phases, but the actual time period and titer depend on the characteristics of the antigen and the individual. The four phases of an antibody response are the lag, log, plateau, and decline phases. Subsequent exposure to the same antigenic stimulus produces an anamnestic antibody response that exhibits the same four phases as the primary responses. An anamnestic response differs from a primary response in the length of time of the response and the type and titer of antibody produced.

Each immunoglobulin molecule is bifunctional. One region is concerned with binding to antigen and a different region mediates binding of the immunoglobulin to host tissues, including cells of the immune system and the first component (C1q) of the classical complement system. A typical monomeric IgG molecule consists of three globular regions (two Fab regions and an Fc portion) linked by a flexible hinge region. If the molecule is digested with certain proteolytic enzymes, it splits into three approximately equal-sized fragments. Two of these fragments retain the ability to bind antigen and are called the antigen-binding fragments (Fab fragments). The third fragment is referred to as the Fc portion.

Each of the five major immunoglobulin classes is unique and possesses its own characteristic antigenic determinants. IgG accounts for 70 to 75% of the total immunoglobulin pool. The subclasses of IgG differ in their heavy chain composition and in some of their characteristics and biologic activities. IgM accounts for about 10% of the immunoglobulin pool. It is the largest molecule and the predominant antibody found in a primary immune response. IgA represents 15 to 20% of the total circulatory immunoglobulin pool. It is the predominant immunoglobulin in secretions, such as tears, saliva, colostrum, breast milk, and intestinal secretions. Secretory IgA is of critical importance in protecting body surfaces against invading microorganisms. IgD is found in very low concentrations in plasma and accounts for less than 1% of the total immunoglobulin pool. This immunoglobulin is primarily a cell membrane immunoglobulin found on the surface of B lymphocytes in association with IgM. IgE is a trace plasma protein in the blood plasma of unparasitized individuals. It is of major importance because it mediates some types of allergic reactions, allergies, and anaphylaxis, and is generally responsible for an individual's immunity to invading parasites.

Immunoglobulins themselves can function as effective antigens when used to immunize mammals of a different species because they are proteins. When the resulting antiimmunoglobulins are analyzed, three principal categories of antigenic determinants can be recognized: isotype, allotype, and idiotype determinants.

The principal function of an antibody is to bind antigen, but antibodies may exhibit secondary effector functions as well as behaving as antigens. The significant secondary effector functions of antibodies are complement fixation and placental transfer. Monoclonal antibodies are purified antibodies that are cloned from a single cell. These antibodies are engineered to bind to a single specific antigen. The greatest impact of monoclonal antibodies in blood banking has been on the analysis of cell membrane antigens.

The Molecular Basis of an Antigen-Antibody Reaction

The basic Y-shaped immunoglobulin molecule is a bifunctional structure. The V domains are primarily concerned with antigen binding. When an antigenic determinant and its specific antibody combine, they interact through the chemical groups found on the surface of the antigenic determinant and on the surface of the hypervariable regions of the immunoglobulin molecule. Although the C domains do not form the antigen-binding sites, the arrangement of the C domains and hinge region give the molecule segmental flexibility that allows it to combine with separated antigenic determinants.

Bonding of an antigen to an antibody takes place because of the formation of multiple reversible intermolecular attractions between an antigen and amino acids of the binding site. Various types of noncovalent bonds are formed in antigen-antibody reactions. These bond types include hydrophobic bonds, hydrogen bonding, Van der Waals forces, and electrostatic forces. Hydrophobic bonds are the most common.

In Vitro Detection of Antigen-Antibody Reactions

Agglutination tests are the most commonly used technique to detect and measure the consequences of antigen-antibody interaction. Agglutination is the clumping of particles that have antigens on their surface, such as erythrocytes, by antibody molecules that form bridges between the antigenic determinants. Agglutination is believed to occur in two stages: sensitization and lattice formation. Sensitization represents the physical attachment of antibody molecules to antigens on the erythrocytic membrane. Lattice formation or the establishment of crosslinks between sensitized particles such as erythrocytes, and antibodies results in clumping.

Antibodies differ in their ability to agglutinate. IgM-type antibodies or complete antibodies are considerably more efficient than IgG or IgA antibodies in exhibiting in vitro agglutination when the antigen-bearing erythrocytes are suspended in physiologic saline. Antibodies that do not exhibit visible agglutination of saline suspended erythrocytes even when bound to the cell's surface membrane are considered nonagglutinating or incomplete antibodies.

Several methods are commonly used in routine blood banking to enhance the agglutination of erythocytes. These procedures include centrifugation, treatment with proteolytic enzymes, the use of colloids and other enhancement agents, such as low ionic strength saline solution, and the anti-human globulin (AHG) test. The AHG test is frequently incorporated into the protocol of many blood banking techniques to demonstrate that erythrocytes have been sensitized but have failed to produce visible agglutination in saline. In the blood bank, it is important to observe the strength of agglutination when it occurs. The strength of agglutination or grading uses a scale of 0 or negative (no agglutination) to 4+ (all of the erythrocytes are clumped). Pseudoagglutination is rare but may occur due to the presence of rouleaux formation.

The Complement System

Complement is a complex series of proteins, many of which are enzymes. Complement enzymes and products formed during the reaction chain, referred to as the complement cascade, have various physiologic and cellular consequences. The most important biologic role of complement in blood bank testing is the production of cell membrane lysis of antibody-coated cells.

REVIEW QUESTIONS

1. Production of antibodies depends on:
   A. An individual's immunologic ability to recognize an antigen as non-self
   B. An individual's immunologic ability to respond to a foreign antigen
   C. The physical nature of an antigen
   D. The chemical nature of an antigen
   E. All of the above
2. The hematologic cells of importance in an immunologic response are:
   A. Lymphocytes, plasma cells, and macrophages
   B. Plasma cells, neutrophils, and macrophages
   C. Macrophages, neutrophils, and monocytes
   D. Neutrophils, lymphocytes, and monocytes
   E. Neutrophils, macrophages, and monocytes
3. Erythrocytes can be antigenic if their membrane contains:
   A. Foreign antigenic determinants
   B. Epitopes
   C. Lipid-rich surface areas
   D. Complement
   E. Both A and B
4. In blood banking, cellular antigens of importance include:
   A. Blood group antigens
   B. Histocompatibility (HLA) antigens
   C. Interferon
   D. Interleukin 2
   E. Both A and B
5. The Lewis blood group antigens are unique among blood group antigens because they:
   A. Are generally restricted to erythrocytes
   B. Are absorbed on the red cells from the plasma
   C. Are an integral part of the red cell membrane
   D. Result in hemolytic anemia if they are missing from the red cell membrane
   E. Both C and D

6. The histocompatibility (HLA) antigens are important in:
   A. Production of IgM antibodies
   B. Production of IgG antibodies
   C. Survival of transplanted organs
   D. Activation of complement
   E. Structural composition of the RBC membrane

7. One of the characteristics of proteins that makes them excellent antigens is their:
   A. Structural simplicity
   B. Structural stability
   C. Molecular flexibility
   D. Rapid destruction
   E. High molecular weight

8. In the primary antibody response to a foreign antigen, the type of antibody initially formed is:
   A. IgM
   B. IgG
   C. IgD
   D. IgA
   E. IgE

9. In a secondary (anamnestic) response, the predominant type of antibody formed is:
   A. IgM
   B. IgG
   C. IgD
   D. IgA
   E. IgE

10-13. Match the following phases of an antibody response with the appropriate description:
10. Plateau
11. Lag
12. Decline
13. Log
   A. No detectable antibody is present
   B. Antibody titer stabilizes
   C. Antibody titer rises
   D. Antibody is catabolized

14-15. Match the following antibody characteristics (use an answer only once).
14. IgM
15. IgG
   A. Molecular weight of 900,000
   B. Half-life of 3 days
   C. 11S (sedimentation coefficient)
   D. Four subclasses
   E. Serum concentration (1.5-40 mg/ 100mL)

16-20. Match the following antibody characteristics (use an answer only once):
16. IgM
17. IgG
18. IgA
19. IgD
20. IgE
   A. Predominant immunoglobulin in secretions
   B. Primarily a cell membrane immunoglobulin found on the surface of B lymphocytes
   C. Mediates some types of allergic reactions
   D. A pentamer configuration
   E. Important in immune responses

21-23. Match the following antigenic determinants with their respective descriptors:
21. Isotype
22. Allotype
23. Idiotype
   A. Determinants found on the immunoglobulins of some, but not all, animals of a species
   B. Result from unique structures on light and heavy chains
   C. The heavy chain constant region structures associated with the different classes and subclasses

24. The principal function of an antibody is to:
   A. Bind antigen
   B. Fix complement
   C. Pass through the placenta to provide passive immunity to the newborn infant
   D. Stimulate the inflammatory response
   E. Differentiate one species from another

25. The term "avidity" refers to:
   A. The bond between a single antigenic determinant and an individual combining site
   B. The strength of an AHG reaction
   C. The pattern of agglutination displayed by HTLA antibodies
   D. The strength with which a multivalent antibody binds to a multivalent antigen
   E. The fact that the binding sites of antibodies directed against determi-

nants of one antigen are not complementary to determinants of another dissimilar antigen

26. The major bond(s) formed between antigens and antibodies is/are:
    A. Hydrophobic
    B. Hydrogen bonding
    C. Van der Waals forces
    D. Electrostatic forces
    E. Both B and C
27. Which of the following is *not* a factor that influences antigen-antibody association?
    A. The number of antibody molecules in relation to the number of antigen sites per cell
    B. The subclass of IgG molecules
    C. pH
    D. Temperature and length of time of incubation
    E. Ionic strength
28. The *prozone phenomenon* can:
    1. Result from excessive antibody concentration
    2. Result in a false positive reaction
    3. Result in a false negative reaction
    4. Be overcome by serially diluting the antibody-containing serum
    5. Be influenced by the length of incubation
    A. 1 only
    B. 1 and 2
    C. 2 and 3
    D. 1, 3 and 4
    E. 2, 4 and 5
29. Lattice formation is the establishment of crosslinks between _____ and antibodies.
    A. Antigens
    B. Erythrocytes
    C. Leukocytes
    D. Sensitized erythrocytes
    E. Plasma proteins
30. Zeta potential is:
    A. The same as the ionic cloud around a particle (e.g., RBC)
    B. The outer edge of the ionic cloud surrounding an RBC in solution
    C. The difference between net charge at the cell membrane and the charge at the surface of shear
    D. Net surface charge density at the surface of the cell membrane

    E. Release of antibody into surrounding medium from an antigen-antibody complex
31. The term "complete antibody" is sometimes used to refer to:
    A. IgM
    B. IgG
    C. IgD
    D. IgA
    E. IgE
32. Which of the following genotypic expressions could produce a "dosage effect?"
    A. Mm
    B. Le^aLe^b
    C. Cc
    D. cc
    E. Kk
33. Which of the following methods would *not* potentially enhance agglutination?
    A. Increasing the speed of centrifugation
    B. Decreasing the speed of centrifugation
    C. Treatment with proteolytic enzymes
    D. Extended incubation time
    E. The use of AHG sera
34-37. Match each of the following grading of agglutination reactions with the appropriate description:
34. Mixed field
35. Weak (+/−)
36. 1+
37. 3+
    A. Medium-sized aggregates, some free erythrocytes, clear supernatant
    B. Few isolated aggregates, mostly free floating cells, supernatant appears red
    C. Several large aggregates, some free erythrocytes, clear supernatant
    D. Tiny aggregates that are barely visible macroscopically, many free erythrocytes, turbid and reddish supernatant.
    E. A few small aggregates just visible macroscopically, many free erythrocytes, turbid and reddish supernatant.
38. The direct antiglobulin test (DAT) detects:
    A. In vivo sensitization of erythrocytes
    B. In vivo sensitization of leukocytes
    C. In vitro sensitization of erythrocytes

D. A or C

39. A polyspecific antiglobulin sera contains:
  A. Anti-IgG
  B. Anti-C3d
  C. Anti-IgE
  D. Anti-IgD
  E. Both A and B

40. To disperse pseudoagglutination, which of the following can be done?
  A. Add a few drops of albumin
  B. Add a few drops of saline
  C. Add a few drops of proteolytic enzyme
  D. Shake the reaction tube vigorously
  E. A or B

41. To inactivate complement in serum, the serum should be:
  A. Frozen at $-18°C$
  B. Incubated at 37°C for 15 minutes
  C. Incubated at 37°C for 30 minutes
  D. Incubated at 56°C for 15 minutes
  E. Incubated at 56°C for 30 minutes

42. The physiologic or cellular components of complement activation produce all of the following except:
  A. Blood vessel dilation
  B. Increased vascular permeability
  C. Cell membrane lysis
  D. Initiation of antibody production
  E. Promotion of opsonization

43. The classical pathway of the complement system is initiated by:
  A. The complexing of antigen and its specific antibody
  B. The presence of IgM in the circulation
  C. The presence of IgG in the circulation
  D. Contact with a foreign surface, e.g., the polysaccharide coating of a microorganism
  E. Either B or C

44. The classic complement pathway is characterized by:
  A. Recognition
  B. Enzymatic activation
  C. Membrane attack
  D. Cellular destruction
  E. All of the above

45. Which classes of immunoglobulin can fix complement?
  A. IgM
  B. IgG

C. IgD
D. IgA
E. Both A and B

46. The membrane attack unit is composed of:
  A. C5b, C6, C7, C8, and C9
  B. C5, C6, C7, C8, and C9
  C. C5, C6, and C7
  D. C1r, C1s, C1q, C4, and C2
  E. C1s, C4b, C2, and Mg^{++}

47. Which complement components *do not* participate in the alternate (Properdin) pathway?
  A. C1r, C1s, and C1q
  B. C1, C4, and C2
  C. C4, C2, and C3
  D. C3, C5, and C6
  E. C7, C8, and C9

ANSWERS

1. E		25. D	
2. A		26. A	
3. E		27. B	
4. E		28. D	
5. B		29. D	
6. C		30. C	
7. E		31. A	
8. A		32. D	
9. B		33. B	
10. B		34. B	
11. A		35. D	
12. D		36. E	
13. C		37. C	
14. A		38. A	
15. D		39. E	
16. D		40. B	
17. E		41. E	
18. A		42. D	
19. B		43. A	
20. C		44. E	
21. C		45. E	
22. A		46. A	
23. B		47. B	
24. A			

BIBLIOGRAPHY

Auffray, C., and Strominger, J. L.: Molecular genetics of the human major histocompatibility complex, Adv. Hum. Genet., *15:*197-247, 1986.

Barrett, J. T.: Textbook of Immunology (4th ed). St. Louis, Mosby, 1983, pp. 29-40.

Beck, M. L., Hardman, J. T., and Henry, R.: Reactivity of a licensed murine monoclonal anti-A reagent with group B cells, Transfusion, 26(6):572, 1986.

Callicoat, P. A., Hall, C., and Brenner, N.: Evaluation of monoclonal anti-A and anti-B for routine ABO grouping in microplates, Transfusion, 26(6):549, 1986.

Carpenter, P. L.: Immunology and Serology. Philadelphia, W. B. Saunders, 1975, 8, 20-22, 38, 239-245.

Dannenberg, A. M., Jr. Macrophages and Monocytes. In Fundamentals of Clinical Hematology. Edited by Jerry L. Spivak. Hagerstown, Md., Harper and Row, 1980, pp. 137-153.

Dunstan, R. A.: Status of major red cell blood group antigens on neutrophils, lymphocytes and monocytes, Br. J. Haematol., 62:301-309, 1986.

Duran, L. W., and Pease, L. R.: Relating the structure of major transplantation antigens to immune function, Transplantation, 41(3):279-285, 1986.

Epley, K. M., Line, L. M., and Severns, M. L.: Evaluation of a monoclonal anti-D for Dᵘ testing, Transfusion, 26(6):549, 1986.

Ersley, A. J., and Gabuzda, T. G.: Phagocytes. In Pathophysiology of Blood. Philadelphia, W.B. Saunders, 1975, pp. 100-118.

Gaidulis, L., Branch, D. R., Lazar, G. S., et al.: The red cell antigens A, B, D, U, Ge, Jk3 and Ytᵃ, are not detected on human granulocytes, Br. J. Haematol., 60:659-668, 1985.

Hall, S., Olekna, D., and Davies, D.: Production of unique monoclonal ABO blood grouping antisera, Transfusion, 25(5):448, 1986.

Hubbard, M.: Paternity testing. In Complements, edited by William G. Cannady Rogers, Arkansas, Pel-Freeze Biologicals, 2(1):1-2, June, 1982.

Keller, R. H., et al.: Monoclonal antibodies: Clinical utility and the misunderstood epitope, Lab. Med. 15(12):795-802, 1984.

Kelton, J. G., and Bebenek, G.: Granulocytes do not have surface ABO antigens, Transfusion, 25(6):567-569, 1985.

McElligott, M. C., Menitove, J. E., and Aster, R. H.: Recruitment of unrelated persons as bone marrow donors, Transfusion, 26(4):309-314, 1986.

Meyers, M. A., Walker, R. H., and Phillips, L. M.: The usefulness of histocompatibility antigens (HLA-A,B) in parentage testing, Transfusion, 25(5):481, 1985.

Moheng, M. C.: Blood banking: State of the art. In Approaches to Serological Problems in the Hospital Transfusion Service. Edited by Pierce, S. R., and Wilson, J. K., Arlington, Va., American Association of Blood Banks, 1985, pp. 1-27.

Monoclonal Antibodies, St. Louis, Sigma Diagnostics, 1985.

Nehlsen-Cannarella, S.: The wonderment of HLA. In Complements, edited by Nehlsen-Cannarella, S. Brown Deer, Wisconsin, Pel-Freeze Biologicals, 4(1):2-4, April, 1984.

Ortho Product Brochure: Anti-Human Globulin (Rabbit and Murine Monoclonal BioClone®) (Clear or Green) Anti-OgG, —C3d, Polyspecific, Ortho Diagnostic Systems Inc, Raritan, NJ, revised June 1986.

Ortho Product Brochure: Ortho Bovine Albumin Solution 22% Protein Concentration pH 7.2, Ortho Diagnostic Systems Inc., Raritan, NJ, revised November 1985.

Pliska, C.: Low ionic strength solution, Lab. Med. 11(3):159-164, 1980.

Rivera, R., and Scornik, J. C.: HLA Antigens on Red Cells, Transfusion, 26(4):375-381, 1986.

Roitt, I.: Essential Immunology (Fifth Edition). Oxford, England, Blackwell Scientific Publications, 1984, pp. 76-85.

Sebring, E. S., Polesky, H. F., and Schanfield, M. S.: GM and KM allotypes in disputed parentage, A. J. C. P., 71(3):281-285, 1979.

Snyder, E. L., and Falast, G. A.: Significance of the direct antiglobulin test, Lab. Med., 16(2):89-96, 1985.

Spitalnik, P. F., and Spitalnik, S. L.: Selective uptake by erythrocytes of Lewis antigens based on ceramide composition, Abstract of papers presented at AABB 39th Annual Meeting, Nov., 1986.

Standards for Blood Banks and Transfusion Services, 12th ed., Arlington, Va., American Association of Blood Banks, 1987, pp. 21, 87, 103, 181.

Steane, E. A., et al.: A proposal for compatibility testing incorporating the manual hexadimethrine promide (Polybrene) test, Transfusion 25(6):540-544, 1986.

Tizard, I. R.: Immunology: An Introduction. Philadelphia, W.B. Saunders, 1984, pp. 14, 22, 93, 97, 105, 127, 197.

Turgeon, M. L.: Clinical Hematology: Theory and Procedures. Boston, Little, Brown and Co., 1988, pp. 97-105.

Vengelen-Tyler, V., and Choy, C.: A comparative study of antibody enhancement techniques, Transfusion, 26(6):570, 1986.

Wenk, R. E., and Brooks, M.: Paternity probabilities of biologic fathers and unexcluded falsely-accused men, Transfusion, 26(6):548, 1986.

Zmijewski, C. M.: Immunohematology. 2nd ed., New York, Appleton Century Crofts, 1972, pp. 20, 38-40.

PART TWO

Erythrocyte Blood Group Systems

4

The ABO Blood Group System

At the conclusion of this chapter, the reader will be able to:
- Describe the history of the discovery of the ABO system.
- Contrast the antigens and antibodies found in the blood in the ABO system.
- Discuss the patterns of inheritance of A and B genes.
- State the phenotypic frequencies of groups A, B, and O.
- Name the specific transferase for the A, B, and H genes.
- Identify the immunodominant monosaccharide residual for A, B, and H genes.
- Describe the synthesis of H, A, and B antigens.
- State the percentage of persons in the United States who are secretors of water-soluble ABH substances.
- Identify the product or products found in the saliva of persons of various ABO groups.
- State the characteristic genotype of a nonsecretor.
- Describe the subgroups of group A.
- Explain the importance of A subgroups in the clinical situation.
- Describe the purpose of absorbed anti-A_1.
- Name the ethnic population with the highest frequency of the superactive B gene.
- State the genotype of individuals with the Bombay phenotype.
- Explain the causes of acquired A antigen and acquired B antigen.
- Describe the characteristics of anti-A and anti-B.
- Analyze some of the types of problems that can be encountered in ABO grouping.

Chapter Outline

HISTORICAL ASPECTS OF THE ABO SYSTEM

In the early 1900s, Landsteiner recognized the presence of two separate erythrocyte antigens, the A and B antigens. Based on his observations of the agglutination reaction of erythrocytes and the presence of serum antibodies in the serum of individuals directed against these antigens, he established the existence of the first known blood group system, the ABO system. He proposed three separate groups: A, B, and O. Shortly hereafter, von Decastello and Sturli identified a fourth group, AB. The serologic reactions of the ABO blood groups are presented in Table 4-1.

GENETIC INHERITANCE

As early as 1908, Epstein and Ottenberg suggested that the ABO blood groups were inherited. It was not until 1924 that Bernstein postulated the existence of three allelic genes, A, B, and O. He proposed that an individual inherited two genes, one from each parent, and that these genes determined which ABO antigens would be present on a person's erythrocytes. The O gene was defined as *amorphic* because no detectable antigen is produced in response to the inheritance of this gene. In 1930, Thompson proposed a four-allele theory of inheritance based on the discovery of von Dungern and Hirszfeld in 1911, which demonstrated that the A antigen could be divided into A_1 and A_2 subgroups. Thompson's four-allele theory encompassed the four allelic genes, A_1, A_2, B and O.

Expression of A and B genes in erythrocytes or body fluids results from the independently inherited Hh, Sese, and A and B genes. The ABO locus is known to reside on chromosome 9 in humans; the loci of the H and Se genes are unknown. Under normal circumstances, if either the A or B genes are present on either chromosome, the gene can be phenotypically demonstrated on erythrocytes. Examples of exceptional cases of expression of A or B genes on erythrocytes and other alterations of genetic expression are discussed later in this chapter.

The four allelic genes of the ABO system (A_1, A_2, B and O) and resulting phenotypes are presented in Table 4-2. Inheritance of the ABO genes follows Mendelian principles, with the A and B genes being codominant. Two examples of genetic crosses involving the ABO system, with the resultant genotypes and phenotypes of the offspring, are given in Tables 4-3 and 4-4.

Table 4-1. Classification of the ABO Blood Types

Blood Group	Erythrocyte Antigens	Serum Antibodies
A	A	Anti-B
B	B	Anti-A
AB	A and B	None
O	None	Anti-A and anti-B

Table 4-2. The Major ABO Genotypes and Phenotypes

Phenotype	Possible Genotypes
A_1	A_1/A_1, A_1/A_2, A_1/O
A_2	A_2/A_2, A_2/O
A_1B	A_1/B
A_2B	A_2/B
B	B/B or B/O
O	O/O

Table 4-3. A Representative ABO Mating

Female: Phenotype A_1, Genotype A_1/O
Male: Phenotype B, Genotype B/O

Female gametes: 50% A_1, 50% O
Male gametes: 50% B, 50% O

		Female gametes	
		A_1	O
Male gametes	B	A_1B	BO
	O	AO	OO

Probability of ABO groups of offspring:
Genotypes: 25% A_1/B; 25% B/O; 25% A_1/O; 25% O/O
Phenotypes: 25% A_1B; 25% B; 25% A_1; 25% O

Table 4-4. A Representative ABO Mating

Female: Phenotype A_2B, Genotype A_2/B
Male: Phenotype A_1, Genotype A_1/A_2

Female gametes: 50% A_2, 50% B
Male gametes: 50% A_1, 50% A_2

		Female gametes	
		A_2	B
Male gametes	A_1	A_1A_2	A_1B
	A_2	A_2A_2	A_2B

Probability of ABO groups of offspring:
Genotypes: 25% A_1/A_2; 25% A_1/B; 25% A_2/A_2; 25% A_2/B
Phenotypes: 25% A_1; 25% A_1B; 25% A_2; 25% A_2B

DEVELOPMENT AND DISTRIBUTION OF THE ABO GROUPS

Development of the A and B Antigens

The A and B antigens are not fully developed in newborn infants, but some antigenic development can be detected on embryonic erythrocytes as early as 5 weeks of gestational age. Although the strength of A and B antigens does *not* increase during fetal life, these antigens do gain strength shortly after birth. Weaker agglutination reactions are observed with fetal and newborn infants' erythrocytes compared to the mature erythrocytes of adults because the number and strength of A and B antigen sites are less (Table 4-5). Group A infants may type as A_2 at birth, but subsequently demonstrate type A_1 reactions by the time

they are 6 to 18 months old. It should also be noted that A and B antigens as well as H, P_1, and D antigens product significantly weaker or negative reactions in reticulocyte-rich blood preparations.

Distribution of ABO Groups

In 1919, Hirszfeld and Hirszfeld discovered that the distribution of ABO blood groups differed for various populations. Mourant conducted a comprehensive survey of the world blood type distribution (Table 4-6). Although this information is mostly of academic interest, an awareness of these differences is a helpful guide to blood bank inventory management.

BIOCHEMICAL ACTIVITIES RELATED TO THE DEVELOPMENT OF A, B, AND H ANTIGENS

Inheritance of A and B genes usually results in the expression of A and B gene products (antigens) on erythrocytes, but H, A, and B antigens are *not* the direct products of the H, A, and B genes, respectively. Each gene codes for the production of a specific *transferase* enzyme (Table 4-7), which catalyzes the transfer of a monosaccharide molecule from a donor substrate to the precursor substance.

Expression of H, A, and B Antigens

The H gene codes for the production of α-L-fucosyl transferase that catalyzes the addition of L-fucose, the immunodominant structure of H antigen, to two slightly different structures known as the type 1 and 2 precursor chains. Once the H gene-specified transferase has acted and L-fucose has been added to the chains, the A and B gene-specified products can then act to add a monosaccharide to these preformed H-bearing chains (Fig. 4-1). If a person does not inherit at least one H gene, L-fucose is *not* transferred to the precursor substance and the A and B immunodominant sugars *cannot* be added subsequently. This is the

Table 4-5. Examples of the Number of A and B Antigen Sites on Eythrocytes

	Antigen	Number of Sites
Adult blood		
	A_1	810,000 to 1,170,000 A antigen sites
	A_2	240,000 to 290,000 A antigen sites
	A_3	35,000 A antigen sites
	A_x	4,800 A antigen sites
	A_m	700 A antigen sites
	A_1B	460,000 to 850,000 A antigen sites
		310,000 to 560,000 B antigen sites
	A_2B	120,000 A antigen sites
	B	610,000 to 830,000 B antigen sites
Newborn cord blood		
	A_1	250,000 to 370,000 A antigen sites
	A_2	140,000 A antigen sites
	A_1B	220,000 A antigen sites
	B	200,000 B antigen sites

Economidous, J., Hughes-Jones, N.C., and Gardner, B.: Quantitative measurements concerning A and B antigen sites. Vox Sang. *12*:321, 1967.

Table 4-6. Representative ABO Frequencies

Phenotype	Genotype	White (%)	Black (%)	Oriental (%)
A_1	A_1A_1, A_1A_2, A_1O	32	19	27
A_2	A_2A_2, A_2O	9	8	(Rare)
B	BB, BO	9	19	25
A_1B	A_1B	3	3	5
A_2B	A_2B	1	1	(Rare)
O	OO	45	49	40

Table 4-7. ABH Genes and Their Enzymatic Products

Gene	Enzyme
H	α-L-fucosyltransferase
A	α-3-N-acetyl-D-galactosaminyl transferase
B	α-3-D-galactosyl transferase
O	None

galactosyl transferase, which attaches D-galactose to the acceptor molecule. Because the A and B transferases convert the same acceptor molecule, they compete with one another for the substrate. Both A_1 and B cells have many immunodominant sugars added, resulting in a low level of detectable H antigen on A_1 and B erythrocytes.

Variations in Transferase Enzymes

The level of A_1-specified transferase enzyme is higher in serum from cord blood than in the sera of A_1 (nonpregnant) adults. In pregnancy, the level of A_1 specified transferase enzyme in the serum drops to less than half the amount present in the sera of nonpregnant A_1 adults.

Although they are specific for the same monosaccharide and use the same acceptor molecule, the transferases produced by the

basis of explanation for the Bombay or O_h phenotype.

Specific transferase enzymes are the products of A or B genes. The A and B antigens result from the actions of these transferases, which attach specific monosaccharides to the H substrate. The immunodominant monosaccharides of the A and B antigens are shown in Figure 4-2. The A gene produces an α-3-N-acetyl-D-galactosaminyl transferase that attaches N-acetyl-D-galactosamine to the acceptor molecule; the B gene produces an α-3-D-

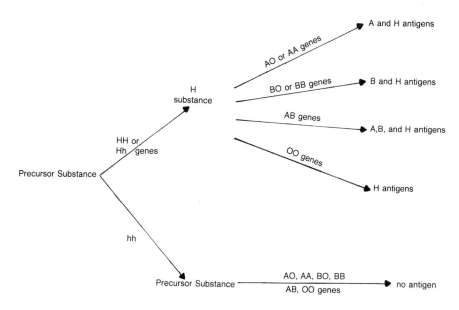

Figure 4-1. Genetic pathway of expression of ABH substances on erythrocytes.

A^1 and A^2 genes are both quantitatively and qualitatively different. It has been demonstrated that the levels of transferase are 5 to 10 times higher in A_1 persons than in A_2 individuals and the transferases differ in their chemical requirements, such as optimum pH.

Studies of transferase indicate that in two individuals with an A_2B erythrocyte phenotype but an A_1B genotype, each has a strong B transferase capable of incorporating more ^{14}C-labelled galactose onto structures with H activity and attaching more galactose onto group O cells at a rate more rapid than normal. Previous investigations provided evidence for the existence of an atypical "superactive" B gene. It has also been suggested that in A_1B persons, a hybrid AB gene-specified transferase may also be made.

Detection and measurement of H, A, and B gene-specified transferases in sera are often important in the investigation of complex problems involving the ABO system.

The Molecular Configuration of A, B, and H

Although there has been considerable debate as to whether the terminal carbohydrates of H, A, and B on erythrocytes were carried on glycoproteins or glycolipids, it is currently believed that most H, A, and B antigens synthesized an the erythrocytic membrane are attached to glycoprotein, while others are attached to glycolipids. Of all the membrane-associated ABO system antigens, about 5% are carried on simple glycosphingolipids, between 10 and 15% on polyglycosylceramides, between 5 to 15% on alkali-labile glycoconjugates, and the remaining 65 to 75% on alkali-stable glycoproteins. In glycoprotein structures, N-acetyl-galactosamine joins the oligosaccharide to the peptide; in the glycolipid structures, glucose is the sugar that links the oligosaccharide to the lipid (ceramide) backbone.

TYPE 1 AND TYPE 2 CHAINS

Two different precursor chain configurations, known as type 1 and type 2 (Table 4-8), are found in blood group active secretions, other body fluids, and various tissues. The chains differ only in the linkage of B-galactose to a terminal β-N-acetylglucosamine residual. The carbon 1 of galactose can be attached to either carbon 3 or carbon 4 of β-N-acetylglucosamine (Fig. 4-3). The beta-1,3 linkage represents a type 1 chain; the beta-1,4 linkage represents a type 2 chain. The H, A, and B immunodominant

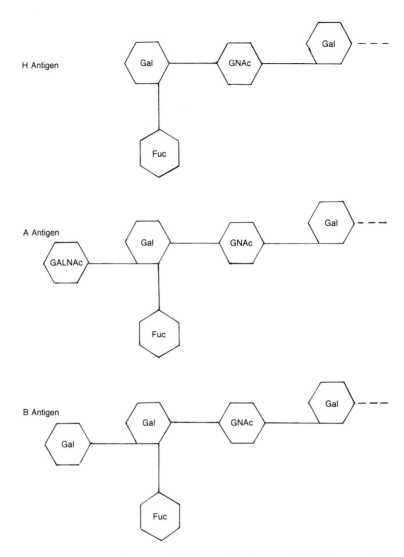

Figure 4-2. Biochemical configurations conferring antigenic specificity. The carbohydrate residual attached to the third carbon of galactose determines antigenic activity. N-acetyl-galactosamine confers A specificity and galactose confers B specificity. If the fucose residual that confers H specificity is not attached to the 2nd carbon, the galactose residual cannot react with either galactose or N-acetyl-galactosamine at the third carbon. Gal = Galactose, GNAc = N-acetyl-glucosamine; Fuc = Fucose; GALNAc = N-acetylgalactosamine.

Table 4-8. Comparison of Type 1 and Type 2 Chains

	Type 1	Type 2
Linkage	Beta 1, 3	Beta 1, 4
Origin	Plasma	Synthesized on erythrocytic precursors
Controlling genes	H, A, B, Se, and Lewis	H, A and B genes

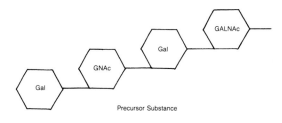

Precursor Substance

Type 1 Chain beta (1-3) Linkage

Type 2 Chain beta (1-4) Linkage

Figure 4-3. Chain types. Gal = Galactose; GNAc = N-acetylglucosamine; GALNAc = N-acetylgalactosamine.

sugars can be added to either of these chains.

ANTIGEN ACQUISITION

Most of the H, A, and B antigens of erythrocytes are synthesized by the erythrocytic precursors; some are acquired from the plasma. The antigens acquired from the plasma are of the type 1 variety and are glycosphingolipids. This attachment of A, B, and H antigens to erythrocytes from the plasma occurs because glycolipids can be

inserted into the membrane of the cells. The H, A, and B structures synthesized on erythrocytic precursors are exclusively of the type 2 variety, which are attached to both glycoproteins and glycosphingolipids. The H, A, and B, as well as Lewis determinants on type 1 chains that reach the erythrocytes by way of the plasma, are dependent on the H, A, B, Lewis, and secretor genes. The site of synthesis of plasma H, A, B, and Lewis antigens is not known. The type 2 chains are controlled (in terms of both presence and quantity) simply by the H, A, and B genes.

Lymphocytes and platelets acquire H, A, and B antigens from the plasma by insertion of preformed glycosphingolipids into the membrane. It is currently believed that little, if any, H, A, or B is synthesized during lymphocyte development. Therefore, all the lymphocyte membrane-borne H, A, and B antigens are acquired from the plasma. There is less agreement about the source of H, A, and B on platelets. However, there is disagreement as to whether all the platelet-borne H, A, and B antigens are acquired from plasma or some acquired and some synthesized during platelet development.

SECRETORS AND NONSECRETORS

Approximately 80% of persons in the United States secrete water-soluble H, H and A, or H and B antigens into saliva and other body fluids such as tears and semen. These secretions have the same specificity as the ABH antigens on the person's erythrocytes (Table 4-9). Lewis system antigens

Table 4-9. ABH Antigens in Secretions

ABO Group	Secretor Status	Secretion
O	Se/Se or Se/se	H
A	Se/Se or Se/se	A,H
B	Se/Se or Se/se	B,H
AB	Se/Se or Se/se	A,B,H
O	se/se	None
A	se/se	None
B	se/se	None
AB	se/se	None
O_h (Bombay)	Se/Se	None
O_h (Bombay)	Se/se	None
O_h (Bombay)	se/se	None

(see Chapter 5) can also be found in saliva. A second alcohol-soluble form of these antigens is present in all body tissues (except the brain) and on the erythrocytes, but is not present in secretions.

The production of A, B, and H antigens in saliva or other body fluids is controlled by the secretor gene, which is inherited independently of the ABO and H genes. Both the locus of the secretor gene (Se) and its allele (se), which is amorphic, and the exact mechanism of inheritance are unknown. At least one Se gene (genotype SeSe or Sese) is essential for the expression of the ABH antigens in secretions. Individuals who are homozygous for se (sese) do *not* secrete H, A, or B antigens regardless of the presence of H, A, or B genes, and at least one H gene is necessary for H, A, or B antigens to be manufactured. Alcohol-soluble antigens are not influenced by the secretor gene.

The suggested role for the Se-specified transferase (L-fucosyltransferase) is transfer of L-fucose to the terminal galactose of type 1 chains, which forms H substance into the secreted material. It is the presence of L-fucosyltransferase that subsequently determines whether ABH soluble substances will be secreted, because H substance must be synthesized before the formation of A or B substances. The Se gene does *not* bring about the formation of A, B, or H antigens on erythrocytes, nor does it control the presence of A, B, or H transferases in hematopoietic tissue. In contrast, the A or B transferase enzymes, unlike A or B antigens, are found in the secretions of A_1 or B persons regardless of secretor status.

Secretor status can be determined by the inhibition (neutralization) test described in Chapter 14. Testing for ABH secretion is helpful in establishing the true ABO group of an individual. The detection of small amounts of A or B antigens in the saliva of a secretor can be a useful confirmatory test when establishing a phenotype that involves a subgroup of A or B.

TYPE A

The A_1 and A_2 Subgroups

Group A antigens can be differentiated into two principal subgroups, A_1 and A_2.

Approximately 78% of group A individuals are A_1, with most of the others belonging to the A_2 subgroup. Inheritance patterns of A_1 and A_2 phenotypes, as well as A_1B and A_2B phenotypes, suggest that the A^1 and A^2 genes code for different transferases. Some biochemical studies appear to have produced evidence that there are different patterns of N-acetyl-D-galactosamine attachment on A_1 and A_2 erythrocytes, which suggests that the acceptor sites for the A_1 and A_2 gene-specified transferases might be different.

Four different types of A-active and H-active glycolipids have been isolated from erythrocytes. The H-bearing chains are classified as H_1, H_2, H_3, and H_4; the A-bearing chains are referred to as A_a, A_b, A_c, and A_d. These chains vary considerably in length and complexity of branching (Table 4-10).

The A-immunodominant carbohydrate and the H_1 and H_2 glycolipids are converted to A_a and A_b glycolipids by the transferase produced by the A^1 or A^2 genes. The H_3 and H_4 glycolipids are converted to A_c and A_d when the A_1 gene-specified transferase is made. Some A_2 cells may lack A_d altogether and carry only small amounts of A_c. This means that H_3 and H_4 are much more readily available when A_2 erythrocytes are tested with anti-H. Thus, the high level of A and low level of H on A_1 cells and the lower level of A and higher level of H on A_2 cells are demonstrable.

Immunodominant sugars are attached to erythrocyte membrane-borne glycoproteins and glycolipids. On the erythrocytes of adults, some of the glycoproteins and glycolipids are straight chains; others are complex branched chains with several different sites at which the H, A, and B, specific carbohydrates can be added. On erythrocytes from cord blood samples, the complex branched chains are not well developed, so that the number of sites to which immunodominant carbohydrates can be added

Table 4-10. A and H Chain Complexity

Straighter Chains	More Branched Chains
H_1 and H_2	H_3–H_4
A_a and A_b	A_c and A_d

are fewer than on the erythrocytes of adults. The decreased number of A and B antigens on fetal erythrocytes acts as a defense against hemolytic disease of the newborn (HDN) even when large amounts of maternal antibody enter the fetal circulation.

The serologic distinction between A_1 and A_2 antigens is based on the reactions of erythrocytes with various antisera. Reagent anti-A sera from human sources rarely differentiates A_1 from A_2 subtypes but anti-A,B sera of human origin can detect common subgroups of A and B and IgM antibodies produced by individual murine hybridomas (monoclonal antibodies) can detect weak subgroups of A.

If anti-A from a group B person is adsorbed with A_2 cells, a typing serum (adsorbed anti-A_1) can be prepared that will agglutinate A_1 but not A_2 erythrocytes. Probably the most practical way to differentiate between A_1 and A_2 subgroups is by use of lectin anti-A_1, which is made from Dolichos biflorus seeds. Lectin anti-A_1 agglutinates A_1 but not A_2 erythrocytes. Dolichos lectin is not totally specific for A_1 because it also agglutinates some group O or group B erythrocytes that carry Cad and other antigens that are polyagglutinable. Such reactions, are rare enough that they do not significantly reduce the usefulness of Dolichos lectin as an anti-A_1 reagent.

For routine transfusion, it is not necessary to distinguish between patients or donors as A_1 or A_2 except when working with an A_2 or A_2B individual whose serum contains anti-A_1. Estimates of the frequency of anti-A_1 in sera vary between 1 and 8% of A_2 persons and 22 and 35% of A_2B persons. Although anti-A_1 is considered clinically insignificant unless it reacts at 37° C, it can cause ABO discrepancies between cell and serum tests and may also cause crossmatch incompatibilities.

Infrequent Subgroups of A

Genetically controlled subgroups of A result from the inheritance of rare alleles at the ABO locus. The distribution and characteristics of the uncommon subgroups of the A antigen, from the strongest A_3 to the weakest A_{end}, comprise a continuum.

Classification of these subgroups of A is based on the reactivity of erythrocytes with anti-A, anti-A,B, anti-H, and anti-A_1 (Dolichos biflorus); the presence or absence of anti-A_1 in the serum; and the secretion of A and H substance by secretors (Table 4-11). Failure to detect a weak A antigen usually results in the blood being mistakenly typed as group O. If a unit of erythrocytes of a weak subgroup of A is transfused to a group O recipient, a transfusion reaction is possible, although significant in vivo erythrocyte destruction may not occur. Factors producing false test results that resemble subgroups of A are discussed later in this chapter.

The Subgroup A_{int}

Originally, this subgroup of A was described as being intermediate between A_1 and A_2 in terms of its reactions with anti-A and anti-A_1. In 1970, it was agreed that blood would be classified as A_{int} based on the reaction with anti-A_1 (Table 4-12) but A_{int} erythrocytes react more strongly with anti-H than either A_1 or A_2 cells. This is indicative of the genetic control of H antigen production that is independent of the effects of the ABO genes.

Additional Subgroups of A

A variety of subgroups of A have been identified but are rare in occurrence. Serologic reactions of these groups are presented in Table 4-13. It is important to rule out conditions such as *chimeras* or weakening of the A antigen before considering these subgroups during laboratory testing.

Many subgroups are believed to result from the inheritance of a specific allele; others are considered to result from genetic interaction (Table 4-14).

TYPE B

Subgroups of variants of type B blood, such as the B_3 phenotype, are much rarer than subgroups of A, but the incidence of B antigen subgroups is more frequent in

Table 4-11. Serologic Reactions of A_1, A_2, A_1B and A_2B Phenotypes

		Reactions			
		A_1	A_2	A_1B	A_2B
Erythrocyte Reactions	Anti-A	+	+	+	+
	Anti-A_1	+	0	+	0
	Anti-B	0	0	+	+
	Anti-A,B	+	+	+	+

		A_1	A_2	A_2 with anti-A_1	A_1B	A_2B	A_2B with anti-A_1
Serum Reactions	A_1 cells	0	0	+	0	0	+
	A_2 cells	0	0	0	0	0	0
	B cells	+	+	+	0	0	0
	O cells	0	0	0	0	0	0

Table 4-12. A Comparison of the Serologic Reactions of A_1, A_{int}, and A_2 Phenotypes

Phenotype	Erythrocyte Reactions*				Serum Reactions†					Saliva of Secretors
	A	B	A,B	H	A_1	A_1	A_2	B	O	
A_1	4+	0	4+	0	4+	0	0	4+	0	A & H
A_{int}	4+	0	4+	3+	2+	0	0	4+	0	A & H
A_2	4+	0	4+	2+	0	‡	0	4+	0	A & H

* Reactions of patient's erythrocytes with reagent antiserum
† Reactions of patient's serum with reagent erythrocytes
‡ The occurrence of anti-A_1 is variable in these phenotypes

Table 4-13. Serologic Reactions of Uncommon A Phenotypes

Phenotype	A_{int}	A_3	A_x	A_m
Anti-A	4+	2+*	Weak/0	+/weak
Anti-A,B	4+	2+*	2+	+/weak
Anti-A_1	2+	0	0	0
Anti-H	3+	4+	4+	4+
Saliva (secretor)	A,H	A,H	H	A,H

REACTIONS OF SERUM AGAINST KNOWN REAGENT ERYTHROCYTES

Phenotype	A_{int}	A_3	A_x	A_m
A_1 cells	0	*†	2+	0
A_2 cells	0	0	0/+	0
B cells	4+	4+	4+	4+
O cells	0	0	0	0

REACTIONS OF ERYTHROCYTES AGAINST KNOWN ANTISERA

Phenotype	A_{end}	A_{el}	A_{bantu}	A_{lae}	A_{finn}
Anti-A	Weak	0	1–2+*	0	Weak
Anti-A,B	Weak	0	1–2+*	0	Weak
Anti-A_1†	0	0	0	3+	0
Anti-H	4+	4+	4+	4+	4+
Saliva (secretor)	H	H	H	H	H

* Mixed field
† Dolichos biflorus

Table 4-14. Characteristics of Uncommon A Subgroups

Phenotype	Date Identified	Characteristics
A_x	1935	Some are possibly inherited as an allele, A_x, at the ABO locus. Others appear to result from modifying genes
A_3	1936	Believed to be an allele, A_3, at the ABO locus
A_m	1942	Originally called A_x. Some result from inheritance of a gene A_m, an allele at the ABO locus. Others demonstrate that the phenotype can result from a double dose (homozygous state) of a rare, recessive, modifying gene, y. Serologically, RBCs of the A_y phenotypes are indistinguishable from the A_m phenotype
A_{end}	1959	Results from the inheritance of an allele at the ABO locus
A_{el}	1964	Thought to result from inheritance of an allele at the ABO locus
A_{bantu}	1966	Controlled by a variant gene that resides at the ABO locus.
A_{finn}	1973	This subgroup is very likely A_{end}

some racial groups. For example, 24% of the Chinese population of Taiwan have type B blood and the frequencies of B_3 and A_1B_3 blood are about 1:900 and 1:1800, respectively.

The proposed terminology based on the percentage of erythrocytes in the sample that are agglutinated by a human anti-B antiserum is conventionally divided into 3 major subgroups: B_3, B_m, and B_x (Table 4-15). The classification of B subgroups by Race and Sanger is divided into three categories (Table 4-16) based on serologic characteristics.

Subgroups of B are usually recognized by variations in the strength of the reaction using human anti-B and anti-A,B reagent antisera. It has been suggested that qualitative as well as a quantitative differences exist in the B antigen of B_3 erythrocytes. These differences have been noted because of the significantly lower avidity of subgroup B_3 and subgroup A_1B_3 with both polyclonal and monoclonal anti-sera, compared to normal group B cells.

ABNORMALITIES ENCOUNTERED IN THE EXPRESSION OF ABH ANTIGENS ON ERYTHROCYTES

The expression of ABH antigens on erythrocytes may be altered by a variety of factors, which include

1. Modifying genes
2. Acquired antigens
3. Altered antigens
4. High levels of soluble ABH substances
5. Depression of A, B, and H antigens in disease
6. Mixtures of blood

Modifying Genes

A SUPERACTIVE B GENE

In some AB people with relatively few A antigen sites on their erythrocytes, the deficit of A antigen is believed to be caused by the presence of a superactive B transferase, coded for by a superactive B gene, that competes with normal A_1 or A_2 trans-

Table 4-15. Characteristics of B Subgroups

Phenotype	Erythrocyte				Serum Reactions				Saliva
	A	B	A,B	H	A_1	A_2	B	O	
B	0	4+	4+	0	4+	4+	0	0	B & H
B_3	0	+mf	+ + mf	4+	4+	4+	0	0	B & H
B_m	0	0	*	4+	4+	4+	0	0	B & H
B_x	0	*	†	4+	4+	4+	0	0	H

* Negative (no agglutination) or ± reaction.
† Negative or 2+.

Table 4-16. Race and Sanger Classification of Erythrocyte Reactions of B Subgroups

	Category I	Category II	Category III
Anti-B	Weak	Weak	Weak
Anti-A,B	Weak	Weak	Weak
Serum	Anti-B	Absent	Absent
Saliva (of secretors)	B,H	B,H	H
			B*

* B may be present in decreased amounts but is usually negative.

ferase. Predominantly Black populations have the highest frequency of this atypical B gene.

Oₕ: THE BOMBAY PHENOTYPE

In 1952, a new phenotype within the ABO system was recognized. It was initially believed that in normal persons an additional gene was necessary for the A or B gene to be expressed as A or B antigen. This gene, originally called X by Levine, was viewed as possibly acting as a suppressor. In Bombay, it was hypothesized that the X (H) gene was not present, but its allele x (h) (in a homozygous state) prevented the production of A or B antigenic expression.

Defining the biochemical composition of the H, A, and B antigens was essential to interpreting the identity of the X and H genes. When the roles of H gene-specified transferase in adding L-fucose to precursor substance and A and B gene-specified transferase in adding the immunodominant monosaccharides of A and B antigens were understood, it was concluded that the X and H genes were the same.

The gene was designated Bombay. Afflicted persons of the Bombay type have an hh genotype and an O_h phenotype. The alleles Hh and ABO have been demonstrated to segregate independently. The O_h phenotype can carry A or B genes, but these genes do not express themselves as A or B antigens on the erythrocytes of the O_h persons because of the lack of H gene and consequent lack of H-bearing structures on the erythrocytic membrane. Therefore, the lack of demonstrable A or B antigens on O_h erythrocytes is a function of the lack of a suitable acceptor site. If, however, an A or B gene is transmitted to offspring with an H gene being received from the other par-

ent, the offspring can have normal A or B antigenic expression (see Fig. 4-1).

The O_h phenotype erythrocytes have normal in vivo survival. There is also no reason to assume that O_h erythrocytes lack anything but the terminal carbohydrates normally attached to the erythrocytic membrane-borne glycolipids and glycoproteins.

In the laboratory, the erythrocytes of the O_h phenotype are not agglutinated by anti-A, anti-B, anti-A,B, or anti-H reagent antisera. The H gene-specified fucosyl transferase is not present in the sera of O_h persons. If anti-H is produced by O_h persons, it is usually more potent at 37° C, in comparison to anti-H produced by A_1 or B persons, which is typically a cold-reacting antibody of no clinical significance. Group O erythrocytes must *never* be transfused to an O_h person.

Aₕ and SIMILAR PHENOTYPES

A or B antigens may, on rare occasions, develop in the absence of H. Different groups of investigators claim to have found hidden H (and/or A and B) antigens on O_h erythrocytes with traces of A and B antigens that are detectable in direct tests.

In 1961, Levine et al. described a person in whom the erythrocytes failed to react with anti-H, but did react weakly with anti-A. The serum contained anti-B and an anti-H antibody that was active at 37° C, but the saliva did not contain ABH substances. Other family members were secretors. The name A_h was applied to this phenotype as parallel to O_h.

Levine hypothesized that the A_h phenotype was caused by a partial suppressor at the Hh locus that prevented normal quantities of H substance from being produced. He concluded that whatever H substance was produced was converted to A substance by action of the A gene. This theory provided an explanation for the absence of, or decreased amount of detectable H substance. Most transferase assays have supported this line of reasoning, but a deficiency of erythrocytic membrane-borne H antigen can occasionally occur even though a person has a normal level of H gene-specified transferase enzyme in the serum. It is possible that variants in the H gene also exist.

Some investigators theorize that an alternative pathway exists for the formation of A (and perhaps B) antigens on the erythrocyte membrane. It is believed that in the absence of H substance, the A and perhaps B gene-specified transferases can add small quantities of A- and perhaps B-immunodominant monosaccharides.

A_m PHENOTYPE

Families have been identified that are believed to be genetically A_1 or A_2 but do not express the A_1 or A_2 phenotype. Individuals from these families have been classified as A_m phenotype, which results from a homozygous state of a rare, recessive, modifying gene, y. This modifying gene is inherited independently of the ABO genes. The common gene, Y, is necessary for normal expression of the A antigen, and the absence of a Y gene (yy) results in decreased expression of A antigen on erythrocytes. The absence of a Y gene does not usually affect the secretion of A substance, nor is the expression of B antigen on erythrocytes usually altered.

A DOMINANT SUPPRESSOR GENE

In 1973, the presence of a dominant suppressor of A and B was noted. In the presence of this dominant suppressor, erythrocytes were typed as group O, but the serum lacked anti-A. Saliva of secretors contained both A and H substances. It is believed that afflicted persons are genetically A_1O.

THE AB CIS GENE

Individuals carrying an AB-cis gene were first observed because of an anomaly of

inheritance of the ABO groups. In these cases, the A and B genes seem to have been inherited on a single chromosome (Fig. 4-4). The term AB-cis gene is used to describe this rare situation, which is believed to result from unequal crossing over at the ABO locus. Both an A gene on one chromosome and a B gene on the other are involved. The resultant new AB cis gene is composed of part of the genetic information normally carried by the A gene and part of the B gene. AB cis gene products include the transferases normally expected as products of A and B genes.

The A and B antigens on erythrocytes of persons genetically AB/O are not as strong as those on the erythrocytes of persons genetically A/B. Many of the phenotypes resulting from the AB cis gene have been characterized as A_2B, with the B antigen reacting more weakly than usual.

Other instances of similar phenotypes caused by AB cis can include an $A_{weak}B$ phenotype, in which a B gene-specified transferase enzyme was so productive that it added galactose to most of the H-bearing receptors before the slower-acting A_2 gene-specified transferase could add galactosamine.

Acquired Antigens

ACQUIRED A ANTIGEN

Acquired A antigen has been reported in persons of type O or type B in association with severe infections caused by *Proteus mirabilis*. In these conditions, reactions with anti-A reagent are visible microscopically as mixed-field agglutination.

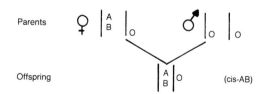

Figure 4-4. Cis-AB phenotype. The cis-AB phenotype results from the inheritance of both A and B genes from one parent and a normal gene from the other parent.

Tn-activated erythrocytes can demonstrate the presence of an acquired A antigen. The reason that group O or group B Tn-activated erythrocytes react with some anti-A reagents is that, like the A antigen, the immunodominant monosaccharide of Tn is N-acetyl-galactosamine. This phenomenon is rare and represents a type of polyagglutinability. Tn activation of erythrocytes is permanent and not associated with bacterial or viral infections.

Acquired B Antigen

Acquired B-like antigen was first recognized in 1959 in association with conditions such as carcinoma of the colon or rectum, intestinal obstruction, massive infection of the lower gastrointestinal tract, and septicemia caused by *Proteus vulgaris.* After recovery from the condition or infection, the acquired B-like antigen is lost and the patient reverts to normal blood status. This phenomenon is infrequently observed in healthy individuals.

The acquisition of B antigen usually occurs in persons of the A_1 phenotype. It is infrequent in those of the A_2 phenotype, and is not known to occur in type O persons. One theory of acquisition of the acquired B antigen is that deacetylation of the A_1 antigen by bacterial enzymes takes place and causes a change in the antigen. The number of A receptor sites diminishes as the number of B receptor sites increases. Acetylation of the acquired B antigen results in the loss of B activity and the reappearance of the A_1 antigen that had been deacetylated. Because the difference between the A and B antigens involves the substitution of only the terminal immunodominant monosaccharide, the change from A_1 antigen to B antigen, by deacetylation can be explained. The greater number of antigen sites on A_1 compared to A_2 erythrocytes explains why acquired B antigens are almost always found in group A_1 individuals.

A second mechanism of antigen formation may exist. An acquired B antigen can result from increased permeability of the intestinal wall and subsequent adsorption of the bacterial polysaccharide (*Escherichia coli* O_{86}) on the erythrocyte. Some types of bacteria produce lipopolysaccharides that

include B-like structures. The passive adsorption of these materials by erythrocytes can result in the cells acquiring a B-like antigen with no reduction of A antigen in the case of A_1 and A_2 erythrocytes. It should be noted that this mechanism has never been established as a route for the in vivo acquisition of B antigen.

The presence of acquired B-like antigen is occasionally associated with polyagglutination of erythrocytes. A state of polyagglutination involving acquired B-like antigen may be restricted to cases in which the acquired antigen represents deacetylation of A. B-like antigen can be suspected when observing a very slowly-reacting and weak appearing agglutination pattern with anti-B typing sera compared to true group B erythrocytes. In these cases, the patient's serum contains a form of anti-B that fails to react with autologous cells or with those from others with an acquired B-like antigen, but reacts with all normal group B erythrocytes. Eluates made from erythrocytes that have acquired B-like antigen do not usually contain anti-B. An anti-B lectin, Bandeirae simplicifolia (modified BS-1 lectin), has the ability to differentiate true B antigens from acquired B-like antigens on erythrocytes. Modified BS-1 lectin does not agglutinate acquired B antigens but does agglutinate true B antigens. This lectin is not widely available. If anti-B typing sera is acidified to pH 6.0, it agglutinates only true B antigens.

Altered Antigens

Erythrocytes may have inherited or acquired surface abnormalities that produce polyagglutination. Polyagglutination is defined as the agglutination of erythrocytes by most normal human sera. Three types of polyagglutination include the following:

1. T-activation
2. Tn-activation
3. Cad polyagglutinability

T Activation

All normal erythrocytes possess antigens that are not usually detectable by routine blood banking methods. T activation or the unmasking of these "hidden antigens" is usually a temporary condition caused by the removal of sialic acid and exposure of the T antigen because of the action of microbial neuraminidase. Organisms that produce neuraminidase include bacteria, particularly *bacteroides* and *clostridium,* as well as protozoa, yeast, and viruses (predominantly influenza). When the causative infection subsides, the erythrocytes are usually no longer T-activated or polyagglutinable.

All normal adult sera contain anti-T; therefore T-activated erythrocytes are polyagglutinable. The reaction of T-activated erythrocytes and serum demonstrates a pattern of mixed-field agglutination. T-activated erythrocytes are not agglutinated by cord serum because the latter lacks anti-T; nor are they agglutinated by the person's own serum, because the serum antibody is not an autoantibody. Additionally, T-activated erythrocytes fail to be aggregated by polybrene. It is possible to obtain a correct ABO typing by preparing T-activated cells and allowing them to absorb the anti-T from the typing sera.

TN ACTIVATION

The Tn antigen is not demonstrated on normal erythrocytes, and all normal sera contain the corresponding antibody. The activation of the Tn antigen is rather uncommon and possibly results from insufficient addition of sialic acid during erythrocyte maturation. Conditions associated with Tn activation include hematologic abnormalities such as hemolytic anemia, leukocytopenia, and thrombocytopenia.

Tn activation of erythrocytes is a permanent alteration and cannot be simulated in vitro. Although these altered cells are agglutinated by *Dolichos biflorus* extract, Tn activation can be identified by using extracts for *Salvia sclarea* or *Salvia haematodes* seeds.

Tn-activated cells and T-activated cells share the following characteristics

1. Reduced erythrocytic membrane sialic acid content

2. A mixed-field agglutination pattern with all normal adult sera
3. No agglutination with cord serum
4. No agglutination with polybrene
5. Reduced M and N surface antigen

The correct ABO status of a person can be determined by treating the Tn-activated cells with 1% ficin or papain to destroy the Tn receptor sites.

CAD POLYAGGLUTINABILITY

Cad cells are polyagglutinable because they carry an extraordinary quantity of the Sd^a antigen; most cells have a much smaller amount of this antigen. Most sera contain trace amounts of anti-Sd^a; therefore, Cad cells are readily agglutinated because of the large quantity of Sd^a surface antigen present. Cad cells are more strongly agglutinated by *Dolichos biflorus* extract than group A$_1$ erythrocytes. Unlike Tn-activated cells, the Cad receptor is not destroyed by enzyme treatment, but may actually be enhanced. The diagnosis of Cad polyagglutination is made by exclusion, aided by the reaction of the seed extract of *Salvia horminum.* This extract agglutinates both Tn and Cad polyagglutinable erythrocytes.

High Levels of Soluble ABH Substances

Rarely, in conditions such as ovarian cysts, carcinoma of the stomach or pancreas, or intestinal obstruction, excess amounts of blood group-specific substances can be observed. The level of ABH substance in a person's serum may be so high that it inhibits the anti-A or anti-B reagent serum. This interference with ABO grouping is caused by neutralization of the reagent anti-A or anti-B by the specific soluble substances, which leaves no unbound antibody to react with the person's erythrocytes. This situation can produce false-negative or weak reactions in the antigen typing of erythrocytes.

Depression of A, B, and H Antigens

ANTIGENIC WEAKENING CAUSED BY DISEASE

Weakening of the A antigen has been noted in patients with leukemia or lymphoma. The subscript g as in A_g has been used to indicate an antigen weakened by the leukemic process. The B and H antigens can also be depressed, but, in some cases, as the level of A or B antigen has decreased, the level of H antigen detectable on erythrocytes has been seen to increase. In addition to antigenic alteration associated with leukemia, similar findings have been observed in Hodgkin's and non-Hodgkin's lymphoma and in refractory anemias associated with abnormal erythrocytic enzymes.

ANTIGENIC WEAKENING IN GROUP AB

Errors of interpretation can occur in cases of subgroups of A antigen in association with the B antigen in the AB phenotype. The phenotype A_2B is sometimes mistakenly designated as A_3B because of the weakening of the A antigen in the presence of B.

The weakened form of A in A_2B blood is caused by transferase activity. It has been found that in the genotype A_1B, the A_1 and B gene-specified transferases are about equal in terms of efficiency in adding immunodominant sugars to H-bearing chains. In the genotype A_2B or other weak forms of A and B, (A_xB) the B gene-specified transferase is more efficient than A. Consequently, more H-bearing chains receive galactose (the B immunodominant monosaccharide) than receive galactosamine (the A immunodominant monosaccharide). In the absence of B gene-specified transferase such as the genotype A_2O, no competition exists and more galactosamine is added to H chains. Therefore, A_2 erythrocytes carry more A antigen sites than the A_2B phenotype.

The most reliable way of correctly determining affected AB persons is to carry out family studies. In some of these cases, the products of the A gene may be found in a family member who lacks the B gene.

MIXTURES OF BLOOD

In 1975 it was found that some individuals who were not genetic blood group *chimeras* had two populations of erythrocytes, group O and group A. Alleles at the ABO locus were found to be responsible. The ABO-mos phenotype, as these cases are designated, is transmitted to different generations within the families.

ANTIBODIES OF THE ABO BLOOD GROUP SYSTEM

Landsteiner reasoned from his observations that most individuals possess antibodies directed against the antigens that are absent from their own cells (see Table 4-1). These antibodies were called "naturally occurring," but this term is really a misnomer. Scientific evidence supports the fact that anti-A and anti-B are stimulated by agents such as bacteria, pollen, or other substances present in the internal or external environment that have molecular configurations similar to the A and B antigen. The wide distribution of these agents ensures constant exposure to A, B, and H-like antigens. Consequently, the immune response to noncellular antigenic stimulation results in the production of the complementary IgM antibodies (anti-A and/or anti-B) in immunologically competent individuals. The predictable relationship between antigens and antibodies in the ABO system permits the use of both serum and cell tests in ABO grouping.

Development of Anti-A and Anti-B

Antibody production is initiated at birth by exposure to foreign substances such as bacteria, pollen, and dust. Initially, antibody titers are usually too low for serologic detection and do not increase until the age of 3 to 6 months. If antibodies are detected in a newborn or young infant, they are probably of maternal origin. Serum from newborn infants may contain IgG antibodies passively acquired by placental transfer from the mother if she has IgG anti-A or anti-B. Anti-A and anti-B production increases for the first 5 or 6 years and then remains fairly constant until late in adult life. In elderly people, the titer of anti-A and anti-B is often much lower than in young adults.

The strength (titer) of antibodies varies considerably from sera to sera. In general, the strength of anti-A in group B and group O sera tends to be greater than anti-B in group A and group O sera. With the exception of group AB serum, complete absence of anti-A, anti-B, or both is rare.

Antibody Characteristics

The antibodies of the ABO blood group system have similar characteristics, including the following:

1. Agglutination of saline suspended erythrocytes.
2. Reactivity at room temperature.
3. Production of hemolysis in vivo and in vitro. Both IgM and IgG anti-A and anti-B are capable of binding complement. All examples of IgG anti-A and about 90% of IgM anti-A have been demonstrated to be hemolytic.
4. Inactivation of IgM anti-A and anti-B with 2-mercaptoethanol (2-ME).

Antibodies to the A and B antigens are generally divided into two classes: IgM, if environmentally stimulated, and IgG, if stimulated by foreign erythrocytes. IgG stimulation can result from the transfusion of ABO-incompatible erythrocytes, receipt of plasma containing blood group substances, or maternal-fetal ABO incompatibility. Examples of anti-A have been identified that consist of partly IgM and partly IgG; partly IgM and partly IgA; a mixture of IgM, IgG, and IgA. Group O individuals normally have anti-A and anti-B of both immunoglobulin classes in their serum in addition to anti-A,B. The presence of IgG anti-A and anti-B is more frequent in group O than in group A or B persons.

If complement is present, erythrocytes may be hemolyzed because of the presence of A or B antigens and their corresponding antibodies. ABO antibodies that produce hemolysis bind to short-chain structures on the erythrocytic membrane and act as hemolysins both in vivo and in vitro. Anti-A and anti-B efficiently activate complement because complement is activated close to the cell membrane, which facilitates the binding of many of the activated complement components to the membrane before they decay.

In vitro hemolysis can produce either a pink discoloration of the supernatant fluid or total destruction of the erythrocytes after centrifugation. Because hemolysis requires complement, it will not occur if an anticoagulant such as calcium-chelating EDTA is present.

Anti-A and anti-B can coat erythrocytes without producing agglutination. Coating antibodies are usually IgG. When a patient's serum contains both coating and agglutinating antibodies of the same specificity, agglutination is the only detectable end point unless the agglutinating antibodies are neutralized or inactivated.

Anti-A,B (Group O)

Serum from type O persons contains the antibody anti-A,B. When type A erythrocytes are used for absorbing anti-A from type O serum, the eluate contains anti-A and anti-A,B, which reacts with both A and B erythrocytes. Similar reactions are observed when B cells are used for absorption. Saliva from group A or group B secretors inhibits the reaction of this antibody with either A or B erythrocytes.

Anti-A,B from group O serum reacts more strongly than anti-A or anti-B with erythrocytes of some A and B subgroups. Although AABB standards do not require the use of anti-A,B or any other procedure to detect weak A or B phenotypes, some laboratories use reagent anti-A,B to check ABO groupings. This procedure is performed to avoid labelling blood as group O when it is a subgroup of A or B. Anti-A,B can be used alone as the required procedure to reconfirm the ABO status of group O erythrocytes before transfusion.

Anti-A$_1$

The anti-A in group O and group B sera has been observed to contain separable anti-A and anti-A$_1$. By absorbing anti-A serum with A$_2$ erythrocytes, reactivity against A$_1$, but no A$_2$ cells remains. The apparent anti-A$_1$ remaining in serum after absorption with A$_2$ erythrocytes is believed to be a weakened form of anti-A. It is believed that individuals with A$_2$ cells that carry A$_a$ and A$_b$, but no or only low levels of A$_c$ and A$_d$, might form anti-A$_1$. Anti-A$_1$ might possibly have an anti-A$_{cd}$ specificity, and A$_c$ and A$_d$ might be missing or present in small amounts more often in A$_2$B erythrocytes than in A$_2$ cells. This theory might explain the higher incidence of anti-A$_1$ in persons who are A$_2$B than in persons who are A$_2$.

Anti-H

There are two kinds of human anti-H. One type is a cold-reacting type antibody in the serum of persons with small amounts of H on their erythrocytes, usually group A$_1$ or AB. The other type is produced by individuals with the rare O$_h$ (Bombay) phenotype whose erythrocytes have no H antigen.

Cold-reactive anti-H is uncommon. Although all blood groups have some H substance on the erythrocytes, it is believed to be blocked by the added sugars of the A and B antigens. Group O and A$_2$ phenotypes are not associated with the production of anti-H. Occasionally, group A$_1$, A$_1$B or, less commonly, group B erythrocytes have such a small amount of unconverted H substance that individuals with this phenotype can produce weakly reacting anti-H. The concept that H is covered on A$_1$ and B cells is supported by the finding that erythrocytes of the subgroups of A lower than A$_2$ have levels of H roughly similar to those on O cells, which have none of the H chains covered by other carbohydrates. As expected, group O erythrocytes react more strongly with anti-H reagent sera than do group A$_2$ cells.

In the case of O$_h$ persons, who completely lack the H antigen, anti-H is a frequent alloantibody. This form of anti-H reacts between 4 and 37° C and agglutinates all erythrocytes other than O$_h$. This type of anti-H binds complement and causes hemolysis. O$_h$ persons *must* be transfused with O$_h$ blood because their anti-H rapidly destroys normal group O erythrocytes.

QUANTITIES OF H ANTIGEN IN DIMINISHING ORDER

$$O > A_2 > A_2B > B > A_1 > A_1B$$

EXAMPLES OF DISCREPANCIES IN ABO FORWARD AND REVERSE GROUPING

Technical errors and various clinical conditions or diseases can contribute to a discrepancy between erythrocyte and serum results in ABO grouping. When the expected *forward grouping,* using known sources of reagent antisera (antibodies) to detect antigens on erythrocytes, or *reverse grouping,* using known reagent erythrocytes to test patient serum, do not produce the complementary matching of ABO antigens and antibodies, the possibility of technical error must first be excluded. If carefully controlled repeat testing yields the same agglutination patterns, the variation can be assigned to one of four categories:

1. Weak or missing antigen reactions
2. Unexpected antigen reactions
3. Weak or missing antibody reactions
4. Unexpected antibody reactions

In this section, conditions that can produce discrepancies and examples of the laboratory findings in these discrepancies are presented. This section reviews previously presented material; however, technical information and laboratory findings that have not been previously discussed are also presented. The protocol for conducting further investigations of each of these problems is presented in Chapters 13 and 14.

Missing or Weak Antigen Reactions

Examples of conditions contributing to missing or weak antigen (Table 4-17) expression on erythrocytes include the following:

1. Subgroups of A or B antigens
2. Disease states such as leukemias
3. Excess blood group-specific soluble substances

Weak antigen reactions may be caused by the inheritance of a subgroup of A or B. Weakened A antigen expression may also result from acquired characteristics such as the changes observed in acute leukemias. The weakening of antigenic strength can occur with B and H antigens as well as antigens of other blood group systems.

Unexpected Antigen Reactions

Examples of conditions (Table 4-18) producing unexpected reactions on forward grouping can be caused by the following:

1. Acquired A or B antigen
2. Altered antigens (T-activation, Tn-activation; Cad polyagglutinability)
3. Erythrocytes coated with antibody

4. Additives to antisera (acriflavin)
5. Mixtures of blood
6. Low incidence antigen and antibody reaction

ACQUIRED A ANTIGEN

Group O or group B persons with Tn-activated erythrocytes can manifest an acquired A antigen.

ACQUIRED B-LIKE ANTIGEN

The characteristics of an acquired B-like antigen are that the erythrocytes react as a group AB, while the serum contains only anti-B. The strength of the forward grouping reaction is much greater for A than B antigen, an autocontrol (patient's serum + patient's cells) is negative, and A substance is present in the saliva of secretors but B substance is not.

ALTERED ANTIGENS

In testing with *Dolichos biflorus* extract, it should be noted that lectin agglutinates Cad Sd (a^{++}) and Tn-activated Sd(a^+) erythrocytes irrespective of ABO group.

Table 4-17. Example of a Weak or Missing Antigen Reaction

Forward Grouping			Reverse Grouping			
Patient's erythrocytes			Patient's serum			
+			+			
Reagent antisera			Reagent erythrocytes			
Anti-A	Anti-B	Anti-A,B	A_1	B	O	Autocontrol
0	0	1+	0	3+	0	0

In contrast to the strong reactions normally observed on forward typing, this patient demonstrated a weak reaction. Based on the reverse grouping, the patient would be expected to demonstrate A antigen activity. The weak agglutination of erythrocytes with anti-A,B, and the absence of agglutination with anti-A suggest a weak subgroup of A.

ADDITIONAL LABORATORY TESTING.

Absorption and elution tests produced anti-A from the erythrocytes. The patient's saliva contains A and H substances, although the ratio of A to H is significantly reduced.

The conclusion derived from these results is that this patient is a subgroup of A (A_2 phenotype).

Table 4-18. Example of a Typical Unexpected Antigen Reaction

Forward Grouping			Reverse Grouping			
Patient's erythrocytes			Patient's serum			
+			+			
Reagent antisera			Reagent erythrocytes			
Anti-A	Anti-B	Anti-A,B	A_1	B	O	Autocontrol
4+	2+	4+	0	4+	0	0

Observation of the 4^+ forward and reverse grouping reactions is typical in a group A person. However, the 2+ reaction of erythrocytes with anti-B cannot be ignored. Note that the autocontrol (patient's serum + patient's cells) is negative.

ADDITIONAL LABORATORY TESTING

A substance but not B substance was present in the saliva of the patient. Additionally, this patient had been admitted to the hospital for a severe gastrointestinal infection.

The conclusion was that the patient was group A with an acquired B-like antigen.

ERYTHROCYTES COATED WITH ANTIBODY

Erythrocytes that are heavily coated with antibody exhibit a positive direct anti-human globulin reaction. This may produce mixed-field or weak agglutination in the forward grouping. Conditions causing this situation include autoimmune hemolytic anemia, drugs such as alpha-methyldopa, transfusion reactions, and hemolytic disease of the newborn.

This type of spontaneous agglutination reacts more weakly at room temperature during ABO testing. It is possible to remove the antibody by elution techniques, after which anti-A and anti-B can reliably be used for ABO grouping.

ADDITIVES TO ANTISERA

Acrifavin, the yellow dye used in some commercial anti-B reagents, can produce agglutination in some persons. This false agglutination results from antibodies against acriflavin in the serum combining with the dye and attaching to the erythrocytes of the individual.

MIXTURES OF BLOOD

Mixture of cell types in recently transfused patients or recipients of bone marrow transplants can produce unexpected reactions in forward typing.

LOW-INCIDENCE ANTIGENS–ANTIBODY REACTION

Antibodies to low-incidence antigens may be present in reagent antisera such as anti-A or anti-B. A low-incidence antibody in antisera rarely reacts with the corresponding low-incidence antigen present on a patient's or donor's erythrocytes; however, this situation should be considered when an unexpected reaction mimics the presence of a weak antigen.

Weak and Missing Antibody Reactions

Missing or weak isoagglutinins result from depressed or absent antibody production. Missing antibody reactions (Table 4-19) on reverse grouping can be caused by the following:

1. Age
2. Hypogammaglobulinema
3. Agammaglobulinemia
4. Chimerism

Table 4-19. Example of a Typical Missing Antibody Reaction

Forward Grouping			Reverse Grouping			
Patient's erythrocytes			Patient's serum			
+			+			
Reagent antisera			Reagent erythrocytes			
Anti-A	Anti-B	Anti-A,B	A₁	B	O	Autocontrol
0	0	0	1+	0	0	0

The absence of agglutination in forward grouping suggests a group O; however, the reverse grouping suggests a group B.

ADDITIONAL LABORATORY TESTING

Incubation of the forward and reverse typing for 30 minutes at room temperature and at 4°C demonstrated additional agglutination in the A₁ reverse grouping cells. The autocontrol remained negative.

The conclusion of this testing was that the patient was a group O with a low titer anti-A isoagglutinin.

AGE

Newborn and young infants and the elderly may exhibit weak or missing isoantibodies. Reverse grouping is not routinely performed on serum from newborn infants because it is unlikely that they have started to produce antibodies. Detectable antibodies in newborn or young infants are acquired in utero from the mother.

HYPOGAMMAGLOBULINEMIA

Decreases in the gamma globulin fraction of plasma protein, (hypogammaglobulinemia) can lead to weak or missing antibodies. Conditions in which hypogammaglobulinemia may be demonstrated include the use of immunosuppressive drugs, lymphomas, leukemias, immunodeficiency disorders, and following bone marrow transplantation.

AGAMMAGLOBULINEMIA

Agammaglobulinemia (absence of plasma gamma globulins) can be either congenital or acquired. Disorders such as Bruton's agammaglobulinemia, immune deficiency disorders, and the effects of physical agents such as radiation exposure and cytotoxic drugs can all contribute to a state of agammaglobulinemia.

CHIMERISM

Chimerism is an infrequent cause of a weak or missing ABO isoagglutinin. True chimerism is rarely found and occurs mostly in twins in whom two cell populations exist in one individual throughout his lifetime. The two cell populations are both recognized as self; consequently, these individuals do not make anti-A or anti-B and no detectable isoagglutins are present in the serum. Chimerism in a person who has no twin may be caused by dispermy (two sperm fertilizing one egg) and indicates *mosaicism*.

Artificial or transient chimeras can be detected when group O erythrocytes are transfused to a group A or B patient after bone marrow transplant, exchange transfusion, or fetal-maternal bleeding.

Unexpected Antibody Reactions

Conditions producing unexpected reactions on reverse grouping (Tables 4-20 through 4-22) can be caused by

1. Rouleaux formation
2. Cold autoantibodies
3. Unexpected ABH isoagglutinins
4. Unexpected alloantibodies

Table 4-20. Example 1 of a Typical Unexpected Antibody Reaction

Forward Grouping			Reverse Grouping			
Patient's erythrocytes +			Patient's serum +			
Reagent antisera			Reagent erythrocytes			
Anti-A	Anti-B	Anti-A,B	A_1	B	O	Autocontrol
4+	0	4+	1+	4+	0	0

The strong (4+) forward agglutination with anti-A and anti-A,B and reverse agglutination with B cells represents a typical group A reaction. The reaction with A_1 cells suggests the presence of an additional weakly reacting antibody.

ADDITIONAL LABORATORY TESTING

The serum was tested against three examples each of A_1, A_2, and O red cells. Agglutination was observed in all of the A_1 erythrocytes but none of the A_2 or O cells. Additionally, the patient's erythrocytes were tested with anti-A lectin. The anti-A_1 lectin was negative.

The conclusion was that this patient was a group A_2 phenotype with an anti-A_1 antibody.

Table 4-21. Example 2 of a Typical Unexpected Antibody Reaction

Forward Grouping			Reverse Grouping			
Patient's erythrocytes +			Patient's serum +			
Reagent antisera			Reagent erythrocytes			
Anti-A	Anti-B	Anti-A,B	A_1	B	O	Autocontrol
4+	0	4+	0	4+	3+	0

Based on the 4+ agglutination pattern, a group A_1 blood is suspected; however, a slightly weaker reaction with Group O cells suggests the presence of an additional antibody.

ADDITIONAL LABORATORY TESTING

Testing of the patient's erythrocytes with anti-A_1 lectin yielded a positive reaction. The patient's serum was tested with additional group O, A_2, A_1 cells and group O cord cells. All of the group O cells and the A_2 cells demonstrated agglutination. The additional A_1 cells were negative.

The conclusion was that the patient was a group A_1 phenotype with anti-H.

ROULEAUX FORMATION

If erythrocytes are suspended in their own serum, rouleaux formation or aggregation of erythrocytes may simulate agglutination. A variety of conditions can produce rouleaux, including abnormal concentrations of serum proteins, elevated globulin levels in diseases such as multiple myeloma, Waldenstrom's macroglobulinemia, increased fibrinogen levels, the presence of plasma expanders such as dextran, and Hodgkin's lymphoma. In cord blood samples from newborn infants, the presence of Wharton's jelly can also cause rouleaux formation.

COLD AUTOANTIBODIES

There may be unexpected autoantibodies in the serum that reacts with antigens other than the A_1 or B cells used for reverse grouping. Anti-I is the most commonly encountered autoantibody in reverse group-

Table 4-22. Example 3 of a Typical Unexpected Antibody Reaction

Forward Grouping			Reverse Grouping			
Patient's erythrocytes + Reagent antisera			Patient's serum + Reagent erythrocytes			
Anti-A	Anti-B	Anti-A,B	A_1	B	O	Autocontrol
4+	4+	4+	2+	2+	2+	2+

The presence of a positive autocontrol (patient's serum + patient's erythrocytes) invalidates the initial testing results.

ADDITIONAL LABORATORY TESTING

A cold autoabsorption method was performed and the absorbed serum was tested against A_1, B, and group O cells. No agglutination was observed with the absorbed serum and these reagent cells. The conclusion was that the patient was a group AB phenotype with an auto anti-I.

ing. Anti-I usually agglutinates all erythrocytes from adult donors, including the patient's own and those used in reverse grouping. Except in fulminant cold hemagglutinin disease, the agglutination caused by anti-I is usually weaker than that caused by anti-A and anti-B. Cord cells that have less I antigen development are generally not agglutinated.

UNEXPECTED ISOAGGLUTININS

Unexpected isoagglutinins in the serum can react at room temperature with the corresponding antigen present on the reagent erythrocytes. Examples of this include A_2 and A_2B individuals who can produce "naturally occurring" anti-A_1 or A_1, and A_1B individuals who may produce "naturally occuring" anti-H. Anti-A_1 in serum from A_2 or A_2B persons may strongly agglutinate A_1 erythrocytes. Anti-H in serum from A_1 or A_1B persons rarely causes a problem in reverse grouping because A_1 and B cells used for serum grouping have relatively little H.

The serum of most cis-AB persons contains a weak anti-B, which leads to an ABO discrepancy in the reverse grouping. The anti-B formed reacts with all ordinary B erythrocytes, but not with cis-AB erythrocytes.

UNEXPECTED ALLOANTIBODIES

Unexpected alloantibodies other than ABO isoagglutinins in a person's serum may cause a discrepancy in the reverse grouping. Reverse grouping erythrocytes possess antigens in addition to the A, B, and I antigens previously discussed. It is possible that other unexpected antibodies present in the serum will react with reagent cells. In these cases, if the screening test for alloantibodies with group O erythrocytes (see Chapter 6) is negative, the reverse grouping with several other examples of A_1 and B cells should be repeated. If the antibody reacts with an antigen so uncommon that the group O cells do not possess it, randomly selected A_1 and B cells can also be expected to lack the antigen.

CHAPTER SUMMARY

Historical Aspects of the ABO System

Landsteiner identified two erythrocyte antigens, the A and B antigens, and established the first blood group system, proposing three groups, A, B, and O. Von Decastello and Sturli identified a fourth group, AB.

Genetic Inheritance

As early as 1908, Epstein and Ottenberg suggested that the ABO blood groups were inherited. In 1924 Bernstein postulated the existence of three allelic genes, A, B, and

O. In 1930 Thompson proposed a four-allele theory of inheritance, encompassing the four allelic genes A1, A2, B and O.

Expression of A and B genes in erythrocytes or body fluids results from the independently inherited Hh, Sese, and A and B genes. Under normal circumstances, if either the A or B gene is present on either chromosome, the gene can be phenotypically demonstrated on erythrocytes. Inheritance of the ABO genes follows Mendelian principles with the A and B genes codominant.

Development and Distribution of the ABO Groups

The A and B antigens are not fully developed in newborn infants but gain in strength shortly after birth. Although group O is the most common blood type, the distribution of groups A and B varies according to racial groups. For example, group B is much more common in Black and Oriental populations than in the White population.

Biochemical Activities Related to the Development of A, B, and H Antigens

Inheritance of the A and B genes usually results in their expression on erythrocytes, but the H, A, and B antigens are not direct products of the H, A and B genes respectively. Each gene codes for the production of a specific transferase enzyme that catalyzes the transfer of a monosaccharide molecule from a donor substrate to the precursor substance.

The H gene codes for the production of (alpha)-L-fucosyl transferase, which catalyzes the addition of L-fucose, the immunodominant structure of H antigen, to two slightly different precursor chains. Once the H gene-specified transferase has acted and L-fucose has been added to the chains, the A and B gene-specified products can then act to add a monosaccharide to these preformed H-bearing chains. If at least one H gene is not inherited, L-fucose is not transferred to the precursor substance and the A and B immunodominant sugars cannot be

added. This is the basis of explanation for the Bombay or O_h phenotype.

Specific transferase enzymes are the products of A or B genes. The A and B antigens result from the actions of the transferases that attach specific monosaccharides to the H substrate. The A gene produces an (alpha)-3-N-acetyl-D-galactosaminyl transferase that attaches N-acetyl-D-galactosamine to the acceptor molecule; the B gene produces an (alpha)-3-D-galactosyl transferase that attaches D-galactose to the acceptor molecule. A and B transferases convert the same acceptor molecule and compete with one another for the same substrate. Both A_1 and B cells have many immunodominant sugars added; therefore, a low level of detectable H antigen is present on A_1 and B erythrocytes.

Although there was considerable debate as to whether the terminal carbohydrates of H, A, and B on erythrocytes were carried on glycoproteins or glycolipids, it is currently believed that most are attached to glycoproteins, but some are attached to glycolipids. Two different precursor chain configurations, known as type 1 and type 2, are found in blood group active secretions, other body fluids, and various tissues. Most of the H, A, and B antigens of erythrocytes are synthesized by the erythrocytic precursors; some are acquired from the plasma. The H, A, and B as well as the Lewis determinants on type 1 chains that reach the erythrocytes by way of the plasma depend on the H, A, B, Lewis and secretor genes. The type 2 chains are controlled by the H, A, and B genes. Lymphocytes and platelets acquire H, A, and B antigens from the plasma by insertion of preformed glycosphingolipids into the membrane.

Secretors and Nonsecretors

Approximately 80% of persons in the United States secrete water-soluble H, H and A, or H and B antigens. Lewis system antigens can also be found in saliva. A second alcohol-soluble form of these antigens is present in all tissues of the body except the brain, and on erythrocytes. The manifestation of A, B, and H antigens in saliva or other body fluids is controlled by a secretor gene that is inherited independently of the A, B, and H genes. At least one Se gene is essential for the expression of ABH antigens in secretions. Individuals who are homozygous for se do not secrete H, A, or B antigens, regardless of the presence of H, A and B genes. At least one H gene is necessary for H, A, or B antigens to be manufactured. Alcohol-soluble antigens are not influenced by the secretor gene.

The Se gene does not affect the formation of A, B, or H antigens on erythrocytes, nor does it control the presence of A, B, or H transferases in hematopoietic tissue. In contrast, the A or B transferase enzymes, unlike A or B antigens, are found in the secretions of A_1 or B persons regardless of secretor status.

The detection of small amounts of A or B antigens in the saliva of a secretor can be a useful confirmatory test in establishing a phenotype that involves a subgroup of A or B.

Group A

Group A antigens can be differentiated into two principal subgroups, A_1 and A_2. Approximately 78% of type A individuals are A_1, with most of the others belonging to the A_2 subgroup. Some biochemical studies appear to have produced evidence that there are different patterns of N-acetyl-D-galactosamine attachment on A_1 and A_2 erythrocytes, suggesting that the acceptor sites for the A_1 and A_2 gene-specified transferases might be different.

The serologic distinction between A_1 and A_2 is based on the reactions of erythrocytes with various antisera. Reagent anti-A serum from human sources rarely differentiates A_1 and A_2 subtypes, but Anti-A,B serum of human origin can detect common subgroups of A and B. IgM antibodies produced by individual murine hybridomas can also detect weak subgroups of A. A common way of differentiating between A_1 and A_2 subgroups is by use of the lectin anti-A_1, which is made from *Dolichos biflorus* seeds.

The distribution and characteristics of the uncommon subgroups of the A antigen, from the strongest A_3 to the weakest A_{end},

comprise a continual curve. Classification of these subgroups of A is based on the reactivity of erythrocytes with anti-A, anti-A,B, anti-H, and anti-A_1, the presence or absence of anti-A_1 in the serum; and the secretion of A and H substance by secretors. Failure to detect a weak A antigen usually results in the erythrocytes being mistyped as group O. A variety of subgroups of A have been identified but are rare. Many of these subgroups are believed to result from the inheritance of a specific allele; others are considered to result from genetic interaction.

Group B

Subgroups or variants of group B are less common than subgroups of A. The incidence of B antigen subgroups is more frequent in certain racial groups. Subgroups of B are usually recognized by variations in the strength of the reaction using human anti-B and anti-A,B reagent antisera. It has been suggested that qualitative as well as quantitative differences exist in the B antigen of B_3 erythrocytes.

Abnormalities Encountered in the Expression of ABH Antigens on Erythrocytes

The expression of ABH antigens on erythrocytes may be altered by various factors. In some AB individuals, the deficit of A antigen is believed to be caused by the presence of a superactive B transferase that competes with normal A^1 or A^2 transferase. In the rare Bombay O_h phenotype, individuals can carry A or B genes, but these genes do not express themselves as A or B antigens on the erythrocytes because of the lack of H gene and consequent lack of H-bearing structures on the erythrocytic membrane.

A or B antigens may rarely develop in the absence of H. Different groups of investigators claim to have found hidden H (and/or A and B) antigens on O_h erythrocytes with traces of A and B antigens that are detectable in direct tests. The name A_h was applied to this phenotype as parallel to O_h. Families have been identified who are believed to be genetically either A_1 or A_2 but do not express the A_1 and A_2 phenotype. Persons from these families have been classified as Am phenotype, which results from a homozygous state of a rare, recessive, modifying gene, y. The presence of a dominant suppressor of A and B represents another example of an abnormality encountered in the expression of ABH antigens on erythrocytes. A rare anomaly of inheritance that represents crossing over at the ABO locus is AB cis. The term AB cis gene is used to describe the condition of expressing gene products normally expected as products of A and B genes.

Examples of acquired A antigen have been reported in persons of group O or B in association with severe infections caused by *Proteus mirabilis.* Tn-activated erythrocytes can also demonstrate the presence of the acquired A antigen. Acquired B-like antigen has been observed in association with conditions such as carcinoma of the colon or rectum, intestinal obstruction, massive infection of the lower gastrointestinal tract, and septicemia caused by *Proteus vulgaris.* Erythrocytes may have inherited or acquired surface abnormalities that produce polyagglutination. The three types of polyagglutination are T activation, Tn activation, and Cad polyagglutinability.

Weakening of the A antigen has been noted in leukemia. The B and H antigens can also be depressed but, in some cases, as the level of A or B antigen has decreased, the level of H antigen detectable on erythrocytes has been seen to increase. Errors of interpretation can occur in cases of subgroups of A antigen in association with the B antigen in the AB phenotype. The weakened form of A in A_2B blood is caused by transferase activity.

Antibodies of the ABO Blood Group System

Landsteiner observed that most individuals possess antibodies directed against the ABH antigens that are absent from their own cells. Although these antibodies were named "naturally occurring," scientific evidence supports the fact that anti-A and anti-B are stimulated by agents such as bacteria,

pollen, or other substances present in the internal or external environment that have molecular configurations similar to the A and B antigens. The immune response to noncellular antigenic stimulation results in the production of the complementary IgM antibodies (anti-A and/or anti-B) in immunologically competent individuals, and a predictable relationship between antigens and antibodies in the ABO system permits the use of both serum and cell tests in ABO grouping.

The antibodies of the ABO blood group system are characterized by agglutination of saline-suspended erythrocytes, reactivity at room temperature, and production of hemolysis in vivo and in vitro. Antibodies to the A and B antigens are generally divided into two classes: IgM, if environmentally stimulated, and IgG, if stimulated by foreign erythrocytes in situations such as post-transfusion of ABO-incompatible erythrocytes or plasma-containing blood group substances or pregnancy with an ABO-incompatible fetus. Serum from type O persons contains the antibody anti-A,B, which reacts more strongly than anti-A or anti-B with erythrocytes of some A and B subgroups.

The anti-A in group O and group B sera has been observed to contain separable anti-A and anti-A_1. The apparent anti-A_1 remaining in serum after absorption with A_2 erythrocytes is believed to be a weakened form of anti-A.

There are two kinds of human anti-H. One is a cold-reacting type antibody in the serum of persons with relatively little H on their erythrocytes, usually group A_1 or AB. The other type is produced by individuals with the rare O_h (Bombay) phenotype whose erythrocytes have no H antigen.

Technical errors and various clinical conditions or diseases can contribute to a discrepancy between erythrocyte and serum results in ABO grouping. When the expected forward and reverse results do not produce the complementary matching of ABO antigens and antibodies, the possibility of technical error must first be excluded. If technical error is excluded, the discrepancy may be due to weak or missing antigen reactions, unexpected antigen reactions, weak or missing antibody reactions, or un-expected antibody reactions.

Examples of Discrepancies in ABO Forward and Reverse Grouping

Examples of conditions contributing to missing or weak antigen expression on erythrocytes include subgroups of A or B antigens, disease states, and excess blood group-specific soluble substances. Unexpected antigen reactions can be due to acquired A or B antigen, altered antigens, erythrocytes coated with antibody, additives to antisera, mixtures of blood, and low-incidence antigen and antibody reactions.

Weak or missing antibody reactions can be caused by depressed or absent antibody production. Conditions producing missing antibody reactions include age, hypogammaglobulinemia, agammaglobulinemia, and chimerism.

Unexpected antibody reactions can be caused by rouleaux formation, cold auto-antibodies, unexpected ABH isoagglutinins, and unexpected alloantibodies.

REVIEW QUESTIONS

1. The discoverer of the ABO system was:
   A. Weiner
   B. Landsteiner
   C. von Decastello
   D. Sturli
   E. Epstein

2–5. Match the following blood types with the respective erythrocytic antigens:

Blood Type	Antigen(s)
2. A	A. Both A and B antigens
3. B	B. A antigen
4. AB	C. Neither A nor B antigens
5. O	D. B antigen

6–9. Match the following blood types with their complementary antibodies:

Blood Type	Antibody/Antibodies
6. A	A. anti-A
7. B	B. anti-B
8. AB	C. Both anti-A and anti-B
9. O	

Blood Type	Antibody/Antibodies
	D. Neither anti-A nor anti-B

10–12. Match the given phenotypes with their respective genotypes:

Phenotype	Genotype
10. A_1	A. A_2/A_2
11. A_2	B. A_1/A_2
12. O	C. A_1/O
	D. O/O

13. From the following ABO mating, what are the probabilities of the ABO phenotypes of potential offspring? Mother: Group O; Father: Group B (heterozygous)
   A. 50% BO, 50% OO
   B. 100% BO
   C. 50% B, 50% O
   D. 50% BO, 50% AO
   E. 50% B, 50% O

14. The greatest number of antigen sites on erythrocytic membranes is found in ____ phenotype.
   A. Cord blood A_1
   B. Cord blood B
   C. Adult A_1
   D. Adult A_2
   E. Adult B

15. The most frequent phenotype in all races is type:
   A. A
   B. B
   C. O
   D. A_1B
   E. A_2B

16. The frequency of phenotype B is more than 15% in:
   A. Whites
   B. Blacks
   C. Orientals
   D. Both A and B
   E. Both B and C

17–20. Match the genes with their specific transferase.

Genes	Enzymes
17. H	A. (α)-L-fucosyltransferase
18. A	B. (α)-N-acetylgalactosaminyltransferase
19. B	C. (α)-Galactosyltransferase

20. O   **D.** None

21–23. Referring to the figure below, match the immunodominant monosaccharide residual with the appropriate antigen.

Immunodominant monosaccharides

Antigen	Immunodominant monosaccharide
21. H	**A.** N-acetyl-D-galactosamine
22. A	**B.** D-galactose
23. B	**C.** L-fucose

24. Most of the H, A, and B antigens that are synthesized on the erythrocytic membrane are attached to:

A. Glycosphingolipids
B. Polyglycosyberamides
C. Glycoconjugates
D. Glycoproteins
E. Both B and C

25. Referring to the figure on p. 123, identify the type 1 chain present in blood group active substances.

26. A, B, and H antigens are acquired by:
A. Synthesis by erythrocytic precursors
B. Synthesis during lymphocytic development
C. Insertion into the erythrocytic membrane from the plasma

Figure for Questions 21-23:

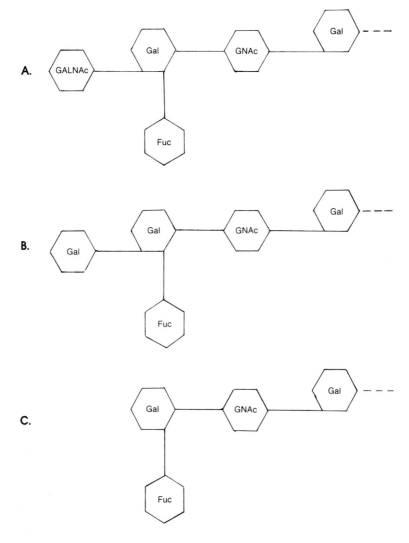

Figure for Question 25:

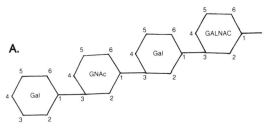

A.

Type 1 Chain beta (1-3) Linkage

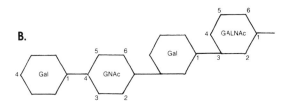

B.

Type 2 Chain beta (1-4) Linkage

    D. Insertion into the lymphocytic membrane from the plasma
    E. Both A and C

27. Approximately ____% of persons in the United States are secretors of water soluble ABH substances.
    A. 10%
    B. 20%
    C. 50%
    D. 80%
    E. 100%

28. Which of the following genotypes is characteristic of a nonsecretor?
    A. SeSe
    B. Sese
    C. sese
    D. Both A and B
    E. Both B and C

29–32. Identify the product(s) found in the saliva of the following:
    A. A, H
    B. B, H
    C. A, B, H
    D. H only
    E. No A, B, or H

ABO Group	Secretor Status	Secretion
O	SeSe or Sese	No. 29
A_1	sese	No. 30
AB	SeSe or Sese	No. 31
O_h	SeSe	No. 32

33. The A_1 phenotype comprises approximately ____% of all A phenotypes.
    A. 15%
    B. 35%
    C. 56%
    D. 78%
    E. 98%

34. Adsorbed anti-A_1 will agglutinate ____ erythrocytes.
    A. A_1
    B. A_2
    C. Weak subgroups of A
    D. Both A and B
    E. All of the above

35. The frequency of anti-A_1 is highest in type:
    A. A_1
    B. A_2
    C. B
    D. A_1B
    E. A_2B

36. With a few exceptions, secretors of the infrequent subgroups of A have _____ in their saliva.
    A. Only H
    B. A and H
    C. A, B and H
    D. A, B, H, and Se
    E. None of the A, B, or H antigens

37. A mixed-field agglutination pattern is characteristic of type:
    A. B
    B. B_3
    C. B_m
    D. B_x
    E. Both B and B_3

38. The highest frequency of the superactive B gene occurs in the _____ population.
    A. Oriental
    B. Oriental in Taiwan
    C. Black
    D. Caucasian
    E. Both A and C

39. Individuals with the Bombay phenotype have the following genotype:
    A. HH
    B. Hh
    C. hh
    D. Either HH or Hh
    E. Either Hh or hh

40. The A_m phenotype is believed to result from:
    A. Absence of an H gene
    B. Absence of a Y gene

C. Inheritance of the hh genotype
D. Inheritance of the yy genotype
E. Both B and D

41. The AB cis genotype is:
A. AB
B. $A_x B$
C. $A_3 B$
D. ABO
E. $A_x BB$

42–46. Match the following conditions with answer **A** or answer **B**.
A. Acquired A antigen
B. Acquired B antigen

42. Demonstrated by Tn-activated erythrocytes

43. Can be associated with *Proteus vulgaris*

44. Can be associated with *Proteus mirabilis*

45. Usually associated with the A_1 phenotype

46. Represents deacetylation of A antigen

47–50. Match the following characteristics with the respective altered antigen condition. An answer may be used more than once.
A. T activation
B. Tn activation
C. Both T and Tn activation

47. Is a permanent alteration

48. Fails to react with cord serum

49. Demonstrates a mixed-field agglutination with all normal sera

50. Produced by bacteria or viruses

51. The Cad receptor is:
A. Not destroyed by enzyme treatment
B. Possibly enhanced by enzyme treatment
C. Not agglutinated by *Dolichos biflorus*
D. Not agglutinated by *Salvia horminum*
E. Both A and B

52. Weakening of the A antigen may be observed in:
A. Leukemia
B. Tn-activated erythrocytes
C. Cad polyagglutinability
D. Bacterial infections
E. Parasitic infections

53–56. Match the following characteristics:
53. "Naturally occurring" antibodies
54. Infants up to 6 months of age
55. IgG
56. Group O persons
A. Low antibody titer

B. Anti-A titer higher than anti-B titer
C. Dust, pollen, bacteria
D. Stimulated by foreign erythrocytes

57–61. Select either answer **A** (true) or **B** (false) for whether the following are characteristics of Anti-A *and* anti-B.

57. Agglutinate in saline-suspended erythrocytes

58. Require 37° C to agglutinate

59. Do not produce in vivo or in vitro hemolysis

60. Are capable of binding complement

61. Can be inactivated by treatment with 2-mercaptoethanol (2-ME)

62. The phenotype with the greatest amount of H antigen on the erythrocytic membrane is:
A. O
B. A_2
C. $A_2 B$
D. B
E. A_1

63–66. Match the following conditions with the reaction they can produce:

63. Additives to antisera — A. Missing or weak antigen

64. Hypogammaglobulinema — B. Unexpected antigen

65. Rouleaux formation — C. Missing or weak antibody

66. Subgroups of A — D. Unexpected antibody

67. Tn activation — A. Missing or weak antigen

68. Related to age — B. Unexpected antigen

69. Excess blood group specific soluble substances — C. Missing or weak antibody

70. Cold autoantibodies — D. Unexpected antibody

ANSWERS

1.	B	10.	B
2.	B	11.	A
3.	D	12.	D
4.	A	13.	C
5.	C	14.	C
6.	B	15.	C
7.	A	16.	E
8.	D	17.	A
9.	C	18.	B

19. C	45. B
20. D	46. B
21. C	47. B
22. A	48. C
23. B	49. C
24. D	50. A
25. A	51. E
26. E	52. A
27. D	53. C
28. C	54. A
29. D	55. D
30. E	56. B
31. C	57. A
32. E	58. B
33. D	59. B
34. A	60. A
35. E	61. A
36. A	62. A
37. B	63. B
38. C	64. C
39. C	65. D
40. E	66. A
41. D	67. B
42. A	68. C
43. B	69. A
44. A	70. D

BIBLIOGRAPHY

Drozda, E.A., Jr., and Dean, J.D.: Another example of the rare A_y phenotype. Transfusion, 25(3):280-281, 1985.

Economidous, J., Hughes-Jones, N.C., and Gardner, B.: Quantitative measurements concerning A and B antigen sites. Vox Sang., 12:321, 1967.

Eversole, M.B., Nonemaker, K., Zurek, S., and Simon, T.: Uneventful administration of plasma products in a recipient with T-activated red cells. Transfusion, 26(2):182-185, 1986.

Frederick, J., Hunter, J., Greenwell, P., et al.: The A^1B genotypes expressed A^2B on the red cells of individuals with strong B gene-specific transferases. Transfusion, 25(1):30-33, 1985.

Gergal, A., Maslet, C., and Salmon, C.: Immunological aspects of the acquired B antigen. Vox Sanguin. 28:398-403, 1975.

Hall, S., Olekna, D., and Davies, D.: Production of unique monoclonal ABO blood grouping antisera. Transfusion, 25(5):448, 1985.

Lin-Chu, M., Broadberry, R.E., and Chiou, P.W.: The B_3 phenotype in Chinese. Transfusion, 26(5):428-430, 1986.

Mallory, D.M.: Problems in the hemagglutination reactions. Part 1: False positive reactions due to drugs, dyes, and interfering substances. In A Seminar on Polymorphisms in Human Blood. Washington, D.C., American Association of Blood Banks, 1975. pp. 129-141.

Mollison, P.L.: Blood Transfusion in Clinical Medicine. 7th Ed. Oxford, Blackwell Scientific Publications, 1983.

Vengelen-Tyler, V., and Gonzalez, B.: Reticulocyte rich RBCs will give weak reactions with many blood typing antisera. Transfusion, 25(5):476, 1985.

Wittels, E.G., and Lichtman, H.C.: Blood group incidence and Escherichia coli bacterial sepsis. Transfusion, 26(6):533-535, 1986.

The Rh, Lewis, and Other Blood Group Systems

At the conclusion of this chapter, the reader will be able to:

- Describe the history of the development of the Rh system.
- List the most common Rh antigens.
- Compare the Rh genotypes in Wiener and Fischer-Race nomenclature.
- State the most common Rh haplotype in Whites and Blacks.
- Explain the chromosomal arrangement of the Rh antigens.
- Define the terms "cis" and "trans."
- Explain variants of the D antigen, including clinical detection and significance.
- State the common variants of C, E, and c antigens.
- Define the term "compound antigen."
- Explain the detection and clinical significance of VS and G antigens.
- Discuss missing Rh antigens, including Rh null.
- State the frequency of the L-W antigen.
- Explain the characteristics of Rh antibodies.
- Describe the mode of inheritance of Lewis and secretor genes.
- Compare the phenotypes and genotypes in the Lewis blood group system.
- Describe the relationship of H, A, and B genes and their expression in secretions and on erythrocytes.
- Diagram the mode of inheritance of the Lewis phenotypes.
- Explain the clinical significance of the Lewis system.

- State the most common Lutheran phenotype or phenotypes.
- Describe the mode of inheritance within the M, N, S, and P blood group systems.
- List the incidence of the most frequent genes within the M, N, S, and P systems.
- Describe the significance of the M, N, S, and P systems.
- Explain the physical and chemical properties of the M, N, S, and P blood group systems.
- Explain the inheritance and development of the Ii blood group system.
- Describe the techniques used in working with "non-specific antibodies."
- Cite the major antigens of the Kell blood system.
- List the incidence of Kell antigens.
- Describe the characteristics of Kell antibodies.
- Discuss the clinical significance of the Kell system.
- Explain the mode of reaction of the Duffy and Kidd systems.
- Describe the clinical significance of Duffy and Kidd antigens and antibodies.
- Cite the incidence of Duffy and Kidd antigens.
- Briefly explain the characteristics of other blood group system antigens and antibodies.
- Name the HLA antigen that is not uncommonly detected on erythrocytes.
- List at least four antigens that are associated with HTLA antibodies.

Chapter Outline

Many of the blood group systems in humans are highly complex. The purpose of this chapter is to present and discuss these systems at the level of general use. More in-depth discussions and theoretical considerations of blood group systems are presented in books such as *Blood Groups in Man* by R.R. Race and R. Sanger (Blackwell Scientific Publications) and *Blood Transfusion in Clinical Medicine* by P.L. Mollison (Blackwell Scientific Publications).

THE Rh SYSTEM

The Rh system was identified in 1940 by Landsteiner and Wiener. This discovery followed the detection of an antibody by Levine and Stetson in 1939 in the mother of a stillborn infant who had been transfused with her husband's blood during pregnancy. Originally, Landsteiner and Wiener found that human erythrocytes were agglutinated by an antibody, apparently common to all rhesus monkeys and 85% of humans. This factor was named the Rh factor. Later the antigens detected by the rhesus antibody and by the human antibody were established as dissimilar, but the system had already been named. This contribution to medical science was the most significant event in blood group systems research since the discovery of the ABO system 40 years before.

The Rh-hr blood group system is probably the most complex of all erythrocyte blood group systems, with more than 40 different Rh antigens. The descriptive terms Rh positive and Rh negative refer *only* to the presence or absence of the red cell antigen D. The early name given to the D antigen, Rh_o, is less frequently used.

Four additional genes (*C, E, c,* and *e*) are recognized as belonging to the Rh system. The major allelic pairs are *C/c* and *E/e*. Many variations or combinations of the five principal genes and their products (antigens) have been recognized. These antigens and their corresponding antibodies characterize the Rh blood group system and account for the majority of Rh antibodies encountered in blood banking.

Genetic Basis of the Rh System

Five major antigens have been observed in the Rh system: D, C, c, E, and e. C and c, as well as E and e, are antithetical but the antithetical antigen for D has never been demonstrated. The term *antithetical* refers to two antigens controlled by a pair of allelic genes. For convenience, the allelic gene to D is expressed as d.

The Rh genes reside on chromosome 1 with the *D* gene acting as an autosomal dominant. The Fisher-Race theory states that there are three closely-linked loci, inherited as a unit, that rarely exhibit crossing over. Each of these loci contains a primary set of codominant allelic genes: *D* and the theoretic *d, C* and *c,* or *E* and *e* (Fig. 5-1). The gene complex of an individual or pop-

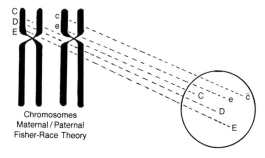 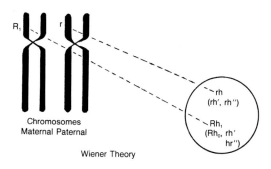

Figure 5-1. Theories of Rh inheritance.

ulation may be referred to as the *haplotype,* which produces an antigen complex with multiple specificities.

An alternate proposal of Rh gene inheritance by Wiener remains controversial. He proposed that multiple alleles were positioned at a single complex locus.

Nomenclature of the Rh System

The CDE and Rh-hr systems of nomenclature in the Rh system are equivalent (Table 5-1). The CDE nomenclature of Fisher and Race is used almost exclusively, but it is sometimes necessary to use a combination of CDE and Rh-Hr terminology. In the CDE terminology of Fisher and Race, the same letter is used for both gene and gene product, but the symbols for genes are printed in italics. Traditionally, the Rh genes (and phenotypes) are expressed in the sequence *CDE*. Although the subloci sequencing is almost certainly *DCE*, both

expressions of the *CDE* arrangements are acceptable.

The Rh-Hr terminology is based on Wiener's concept that the immediate gene product is a single entity, *an agglutinogen,* with each agglutinogen characterized by numerous individual serologic specificities called *factors.* Each factor is recognized by its own specific antibody. What Wiener called agglutinogens are now called haplotypes and what he called factors are now called antigens. In the Wiener terminology, R is used for haplotypes that include D (Rh_o) among their products and r is used for haplotypes that do not include D (Rh_o). The various superscript symbols R^1, R^2, R^o, R^z, r', r'', r and r^y denote different alleles. The shorthand phenotypic notations use the single letters R and r in roman type, with subscripts or occasionally superscripts, to indicate antigenic combinations. For example, R_1 symbolizes the presence of C, D, and e, whereas R_2 indicates the presence of c, D, and E. The combinations of the major Rh genes using both the Fisher-Race and Wiener systems, their shorthand notations, and their respective frequencies are presented in Table 5-2. In most populations, the *Rh* genes R^1 (*CDe*), R^2 (*cDE*) and r (*cde*) are common, while r' (*Cde*), R'' (*cdE*), r^y (*CdE*), and R^z (*CDE*) are rare. R^o is considerably more common in Blacks than in Whites.

Rosenfield proposed a system of nomenclature based only on serologic (agglutination) reactions. Antigens are numbered in order of their discovery or recognition of the antigen as belonging to the Rh system. This system designates the antigen with a

Table 5-1. Examples of Equivalent Nomenclature

Fisher-Race	Wiener	Rosenfield
CDE	Rh-Hr	
D	Rh_o	Rh1
C	rh'	Rh2
E	rh''	Rh3
c	hr'	Rh4
e	hr''	Rh5
f	hr	Rh6
C^w	rh^{w1}	Rh8
G	rh^G	Rh12

Table 5-2. Rh Nomenclature

Fisher-Race Terms	Genes Rh-Hr Terms	Shorthand Symbols	Freq. (U.S.) White	Black	Gene Products Shorthand Symbols	Antigens Expressed
CDe	Rh^1	R^1	0.42	0.17	R_1	C, D and e
cDE	Rh^2	R^2	0.14	0.11	R_2	c, D and E
cDe	Rh°	R°	0.04	0.44	R_o	c, D and e
CDE	Rh^z	R^z	rare	rare	R_z	C, D and E
cde	rh	r	0.37	0.26	r	c and e
Cde	rh'	r'	0.02	0.02	r'	C and e
cdE	rh''	r''	< 0.01	rare	r''	c and E
CdE	rh^y	r^y	rare	rare	r^y	C and E

numeric citation preceded by the prefix Rh, for example, Rh1.

Rh Phenotypes

In the clinical laboratory, only five reagent antisera are commonly available. Routine testing involves only the use of anti-D, although other antisera are used to resolve antibody problems or conduct family studies. The agglutination reactions of an individual's erythrocytes with specific Rh antisera produce a variety of patterns. These reactions represent the Rh phenotype (Table 5-3).

Identification of antigens does not always allow the haplotype to be deduced with certainty. No reliable serologic method exists to distinguish between red cells with D antigen resulting from one gene and those with D antigen as the product of two genes.

A person whose erythrocytes are D positive can be assigned a genotype only by inference from the frequencies with which the individual Rh gene complexes occur in the population. The racial origin of the person in question should influence deductions regarding the genotype because the frequencies of the Rh genes differ based on ethnic origin. The frequencies of the common Rh phenotypes estimated from haplotype frequencies are presented in Table 5-4. The patient's agglutination reactions allow estimations of the probabilities of an individual Rh genotype (Table 5-5).

Biochemical Composition of Rh Antigens

Multiple research studies agree that the Rh antigens are present on a protein structure and are probably all on the same poly-

Table 5-3. Rh Phenotypes Based on Reactions of Antisera with Erythrocytes

Anti-D	Anti-C	Antisera Anti-E	anti-c	anti-e	Phenotypes Wiener	Fisher-Race
+	+	0	+	+	Rh_1rh	CcDe
+	+	0	0	+	Rh_1	CDe
+	+	+	+	+	Rh_1Rh_2	CcDEe
+	0	0	+	+	Rh_o	cDe
+	0	+	+	+	Rh_2rh	cDEe
+	0	+	+	0	Rh_2	cDE
+	+	+	0	+	Rh_zRh_1	CDEe
+	+	+	+	0	Rh_zRh_2	CcDE
+	+	+	0	0	Rh_z	CDE
0	0	0	+	+	rh	ce
0	+	0	+	+	rh'rh	Cce
0	0	+	+	+	rh''rh	cEe
0	+	+	+	+	rh'rh''	CcEe

Table 5-4. Selected Rh Genotypes

Genes	Present	Probable	Haplotype
Rh_1rh	CcDee	R^1R^o	CDe/cDe
		R^1r	CDe/cde
Rh_o	ccDee	R^oR^o	cDe/cDe
		R^or	cDe/cde
Rh_2rh	ccDEe	R^2R^o	cDE/cDe
		R^2r	cDE/cde
Rh_1Rh_1	CCDee	R^1R^1	CDe/CDe
		R^1r'	CDe/Cde
Rh_2Rh_2	ccDEE	R^2R^2	DcE/DcE
		R^2r''	cDE/cdE
Rh_2Rh_1	ccDEE	R^1R^z	cDE/cDE
Rh_zRh_2	CcDEE	R^zR^2	cDE/CDE
Rh_zrh	CcDEe	R^1R^2	CDe/cDE
		R^1r''	CDe/cdE
		R^2r'	cDE/Cde
rh	ccdee	rr	cde/cce
rh'rh	Ccdee	rr'	cde/Cde
rh''rh	ccdEe	rr''	dce/dcE

r make separate polypeptides for the same cell membrane. The Rh antigens exhibit numerous serologic complexities that undoubtedly represent an extremely complicated polypeptide.

Expression of CDE Antigens

The production or nonproduction of D, as well as the production of either C or c and E or e antigens, is genetically determined. Rh antigen sites are believed to be randomly distributed on the red cell membrane. Based on computer analysis, the distance between sites appears to be orderly, but the number of Rh antigen sites varies with genotype (Table 5-6). The number of antigen sites can potentially influence the strength of antigenic expression. The number of D antigen sites varies from 10,000 to 33,500 per erythrocyte.

ALTERATION OF GENETIC EXPRESSION

The expression of an inherited gene can be affected by the interaction between genes. When an Rh gene on one chromosome affects the action of another Rh gene on the same chromosome (in terms of increased or decreased antigen production), it is referred to as a *cis* effect. When an Rh gene on one of the chromosomes of a homologous pair affects the action of an Rh

peptide chain. It appears probable that membrane lipids are restricted to a supporting role at the phenotypic level. Simple antigens such as D, C, and E presumably represent certain amino acid sequences; however, antigens like G represent some of the amino acids of D and some others. Antigens such as rh are thought to represent repressed amino acids of C and e that are located adjacent in the R^1 and r' specified folded polypeptide, but apart when R^2 and

Table 5-5. Estimation of Probabilities in Rh Genotyping

Anti-D	Anti-C	Antisera Anti-E	Anti-c	Anti-e	Possibilities 1st Choice	2nd Choice
+	+	0	+	+	CDe/cde (R^1r)	CDe/cDe (R^1R^o)
+	+	0	0	+	CDe/CDe (R^1R^1)	CDe/Cde (R^1r')
+	+	+	+	+	CDe/cDE (R^1R^2)	CDe/cdE (R^1r'')
						CDE/cde (R^zr)
						cDE/cDe (R^2R^o)
+	0	0	+	+	cDe/cde (R^or)	cDe/cDe (R^oR^o)
+	0	+	+	+	cDE/cde (R^2r)	cDE/cDe (R^2R^o)
+	0	+	+	0	cDE/cDE (R^2R^2)	cDE/cdE (R^2r'')
+	+	+	0	+		
+	+	+	+	0		
+	+	+	0	0		
0	0	0	+	+	cde/cde (rr)	—
0	+	0	+	+		
0	0	+	+	+		
0	+	+	+	+		

Table 5-6. Representative Examples of the Number of Antigen Sites on Erythrocytes*

Phenotype	D	C	E	c	e
CDe / CDe	14,500 to 19,500	46,000 to 56,500	0	0	18,000 to 24,500
CDe / cde	10,000 to 15,000	21,500 to 40,000	0	37,000 to 53,000	18,000 to 24,500
cDE / cDE	16,000 to 33,500	0	25,500	70,000 to 85,000	0
cde / cde	0	0	0	70,000 to 85,000	18,000 to 24,500

* Modified from Issitt, P.D.: Applied Blood Group. Serology, 3rd ed. Miami, FL, Montgomery Scientific, 1985.

gene on the other homolog, it is called a *trans* effect.

The cis effect produces a weaker expression of the E antigen in the genotype cDE/cde than in cdE/cde. The most dramatic Rh trans position effect known occurs when C is trans to D (CDe/Cde), which weakens the D antigen.

The D^u Phenotype. D^u is not considered to be an antigen separate from D. It is now recognized that the D^u phenotype can arise in 3 different ways:

1. Suppression of D antigen expression because of genetic interaction.
2. Inheritance of a gene that codes for less D antigen, weak D.
3. Absence of a portion of portions of the total material that comprises the D antigen, the D mosaic.

Gene Suppression. One form of the D^u phenotype results from an alteration in genetic expression, gene suppression. It occurs when a person has a C gene on one chromosome that affects the expression of the D gene on the other. The effect of this trans position, whereby a gene on one chromosome affects the expression of a gene on the paired autosome, was discussed in the preceding section.

Weak D. Some Rh genes appear to code for a weakly reactive D antigen. This form of D^u is the least frequent type and simply codes for the production of less D antigen. Weak D antigen expression exhibits a pattern of Mendelian dominance. It is fairly common in Blacks. Transmission of a weak form of D is considerably less common in

Whites. When it does occur, however, it is more often the product of a deviant R^1 (CDe) or R^2 (cDE) gene. A genetically determined weak D antigen, sometimes referred to as low-grade D^u, exhibits negative or very weak reactions in direct agglutination tests with most anti-D sera but is readily detectable with anti-human globulin (AHG).

The D Mosaic. The concept of the D mosaic was advanced to explain the fact that some people with D positive erythrocytes produced anti-D that was nonreactive with their own cells. Wiener originally proposed that the D antigen on normal D positive erythrocytes included all of the components of the mosaic: A, B, C, D. If one or more components are missing from D positive cells, some demonstrate a positive reaction with anti-D sera and others may react weakly with anti-D and be classified as D^u. Phenotypically, erythrocytes of the D mosaic type are similar to low-grade D^u and often indistinguishable. The distinction, however, is qualitative. This true variant of D is sometimes called D mosaic to distinguish it from other D^u phenotypes.

Another antigen, Go^a, is part of the Rh system of antigens and is found on erythrocytes that lack part of the D mosaic. This antigen was originally discovered in 1955 and named D^{cor}. When anti-Go^a was described in 1967, it was not immediately recognized that the D^{cor} and Go^a antigens were the same and the Go^a terminology persisted. The Go^a antigen, which probably represents a single point mutation, is found in 1.9 to 2.8% of American Blacks. In instances of anti-Go^a formation, the antibody may cause severe hemolytic disease of the newborn.

Rh$_o$ (D)

Rh positive blood very rarely lacks any of the mosaic components. A different system of classifying D positive persons who produce anti-D, however, was devised in 1962. The six categories of antibody formers are referred to as I, II, III, IV, V, and VI based on the reactions of erythrocytes with anti-D from these individuals, as well as the specificity of the anti-D produced. The serologic characteristics of the original classification of the categories and the frequency of occurrence are presented in Table 5-7. Heterogeneity exists within some categories and subdivisions exist within categories III, IV, and V.

Representative properties of each of the six categories are as follows:

I. The anti-D produced by persons in this category is always very weak. Erythrocytes from individuals in this category react with all anti-D sera, except their own.

II. Rare cases have been reported in this category.

III. The serum used to describe this category is the original anti-Rh^D. Individuals in this category are classified as Rh^d_o; most are Black; many are cDe, VS+, V−.

IV. Some examples of anti-D sera show Go(a+) category IV persons to have elevated D. Black category IV members are Go(a+); White category IV members are Go(a−).

V. The original case in this category formed anti-RH^c. The erythrocytes of all members react with anti-D^w. The

D^w gene segregates with the unusual D gene. This category has both Black and White members.

VI. Only a very small proportion of anti-D antisera reacts with the erythrocytes of individuals belonging to category VI. These red cells are often called Rh^B (or D^B); however, the classification is a misnomer because Rh^B has been shown to be a normal component of the D antigen. All of the many members of this category are White.

Rh Deletion Phenotypes

There are some rare *Rh* genes that behave as if portions of the genetic material have been deleted or rendered nonfunctional. The first recognized case was the D-deletion gene (D--). Since the first example, many others have been reported. Presumably the multitude of Rh genes arose from mutation. In some cases, it is assumed that some mutations arose as new mutations of previous mutants. It is also commonly believed that even the most bizarre-acting Rh genes have a close relative, or a series of predecessors, among the more common Rh genes.

The D Deletion Gene (D--). D-- genes do not code for the production of some common Rh antigens such as the Cc or Ee series, but they do code for the production of D and G antigens. Homozygous individuals immunized to antigen-positive erythrocytes by means of transfusion or pregnancy can and do form anti-Hr and anti-Hr$_o$, that are probably group names for antibodies of

Table 5-7. Classification of D+ Red Cells of Individuals who Produce Anti-D*

Red Blood Cell Category	Reactions of Anti-D Produced by Individuals with Red Cells of the Following Categories:					Percent of Anti-D Produced by D Negative Individuals of Each Category
	II	III	IV	V	VI	
I	+	+	+	+	+	100
II	0	+	+	+	+	100
III	+	0	+	+	+	100
IV	+	(+)	0	+	+	96
V	+	0	+	0	(+)	74
VI	0	0	+	0	0	35

* From Issitt, P.D.: Applied Blood Group Serology, 3rd ed. Miami, FL, Montgomery Scientific, 1985.

similar but not identical specificity. The rare nondeleted Rh genes are most often found in Blacks and code for the production of Hr with Hr. Because of this, rare individuals with the genes can and do form anti-Hr without anti-Hr. Most often, the -D-phenotype is identified as the result of alloantibody investigations. Evans, a low-frequency antigen, is also present on the erythrocytes of individuals who inherit genes somewhat similar to D--.

Other Gene Deletions. Rare genes exist that code for Rh polypeptides lacking activity at the E/e site, or at the sites of both C/c and E/e. In some cases, only D (or D and C/c) are detectable. In addition to -D-, examples of this situation are seen in the haplotypes C^wD-, $cD-$, and .D. These haplotypes are extremely uncommon. Recognition of erythrocytes that lack Rh antigens may be detected during routine testing because the D antigen may show exceptionally strong D reactivity.

Rh Null Syndrome and Rh Mod. When no Rh antigens are expressed on the erythrocyte membrane, the term Rh null is used to describe this phenotype. If a less complete type of suppressed Rh gene expression is observed, the term Rh mod is used. In both of these situations, erythrocytes lacking Rh antigens have membrane abnormalities that shorten the in vivo red cell survival time. The severity of the hemolytic anemia resulting from the production of red cells with a defective protein portion of lipoprotein in the lipoprotein molecule in the membrane varies, but Rh null persons exhibit stomatocytosis (cup-shaped red cells), and have different reaction patterns with other blood group antigens, such as S, s, and U.

RH NULL SYNDROME. This condition has been observed in at least 22 persons in 14 different families. It is produced by two different genetic mechanisms. In the more common regulator-type of Rh null, the absence of a very common regular gene X^1r prevents expression of normal Rh genes. Rh null persons are thought to be homozygous for X^Qr, a rare allele of X^1r that segregates independently of genes of the Rh system. In these cases, individuals appear to transmit normal Rh genes to their offspring, but, in some cases, parents or children of indi-

viduals with the regulator-type of Rh null show overall depression of their Rh antigens.

The other, extremely rare form of Rh null occurs in persons homozygous for an amorphic gene (/r) at the Rh locus. The gene appears to have no detectable gene product with Rh antisera. In these cases, parents and children are heterozygous for the amorph. Their phenotypes invariably reflect the presence of a single Rh haplotype, the one inherited from the parent with normal Rh antigens.

The erythrocytes of both types of Rh null are never both C positive and c positive, or E positive and e positive.

RH MOD. The Rh mod phenotype shares a similar genetic basis with the regulator Rh null. The term X^Qr has been given to the unlinked recessive modifier gene thought to be responsible for the condition. Unlike Rh null cells, those classified as Rh mod do not completely lack Rh and LW antigens (to be discussed later in this chapter); expression, however, is reduced and sometimes variable in expression.

THE E MOSAIC

The e antigen of some Blacks may be a mosaic-type structure. The appearance of e-like antibodies made by e positive individuals is analogous to the anti-D made by individuals with the D mosaic.

The e antigen is of high incidence and, in most cases, the relationship of e and anti-e is straightforward. If antibody is formed by E +e- (usually R^2R^2) persons, it typically reacts with all e positive erythrocytes. In Blacks, however, the situation is different; some have red cells that type as e+ but make antibodies that closely resemble anti-e (or anti-f or anti-rh_1) but do not react with the person's own red cells. The e, hr^S, Hr^B, and hr^S-like (Santiago antibody defined) portions of the e mosaic have been studied and characterized, but do not fully explain the complexity of the e mosaic.

Other Rh Antigens

Of the more than 40 identified Rh antigens (Table 5-8), only a few additional and

Table 5-8. Summary of Selected Rh Antigens and Variants

CDE Term	Year Antigen Reported	Whites Positive for the Antigen (%)
D	1939	85
C	1941	70
C^w	1946	1–2
C^x	1954	<1
E	1943	30
c	1941	80
e	1945	98
f	1953	64
CE	1961	<1
Ce	1958	70
cE	1961	30
E^w	1955	<1
E^T	1962	30
G	1958	85
Go^a		
D^{Cor}	1958	<1
C^B	1961	70
V	1955	2
VS	1960	2

variant antigens will be discussed in this section.

THE G ANTIGEN

In 1958, the G antigen, which does not fit neatly into the concept of three subloci of the Rh system, was defined. Almost all genes that make C or D antigens make G antigen as well. Conversely, the genes that do not make C or D usually do not make G. Some examples of erythrocytes that express at least a part of the D antigen but lack G antigen have been demonstrated. Rare cells have been discovered that possess G antigen, but lack D antigen and exhibit diminished or altered expression of C antigen.

Before 1958, questions arose about the production and serologic reactions of antibodies with apparent anti-C plus anti-D (anti-CD) specificity in rr individuals exposed to R_o (cDe) or r′ (Cde) erythrocytes via pregnancy of transfusion. Superficially, these antibodies appeared to be anti-C positive, D but were actually anti-G, which cannot be separated into anti-C and anti-D (Table 5-9). The fact that G appears to exist as an entity common to D and C explains why D− persons immunized by C−, D+ erythrocytes sometimes appear to make anti-C+D. It may also explain why D− persons who are exposed to C+D− erythrocytes may develop antibodies appearing to contain an anti-D component.

The G antigen appears to be no more immunogenic than the C antigen. For potent anti-G to be produced, rr individuals who have already made anti-C and anti-D must be exposed to additional G positive erythrocytes before anti-G is synthesized in significantly detectable amounts.

THE V AND VS ANTIGENS

In 1955, the V antigen was discovered. This antigen is always the product of $R°$, R^{ou} or r genes. V antigen is present on the erythrocytes of almost 30% of random American Blacks and up to 40% of individuals in other Black populations. Very few Whites have the V antigen.

COMPOUND ANTIGENS

The term compound antigen is used to communicate the idea that certain combinations of Rh antigens demonstrate a combined effect, such as the ce or f antigen. Other examples of compound antigens include: rh_1 (Ce), cE (rh 27), and CE (Rh 22). These combined gene products are cis gene products and are expressed when two Rh genes are carried on the same chromosome. The R^1 (CDe) gene creates the C and e antigen and also produces rh_1 (Ce) when located in the cis position. The product of the gene R^1 (CDe) possesses antigenic activity defined as D, C, and e. It also includes Ce (rh^1), a compound product that always accompanies C and e when they are determined by the same gene. Cells having C and e determined by separate genes, for example R^zr (CDE/cde), do not have the Ce antigen.

Antibodies against these compound antigens are not rare but are encountered less frequently than antibodies with single specificities. Antibodies directed against compound antigens may be concealed in serums containing antibodies of the more obvious specificities. Only absorption with erythrocytes of selected phenotypes will demonstrate their presence.

Table 5-9. Adsorption-Elution Technique to Recognize Anti-G

Process	Serum No. 1	Serum No. 2
Antibodies Present:	Anti-D, -C	Anti-D, -C, -G
Phenotype of RBCs for		
first adsorption	cDeG	cDeG
Antibodies in eluate	Anti-D	Anti-D, -G
Phenotype of RBCs for		
second adsorption	CdeG	CdeG
Antibodies in eluate	None	Anti-G

Variant Antigens

Although erythrocytes from most individuals with common alloantibodies give straightforward reactions, some produce atypical reactions and others stimulate the production of alloantibodies that do not react with erythrocytes of common Rh phenotypes. Unexpected reactions in this category usually represent subtle differences in composition among various Rh gene products.

By considering C and c or E and e as expressing antithetical products, the concept can be expanded to include alternate antigenic activities. If the genes are together at the same site but are determined by genes coding for products distinct from the common Rh determinants, variant activity can be observed. In Blacks, atypical activity at the e antigen site is common. Several patterns have been identified (hr^{s-} and hr^{B-}).

The antigen C^w is an example of a variant antigen that usually functions as an allele in the antithetical relationship of C/c. This antigen is expressed in approximately 1 to 2% of some White populations. C^w was first described in 1962 in an R^1R^1 person who had been transfused with blood of the genotype C^wDe/CDe ($R^{1w}R^1$). Characteristics of C^w antibody include demonstration of a "dosage effect." This antibody has the capability of causing hemolytic transfusion reactions and hemolytic disease of the newborn.

The LW Antigen

The LW (LW^a) antigen, which was demonstrated with the original animal antirhesus sera, was named in honor of Landsteiner and Wiener. It is now recognized as distinct from the D antigen. This antigen is present on rhesus monkey erythrocytes and on the majority of human erythrocytes. In human adults, D– individuals display comparatively weaker LW activity, but umbilical cord bloods from both D+ and D– babies are strongly reactive. In general, the amount of LW antigen demonstrated on a person's erythrocytes is related to the presence or absence of D antigen. The classifications LW_1 and LW_2 describe the strong LW reactivity of D^+ erythrocytes and the weaker LW reactivity of adult D– erythrocytes. The category LW_3 represents the phenotype of individuals who produce anti-LW but have nonreactive erythrocytes with the LW antibody. The classification LW_4 (LW a– b–) has been applied to the extremely rare case of having LW^- erythrocytes with serum containing a potent form of anti-LW that agglutinated LW_3 erythrocytes as well as LW_1 and LW_2 erythrocytes.

There is a strong phenotypic association between the Rh and LW blood group systems; but the CDE and LW genes control different blood group antigens and segregate independently. LW is a very high incidence antigen. All erythrocytes of the Rh null phenotype, however, are LW–. Rare cases have been documented in which normal Rh antigens, with or without D antigen, are present but LW antigen is absent. The LW (LW^a) gene appears to require for its expression some product of Rh gene activity.

As the LW subclassifications demonstrate, LW– individuals can form alloanti-LW. The antibody displays the same degree of reactivity with D+ and D– erythrocytes as the animal antisera. Anti-LW has sometimes been identified in the sera of LW positive persons whose erythrocytes at the time of antibody formation were either transiently LW− or exhibited very weak reactivity with anti-LW sera. In these transient cases, the normal LW+ status of the erythrocytes has been documented to return to a positive status as the antibody disappears.

In 1981, a new blood group antigen, Ne^a, was reported with a frequency of approximately 5% in the Finnish population. Anti-Ne^a displayed a variation in the strength of reactivity similar to anti-LW that suggested a relationship between Ne^a and LW. It is now known that Ne^a and LW are products of allelic genes. Therefore, the antigen formerly called LW has become LW^a and Ne^a becomes LW^b.

Rh Antibodies

The Rh antibodies are predominantly of the immunoglobulin class IgG. The production of these antibodies is consistent with the classical immune response that initially elicits IgM antibody followed by IgG. Some examples of IgA have been identified. When IgG antibodies are synthesized, most of them are IgG1 or IgG3. The IgG1 subclass of anti-D is more common if immunization results from pregnancy. Although Rh antibodies are associated with both hemolytic transfusion reactions and hemolytic disease of the newborn, in vitro binding of complement is rare. The lack of in vitro complement fixation is believed to be hampered by the small number of Rh antigen sites, the distance of the antigen from the erythrocyte membrane, and the lack of exposure of the combining site of the complement C1q component on the immunoglobulin molecule.

Antibody Characteristics and Frequencies

Except for some examples that occur without a known red cell stimulus, most Rh antibodies result from erythrocyte immunization subsequent to pregnancy or transfusion. Therefore, the majority of these antibodies are IgG. The characteristics of selected Rh antibodies are presented in Table 5-10. The D antigen is the most potent Rh immunogen. Of D− patients who receive a single unit of D+ blood, 50 to 75% can be expected to develop anti-D; but 25 to 30% of D− individuals are nonresponders, which makes them unable to produce anti-D. Additionally, some D^u recipients can form anti-D if transfused with D+ blood.

In studies of deliberate immunization to induce alloantibody production, the C, c, E, and e antigens were demonstrated to be much less immunogenic than D. Anti-E is the most common antibody associated with these four antigens, followed by anti-c. Anti-E can be found in the absence of erythrocyte antigen exposure. Some examples of anti-E react only with protease-modified erythrocytes, while others are reactive at temperatures below 37° C. Anti-C as a single antibody is rare in both Rh positive and negative persons. Anti-e is rarely found because only about 2 individuals in 100 are able to synthesize anti-e.

Some Rh antibodies commonly occur together. For example, an R_1R_1 person who has made immune anti-E has probably been exposed to the c antigen as well as E. In these cases, anti-c is usually present in addition to anti-E, although the titer of anti-c may be low and not detectable when the anti-E is demonstrated. Anti-c can produce a hemolytic transfusion reaction following the administration of compatible E negative, c positive blood. When selecting blood for transfusion to R_1R_1 recipients with detectable anti-E who might also produce anti-c, transfusing with R_1R_1 blood should be considered. A patient with detectable anti-c may not have a concurrent anti-E because exposure to c antigen is more probable than exposure to E antigen.

Dosage Effects

Anti-D seldom exhibits any difference in reactivity between erythrocytes with homozygous or heterozygous expression of the D antigen. Variably strong reactions, however, may be observed with red cells representing certain genotypes, such as R_2R_2. The (cDE/cDE) dosage effect can be observed with antibodies having specificities

Table 5-10. Characteristics of Selected Rh Antibodies

| Antibody | Mode of Reactivity | | | Usual Immunoglobulin Subclass | | | Usual Form of Stimulation | |
	Sal.	AHG	Enz.	IgM	IgG	IgA	RBCs	Other
Anti-D		X	X	Some	Most	Few	X	Rare
Anti-C		X	X		Most		X	Rare
Anti-E	X	X	X	Some	Most		X	Some
Anti-c		X	X		Most		X	
Anti-e		X	X		Most		X	
Anti-C^w	X	X	X	Some	Most		X	Some

for the E, c, or e antigens. Dosage may occasionally be observed with anti-C.

THE LEWIS SYSTEM

The two common antigens of the Lewis system are Lewis^a (Le^a) and Lewis^b (Le^b). The first antibody of this system, anti-Le^a, was identified in 1946. The antibody to the corresponding allele, anti-Le^b, was recognized in 1948. The Lewis blood group system is unlike other blood group systems in that genetic control of the two antigens, Le^a and Le^b, appear to reside in a single gene, called Le. This system, which represents a complex interaction between the independent Lewis, ABO, and secretor genes, is best understood by thinking of it as a system of genetically determined water-soluble antigens that are present in body fluids and secretions, such as saliva. Under certain circumstances, the Lewis antigens attach themselves to cells such as erythrocytes.

The Lewis system differs from other blood group systems in three significant ways. The differences include the following:

1. Erythrocytes acquire the Lewis phenotype by adsorbing Lewis substances from the plasma, rather than being membrane-bound antigens.
2. Although the Lewis and secretor genes are inherited independently, the Lewis phenotype is influenced by the secretor status. Inheritance of the nonsecretor (sese) genes and Lewis genes results in the phenotype Le(a+b−); while inheritance of at least one secretor gene, Sese or SeSe, and the

Lewis gene results in the phenotype Le(a−b+).
3. The Lewis phenotype may be modified by the ABO phenotype (such as A$_1$), which may interfere with the expression of the Le^a antigen in Le(b+) individuals.

The Secretor Status

The terms secretor and nonsecretor refer only to the presence of water-soluble ABH antigen substances in body fluid. This condition is influenced by the independently inherited regulator Se gene. Approximately 78% of humans possess at least one Se gene and secrete A, B, or H water-soluble antigens (Table 5-11). The presence of the Se gene allows the H gene to function in secretory cells.

These secretions have the property of reacting with their corresponding antibodies to neutralize or inhibit the ability of these antibodies to agglutinate erythrocytes possessing the corresponding antigen. This reaction is termed hemagglutination inhibition and provides a means of assaying the relative activity or potency of these water-soluble blood group substances (see Chapter 14).

Table 5-11. The Relationship of ABH Substances and ABO Group

| ABO Blood Group Secretors | ABH Substances in Saliva | | |
	A	B	H
A	Much	None	Some
B	None	Much	Some
O	None	None	Much
AB	Much	Much	Some

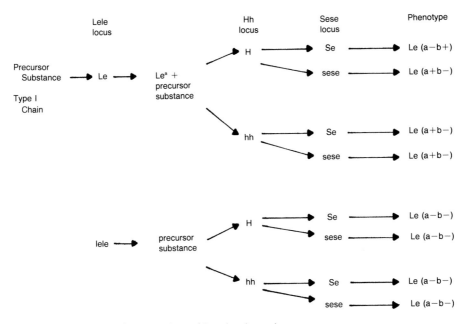

Figure 5-2. Mechanism of expression of Lewis phenotypes.

The water-soluble form of the Le^a and Le^b antigens is present in appropriate saliva. With the exception of the Lewis antigens and another antigen, Sd^a, there is no evidence of the presence of any of the other blood group antigens in saliva and other body secretions. Individuals who possess the Se gene are Le (a−), but these subjects can secrete ABH substance in a water-soluble form. Their erythrocytes type as Le (a−). All Le (a−b−) individuals are nonsecretors of ABH substance (Table 5-12).

Table 5-12. Blood Group Substances

Genes[1]	In Secretions	On Erythrocytes
H, Se, A, Le	H,A, Le^a, Le^b	H, A, Le^b
H, Se, OO, Le	H, Le^a, Le^b	H, Le^{a2}, Le^b
H, Se, A, lele	H, A	H,A
H, sese, A, Le	Le^a	H, A, Le^a
hh[3], Se, A, Le	Le^a	Le^a

[1] The H, Se, A(or B), and Le genes produce their effect when present in either the homozygous or heterozygous state. When the amorphic genes h, O, le and se are present in a homozygous state, no detectable effect is produced.

[2] In some group O (and A$_2$) individuals who have the genes H, Se, and Le. Le^a as well as Le^b can be detected on the erythrocytes.

[3] The H gene is necessary for the formation of H, A, and Le^b substances.

Mode of Inheritance

The inheritance of an Le gene produces Le^a antigen. The inheritance of the amorph gene, le, in a homozygous state (lele) prevents the production of any Lewis antigen and results in the null phenotype. The Le^b antigen is the product of the interaction of the dominant Lewis gene and the H gene in the presence of the Se gene (Fig. 5-2). This explains why an Le^b gene is not required for the formation of the Le^b antigen.

The Lewis gene does not directly code for the production of Lewis antigens. Without the Le gene, no Lewis substances can be formed, and the erythrocytes are Le(a−b−), regardless of the secretor status. If the Le gene is inherited, antigens are produced by the action of a specific glycosyl transferase, L-fucosyl transferase, which adds L-fucose to the basic precursor substance. It should be noted that Lewis genes compete with A and B genes in the addition of L-fucose to the N-acetylglucosamine sugar of the common precursor structure manufactured by tissue cells.

The result of the Lewis gene activity is the production of an α-4-L-fucosyltransferase that catalyzes the transfer of fucose to the carbon-4 position of N-acetylglucosamine produces the Le^a active structure. The Le^a soluble antigen is then secreted and adsorbed onto the erythrocyte membrane. In the absence of the secretor gene, Le^a is not converted to Le^b; therefore, body fluids contain abundant Le^a and no Le^b and the erythrocytes are Le(a+b−).

If both the H and Le gene products are present, the addition of fucose to the carbon-4 position of N-acetylglucosamine results in an Le^b active structure (Fig. 5-3), because the H gene has transferred fucose to the carbon-2 position of galactose. This Le^b substance will be present on erythrocytes as well as in body fluids. The small amount of the initial Le^a that was not converted can be detected in body fluids but is insufficient to attach to erythrocytes. In this case, the phenotype is Le(a−b+).

To further understand the Lewis system,

it is important to realize that there are two types of carbohydrate chains ending in the glycoprotein of the precursor substance. The same sugars are present in each type of chain, although they have different linkages. In Type I chains, the terminal galactose has a β-1,3 linkage with N-acetylglucosamine and in Type II chains, the sugar has a β-1,4 linkage. The fucosyltransferase produced by the Le gene is unable to act on a type II chain because the number 4 carbon atom is already occupied by the galactosyl structure. Two antigens, Le^c and Le^d, are postulated to be derived from the precursor substance of the type II chains.

The Biochemical Nature of Lewis Antigens

The water-soluble Lewis antigens found in secretions are glycoproteins, as are the ABH substances from secretors. These glycoproteins are composed of approximately 80% carbohydrates and 15% amino acids. Lewis specificity that is similar to ABH antigens resides in the carbohydrate portion of the molecule. In the blood plasma, the Lewis antigens as well as the ABH substances are glycosphingolipids.

Le^a and Le^b antigens are absent or extremely weak at birth. Cord blood specimens are essentially Le (a−b−). The Le^a antigen develops more rapidly than Le^b. By 3 months of age, more than 80% of children produce an Le(a+) reaction, but this reactivity, decreases with age, and by about 2 years of age, the adult level of 20% reactivity is established. The expression of the adult frequency of approximately 70% reactivity of Le^b antigen on erythrocytes is reached at about 6 years. Antigenic strength is also known to vary during pregnancy for unknown reasons. In cases of diminished activity, normal reactivity returns after pregnancy.

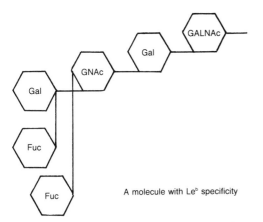

A molecule with Le^a specificity

A molecule with Le^b specificity

Figure 5-3. Molecules with Lewis specificity.
Key:
Gal = D−Galactose
GNAc = N-acetylglucosamine
Fuc = Fucose
GALNAc = N-acetylgalactosamine

Lewis Phenotypes

The expression of Lewis antigens results from the continuous exchange of glycosphingolipids between the plasma and the erythrocyte membrane. Because erythrocytes adsorb Lewis antigens in vivo, the Lewis phenotype depends entirely on the uptake of antigens from the plasma.

Three major Lewis phenotypes exist in adults (Table 5-13):

1. Le(a+b−)
2. Le(a−b+)
3. Le(a−b−)

THE Le(a+b−) PHENOTYPE

Characteristics of this phenotype, Le(a+b−), include the presence of Le^a antigen in plasma and saliva and agglutination of erythrocytes with anti-Le^a reagent sera. Le(a+b−) erythrocytes do not react with anti-Le^b because of the absence of Le^b antigen. Although these individuals produce large amounts of Le^a substance, they do not secrete ABH substances in their saliva. Only saliva from Le(a+b−) individuals forms a precipitate with an anti-Le^a serum produced in rabbits.

THE Le(a−b+) PHENOTYPE

This is the most common phenotype in adults. Individuals of the phenotype Le (a−b+) have the genes H, Se, and Le and their secretions contain H, Le^a and Le^b. If Le(a−b+) individuals have an A (or B gene), they will also have A or B substances, respectively, in their secretions. The plasma of Le(a−b+) individuals contains predominantly Le^b substances, but trace amounts of Le^a may also be detected. The phenotype Le(a+b+) can be observed with erythrocytes of rare O and A$_2$ persons. These anti-Le^a reactions are weak and detectable only with antihuman globulin (AHG) testing. The phenotype Le(a+b+) has not been found in A$_1$ adults, probably because they make less Le^a substance as a result of competition between the A^1 and Le gene products for the basic precursor substance.

THE Le(a−b−) PHENOTYPE

This uncommon phenotype, Le(a−b−), has the genotype lele, which results in erythrocytes with the phenotype Le (a−b−). These erythrocytes react with either anti-Le^c or anti-type I H (previously anti-Le^d). Persons with the genotype lele have traces of Le^a in their serum.

Lewis Antibodies

The Lewis antibodies (anti-Le^a and anti-Le^b) are frequently found in individuals who have never been transfused or received any other known erythrocyte antigen stimulus. As many as 20% of Le(a−b−) individuals have a Lewis antibody. Anti-Le^a and anti-Le^b are especially common in pregnant women. The Lewis antibody incidence in Le(a−b−) persons is 4 times more common in Blacks than Whites. Rare cases of hemolytic disease of the newborn (discussed in Chapter 10) have been attributed to anti-Le^a. Lewis antibodies have been cited as the cause in a few hemolytic transfusion reactions.

Anti-Le^a is more common as an individual antibody than anti-Le^b and is found only in individuals who are genetically Lewis-negative, lele, and have the phenotype Le(a−b−). Anti-Le^b is usually a weakly re-

Table 5-13. Lewis Phenotypes in Adults

Red Cell Phenotype	Genotype	Lewis Substance (Saliva)	H Substance (Saliva)	Frequency (Approximate)	
				White (%)	Black (%)
Le(a+b−)	H, sese, Le	Le^a	Absent	22	23
	very rare hh, Se or sese, Le				
Le(a−b+)	H, Se, Le	Le^b+Le^a	Present	72	55
Le(a−b−)	H, Se, lele	Absent	Present	6	22
	H, sese, lele	Absent	Absent	1	?
	very rare hh, Se or sese, lele				

active antibody in serum which contains a relatively potent anti-Le^a. The incidence of anti-Le^b as a single antibody is infrequent. Producers of anti-Le^b (without anti-Le^a) are nonsecretors of ABH and always of the phenotype Le(a−b−). It is very rare for Le(a+b−) individuals to form anti-Le^b; but there is no theoretic reason why they should not be able to do so, because they are completely lacking in Le^b antigen. Almost all Lewis antibodies are of the IgM variety. Rare examples of anti-Le^a are solely IgG. The in vitro stability of these antibodies in serum is unpredictable, even when they are frozen.

Sera containing anti-Le^a usually agglutinate Le(a+) cells suspended in saline and react more strongly at room temperature or colder temperatures. Erythrocytes agglutinated by anti-Le^a characteristically have a "stringy" appearance. This agglutination may not be obvious with saline-suspended erythrocytes. Hemolysis of erythrocytes, particularly cells treated with a proteolytic enzyme, may be observed at 37° C because the antibody almost always binds complement. Some examples of Le^a, and less frequently anti-Le^b, are detectable only with antihuman globulin (AHG) testing, if complement is presence in the test mixture and a polyspecific antiserum is used.

Some examples of anti-Le^b fail to react with A$_1$ cells but react strongly with group O or A$_2$ erythrocytes. Two kinds of anti-Le^b exist. Those that are neutralized by the saliva of all ABH secretors, including those of Le(a−b−) individuals. These anti-Le^b antibodies are referred to as anti-Le^{bH}. The other form, referred to as anti-Le^{bL}, (true anti-Le^b) is neutralized by the saliva of Le(a−b+) persons. This form of anti-Le^b

reacts with A$_1$ erythrocytes almost as well as with erythrocytes of other blood groups.

Other Lewis Antibodies

Two additional antibodies have been named in the Lewis blood group system, although the products with which they react are not determined by Lewis genes. These antibodies are anti-Le^c and anti-Le^d. Anti-Le^c reacts with the erythrocytes of Le (a−b−) nonsecretors, from individuals of genotype lele, sese, and also with those of genotype lele, hh. This antibody is inhibited by the saliva of individuals of the same genotypes. Anti-Le^d reacts with erythrocytes of Le(a−b−) secretors.

A summary of the typical serologic behavior of Le^a and Le^b is found in Table 5-14.

ADDITIONAL MAJOR BLOOD GROUP SYSTEMS

Other major blood group systems exist in addition to the ABO, Rh, and Lewis blood group systems. A summary of the antigen frequencies and serologic behavior of the antibodies of the blood group systems is presented in Tables 5-15 and 5-16.

For convenience these systems can be divided into the two following categories:

1. The typically IgM antibody systems that are best detected at cold temperatures (MNSsU, P, and I systems).
2. The typically IgG antibody systems that are detectable by antiglobulin (AHG) testing (Kell, Duffy, and Kidd systems).

Table 5-14. In Vitro Serologic Behavior of Le^a and Le^b

Antibody	In Vitro Reactions					
	Saline		Albumin	AGH*	Enzymes	Hemolysis
	4°C	22°C	37°C	—	37°C	—
Anti-Le^a	Most	Most	Few	Many	Most	Some
Anti-Le^b	Most	Most	Few	Some	Some	Occasional

* AGH signifies antihuman globulin (AHG) phase of testing using a broad-spectrum (polyspecific) antisera.

Table 5-15. Summary of Antigen Frequencies

Blood Group	Antigen	Frequency in Population (%)	
		White	Black
Rh-hr	D	85	92
	C	70	33
	E	30	21
	c	80	97
	e	98	99
	C^w	1	< 1
	V	< 1	30
Kell	K	9	2
	k	99.9	> 99.9
	Kp^a	2	Rare
	Kp^b	> 99.9	100
	Js^a	Rare	20
	Js^b	> 99.9	99
Duffy	Fy^a	66	10
	Fy^b	83	23
Kidd	Jk^a	77	91
	Jk^b	72	41
Lutheran	Lu^a	8	—
	Lu^b	99.9	—
MNSs	M	78	70
	N	72	74
	S	55	31
	s	89	97
	U	100	> 99
Lewis	Le^a	22	23
	Le^b	72	55
P	P^1	79	94
	P	100	100
	Tj^a	100	100
Xg^a	Xg^a	66F	66F
		89M	89M
Colton	Co^a	> 99	> 99
	Co^b	10	10
Dombrock	Do^a	67	—
	Do^b	83	—
Diego	Di^a	Rare	—
	Di^b	100	—
Wright	Wr^a	< 1	—
Vel	Vel	100	—
Sid	Sd^a	91	—
HLA	Bg^a	17	17
	Bg^b	9	28
	Bg^c	8	17
Cartwright	Yt^a	> 99	> 99
	Yt^b	8	8

Table 5-15. Summary of Antigen Frequencies

Blood Group	Antigen	Frequency in Population	
		White	Black
HTLA	Ch^A	Ch(a+)	Rg(a+)a
	Rg^a	95	95
	Kn^a	Kn(a+)	McC(a+)
	McC^a	97	95
	Cs^a	Cs(a+)	Yka(+)
	Yk^a	82	96
	JMH	99.9	99.9
I	I	See	See
	i	text	text

References:
  Issitt, P. D.: Applied Blood Group Serology, 3rd Ed. Miami, FL, Montgomery Scientific, 1985.

  Widmann, Frances K. (Ed.): AABB Technical Manual, 9th ed. Arlington, VA, American Association of Blood Banks, 1985.

Typical IgM Antibody Blood Group Systems

THE LUTHERAN SYSTEM

The first antigen of the Lutheran system was recognized in 1945. This antigen, Lu^a, is low in frequency. The antithetical high frequency antigen, Lu^b, was reported in 1956. More than 17 antigens, such as Lu^9 and Lu^6, are known to exist in this system; most are high frequency antigens.

Mode of Inheritance. Initially, the Lewis and Lutheran genes were erroneously believed to be linked; it was later discovered that the Lutheran genes were actually linked to the gene that controls secretor status. The Lutheran and secretor locus had the distinction of providing the first example of autosomal linkage and the first example of autosomal crossing-over in humans.

The Lu^a and Lu^b genes are codominant; however, as in other blood group systems, the expression of these genes is not straightforward (Fig. 5-4).

The rare Lu(a−b−) null phenotype is categorized as either recessive or dominant in type. The recessive null phenotype re-

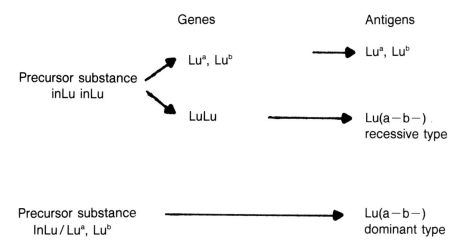

Figure 5-4 Theoretical mechanism of expression of Lutheran antigens.

sults from the homozygous inheritance of an amorphic gene. Consequently, the person lacks all Lutheran antigens. The dominant type of Lu(a−b−) null phenotype results from the inheritance of a single dominant gene that prevents normal Lutheran antigen synthesis. This independently segregating inhibitor gene has been named InLu (Lutheran inhibitor). If a single InLu gene is inherited even in the presence of normal Luª and Luᵇ genes, the resulting phenotype is Lu(a−b−). This rare gene also inhibits the production of other antigens such as P_1, i and Auª.

The Biochemical Nature of Lutheran Antigens. Lutheran antigens are probably glycoproteins in nature and are of questionable immunogenicity. Although the Luª antigen is poorly developed at birth, the strength of the antigen is known to increase until about the age of 15 years. The Luᵇ antigen of an Lu(a−b+) cord blood is also weaker than in adults. Lutheran antigens may occasionally demonstrate dosage, but it is not as evident as in other blood group antigens such as c and M. Enzymes do not usually affect the Lutheran antigens.

Lutheran Phenotypes. The Lu(a−b+) phenotype is the most common and Lu(a−b−) is the rarest (Table 5-17). Racial differences are not apparent.

Lutheran Antibodies. The Lutheran antibodies, particularly Anti-Luª, are infrequently observed; this is partially due to

the fact that a small proportion of individuals possess the Luª antigen. Lutheran antibodies, however, particularly anti-Luª, are known to occur with no known erythrocyte stimulus in the majority of cases. Most examples of anti-Luᵇ are associated with a known exposure to Luᵇ antigen by way of transfusion or pregnancy. Some Lutheran antibodies bind complement, but in vitro reactions are not associated with hemolysis. Anti-Luª has been infrequently associated with mild hemolytic disease of the newborn, and anti-Luᵇ has been noted in decreased erythrocyte survival and transfusion reactions.

The immunologic and in vitro characteristics of anti-Luª and anti-Luᵇ are presented in Table 5-18.

Anti-Luª reactivity is characterized by mixed-field agglutination. Most examples of anti-Luª are IgM, more reactive at lower temperatures, and agglutinate saline suspended erythrocytes. Some dosage effect is exhibited. Anti-Luᵇ occurs as both an IgG and IgA antihuman globulin (AHG) antibody; it is rarely an IgM antibody.

Anti-Lu3 (anti-LuªLuᵇ) is an antibody produced by individuals of the rare Lu(a−b−) phenotype. A person of this phenotype is capable of forming anti-Lu3 as well as any other Lutheran system antibody. It seems as though anti-Lu3 is made by persons of the recessive type and not by those of the dominant type of Lu(a−b−).

Table 5-16. Serologic Characteristics of Blood Group Antibodies

System	Antibody	Reactive Phases				Comments
		R.T.	37° C	A.H.G.	Enzyme	
Rh-hr	Anti-D	Some	Most	Most	Most	
	Anti-C	Few	Most	Most	Most	Often found with anti-D, anti-Ce, or anti-C^w
	Anti-E	Some	Most	Most	Most	Often found with anti-c
	Anti-c	Rare	Most	Most	Most	Often found with anti-E
	Anti-e	Rare	Most	Most	Most	Often found with anti-C
	Anti-C^w	Some	Most	Most	Most	
	Anti-V	Rare	Most	Most	Most	
Lewis	Anti-Le^a	Most	Few	Some	Most	
	Anti-Le^b	Most	Rare	Some	Some	Often found with anti-Le^a
Lutheran	Anti-Lu^a	Most	Few	Few	Few	Produces mixed field type of agglutination
	Anti-Lu^b	Few	Few	Most	Few	
MNSs	Anti-M	Most	Few	Some	0	May exhibit dosage
	Anti-N	Most	Rare	Rare	0	
	Anti-S	Some	Some	Most	Variable	
	Anti-s	Few	Few	Most	Most	
	Anti-U	Rare	Some	Most	Most	
P	Anti-P$_1$	Most	Rare	Rare	Most	
	Anti-P	Most	Some	Some	Most	
	Anti-PP$_1$P^k (Tj^a)	Most	Some	Some	Most	
I	Anti-I	Most	Few	Some	Most	
	Anti-i	Most	Few	Some	Most	
Kell	Anti-K	Few	Few	Most	Most	
	Anti-k	Rare	Rare	Most	Most	
	Anti-Kp^a	Rare	Rare	Most	Most	
	Anti-Kp^b	Rare	Rare	Most	Most	
	Anti-Js^a	Rare	Rare	Most	Most	
	Anti-Js^b	0	0	Most	Most	
Duffy	Anti-Fy^a	Rare	Rare	Most	0	Some exhibit dosage; some may bind complement
	Anti-Fy^b	Rare	Rare	Most	0	Some exhibit dosage; some may bind complement
Kidd	Anti-Jk^a	Rare	Rare	Most	Most	May exhibit dosage; titers can rapidly decline; may require anti-C3 for detection

Table 5-16. Serologic Characteristics of Blood Group Antibodies (continued)

System	Antibody	Reactive Phases				Comments
		R.T.	37° C	A.H.G.	Enzyme	
	Anti-Jk[b]	Rare	Rare	Most	Most	May exhibit dosage; titers can rapidly decline; may require anti-C3
Xg	Anti-Xg[a]	Few	Few	Most	0	
Sid	Anti-Sd[a]	Some	Some	Some	Most	Agglutinates have a refractile, mixed-field appearance
Cartwright	Anti-Yt[a]	0	0	Most	Some	Usually found in combination with other antibodies
	Anti-Yt[b]	0	0	Most		
Colton	Anti-Co[a]	0	0	Some	Most	
	Anti-Co[b]	0	0	Some	Most	
Diego	Anti-Dj[a]	Some	Some	Most	Some	
	Anti-Dj[b]	0	0	Most	Some	
Dombrock	Anti-Do[a]	0	0	Most	Most	
	Anti-Do[b]	0	0	Most	Most	
HLA Related	Anti-Bg[a]	0	0	Most	Some	Usually weakly reactive
	Anti-Bg[b]					
	Anti-Bg[c]					
Vel	Anti-Vel	Some	Some	Some	Some	
Wright	Anti-Wr[a]	Most	Few	Some	Some	
HTLA	Anti-Ch[a]	0	0	Most	Few	All are usually weakly reactive
	Anti-Cs[a]				Most	
	Anti-Gy[a]				Most	
	Anti-Hy				Most	
	Anti-JMH				Few	
	Anti-Kn[a]/Mc[a]				Most	
	Anti-Rg[a]				Few	
	Anti-Yk[a]				Most	

Table 5-17. Frequency of Lutheran Phenotypes

Phenotype	White (%)	Black (%)
Lu(a+b−)	0.1	0.1
Lu(a+b+)	7.0	5.2
Lu(a−b+)	92.9	94.7
Lu(a−b−)	Very rare	Very rare

This antibody is usually IgG or IgA and is capable of destroying incompatible erythrocytes; it reacts best with antihuman globulin (AHG) testing. Anti-Lu3 can react with all Lutheran-positive cells and is only nonreactive with other Lu(a−b−) cells.

Many other antibodies (such as anti-Lu$_4$) have been described. All fail to react with

Table 5-18. Characteristics of Lutheran Antibodies

	IgG	IgM	IgA	Saline Reactivity	AHG Reactivity
Anti-Lu[a]	Rare	Common	Some	Common	Some
Anti-Lu[b]	Some	Rare	Some	Few	Common

Lu(a−b−) erythrocytes, although they do react with the erythrocytes of other rare Lutheran phenotypes. Antibodies that fail to react with Lu(a−b−) erythrocytes of the dominant type may not belong to the Lutheran blood group system.

THE MNSs SYSTEM

The M and N antigens are classically associated with paternity testing. This system was discovered in 1927 by Landsteiner and Levine when anti-M and anti-N were formed by injecting human erythrocytes into rabbits. The S and s antigens were later added to this blood group system. The MNSs system includes a group of mostly low-frequency "satellite" antigens, such as anti-M^g, that are rarely of clinical significance. Several of these low-frequency antigens are considered interrelated and form the Miltenberger subsystem.

Mode of Inheritance. The MNSs system is governed by two closely linked sets of allelic genes, MN and Ss. Because of linkage, one of four possible genetic combinations is inherited from each parent: MS, Ms, NS, or Ns. This results in 10 possible genotypes. Linkage produces disequilibrium and the gene complex Ns is 5 times more common than NS. A small proportion of Blacks are S−s− and most are also negative for the high frequency antigen, U.

The U antigen is found in all Whites and about 98.5% of Blacks. The rare phenotype S−s− is often written S^u and is the product of another allele at the Ss genetic locus.

The Biochemical Nature of MNSs Antigens. M and N are glycoproteins with approximately 60% carbohydrate. The antigens of the MNS system are related to the erythrocyte membrane sialoglycoproteins referred to as glycophorin A and glycophorin B.

M and N antigen activity resides on the glycophorin A molecule. There are approx-imately 500,000 copies of this molecule present on each erythrocyte. This molecule is embedded in the erythrocyte, membrane with the antigenic molecular sequence located on the external portion of the molecule. When glycophorin A carries M antigenic activity, glycophorin A^M, the first amino acid residual is serine and the fifth is glycine. When it carries N activity, glycophorin A^N, leucine, and glutamic acid replace serine and glycine at positions one and five, respectively.

Glycophorin B is a smaller molecule than glycophorin A but possesses a segment, consisting of 26 amino acids, that duplicates the sequence of glycophorin A^N. This characteristic accounts for the presence of an N-like antigen on almost all erythrocytes, regardless of the MN type. Approximately 100,000 copies of this molecule are present on an erythrocyte. Glycophorin B is thought to carry U, S, and s antigen activity.

MNSs Phenotypes. Three phenotypes, MM, NN, and MN, along with 10 genotypes exist in the MNSs blood group system. These phenotypes, genotypes, and the frequencies of each are presented in Table 5-19.

MNSs Antibodies. Antibodies of the MNSs blood group system are usually considered of minor clinical significance. Anti-M can be observed in multiparous women but rarely develops during pregnancy. Anti-N is an infrequently encountered antibody. Examples of anti-N have been observed in dialysis patients. The stimulus to antibody formation in these patients is attributed to a formaldehyde-induced alteration of the N antigens resulting from the reuse of formaldehyde-sterilized dialyzer membranes.

Most examples of anti-M and anti-N are cold-reacting IgM antibodies produced by nonerythrocytic stimuli, but some rare examples are IgG-type antibodies. Because of their IgM nature, anti-M and anti-N react in saline and exhibit stronger reactivity at

Table 5-19. Genotypes and Frequencies in MNSs System

Phenotype	Phenotypic Frequency (%)	Possible Genotype		Approx. Genotype Frequency (%)	Percentage Positive	
					Anti-S	Anti-s
M	30	MS	MS	6	66	80
		MS	Ms	14		
		Ms	Ms	10		
MN	49	MS	NS	4	53	92
		MS	Ns	22		
		Ms	NS			
		Ms	Ns	23		
N	21	NS	NS	0.3	25	99
		NS	Ns	5		
		Ns	Ns	16		

cold temperatures. Enzyme treatment of erythrocytes does not enhance reactivity, but anti-M reacts better at an acid pH level. Some examples of anti-M react in anti-human globulin (AHG) testing; these antibodies should be considered potentially dangerous. When testing sera for the presence of anti-M or anti-N, the dosage effect is frequently observed. A dosage effect pattern of reactivity of suspected anti-M or anti-N displays stronger agglutination reactions with erythrocytes that are homozygous for MM or NN, respectively.

Anti-S and anti-s are usually erythrocyte-stimulated IgG antibodies. Antibodies of this type can produce hemolytic disease of the newborn (HDN) or transfusion reactions. Anti-U is rare but can be formed in S−s− individuals. These antibodies can also cause HDN and transfusion reactions. Although anti-S may react in saline or AHG tests, it does not react with enzyme enhancement. Anti-s and anti-U react in AHG tests. Anti-U is enhanced with enzyme treatment. Anti-s is not destroyed by enzymes.

THE P SYSTEM

The P_1 antigen, originally referred to as P, was discovered in 1927 by Landsteiner and Levine. The original P antigen was reassigned to an antigen present on almost all human erythrocytes. Erythrocytes lacking the P_1 antigen but possessing the P antigen are referred to as P_2. Four antigens are recognized in the P system: P_1, P, P^k, and p.

Mode of Inheritance. The inheritance of antigens in the P blood group system is apparently complex. The P_1 gene is considered to be inherited as a Mendelian dominant, but the P^k locus is separate from the P_1 locus. It is not yet known whether there is actually a p gene that codes for a sialyl transferase.

The P blood group system is related to the ABO, Ii, and Lewis blood group systems. All of the antigens of these systems share a common precursor substance, lactosyl ceramide. Antigens of these systems are synthesized by the sequential addition of carbohydrate residues to the common precursor (Fig. 5-5). In one pathway, synthesis leads to globoside, with the P antigen present on almost all erythrocytes. The other pathway produces paragloboside, which results in the P_1 antigen. It should be noted that sialosylparagloboside, the substance recognized as p antigen, differs from paragloboside only by the addition of sialic acid residue.

Because the P blood group antigens are carbohydrates, they cannot be direct gene products. The gene products are glycosyltransferases that transfer a specific carbohydrate to an oligosaccharide chain. Although antigens of the ABO, Ii, and Lewis systems can be glycolipid or glycoprotein, the P antigens in man have been found to be only glycolipids.

The Biochemical Nature of P Antigens. Each of the antigens of the P blood group system has distinctive characteristics. In addition, the Luke antigen has some relationship to both the ABO and P system.

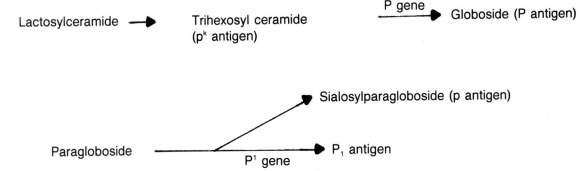

Figure 5-5 Mechanism of expression of selected P blood group system antigens.

P_1. P_1 is a glycosphingolipid on the erythrocyte membrane. This antigen results from the conversion of paragloboside. P_1 is poorly developed on the erythrocytes of newborn infants and may take years to reach adult levels. Antigen strength can be variable. Expression of the antigen can be drastically reduced by the inhibitor gene InLu (a gene of the Lutheran system). The P_1 antigen is known to deteriorate rapidly on stored erythrocytes. P_1 antigen is also found on leukocytes and tissue cells as well as in some secretions, such as hydatid cyst fluid.

P. This antigen is a globoside. Only the p^k and p phenotypes are known to lack P antigen. In addition to the presence of P antigen on almost all erythrocytes, it is also found in plasma, on leukocytes, and on tissue cells.

P^k. This antigen is rare but universal. It is produced by the addition of (α) galactose to lactosyl ceramide. The presence of P^k is undetectable on erythrocytes because of the almost complete conversion of P^k to P antigen. This antigen occurs on some leukocytes and tissue cells, and in plasma. The fibroblasts of all but pp individuals possess P^k antigen.

p. The p gene has been considered an amorphic gene when inherited in a homozygous state. In recent years this hypothesis has been questioned. It has been suggested that a genetic abnormality exists and that an absence of α-galactosyl transferase(s) coding for P^k and P_1 results. Sialosylparagloboside has been designated the p antigen. It should be noted that p (Tj^{a-})

erythrocytes exhibit an excess of sialosylparagloboside as well as paragloboside.

Disorders Associated with P Antigens. In cases of paroxysmal cold hemoglobinuria (PCH), the associated antibody is usually auto-anti-P. A rare example of PCH has been auto-anti-IH-induced.

P System Phenotypes. Four antigens are recognized in the P system: P_1, P, P^k, and p. The P_1 antigen is the most common. These four antigens combine to form one of five phenotypes: P_1, P_2, P_1^k P_2^k, and p (Tj^a negative). The phenotypes, detectable antigens, and phenotypic frequencies are presented in Table 5-20. The p phenotype lacks P, P_1, and P^k and was previously referred to as Tj^{a-}.

P System Antibodies. Anti-P_1 is a common antibody. It is often found in P_2 persons and it is usually a cold-reacting IgM antibody. This antibody is a strong nonagglutinating, complement-binding antibody. Samples containing anti-P_1 that react at 4° C are considered clinically insignificant, but rare examples of IgG anti-P_1 as well as anti-P_1 with a wide thermal range can be hemolytic.

Table 5-20. P Blood Group System Phenotypes

Phenotype	Detectable Antigens	Phenotypic Frequency White (%)	Black (%)
P_1	P_1, P	79	94
P_2	P only	21	6
P_1^k	P_1, P^k	Very rare	
P_2^k	P^k only	Very rare	
p	p only	Very rare	

Anti-P is an extremely rare antibody in pure form. It can be produced only by individuals of the P^k phenotype. Anti-P is usually a potent IgM antibody with a wide thermal range, but it may occur as an IgG antibody. Occasional cases of habitual abortion have been attributed to anti-P.

Anti-P^k has not been reported as a pure antibody. It has been found only as a component of anti-Tj^a using selective absorption with P_1+ cells.

Only a few examples of anti-p have been reported. Anti-p antibodies react at either 4° C or in AHG. Anti-p is neutralized by sialosylparagloboside, but enzymes, such as papain, appear to enhance agglutination reactions.

Anti-Tj^a, a very rare antibody, is also known as anti-PP_1P^k. It can be produced by persons lacking P, P_1, and P^k antigens and has been isolated in the serum of p individuals, often without prior erythrocyte exposure. This antibody can be either IgM or IgG or a combination of both. Anti-Tj^a binds complement, is a potent hemolysin, and has a wide thermal range of activity. This antibody has been associated with hemolytic disease of the newborn and severe hemolytic transfusion reactions. It has also been implicated in chronic abortions and rejection of organs subsequent to transplantation.

Examples of other antibodies encountered in the P blood group system, rarely encountered, include compound, cold-reacting antibodies such as anti-IP_1, iP_1, and anti-I^TP_1.

THE Ii SYSTEM

The Ii system appears to include only two antigens, I and i. This blood group system sometimes interacts with the ABO, I, Lewis, and P systems, to form compound antibodies, such as anti-IP_1, anti-ILe^{bH}, and anti-IH.

Several I and i phenotypes are recognized based on genetically determined differences in the amount of I and i on erythrocytes. These phenotypes tend to be quantitative rather than qualitative; therefore, the terms I+ and I− are relative terms.

Mode of Inheritance. It seems likely that no single I or i gene actually exists but that the presence or absence of many glycosyl transferases that attach carbohydrates result in different carbohydrate sequences. These sequences are subsequently recognized as I or i antigens by the heterogeneous antibodies designated as anti-I and anti-i. The antibody diversity of anti-I and anti-i may represent antibody recognition of a single carbohydrate, a combination of carbohydrates, or perhaps an entire chain.

With the exception of the rare i_{adult} phenotype (approximately 1:10,000 persons), the expression of the I+ antigen status develops along a continuum. The change from the i cord blood and newborn state to the I adult status gradually changes over a period of about 18 months. This transition in Ii status reflects antigen density on the erythrocyte membrane (Table 5-21). Individuals of the O_h phenotype possess the greatest concentration of I antigen in adults.

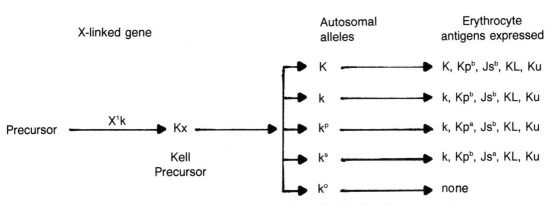

Figure 5-6. Theoretical mechanism of expression of selected Kell antigens.

Table 5-21. Comparative Amounts of Ii Antigen Expressed on Human Erythrocytes

Phenotype	Antigen	
	i	I
i_{cord}	Elevated	Diminished
i_{adult}	Elevated	Trace
I_{adult}	Diminished	Elevated

The Biochemical Nature of Ii Antigens. I antigen activity is located within or below the ABO molecular structure of the erythrocyte membrane. Ii antigen specificity appears to be located on the same chains that determine ABO specificity. These ABH structures exist as either straight or branched glycosphingolipid structures (see Chapter 4).

The type 2 oligosaccharide chains carrying the terminal carbohydrates that determine ABH specificity include multiple β-N-acetylglucosamine (1,3) and β-galactose (1,4) units. The i antigenic activity is thought to be formed by the straight chain oligosaccharides. In comparison, the erythrocytes of adults demonstrate that branched chains predominate. I specificity is associated with the branched chains. The transition of Ii antigenicity in the erythrocytes of a newborn infant to those of an adult is considered a reflection of the change from predominance of straight chains to predominance of branched chains.

The Ii antigens present on erythrocytes are also demonstrated on other blood cells such as leukocytes and platelets, and probably exist on many tissue cells, as do the ABH antigens. Both I and i as soluble glycoproteins are found in plasma, serum, and secretions, such as saliva, of newborn infants and adults. Human milk (colostrum) is known to be rich in I substance.

Disorders Associated with Ii Antigens. It is not uncommon to detect anti-I, as an autoantibody, if the serum of normal healthy adults is tested at room temperature or cooler. However, Anti-I is usually associated with cold agglutinin disease and atypical pneumonia caused by a pleuro-

pneumonia-like organism or *Mycoplasma pneumoniae*. Potent examples of auto-anti-I are rare but may be observed in patients with some forms of autoimmune disorders, such as cold autoimmune hemolytic anemia.

Anti-i antibody is classically associated with certain viral disorders, such as infectious mononucleosis caused by the Epstein-Barr virus and cytomegalovirus. It may also be seen in reticulosis, alcoholic cirrhosis, and myelogenous leukemia.

Rare examples of auto-anti-IH have been observed in cases of paroxysmal cold hemoglobinuria (PCH).

Ii Phenotypes. Except for unusual examples, the Ii phenotypes are straightforward. Cord blood cells demonstrate the lack of I antigen and are therefore referred to as i_{cord} and the erythrocytes of adults are I positive. Intermediate reactions can be observed in young children as the transition from i to I takes place. Rare examples of i and weak forms of I have been noted in adults.

Ii Antibodies. Most examples of anti-I are of the IgM type. This antibody is usually clinically insignificant; but it can be dangerous, if it masks other significant alloantibodies. To determine if other antibodies such as anti-M or anti-Le^a are also present, it is useful to adsorb the patient's serum (see Chapter 14) with the patient's enzyme-treated erythrocytes and then retest the adsorbed serum.

Anti-I reacts best at 4° C. It exhibits activity in saline, albumin, and with enzyme treatment. If an antibody agglutinates all adult cells, including an autocontrol, but fails to agglutinate cord blood cells, anti-I should be suspected.

The anti-I in patients with autoimmune disorders differs from the previously described autoantibody. Individuals who are i_{adult} will often produce an allo-anti-I that reacts at a wider thermal range and is a more potent antibody than auto-anti-I. This antibody could reduce survival of transfused erythrocytes and may warrant the use of I− blood, if transfusion is necessary.

Anti-i shares many of the characteristics of anti-I but reacts strongly with cord blood (Table 5-22).

Table 5-22. Sample Test Results with Typical Cold Antibodies

	I	i	H*	IH
A_1 (Adult)	4+	0–1+	0–1+	0–2+
A_2 (Adult)	4+	0–1+	2–3+	4+
B (Adult)	4+	0–1+	2–3+	4+
O (Adult)	4+	0–1+	4+	4+
O (cord)	0–2+	4+	3–4+	0–2+
Auto	0–4+	0–1+	0–2+	0–2+

* Anti-H is typical of the antibody that may be formed by A_1 and A_1B persons.

Typical IgG Antibody Systems Detectable by AHG Testing

THE KELL SYSTEM

This system was first defined in 1946, when the serum of the mother of a baby with hemolytic disease of the newborn (HDN) was found to contain anti-Kell. In 1949, the Kell antigen was subsequently matched with the hypothetical allele Cellano (k) and a new blood system was established. Two other pairs of antithetical antigens were subsequently identified: Kp^a (Penney, 1957) and Kp^b (Rautenberg, 1958); and Js^a (Sutter, 1958) and Js^b (Matthews, 1963). More than 20 antigens have been identified and incorporated into this blood group system.

Mode of Inheritance. The genes Kp^a and Kp^b, and Js^a and Js^b are believed to be inherited as a complex or cluster together with K/k. It is further believed that Kell antigens are controlled by an inherited gene complex or by one gene that codes for several antigenic determinants. The extremely rare K_O phenotype represents the null phenotype of the Kell system, a condition in which none of the six antigens is expressed. It is important to remember that K_O is not an antigen; it designates a phenotype.

The mode of inheritance of Kell system antigens appears to be complex. It is assumed that a precursor substance, K_x, is coded for by a gene X^1k on the X chromosome. This K_x precursor is then converted, perhaps by enzymatic (transferase) action, to the appropriate gene products of the inherited Kell genes (see Fig. 5-6). A K_O person is negative for all the previously described; but K_O cells are rich in K_x antigens.

The Biochemical Nature of Kell Antigens. Very little is known about the structure of Kell antigens. In addition to the presence of the glycoproteins portion of the antigenic determinant, questions remain about the role that the immunodominant carbohydrate mechanism may be playing in the development of Kell antigen specificity.

The Kell antigens are well-developed at birth. With the exception of K_x, the antigens seem to be restricted to the erythrocyte membrane. K_x is also found on the membranes of macrophages and neutrophilic leukocytes. The number of Kell antigen sites varies according to the phenotype. The KK phenotype has approximately 6000 Kell antigen sites, whereas the K+k+ phenotype has approximately 3500 Kell antigen sites.

Disorders Associated with Kell Antigens. Normal erythrocytes carry trace amounts of the K_x antigen. When a person lacks K_x on the red blood cell membrane, the McLeod phenotype results. In the absence of K_x, normal expression of inherited Kell genes is blocked. If some synthesis does occur, the resulting antigens react weakly, if at all.

The lack of K_x antigen is associated with abnormal erythrocytes (acanthocytes) that are prematurely destroyed, causing chronic hemolytic anemia. A lack of leukocytic K_x produces chronic granulomatous disease (CGD). Two types of CGD exist: Type I and Type II. In the Type I disorder, the usual Kell antigens, including K_x, are of normal strength. In Type II, many of the Kell antigens are weak and K_x is undetectable. Although both types of CGD lack leukocytic K_x, in Type II, the erythrocytes are of the McLeod phenotype.

Kell Phenotypes. The frequency of Kell blood group system antigens varies and racial differences exist. Certain combinations of antigens are common, whereas others are rare (Table 5-23).

Kell Antibodies. Kell (K) antigen has an immunogenicity second only to the D antigen. Because of the potency of the K antigen, anti-K is one of the most common immune erythrocyte antibodies and accounts for almost two-thirds of non-Rh im-

Table 5-23. Phenotypic Frequencies of the Major Kell Antigens

	White (%)	Black (%)
kk	91	96.5
Kk	8.8	3.5
KK	0.2	< 0.1
Js (a−b+)	> 99.9	80.5
Js (a+b−)	0.1	1.1
Js (a+b+)	0.1	18.4
Kp (a−b+)	98	—
Kp (a+b+)	2	—
Kp (a+b−)	< 0.1	—

mune alloantibodies. If a K− individual receives a unit of K+ blood, the chances are 1 in 10 that an alloantibody will be produced. Cases of nonerythrocyte-stimulated anti-K are infrequent. Kell blood group system antibodies have been implicated in both hemolytic transfusion reactions and hemolytic disease of the newborn (see Chapter 10 for a further discussion of HDN).

Anti-K is usually an IgG antibody detectable with anti-human globulin (AHG). Uncommon examples of IgM anti-K can be encountered, but they must be very potent to agglutinate red cells without AHG. Additionally, some examples bind complement and therefore sensitize erythrocytes. In these cases, agglutination can be detected with anti-complement as well as by anti-IgG AHG. Anti-K and anti-Js^b can also react with enzyme-treated cells.

Examples of anti-k are rare because only 2 persons in 1000 are k−. Other Kell blood group system antibodies, anti-Kp^a, anti-Kp^b, anti-Js^a, and anti-Js^b, are rare. Anti-Ku is found only in K$_o$ persons and reacts with all erythrocytes except those of the phenotype K$_o$. Anti-KL has been found in several patients with CGD or symptoms suggestive of it and reacts with the cells of all subjects except those of the McLeod phenotype.

THE DUFFY SYSTEM

The first member of the Duffy blood group system, Fy^a, was identified in 1950 in a multiply transfused hemophiliac named Duffy. The corresponding allele, Fy^b, was described in 1951. In 1965 it was discovered

that the erythrocytes of some Whites, previously assumed to be Fy− (heterozygous Fy^a− Fy^b−), were actually Fy^x. The Fy^x makes a very small amount of Fy^b. The exact relationship between Fy^b and Fy^x is unknown. In 1968, the Duffy locus was the first locus to be linked to an inherited visible abnormality, congenital cataract, on chromosome 1. The Duffy locus has the distinction of being the first locus in humans to be assigned to a particular autosome. The Fy^a and Fy^b genes are alleles at the same locus. Since 1970, three additional antigens, anti-Fy:3 (Fy:3), anti-Fy-4 (Fy:4), and anti-Fy:5 (Fy:5) have been identified. It is suspected that Fy:3 and Fy:4 are alleles at a different locus on the same gene.

Mode of Inheritance. The development of Duffy antigens is speculative. A proposed model (Fig. 5-7) suggests that a basic precursor substance is converted into an Fy precursor by the action of the hypothetical F gene. The locus of this gene is unknown, but it is believed to be independent of the Fy^a, Fy$^{b/x}$, Fy^3, and Fy^4 genes.

The Fy precursor substance can be acted on by inherited Fy blood group system genes (most Whites have Fy^a, Fy^b, or Fy^x genes) to produce their respective gene products. Another mechanism, possibly using the same genes, produces the simultaneous production of Fy:3 antigen. Fy:3 seems to be present on all erythrocytes, except Fy (a−b−) phenotypes. Fy:4 is of high antigen frequency in Blacks, most of whom have the Fy4Fy4 genotype and only produce Fy:4. If the F gene is absent, basic precursor substance fails to be converted; therefore, inherited Duffy genes cannot be expressed but an f individual is able to transmit Fy^a and Fy^b genes normally.

It is speculated that production of Fy:5 antigen results from interaction between normal Rh genes and normal Fy genes (Fy^a, Fy^b, Fy^x). If a person possesses a normal Rh phenotype and has either Fy^a or Fy^b genes, Fy:5 antigen is produced, even the Fy (a−b−) type produces the Fy:5 antigen. Fy:5 antigen is absent in the Fy:4 type Fy(a−b−), who has neither Fy^a nor Fy^b genes, and an Rh$_{null}$ person who has no Rh antigens. A person of the Rh gene deletion types, D--, produces a limited quantity of Fy:5. Fy:5 is found on the erythrocytes of

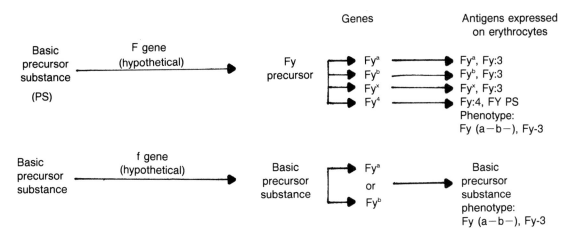

Figure 5-7. Theoretical mechanism of expression of Duffy antigens.

most Whites, but is not as widespread in Blacks.

The Fy^a, Fy^b, Fy:3 and Fy:5 antigens are significantly developed at birth. The appearance of Fy:4 has not been as well documented.

The Biochemical Nature of Duffy Antigens. The Duffy antigens are well developed on fetal cells. The number of Fy^a antigen sites on Fy^aFy^a erythrocytes is estimated at 12,000. These antigens are probably protein in nature and are destroyed by in vitro treatment with proteolytic enzymes, such as ficin and papain. Dosage effects are common, but not all antibodies detect the dosage effect.

Disorders Associated with Duffy Antigens. It is believed that, for certain malarial parasites (*Plasmodium vivax*) to enter erythrocytes, Fy^a or Fy^b antigens must be present. In Africa, where malaria is endemic, natives have been found to be resistant to *Plasmodium vivax*. This resistance is undoubtedly related to the fact that almost all the native population has the Fy(a−b−) phenotype. This phenomenon may reflect a natural defense mechanism that has persisted through natural selection. American Blacks have partially lost this characteristic because of interracial genetic mixing and the lack of need for such a defense mechanism.

Duffy Phenotypes. The frequency of Duffy blood group system antigens (Fy^a and Fy^b) exhibits more racial differences between Whites and Blacks than any of the other major blood group systems, but these differences are less pronounced among Blacks in the United States than in Africa. The most predominant antigen in Whites is Fy^a. Many Blacks lack both Fy^a and Fy^b antigens. The phenotypic distribution in the United States is presented in Table 5-24.

Duffy Antibodies. Compared to the D and Kell antigens, Fy^a and Fy^b do not appear to be strongly antigenic; therefore the Duffy antibodies are seen about three times less frequently than anti-K. Duffy antibodies tend to occur more frequently in Whites than in Blacks. When Duffy antibodies are observed, anti-Fy^a is more frequent. Anti-Fy^b usually occurs in sera with multiple antibodies rather than as a single antibody. Duffy antibodies are almost always stimulated by erythrocyte antigen exposure through transfusion or pregnancy. Anti-Fy^a occasionally causes hemolytic disease of the newborn, but has frequently been im-

Table 5-24. Phenotypic Distribution of Duffy Antigens in the American Population

Phenotype	Frequency White (%)	Black (%)
Fy (a+b−)	18	14
Fy (a+b+)	49	2
Fy (a−b−)	33	19
Fy (a−b−)	0	65

plicated as a cause of hemolytic transfusion reactions. Fy^b can be a cause of fatal transfusion reactions.

Anti-Fy^a and anti-Fy^b are found mostly as IgG immunoglobulins. The most sensitive method of detecting these antibodies is AHG testing. If enzyme testing is employed, anti-Fy^a may bind complement. It is important to note that the Fy^a antigen is destroyed by most enzymes.

An individual with the phenotype Fy(a−b−),Fy:3−, Fy:4 does not produce antibodies to the antigens he lacks because Duffy precursor substance is a similar structure. These antigens are not recognized as foreign. Anti-Fy:3 reacts with all human erythrocytes except those of the phenotype Fy(a−b−). Individuals with the phenotype Fy(a−b−),Fy:3− have been rarely noted to produce anti-Fy:3 because of the lack of Fy precursor. All Fy antigens, however, are recognized as foreign.

Anti-Fy:3 is not deteriorated by enzyme treatment and reacts with all Fy^a+ and Fy^b+ cells. It does not react with Fy(a−b−) cells. This antibody has been consistently observed in the serum of non-Black Fya−b− individuals.

Anti-Fy:4 was first identified in the serum of a multiply transfused Fy(a+b+) child. It reacts with all Fy(a−b−) erythrocytes and some Fy^a or Fy^b+ erythrocytes but not with Fy(a+b+) erythrocytes. If enzyme-treated erythrocytes are used in antibody detection, the antigen resists degradation by proteolytic enzymes.

Anti-Fy:5 has been identified. The antibody reacts with AHG and enzyme-treated erythrocytes. Reactivity of the antibody is similar to anti-Fy:3, except that it also reacts with Fy(a−b−) erythrocytes, does not react with Rh null erythrocytes of the usual Duffy phenotypes, and reacts weakly with -D-/-D- erythrocytes.

THE KIDD SYSTEM

The first example of the Kidd blood group system, Jk^a, was identified in 1951. The antithetical gene, Jk^b, was found in 1953. In 1959, Jk3, which is apparently a universal antigen, was discovered. Examples of the rare phenotype Jk(a−b−) Kidd null have also been recognized. It has been suggested that Jk^aJk^b is a distinct specific antigen in this system and probably a fundamental one in the Kidd system.

Mode of Inheritance. The Jk^a and Jk^b genes are known to be codominant alleles, but the mechanism of antigen expression in the Kidd system has not been well defined. In the case of the rare Kidd null phenotype, it is believed that it may arise from one of two mechanisms. Homozygous inheritance of an amorphic Jk gene is one explanation, and the inheritance of a suppressor gene that prevents Jk^a/Jk^b expression on erythrocytes is the other.

The Biochemical Nature of Kidd Antigens. Only a limited amount of information is known about the nature and structure of the Kidd antigens, which are known to be well developed at birth. They are also low in immunogenicity. In laboratory testing, the antigens are not destroyed by enzyme treatment; in fact, ficin and trypsin have been observed to enhance reactions. Questions remain as to whether Jk^a and Jk^b exist on cells other than erythrocytes.

Kidd Phenotypes. The phenotypes and frequencies of the two antigens of the Kidd system are given in Table 5-25. The phenotype lacking both antigens is rare.

Kidd Antibodies. Kidd antibodies are infrequently encountered. Anti-Jk^b is rarer than anti-Jk^a and is usually found in sera with other immune alloantibodies. Although Kidd antibodies have been known to cause mild hemolysis, they are extremely dangerous because they disappear from the circulation rapidly and may produce violent delayed hemolytic transfusion reactions. Anti-Jk^a has the reputation of causing in vivo destruction, which is much greater than might be expected from the reactions produced in vitro.

Table 5-25. Phenotypes of Kidd System

Phenotype	Genotype	Frequency White (%)	Black (%)
Jk (a+b−)	Jk^aJk^a	25	75
Jk (a+b+)	Jk^aJk^b	50	34
Jk (a−b+)	Jk^bJk^b	25	9
Jk (a−b−)*	JkJk	0	0

* Rare individuals of this type have been found among South American Indians and Chinese.

Kidd antibodies are usually of the IgG type, but may also be either IgM or a combination of both types. These antibodies are often complement-dependent, very labile on storage, and most easily detected in fresh serum. All the examples of Kidd antibodies have been shown to react in AHG and not in saline, and all react with enzyme treatment. AHG reactions with anticomplement are distinctly stronger, and in some cases positive reactions are observed only with anticomplement antisera. Dosage effects may be observed. Anti-JK^a frequently exhibits dosage effects and may be positive only with Jk^{a}Jk^a erythrocytes.

OTHER BLOOD GROUP SYSTEMS

Xg

One of the most unique blood groups is the sex-linked Xg system. The Xg^a antigen is the only presently recognized antigen in this system. An antithetic allele (Xg) has not been identified. Individuals are of either the Xg(a+) or Xg(a−) phenotype. Because the Xg^a antigen is X-linked, it is more likely to occur in women than in men.

The frequency of the phenotype Xg(a+) is approximately 88% in women and 64% in men. The genotype of women may be Xg^{a}Xg^a, Xg^{a}Xg, or XgXg, but men can be only Xg^a or Xg. Men who are Xg(a+) pass on Xg^a to all their daughters but transmit no Xg genes to their sons. The mating of an Xg(a+) man with an Xg(a−) woman must produce all Xg(a+) daughters and Xg(a−) sons.

Anti-Xg^a is an uncommon antibody. Rare examples of auto anti-Xg^a in Xg(a+) individuals have been reported. Some examples of the antibody react at room temperature or 37° C, but most of these antibodies react in the AHG phase of testing. Anti-Xg^a has not been associated with either hemolytic transfusion reactions or hemolytic disease of the newborn.

Sid

Sd^a, the only defined antigen in this system, is inherited as an autosomal dominant character and appears to be genetically independent of most other blood group systems. Rare cases have demonstrated an enhanced erythrocyte antigen, called Sd(a++) or "Super Sid," and another form of Sd^a, named Cad, was originally thought to be a form of inherited polyagglutinability. The incidence of Sd^a antigen is <90%. This antigen is often difficult to work with because of a wide variation in antigenic expression; it is known to be weaker during pregnancy. A possible relationship exists between Sd^a and Cad antigens and the ABO system.

Sd^a substance is present in most body secretions. Four times as much Sd^a is found in the saliva of newborn infants as in the saliva of adults. Because the greatest concentration of Sd^a occurs in the urine, it is sometimes easier to categorize apparent weak Sd(a+) persons by testing their urine.

Anti-Sd^a is characteristically weakly reactive. Some Sd^a antibodies react at room temperature, 37° C, and AHG. Most examples of anti-Sd^a are demonstrable with enzyme-treated red cells and cells enhanced with LISS. Observable agglutinates have a characteristic refractile, mixed-field appearance.

Although a hemolytic transfusion reaction caused by anti-Sd^a was reported in 1970, the antibody is not generally associated with hemolytic transfusion reactions, even if incompatible blood is transfused, or with HDN.

An autoantibody, Sd^x, has been described which seems to define an erythrocyte receptor related to Sd^a. The antibody, which is inhibited by Sd(a+) urine but not by Sd(a+) urine, has been responsible for rare cases of cold antibody autoimmune hemolytic anemia.

Cartwright

Yt^a is a common antigen, found on the erythrocytes of <99% of both the White and Black population. The Yt^b antigen has a frequency of about 8% in both Whites and Blacks. The Yt^a antigen was defined in 1956 and the allele, Yt^b, in 1964.

Anti-Yt^a is not uncommon in Yt(a−) persons with a history of pregnancy or transfusion. In contrast, anti-Yt^b is a rare antibody usually found in combination with other antibodies. Both anti-Yt^a and anti-Yt^b are usually reactive in AHG and with LISS enhancement. Some examples are reactive in enzyme-enhanced red cell suspensions.

Anti-Yt^a has been implicated in both hemolytic transfusion reactions and HDN. Anti-Yt^b has also been associated with HDN.

Colton

Two antigens, Co^a and Co^b, have been identified in this system. About 99.8% of the White population are Co(a+) and about 10% are Co(b+). American Blacks may have a lower incidence of Co(a−).

Anti-Co^a and anti-Co^b were identified in 1974. These antibodies are IgG in nature and have been associated with pregnancy with an incompatible fetus. Both Co^a and Co^b can be detected in the AHG phase of testing. Enzyme enhancement of erythrocytes allows most examples of both antibodies to be demonstrated. Anti-Co^a can cause both hemolytic transfusion reactions and hemolytic disease of the newborn. Anti-Co^b has been implicated in hemolytic transfusion reactions.

Dombrock

The antigens Do^a and Do^b are the two demonstrable antigens of this system. Approximately 67% of Whites are Do(a+) and about 83% are Do(b+). The incidence of Do^a is lower in Blacks, American Indians, and Orientals.

Both anti-Do^a and anti-Do^b are infrequently encountered. Most examples of both antibodies are reactive in AHG and in enzyme and LISS enhancement. Anti-Do^a has been associated with hemolytic transfusion reactions.

Diego

Di^a was identified in 1955. All Whites are Di(a−), and approximately 36% of certain South American Indians are Di(a+). Five to 15% of Japanese and Chinese are Di(a+). The Di^b antigen was identified in 1967, when the first two examples of anti-Di^b were described. The frequency of Di^b is 100% in Whites and undetermined in other racial groups.

Some examples of anti-Di^a react at room temperature, 37° C, and with enzyme enhancement. Most Di^a antibodies react in the AHG phase. Anti-Di^b generally reacts in AHG, but some examples are reactive with enzyme-enhanced erythrocytes. Both antibodies have been implicated in hemolytic transfusion reactions and HDN.

Scianna

The Scianna (SC) blood group is inherited in a dominant Mendelian manner and occupies a locus on chromosome 1. SC1, a very high-frequency antigen, was originally called Sm^1. SC2, a very low-frequency antigen, was initially referred to as Bu^a before it was realized that Sc^1 and Sc^2 were, in all probability, alleles. Sc1 and Sc2 are now considered antithetic antigens. The most frequent phenotype is Sc:1,−2, but the incidence of Sc 2 antigen is higher in the Mennonite population than in other Whites. Both anti-Sc1 and Sc2 are uncommon antibodies and have not been implicated in transfusion reactions or HDN.

In 1980, the existence of a third antigen in the Scianna blood group system was suggested after an alloantibody directed against a high-frequency red cell antigen was identified in a Sc:−1,−2 patient. The Sc:−1,−2 phenotype is rare. The findings in three cases of patients who developed IgG alloantibodies directed against red blood cell antigens that were not present on Sc null cells suggest that red cells of this phenotype may lack additional Sc antigens or have no expression of other unrelated high-frequency antigens. It is possible, however, that Sc:−1,−2 red cells represent an Sc null phenotype similar to the Rh$_{null}$ phenotype of the Rh blood group system or the K$_o$ of the Kell blood group system.

HUMAN LEUKOCYTE ANTIGENS (HLA) DETECTABLE ON ERYTHROCYTES

In the late 1950s and early 1960s, researchers identified antibodies that were contaminants in many typing sera. These antibodies were frequently found in multiparous women, often with isoleukoagglutinins. They are enhanced by the enzymes trypsin and papain but destroyed by the enzyme, bromelin, and best detected with fresh erythrocytes collected into ACD anticoagulant.

The corresponding antigens to these antibodies vary within families as well as in individuals over a period of time, and are not fully expressed at birth. These antigens were initially classified as Bg^a and Bg^b with the "Bennett-Goodspeed" group. Later, a third antigen, Bg^c, was defined.

In 1969, the erythrocyte antigen Bg^a was correlated with the leukocyte antigen HLA-B7. This was the first leukocyte antigen to be demonstrated on erythrocytes. The antigen frequency on erythrocytes is about 17% in both White and Black populations. In 1971, the identification of Bg^b as HLA-B17 and Bg^c as HLA-A28 was reported. The frequency of Bg^b is approximately 9% in Whites and 28% in Blacks. Bg^c has a frequency of about 8% in Whites and approximately 17% in Blacks. Most, if not all, HLA antigens may be present on erythrocytes, but the Bg antigens, particularly Bg^a and Bg^c, are remarkable because they give much stronger reactions than other HLA antigens. These antigens, however, cannot be detected on the erythrocytes of all individuals possessing the same antigens on their leukocytes. Enzyme treatment of red cells may depress some Bg reactivity and enhance others. Bg^a is more likely than Bg^b to be weakened by proteolytic enzymes.

The Bg, or hemagglutinating HLA antibodies, may be detected in multiparous or multitransfused patients. The incidence of anti-Bg^a is approximately 1.5%. It is exceedingly difficult to test a high-frequency antibody for accompanying HLA antibodies, and the possibility of such contamination must be considered when discrepant or weaker than expected results are obtain. The identification of low-frequency erythrocyte antibodies is also menaced by the possible presence of HLA antibodies.

HIGH-INCIDENCE ANTIGENS UNRELATED TO THE PRINCIPAL BLOOD GROUP SYSTEMS

Antigens of high frequency are defined as occurring in 99.9% of the population. Ex-

amples of high-frequency antigens that are apparently unrelated to principal blood group systems include Augustine (At^a), Cromer (Cr^a), En^a, Gerbich (Ge), Gregory (Gy^a) and Holley (Hy), Jacobs (Jr^a), Joseph (Jo^a), Langereis (Lan), Ok^a, and Vel (Ve). It should be noted, however, that the At $(a-)$, Cr $(a-)$, and Jo $(a-)$ phenotypes are found predominantly in Blacks. In addition, Ok^a has been found only in one family of Japanese origin.

Antibodies to the high incidence antigens are rarely observed. Some of these, such as anti-Vel, are IgM antibodies and bind complement. Others, such as anti-Ge, are more commonly AHG-reactive. Anti-Vel and probably anti-Ge are considered clinically significant antibodies.

LOW-INCIDENCE ANTIGENS UNRELATED TO THE PRINCIPAL BLOOD GROUP SYSTEMS

Low-incidence antigens unrelated to the principal blood group systems are defined as antigens with an incidence of less than 1%. Examples of this type of antigen include the Wright blood group system, which is independent of all other blood group systems, as well as the Swann (Sw^a), By, Mt^a, and Tr^a antigens. In general, these antigens are unimportant in blood transfusion because it is easy to find compatible blood for patients who develop corresponding antibodies to these antigens.

Wright

The antigen Wr^a is present in about 2 in 1000 blood samples in the White population.

Anti-Wr^a is a frequently occurring antibody; it can be detected in 1 in 100 persons. It has even been identified in men who have never been transfused. Anti-Wr^a is often found in the serum of patients who have formed other blood group antibodies and in the serum of patients with autoimmune hemolytic anemia.

Anti-Wr^a has been reported to occur in both IgM and IgG forms. The phases of reactivity range from room temperature to AHG. Some examples react with enzyme-enhanced erythrocytes. It has been implicated in both hemolytic transfusion reactions and HDN.

HIGH-TITER, LOW-AVIDITY (HTLA) ANTIBODIES

The high-titer, low-avidity (HTLA) antibodies are collectively considered together because they show a similar pattern of serologic reactions. The name HTLA refers to the fact that these antibodies exhibit reactivity at high dilutions of serum but weak agglutination at any dilution. This characteristic differentiates HTLA antibodies from other blood group antibodies that demonstrate progressively weaker reactivity with increased dilution of the antibody-containing serum.

The HTLA antibodies most frequently encountered are those directed at the high-frequency antigens: York (Yk^a) and Cost-Stirling (Cs^a), Knops-Helgeson (Kn^a) and McCoy (McC^a), Chido (Ch^a) and Rodgers (Rg^a), and John Milton Hagen (JMH). The Chido and HLA loci are linked. Rodgers, like Chido, is linked to the HLA-B locus. It has recently been shown that Ch^a and Rg^a are, in fact, antigens on C$_4$ molecules.

Antibodies to these antigens characteristically exhibit varying degrees of reactivity with different samples of antigen-positive erythrocytes. This variability is particularly marked with Ch^a and Rg^a. Most of the HTLA antibodies are reactive in the AHG phase of testing.

Chido antibody is a common cause of difficulty in crossmatching in previously transfused patients. This antibody is absorbed by the leukocytes of Ch(a+) individuals and neutralized by the plasma and serum but not the saliva of Ch(a−) individuals. Anti-Ch^a does not reduce the survival of Ch(a+) erythrocytes in vivo. Both anti-Ch^a and anti-Rg^a react more weakly with enzyme-treated cells than with untreated cells. A characteristic of Rg(a+) erythrocytes is that cells stored as a clot react more strongly than fresh cells.

The clinical significance of the HTLA antibodies is questionable, but there is little evidence that most of them cause hemolytic

transfusion reactions. Anti-McC^a has been associated with such reactions and probably with HDN. It is important, however, to distinguish HTLA antibodies from low-titered antibodies to high-incidence antigens, such as Kp^b, Lan, and Vel.

CHAPTER SUMMARY

The Rh System

The Rh system was identified in 1940 by Landsteiner and Wiener, who originally found that human erythrocytes were agglutinated by an antibody apparently common to all rhesus monkeys and 85% of humans. This factor was named the Rh factor. The Rh-hr blood group system is probably the most complex of all red cell blood group systems, with more than 40 different Rh antigens. The descriptive terms Rh positive and Rh negative refer *only* to the presence or absence of the red cell antigen D. Four additional genes (C, E, c, and e) are recognized as belonging to the Rh system.

The CDE and Rh-hr systems of nomenclature in the Rh system are equivalent. In the clinical laboratory only five reagent antisera are commonly available for the D, C, c, E, and e antigens. Routine testing involves only the use of anti-D, but other antisera are used to resolve antibody problems or conduct family studies.

Multiple research studies agree that the Rh antigens are present on a protein structure and are probably all on the same polypeptide chain. It appears probable that membrane lipids are restricted to a supporting role at the phenotypic level. Simple antigens such as D, C, and E presumably represent certain amino acid sequences. However antigens like G represent some of the amino acids of D and some others. Antigens such as rh are thought to represent repressed amino acids of C and e located adjacently in the R^1 and r^1 specified folded polypeptide, but apart when R^z and r make separate polypeptides for the same cell membrane. The Rh antigens exhibit numerous serologic complexities that undoubtedly represent an extremely complicated polypeptide.

The production or nonproduction of D, as well as the production of either C or c and E or e antigens, is genetically determined. Rh antigen sites are believed to be randomly distributed on the red cell membrane. The expression of an inherited gene can be affected by the interaction between genes. When an *Rh* gene on one chromosome affects the action of another Rh gene on the same chromosome, in terms of increased or decreased antigen production, it is referred to as a *cis* effect. When an Rh gene on one of the chromosomes of a homologous pair affects the actions of an Rh gene on the other homolog, it is called a *trans* effect. The most dramatic *Rh trans* position effect known occurs when C is in *trans* to D (Cde/Cde), weakening the D antigen. This is one reason for the D^u phenotype, but it is now recognized that the D^u phenotype can also arise in two other ways: the inheritance of a gene that codes for less D antigen (weak D), and the absence of a portion or portions of the total material that comprise the D antigen (the D mosaic).

Rh positive blood rarely lacks any of the mosaic components. However, a different system of classifying D positive persons who produce anti-D was devised in 1962. The six categories of antibody formers are referred to as I, II, III, IV, V, and VI, based on the reactions of erythrocytes with anti-D from these individuals, as well as the specificity of the anti-D produced.

The e antigen of some Blacks may be a mosaic-type structure. The appearance of e-like antibodies made by e positive individuals is analogous to the anti-D made by individuals with the D mosaic. More than 40 other Rh antigens have been identified, including the G and V antigens. The term compound antigen is used to communicate the idea that certain combinations of Rh antigens demonstrate a combined effect. An example of a compound antigen is the ce or f antigen. Variant antigens also exist. The antigen C^w is an example of a variant antigen. There are some rare Rh genes that behave as if portions of the genetic material have been deleted or rendered nonfunctional. The first recognized case was the D-deletion gene (D− −). When no Rh antigens are expressed on the red cell membrane, the term Rh null is used to describe this phenotype; if a less complete type of suppressed Rh gene expression is observed, the term Rh mod is used. The LW antigen, which was demonstrated with the original animal anti-rhesus sera, was named in honor of Landsteiner and Wiener. It is now recognized as distinct from the D antigen. This antigen is present on rhesus monkey erythrocytes and on most human erythrocytes.

The Rh antibodies are predominantly of the immunoglobulin class IgG. Most Rh antibodies result from erythrocyte immunization due to pregnancy or transfusion. Some Rh antibodies commonly occur together.

The Lewis System

The two common antigens of the Lewis system are Lewis^a (Le^a) and Lewis^b (Le^b). The Lewis blood group system is unlike the other blood group system in that genetic control of the two antigens Le^a and Le^b appears to reside in a single gene called Le. This system represents a complex interaction between the independent Lewis, ABO, and secretor genes and is best understood by thinking of it as a system of genetically determined water-soluble antigens present in body fluids and body secretions.

The Lewis system differs from other blood group systems in three significant ways. These differences include the fact that Lewis substances are absorbed from the plasma rather than being membrane-bound antigens, the Lewis phenotype is influenced by the secretor status, and the Lewis phenotype may be modified by the ABO phenotype. In addition, the Lewis gene does not code directly for the production of Lewis antigens.

Lewis antibodies are frequently found in individuals who have never been transfused or received any other known erythrocyte antigen stimulus. Anti-Le^a and anti-Le^b are especially common in pregnant women. Rare cases of hemolytic disease of the newborn (HDN) attributed to anti-Le^a and Lewis antibodies have been cited as the cause in a few hemolytic transfusion reactions.

Additional Major Blood Group Systems

In addition to the ABO, Rh, and Lewis blood group systems, other blood group systems also exist. The typically IgM antibody systems that are best detected at cold temperatures include MNSsU, P, and I systems. The typically IgG antibody systems detectable by antiglobulin (AHG) testing include the Kell, Duffy, and Kidd systems.

Initially, the Lewis and Lutheran genes were believed to be linked, but it was later discovered that the Lutheran genes were actually linked to the gene-controlling secretor status. The Lu^a and Lu^b genes are codominant. The $Lu(a-b+)$ phenotype is the most common and the $Lu(a-b-)$ is the rarest. The Lutheran antibodies, particularly Anti-Lu^a, are infrequently observed but are known to occur with no known erythrocyte stimulus in most cases. Most examples of anti-Lu^b are associated with known exposure to erythrocyte antigen through transfusion or pregnancy.

The M and N antigens are classically associated with paternity testing. The MnSs system includes a group of mostly low-frequency "satellite" antigens rarely of clinical significance. Several of these low-frequency antigens are considered interrelated and form the Miltenberger subsystem. Three phenotypes, MM, NN, and MN, and 10 genotypes exist in the MNSs blood group system. Antibodies of the MNSs blood group system are usually considered of minor clinical significance, but anti-S and anti-s are usually erythrocyte-stimulated IgG antibodies and can produce HDN or transfusion reactions. Four antigens are recognized in the P system: P_1, P, P^k, and p. In cases of paroxysmal cold hemoglobinuria, the associated antibody is usually auto-anti-P.

The Ii system appears to include only two antigens, I and i. This blood group system sometimes interacts with the ABO, I, Lewis, and P systems to form compound antibodies such as anti-IP_1, anti-ILe^{bH}, and anti-IH.

The Kell blood group system consists of Kell and its allele, Cellano (k), as well as two other major pairs of antithetic antigens, Kp^a (Penney) and Kp^b (Rautenberg); and Js^a (Sutter) and Js^b (Matthews). More than 20 antigens have been identified and incorporated into this blood group system. The Kell antigen has a strength of immunogenicity second only to the D antigen. Because of the potency of the K antigen, anti-K is one of the most common immune red blood cell antibodies and accounts for almost two thirds of non–Rh-immune red cell alloantibodies.

In the Duffy blood group system, the Fy^a and Fy^b genes are alleles at the same locus. Three additional antigens, anti-Fy3 (Fy:3), anti-Fy-4 (Fy:4), and anti-Fy-5 (Fy:5), have been identified. Compared to the D and Kell antigens, Fy^a and Fy^b do not appear strongly antigenic; therefore the Duffy antibodies are seen about three times less frequently than anti-K. These antibodies are almost always stimulated by erythrocyte antigen exposure through transfusion or pregnancy. Anti-Fy^a occasionally causes HDN, but has more frequently been implicated as a cause of hemolytic transfusion reactions. Fy^b can cause fatal transfusion reactions.

In the Kidd blood group system, the Jk^a and Jk^b genes are known to be codominant alleles. Kidd antibodies are infrequently encountered. Although Kidd antibodies have been known to cause mild hemolysis, they are extremely dangerous because they disappear from the circulation rapidly and produce violent delayed hemolytic transfusion reactions.

Other Blood Group Systems

The category of miscellaneous blood groups represents more than 300 blood group antigens, which may or may not belong to independent blood group systems such as the Xg^a, Wright, Diego, and Colton systems. One of the most unique blood groups is the sex-linked Xg system. Sd^a is the only defined antigen in the Sid system. Rare cases have demonstrated an enhanced erythrocyte antigen, called Sd (a++) or "Super Sid," and another form of Sd^a named Cad, was originally thought to be a form of inherited polyagglutinability. The Cartwright system consists of the high-frequency Yt^a antigen and the low-frequency antigen Yt^b. The Colton system, like the

Cartwright system, consist of two antigens, the high-frequency Co^a antigen and the low-frequency Co^b antigen. In the Dombrock system, Do^a and Do^b are the two demonstrable antigens of the system. Approximately 67% of Whites are Do(a+) and about 83% are Do(b+). The incidence of Do^a is lower in Blacks, American Indians, and Orientals. The first Diego blood system antigen, Di^a, was identified in 1955. All Whites are Di(a−) and approximately 36% of certain South American Indians are Di(a+). Five to 15% Japanese and Chinese are Di(a+). The Di^b antigen was identified in 1967 and the frequency of Di^b is 100% in Whites and undetermined in other racial groups. In the Scianna blood group system, Sc1 and Sc2 are now considered antithetic antigens. The most frequent phenotype is Sc:1, −2.

Human Leukocyte Antigens (HLA) Detectable on Erythrocytes

In 1969, the erythrocyte antigen Bg^a was correlated with the leukocyte antigen HLA-B7. This was the first leukocyte antigen to be demonstrated on erythrocytes. In 1971, the identification of Bg^b as HLA-B17 and Bg^c as HLA-A28 was reported. Most, if not all, HLA antigens may be present on erythrocytes, but the Bg antigens, particularly Bg^a and Bg^c, are remarkable because they give much stronger reactions than other HLA antigens. These antigens, however, cannot be detected on the erythrocytes of all individuals possessing the same antigens on their leukocytes.

High-Incidence Antigens Unrelated to the Principal Blood Group Systems

Antigens of high frequency are defined as occurring in 99.9% of the population. Examples of high frequency antigens apparently unrelated to principal blood group systems include Augustine (At^a), Cromer (Cr^a), En^a, Gerbich (Ge), Gregory (Gy^a) and Holley (Hy), Jacobs (Jr^a), Joseph (Jo^a), Langereis (Lan), Ok^a, Vel (Ve). It should be noted, however, that the At (a−), Cr (a−), and Jo (a−) phenotypes are found predominantly in Blacks. In addition, Ok^a has been found only in one family of Japanese origin.

Low-Incidence Antigens Unrelated to the Principal Blood Group Systems

Low-incidence antigens that are unrelated to the principal blood group systems are defined as antigens with an incidence of less than 1%. Examples of this type of antigen include the Wright blood group system, which is independent of all other blood group systems, and the Swann (Sw^a), By, Mt^a, and Tr^a antigens.

The antigen Wr^a is present in about 2 in 1000 blood samples in the White population. Anti-Wr^a is a frequently occurring antibody.

High-Titer, Low-Avidity Antibodies

The high-titer, low-avidity (HTLA) antibodies are collectively considered together because they show a similar pattern of serologic reactions. The name HTLA refers to the fact that these antibodies exhibit reactivity at high dilutions of serum but weak agglutination at any dilution. The HTLA antibodies most frequently encountered are those directed at the high-frequency antigens, York (Yk^a) and Cost-Stirling (Cs^a), Knops-Helgeson (Kn^a) and McCoy (McC^a), Chido (Ch^a) and Rodgers (Rg^a), and John Milton Hagen (JMH).

REVIEW QUESTIONS

1. The term Rh positive refers to the presence of:
   A. Anti-D
   B. D antigen
   C. C antigen
   D. E antigen
   E. c antigen
2. The symbol R is used for haplotypes that include:
   A. c
   B. Rh_o
   C. r
   D. D
   E. Both B and D

3–7: Match the following examples of equivalent nomenclature:

Fisher-Race	Wiener
3. D	**A.** hr′
4. c	**B.** rh′
5. E	**C.** RH$_o$
6. e	**D.** rh″
7. C	**E.** hr″

8–13. Match the following Fischer-Race terms with their respective shorthand symbols:

8. CDe	**A.** R^2
9. cDE	**B.** R^O
10. cDe	**C.** r
11. CDE	**D.** R^Z
12. cde	**E.** R^1
13. CdE	**F.** r^y

14. The most common Rh haplotype in Whites is:
  A. R^1R^1
  B. R^1R^2
  C. $R'r$
  D. rr
  E. R^2r

15. The most common Rh haplotype in Blacks is:
  A. R^or
  B. R^oR^o
  C. $R'R^o$
  D. $R'r$
  E. rr

16. Based on the following reactions, what is this person's most probable genotype?

Antisera

Anti-D	Anti-C	Anti-E	Anti-c	Anti-e
+	0	+	+	0

  A R^1r
  B. R^2R^2
  C. R^zR^z
  D. R^or
  E. R^1R^1

17. The highest number of D antigen sites is found on erythrocytes of which genotype?
  A. cDE/cDE
  B. CDe/CDe
  C. CDe/cde
  D. cde/cde
  E. *Both C and D*

18. When an Rh gene on one chromosome affects the action of another Rh gene on the same chromosome, in terms of increased or decreased antigen production, it is referred to as:
  A. Cis effect
  B. Trans effect
  C. Either cis or trans effect

19. A D^u phenotype resulting from gene suppression is characterized by:
  A. The action of a C gene
  B. A trans position effect
  C. Low grade D^u activity
  D. Being more common in Whites
  E. Both A and B

20. Phenotypically erythrocytes of the D mosaic type react similarly to:
  A. Low grade D^u
  B. High grade D^u
  C. D positive RBCs
  D. D^u negative RBCs
  E. Both A and D

21. The Go^a antigen is:
  A. Part of the Rh system
  B. Found on D mosaic type of RBCs
  C. Found in 1.9-2.8% of American Blacks
  D. Identical to D^{COR}
  E. All of the above

22. The D____ phenotype does not code for the production of ____ antigen.
  A. D
  B. C
  C. c
  D. E
  E. All of the above, except **A**

23. When no Rh antigens are expressed on the RBC membrane, the term ____ is used to express the phenotype.
  A. Rh mod
  B. Rh null
  C. −D−
  D. CD−
  E. None of the above

24–27. Match the following:

24. G antigen	**A.** Compound antigen
25. V antigen	**B.** Antibodies resemble anti-C + anti-D
26. f antigen	
27. C^W	**C.** Example of a variant antigen
	D. Product of R^o, R^{OU}, or r genes

28. The following is/are true of L-W antigen:

A. Strength is related to the presence or absence of D antigen
B. Is negative in cases of Rh null phenotype
C. Is a high incidence antigen of human RBCs
D. Is the same as the Rho antigen
E. All of the above, except **D**

29. Rh antibodies are predominantly:
    A. IgM
    B. IgG
    C. IgD
    D. IgA
    E. IgE

30–35 are true or false. Indicate A for true, B for false.

30. Most Rh antibodies are stimulated by RBC antigens
31. In vitro binding of complement is common
32. The c antigen is the most potent immunogen of all of the Rh antigens
33. Anti-e is a frequently encountered antibody
34. Anti-E and anti-c are commonly found together
35. Dosage effects may be observed with E, c, or e

36. A person of the genotype rr could potentially produce antibodies of the following Rh specificity, if appropriately stimulated:
    A. Anti-D
    B. Anti-C
    C. Anti-E
    D. Anti-c
    E. All of the above, except **D**

37. Select the appropriate characteristic(s) of the Lewis blood group system:
    A. Antigens are membrane-bound lipoproteins
    B. Expression of antigens is influenced by the secretor status
    C. Antigens are adsorbed from the plasma
    D. Antigen expression may be modified by ABO antigens
    E. All of the above, except **A**

38. Inheritance of sese genes and the Lewis gene produces the following phenotype:
    A. Le a+b−
    B. Le a+b+
    C. Le a−b+

D. Le a−b−
E. None of the above

39. Inheritance of Sese and the Lewis gene produces:
    A. Le a+b−
    B. Le a+b+
    C. Le a−b+
    D. Le a−b−
    E. None of the above

40–44. Complete the following table.

Genes	In Secretions	On Erythrocytes
H, Se, A, _40_	H,A, Le^a, Le^b	H, A, Le^b
H, Se, OO, Le	H, Le^a, Le^b	H, _41_
H, Se, A, lele	H, A	H, A
H, sese, A, Le	H, A, _42_	H, A, _43_
hh, _44_, Le^a A, Le	Le^a	Le^a

A. se
B. Le
C. Le^a
D. no Le^a or Le^b
E. Se

40. ___
41. ___
42. ___
43. ___
44. ___

45–48. Complete the flow diagram on page 164. An answer can be used more than once.

A. Le(a−b−)   45. ___
B. Le(a+b−)   46. ___
C. Le(a−b+)   47. ___
D. Le(a+b+)   48. ___
E. lele

49. The most common Lewis phenotype is:
    A. Le(a+b−)
    B. Le(a−b+)
    C. Le(a+b+)
    D. Le(a−b−)
    E. Both B and C

50. Select the appropriate characteristic or characteristics of the Lewis antibodies:
    A. Predominantly IgG and most frequently anti-Le^b
    B. Anti-Le^a is the most common
    C. Most common in Le(a+b−) persons
    D. May demonstrate in vitro hemolysis
    E. Both B and D

Diagram for Questions 45–48

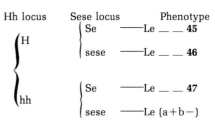

Precursor Substance
Type I Chain   Le——Le^a + precursor substance

lele——precursor substance

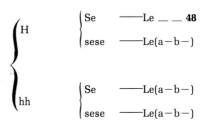

51–56. Match the following:
   A= Typically associated with IgM type antibodies
   B= Typically associated with IgG type antibodies
51. Anti-Le^a
52. Anti-Le^b
53. Anti-M
54. Anti-I
55. Anti-K
56. Anti-Kidd
57. The most common Lutheran phenotype(s) is (are):
   A. Lu a+b+
   B. Lu a+b−
   C. Lu a−b+
   D. Lu a−b−
   E. Both A and B
58. Fill in the blank. The allelic gene to M is ____.
   A. M
   B. N
   C. S
   D. s
   E. U
59. P blood group antigens are:
   A. Proteins
   B. Carbohydrates
   C. Lipoproteins
   D. Glycoproteins
   E. None of the above
60. The most common phenotype of the P blood group system is:
   A. P$_1$
   B. P$_2$
   C. P$_1^k$
   D. P$_2^k$
   E. p
61. The Ii antigen status of newborn cord blood erythrocytes is:
   A. I positive
   B. I negative
   C. i positive
   D. i negative
   E. Both B and C
62. The allelic gene to K is:
   A. J$_s^a$
   B. J$_s^b$
   C. K$_p^a$
   D. K$_p^b$
   E. k
63. The most common Kell phenotype is:
   A. KK
   B. Kk
   C. kk
   D. KJs^a
   E. KJk^b
64. Select the most appropriate characteristic(s) of anti-K:
   A. Usually IgM, rarely IgG
   B. Infrequently encountered in routine blood banking
   C. Stimulated by k antigen
   D. Second in immunogenicity to D antigen
   E. Usually not a cause of hemolytic transfusion reaction
65. Which Duffy phenotype offers the greatest resistance to invasion by malarial parasites?

A. Fy a+b−
B. Fy a+b+
C. Fy a−b+
D. Fy a−b−
E. Both C and D

66. The most common Duffy phenotype in Whites is:
   A. Fy a+b−
   B. Fy a+b+
   C. Fy a−b+
   D. Fy a−b−
   E. A and B are almost equal

67. Which of the following statements is *not* true of the Duffy blood group system antibodies?
   A. Mostly IgG in type
   B. Anti-Fy^b is more frequent than anti-Fy^a
   C. Almost always stimulated by RBCs
   D. Enhanced reactivity if RBCs with corresponding antigen are treated with enzymes
   E. Anti-Fy^a may bind complement

68. The most common Kidd phenotype in Blacks is:
   A. Jk(a+b−)
   B. Jk(a+b+)
   C. Jk(a−b+)
   D. Jk(a−b−)
   E. Both A and B

69–72. Match the following blood group system antigen or antibody with its representative characteristics.

69. Xg^a
70. Sd^a
71. Anti-Yt^a
72. Anti-Co^b
   A. Another form of this antigen is called Cad
   B. Has been implicated in hemolytic disease of the newborn and hemolytic transfusion reactions
   C. Not found in the White population but found in more than one-third of the South American Indian population
   D. Sex-linked
   E. Has only been implicated in hemolytic disease of the newborn

73. The Scianna (SC 1) antigen is ____ in frequency.
   A. High
   B. Low

74. An HLA antigen that is not uncommonly detected on erythrocytes is:
   A. Di^a
   B. Sd^a
   C. Bg^a
   D. Co^a
   E. Fy^a

75. An antigen that is associated with HTLA antibodies is:
   A. Wr^a
   B. Bg^a
   C. York
   D. Co^b
   E. Xg^a

ANSWERS

1. B	26. A	51. A
2. E	27. C	52. B
3. C	28. E	53. A
4. A	29. B	54. A
5. D	30. A	55. B
6. E	31. B	56. B
7. C	32. B	57. C
8. E	33. B	58. B
9. A	34. A	59. B
10. B	35. A	60. A
11. D	36. E	61. E
12. C	37. E	62. E
13. F	38. A	63. C
14. C	39. C	64. D
15. A	40. B	65. D
16. B	41. D	66. B
17. A	42. C	67. B
18. A	43. C	68. A
19. E	44. E	69. D
20. A	45. C	70. A
21. E	46. B	71. E
22. E	47. B	72. B
23. B	48. A	73. A
24. B	49. C	74. C
25. D	50. E	75. C

Bibliography

Albrey, J.A., et al.: A new antibody, anti-Fy^3, in the Duffy blood group system. Vox Sang., *20*:29, 1971.

Allen, F.H., Jr, Diamond, K.L., and Niedziela, B.: A new blood group antigen. Nature, *167*:482, 1951.

Allen, F.H., Lewis, S.J., and Fudenberg, H.: Studies of anti-Kp^b, a new antibody in the Kell blood group system. Vox Sang., *3*:1, 1958.

Allen, F.H., and Lewis, S.J.: Kp[a] (Penney), a new antigen in the Kell blood group system. Vox Sang., 2:81, 1957.

Ballas, S.K., Dignam, C., Harris, M., and Marcolina, M.J.: A clinically significant anti-N in a patient whose red cells were negative for N and U antigens. Transfusion, 25(4):377-380, 1985.

Beattie, K.M.: Perspectives on some usual and unusual ABO phenotypes. In: A Seminar on Antigen in Blood Cells and Body Fluids. Edited by C.A. Bell. Washington, D.C., American Association of Blood Banks, 1980. pp. 97-149.

Berlin, B.S., Chandler, R., and Green, D.: Anti-"i" antibody and hemolytic anemia associated with spontaneous cytomegalovirus mononucleosis. Am. J. Clin. Pathol. 67:459, 1977.

Bezhad, O., et al.: A new anti-erythrocyte antibody in the Duffy system: Anti-Fy[4]. Vox Sang., 24:337, 1973.

Callender, S.T., and Race, R.R.: A serological and genetical study of multiple antibodies formed in response to blood transfusion by a patient with lupus erythematosus diffusus. Ann. Eugen., 13:102, 1946.

Ceppellini, R., Dunn, L.C., and Turri, M.: An interaction between alleles at the Rh locus in man which weakens the reactivity of the Rho factor (D[u]). Proc. Nat. Acad. Sci. USA, 41:283-288, 1955.

Characteristics of Blood Group Antibodies (Product Brochure). Miami, FL, Baxter Healthcare Corporation, Dade Division, 1987.

Chown, B., Lewis, M., and Kaita, H.: The Duffy blood group in Caucasians: Evidence for a new allele. Am. J. Hum. Genet., 17:384, 1965.

Chown, B., Lewis, M., and Kaita, H.: A "new" Kell blood group phenotype. Nature, 180:711, 1957.

Cleghorn, T.E.: MNSs gene frequencies in English blood donors. Nature, 187:701, 1960.

Colledge, K., Pezzulich, M., and Marsh, W.L.: Anti-Fy[5], an antibody disclosing a probable association between the Rhesus and Duffy blood group genes. Vox Sang., 24:193, 1973.

Coombs, R.R.A., Mourant, A.E., and Race, R.R.: In vivo iso-sensitization of red cells in babies with haemolytic disease. Lancet, I (Feb. 23):264-266, 1946.

Crawford, M.N.: HLA and The Red Cell. Malvern, PA, Cooper Bio medical, 1983.

Cutbush, M., Chanarin, I.: The expected blood-group antibody, anti-Lu[b]. Nature, 178:855, 1956.

Cutbush, M., Mollison, P.L., and Parkin, D.M.: A new human blood group. Nature, 165:188, 1950.

Devine, P., et al.: Serologic evidence that scianna null (SC:−1, −2) red cells lack multiple high-frequency antigens. Transfusion, 28(4):346-349, 1988.

Diamond, L.K.: Erythroblastosis fetalis or hemolytic disease of the newborn. Proc. Roy. Soc. Med., 40:546-550, 1947.

Furukawa, K., et al.: Examples of blood groups P and P[k] in Japanese families. Japanese J. Hum. Genet., 12:137, 1974.

Giblett, E.R.: Js, a new blood group antigen found in Negroes. Nature, 181:1221, 1958.

Giblett, E.: Blood group antibodies causing hemolytic disease of the newborn. Clin. Obstet. Gynecol., 7:1044-1055, 1964.

Graham, H.: An overview of the biochemistry of the Lewis, ABH, and P systems. In A Seminar on Antigens on Blood Cells and Body Fluids. 33rd Annual Meeting of the American Association of Blood Banks, 1980.

Horowitz, et al.: Cold agglutinins in infectious mononucleosis and heterophile-antibody-negative mononucleosis-like syndromes. Blood, 50:195, 1977.

Howell, E., and Perkins, H.A.: Anti-N-like antibodies in the sera of patients undergoing chronic hemodialysis. Vox Sang., 23:291-299, 1972.

Ikin, W.E., et al.: Discovery of the expected hemagglutinin, anti-Fy[b]. Nature, 168:1077, 1951.

Huestis, D.W., Bow, J.R., and Case, J.: Practical Blood Transfusion. Boston, Little, Brown and Co., 1988, pp 93-116.

Issitt, P.D.: Applied Blood Group Serology, 3rd ed. Miami, FL, Montgomery Scientific, 1985.

Jenkins, W.J., et al.: Infectious mononucleosis: An unsuspected source of anti-i. Br. J. Haematol. 11:480, 1965.

Landsteiner, K., and Levine, P.: Proc. Soc. Exp. Biol. Med., 24:600, 1927.

Levine, P., et al.: A new human hereditary blood property (Cellano) present in 99.8% of all bloods. Science, 109:464, 1949.

Levine, P.: On Hr factor and Rh genetic theory. Science. 102:1-4, 1945.

Marcus, D.M., and Kundu, S.: Immunochemistry of the P blood group system. In Immunobiology of the Erythrocyte, Progress in Clinical and Biological Research. (Edited by G. Sandler, and J. Nusbacher). New York, Alan R. Liss, 1980.

Marsh, W.L., et al.: Mapping human autosomes: Evidence supporting assignment of rhesus to the short arm of chromosome No. 1. Science, 183:966-968, 1974.

Mollison, P.L.: Blood Transfusion in Clinical Medicine, 7th ed. Oxford, Blackwell Scientific Publications, 1983.

Morton, N.E., et al.: Genetic evidence confirming the localization of Sutter in the Kell blood group system. Vox Sang., 10:608, 1965.

Mournat, A.E.: A new rhesus antibody. Nature, 155:542, 1945.

Naiki, M., and Marcus, D.M.: Human erythrocyte P and P[k] blood group antigens: Identification as glycosphingolipids. Biochem. Biophys. Res. Commun., 60:3, 1974.

Pierce, S.R.: A review of erythrocyte antigens shared with leukocytes. In A seminar on Antigens on Blood Cells and Body Fluids. 33rd Annual Meeting of the American Association of Blood Banks, 1980.

Pinkerton, E.J., et al.: The phenotype Jk(a−b−) in the Kidd blood group system. Vox Sang., 4:155, 1959.

Plant, G., et al.: A new blood group antibody, anti-Jk[b]. Nature, 171:431, 1953.

Pollack, W., et al.: Studies on Rh prophylaxis after transfusion with Rh-positive blood. Transfusion, 11:340-344, 1971.

Race, R.R., and Taylor, G.L.: A serum that discloses the genotype of some Rh-positive people. Nature. 152:300, 1943.

Race, R.R., Taylor, G.L., Cappell, D.F., and McFarlane,

M.M.: Recognition of a further common Rh genotype in man. Nature, *153*:52-53, 1944.

Rosenfield, R.E., et al.: Anti-i, a frequent cold agglutin
in infectious mononucleosis. Vox Sang., *10*(5):631-
634, 1965.

Ruddle, F., et al.: Somatic cell genetic assignment of
peptidase C and the Rh linkage group to chromosome A-1 in man. Science, *176*:1429-1431, 1972.

Schwarting, G.A., Marcus, D.A., Metazas, M.: Identification of sialosylparagloboside as the erythrocyte receptor for an anti-p antibody. Vox Sang.,
32:257, 1977.

Shirey, R.S., et al.: The association of anti-P and early
abortion, Transfusion, *27*(2):189-191, 1987.

Vos, G.H., et al.: A sample of blood with no detectable
Rh antigens. Lancet, *I* (July 7):14-15, 1961.

Walker, R.A., et al.: Js[b] of the Sutter blood group system. Transfusion, *3*:94, 1963.

Watkins, W.M.: Blood group substances in the ABO
system the genes control the arrangement of sugar
residues that determine blood group specificity.
Science, *152*:172, 1966.

Wimer, B.M., et al.: Haematological changes associated with the McLeod phenotype of the Kell blood
group system. Br. J. Haematol. *36*:219, 1977.

Part Three

Transfusion Practices

6

Pretransfusion Testing: Compatibility Testing and Antibody Detection

At the conclusion of this chapter, the reader will be able to:

- Describe the history of the development of crossmatching blood.
- Diagram and explain the constituents of the major and minor crossmatch.
- Describe the rationale of the type and screen protocol.
- State the procedures that are included in the type and screen protocol.
- Cite the major reason for performing a pretransfusion autocontrol.
- Explain the abbreviated crossmatch procedure.
- State the primary purpose or purposes of the major crossmatch.
- Explain the purpose of screening cells in pretransfusion testing.
- Name the patient history factors that are important in the investigation of a blood bank problem.
- List the steps in the preliminary serologic testing of an antibody problem.
- Name the possible causes for a major crossmatch incompatibility at room temperature.
- Discuss the reasons why variable-strength reactions can be encountered in reagent screening cells or crossmatching.
- Describe the types of antibodies that can be encountered in each of the phases of testing with reagent screening cells or in a crossmatch.
- State the characteristics of cold agglutinins produced by various pathologic conditions.
- Describe the steps that can be taken if a weakly reacting antibody is encountered in the AHG phase of antibody testing.
- Name the possible causes of a mixed-field agglutination pattern of patient's serum and donor's cells.
- Discuss the advantages and disadvantages of polybrene-enhancement
- Define the terms "panagglutination," "polyagglutination," "albumin-agglutinating phenomenon," "antibody to a preservative," and "rouleaux formation."
- State the reasons why a patient could have a negative alloantibody screen but one or a few units of incompatible blood.
- List the potential causes of either a false positive or a false negative direct antiglobulin test.
- Name the diseases or disorders that can produce positive DAT results with polyspecific and monospecific antiseras.
- Explain the possible causes of autoimmune hemolytic anemia.
- State the four possible mechanisms that produce positive direct antiglobulin test (DAT) results due to drugs.
- Name at least five common drugs that can produce positive DAT results.
- Name at least three causes of mixed-field agglutination.

Chapter Outline

Historical Development of Crossmatching

The Classic Crossmatch: Procedure and Rationale

Modern Developments in Pretransfusion Testing
 Modern Blood Banking Practices
 Type and Screen Protocol
 Streamlining Compatibility Testing
  The Abbreviated Crossmatch
  Current Mandated Tests for Pretransfusion
   Samples
 Optional Pretransfusion Testing

Antibody Screening (Indirect Antiglobulin Testing
 Basic Screening for Antibodies
 The Two-Cell Screening Procedure
 Preliminary Antibody Identification
 Panel Cell Identification

Solving Antibody Problems
 First Step—Patient History
 Second Step—Preliminary Serologic Testing
 Third Step—Evaluation and Identification of
  Antibodies
 Investigation of Antibodies that React Best
  at Room Temperature

HISTORICAL DEVELOPMENT OF CROSSMATCHING

The first transfusion of human blood took place early in the nineteenth century and numerous transfusions were performed during the following 50 years. Late in the nineteenth century, adverse reactions were common. Experiments in the transfusion of presumed blood substitutes, such as human milk, electrolyte solutions, and animal blood were attempted. With Landsteiner's discovery of the ABO system at the beginning of the twentieth century, blood transfusion became established as a scientific field.

The crossmatching of blood was first described in 1907 and has been modified continually since its inception. The major milestones include the following:

1. Demonstration of the relative importance of red blood cell typing and crossmatching.
2. Development of rapid techniques for crossmatching.
3. Advent of high protein, anti-human globulin (AHG), and enzyme techniques.

Many scientists have contributed to the basic theory and practice of blood transfusion. Table 6-1 lists some of the most significant events in blood transfusion history.

THE CLASSIC CROSSMATCH: PROCEDURE AND RATIONALE

Although the classic crossmatch (Table 6-2) has been modified, the same basic principles are fundamental to contemporary testing. The absence of agglutination is essential to the safety of blood transfusion. Agglutination in any phase (also known as *incompatibility*) is generally an expression of the presence of an antibody and its corresponding antigen. The appearance of agglutination in vitro may be expressed as hemolysis of erythrocytes in vivo. Although incompatibility on either the major or minor side of the crossmatch is not desired, incompatibility on the major side can produce a hemolytic transfusion reaction.

The classic crossmatch consists of a major and minor crossmatch. The major side of the crossmatch contains patient serum and donor erythrocytes; the minor crossmatch consists of the reverse combination, patient erythrocytes and donor plasma. A high-protein substance, usually 22% albumin, is added to one tube of the major and minor sides as an enhancement agent.

These four tubes are centrifuged and examined immediately (immediate spin-IS-room temperature phase). The set is then incubated from 15 to 60 minutes at 37° C. After incubation, the tubes are again centrifuged and examined macroscopically. All of the tubes are washed 3 times with normal physiologic saline. After the final decanting of saline, AHG antisera is added to each tube. The tubes are gently mixed, recentrifuged, and examined for agglutination. In

Table 6-1. Milestones in Blood Transfusion History

Year	Event
1907	*Ottenberg* performed ABO testing before transfusion and predicted that these tests would be important in blood transfusion therapy.
	Hektoen noted that possible danger could be avoided by selecting a donor whose erythrocytes were not agglutinated by the serum of the patient and whose serum was not agglutinated by the donor's erythrocytes. He further advocated that the recipient and donor be of the same blood group. This led laboratory scientists to consider the ABO grouping of the patient and donor as an acceptable alternative to the crossmatching test.
	Crile advocated a 48-hour test between the serum and erythrocytes of the donor and patient. He considered that in vitro hemolysis of the patient's erythrocytes by the donor's serum was more dangerous than destruction of the erythrocytes of the donor by the patient's serum.
1917	*Bernheim and Lee* advocated the use of a matching test. Bernheim supported the use of both a major (patient's serum and donor's cells) and a minor (patient's erythrocytes and donor's serum) crossmatch and recommended testing at 37° C. Lee believed that the only important consideration was that the serum of the patient should not agglutinate or hemolyze the erythrocytes of the donor. He also proposed the use of a slide test for crossmatching, and condoned the use of group O blood for all patients. The philosophy of using group O blood without crossmatching, when facilities were unavailable, predominated throughout World War I.
1918	*Moss* noted that hemolysis paralleled agglutination. This led to ABO blood grouping determination by agglutination rather than by the hemolysis test. All testing at this time was performed at room temperature. *Direct testing* consisted of mixing citrated drops of the patient and donor blood on glass slides and observing them microscopically for agglutination for up to 15 minutes. *Indirect testing* referred to blood grouping of patients and donors.
	Vincent advocated the use of stock test serums preserved with citrate. Direct testing using a slide technique at room temperature and Vincent's grouping procedure were the most widely used methods during the ensuing two decades.
1937	*Hoxworth and Ames* recommended that if the ABO selection of donors could be rigidly restricted to a choice of individuals from the same blood group as the patient, no further testing of compatibility would be required except as a check for possible errors in grouping and the exceptional occurrence of alloantibodies. They proposed a method whereby a 1:5 mixture of donor and patient saline-suspended, defibrinated whole blood was observed for agglutination for 15 minutes, at room temperature in a humid atmosphere.
	The first blood bank was established at Cook County Hospital, Chicago, Illinois.
1939	*Riddell* advocated the use of a major crossmatch. Use of the slide technique continued through the 1940s.
1945	*Diamond and Dentor* described enhancement of agglutination with bovine albumin.
	Coombs, Mourant, and Race reported a new test (Coombs or Anti-human Globulin–AHG) for the detection of weak and incomplete Rh antibodies in the *British Journal of Experimental Pathology*.
1947	*Morton and Pickles* described the effect of proteolytic enzymes as an enhancement technique.
1950s	The American Association of Blood Banks requirements supported saline and high-protein phases of the crossmatch and some form of routine antibody screening.
	Many new blood group antigens and/or systems were described because of the antibodies discovered during compatibility testing and/or associated with hemolytic transfusion reactions.
	In this time period, emphasis was placed on developing tests that would detect any blood group antibodies present in a patient's serum. The reagents and basic techniques for blood grouping and crossmatching remained essentially unchanged.

Table 6-2. Classic Crossmatch Procedure

Major Side		Minor Side	
Saline	High Protein	Saline	High Protein
Patient's serum + donor's cells	Patient's serum + donor's cells + 22% albumin	Patient's cells + donor's plasma	Patient's cells + donor's plasma + 22% albumin

tubes exhibiting no agglutination, coated erythrocytes are added, centrifuged, and examined for agglutination. Agglutination must be observed after the addition of the coated erythrocytes as a positive quality control step.

Testing at different temperatures and the addition of other agents assists in the detection of various antibodies. The detected antibodies at different phases are shown in Table 6-3.

Cases 1 through 3 demonstrate the types of reactivity that might be detected in crossmatching patients.

MODERN DEVELOPMENTS IN PRETRANSFUSION TESTING

Although the terms *crossmatch* and *compatibility testing* are sometimes used synonymously, the crossmatch is presently

Case 1: Examination at Room Temperature

Patient: Group O Rh Positive	Serum: Anti-A, anti-B;	RBCs: No antigens
+		
Donor: Group A Rh Positive	Serum: Anti-B	RBCs: A antigen

	Major Side	Minor Side
Patient	Anti-A Anti-B	No A or B antigens
	+	+
Donor	A antigen	Anti-B
	INCOMPATIBLE	COMPATIBLE

Case 2: Examination at 37 °C

Patient: Group A Rh Negative with Anti-D	Serum: Anti-B, anti-D	RBCs: A antigen
+		
Donor: Group A Rh Positive	Serum: Anti-B	RBCs: A antigen

	Major Side	Minor Side
Patient	Anti-B Anti-D	A antigen
	+	+
Donor	A antigen D antigen	Anti-B
	INCOMPATIBLE	COMPATIBLE

Case 3: Examination after Addition of AHG

Patient: Group A Rh Positive Kell Positive	Serum: Anti-B	RBCs: A antigen
+		
Donor: Group A Rh Positive with Anti-Kell	Serum: Anti-B, Anti-Kell	RBCs: A antigen

	Major Side	Minor Side
Patient	Anti-B	A antigen Kell antigen
	+	+
Donor	A antigen	Anti-B Anti-Kell
	COMPATIBLE	INCOMPATIBLE

Table 6-3. Antibodies Detected at Various Phases

Phase	Antibodies Detected
Immediate spin	IgM antibodies (e.g., anti-A and anti-B, anti-Le^a, anti-Le^b, M, N)
37° C	IgG antibodies–High-titered Rh antibodies (e.g., anti-C, anti-c, anti-E, anti-e); occasionally Anti-Kell)
	High protein (albumin) enhances Rh antibodies.
AHG	IgG antibodies (e.g., anti-Fy^a, anti-Fy^b, anti-Kell, and Rh antibodies

only part of compatibility testing in the United States. Compatibility testing now includes several tests:

1. ABO and Rh typing of the donor and patient
2. Screening of donor and patient serum for alloantibodies
3. Crossmatching

The developments that led to currently accepted testing are listed in Table 6-4.

Modern Blood Banking Practices

During the last 10 years there has been a distinct change in the attitudes about pretransfusion testing. The early 1980s became a time for decisions to eliminate portions of standard testing because of the restricting economic climate. This environment stimulated the philosophy that no testing should be done unless the results are likely to influence patient care. Protocols have

Table 6-4. Milestones in Pretransfusion Testing

Year	Development
1958	*Jennings and Hindman* questioned the value of the minor crossmatch.
1968	Acceptance of pretransfusion antibody screening increased, with the minor crossmatch beginning to be regarded as optional.
1976	The beginning of a change in thinking in regard to crossmatching was initiated by *Giblett* in his classic Karl Landsteiner award lecture. He attacked the use of room temperature testing when screening serums from blood donors and in the more controversial area of compatibility testing. Dr. Giblett's opinions, which were supported by the fundamental work of *Mollison*, included the belief that antibodies reacting only at room temperature but not at 37° C were of no clinical significance. In his opinion, room temperature testing provided no extra protection for the patient and generated extra work and problems. The exception to this opinion was that room temperature testing should continue for the immediate spin crossmatch procedure.
1976	*Friedman et al.* and *Mintz et al.* independently advocated the use of the type and screen protocol in surgical cases that rarely required blood transfusion. The typing of the patient's erythrocytes should include ABO and Rh grouping and the screening of patient's serum for alloantibodies.
	Some laboratory scientists wanted to delete the AHG phase of the crossmatch from all compatibility tests if the alloantibody screen was negative.
1976	*Garratty and Petz* noted that antibodies detectable only through the anticomplement activity of the AHG were rare and that high levels of anti-C3d activity of AHG could result in many nonspecific reactions.
Until the mid-1970s	Tests were performed at room temperature and at 37° C, in the presence of various enhancers (such as albumin, and enzymes). All of these approaches were designed to increase sensitivity and to detect more and more antibodies. The minor crossmatch continued to be retained as a standard procedure by most blood banks.
1980	The Food and Drug Administration and American Association of Blood Banks required an AHG phase of the crossmatch.
1985	The AHG phase of the crossmatch was no longer a required procedure.

been developed based on a balance between the following:

1. Patient safety
2. The number of unwanted reactions eliminated (such as cold agglutinins)
3. The simplicity, sensitivity, and specificity of selected methods
4. The speed with which test procedures can be performed

Type and Screen Protocol

The type and screen procedure has emerged as an acceptable alternative to crossmatching blood. This protocol consists of performing an ABO grouping and Rh typing and an indirect antiglobulin test for alloantibodies. This protocol has been established as a safe and cost-effective measure. It promotes more effective use of the blood supply because it reduces the unnecessary crossmatching of blood for surgical procedures in which blood is rarely used.

Although the amount of blood needed varies according to the technique used, as well as factors such as the condition of the patient, this practice is primarily based on observations of the amount of blood generally used in a specific surgical procedure. (Table 6-5). If unusual complications produce an immediate need for blood by a patient who has had a type and screen, the patient can receive ABO group and Rh type-specific blood without a crossmatch.

Streamlining Compatibility Testing

In the early 1980s, the use of anti-A,B antisera and A_2 erythrocytes in ABO grouping, repeat Rh typing of Rh positive donor units, D^u testing, repeat allo-antibody screening of donor units, direct anti-human globulin (DAT) testing, and the preparation and testing of eluates began to be discussed. Questions were raised as to the clinical significance of antibodies reactive at room temperature or below, the usefulness of albumin in the reaction mixture, and the appropriateness of using AHG in both the alloantibody screening test and crossmatch.

During 1984-1985, the Food and Drug Administration (FDA) and American Association of Blood Banks (AABB) allowed the AHG phase of the crossmatch to be deleted if the antibody screen was negative. Crossmatching was felt to be necessary only to confirm ABO compatibility. In 1984, Judd recommended deleting the autocontrol in pretransfusion testing. The autocontrol was felt to be mainly of value in judging whether a cold antibody was an autoantibody or an alloantibody. Without the room temperature phase, the only reason for using the DAT or autocontrol would be to detect immune hemolytic anemia induced by autoantibody, alloantibody, or drug-induced hemolytic anemia in random patients that was not detectable in the patient's serum by conventional methods. By 1986, the mi-

---

Table 6-5. Surgical Procedures Appropriate for the Type and Screen Protocol

Category	Specific Types of Surgery
General	Breast biopsy, cholecystectomy, colonostomy or closure, exploratory laparotomy, sigmoidectomy, hernia repair (ventral); splenectomy; mastectomy (simple), thyroid lobectomy
Ear, Nose and Throat (ENT)	Caldwell-LUC, tonsillectomy and adenoidectomy, transantral ethmoidectomy
Neurosurgery	Carpal tunnel release, laminectomy for disc removal, shunt procedure, percutaneous chordotomy
OB and GYN	Cesarian section, hysterectomy (simple), laparoscopic tubal ligation, ovarian wedge resection, tuboplasty, Stanley procedure
Orthopedic	Arthrotomy, leg amputation, meniscectomy, minor hand or foot surgery, removal of hip pin, shoulder reconstruction, total knee replacement
Plastic	Augmentation mammoplasty, reduction mammoplasty, skin flap; skin graft (minor)
Urologic	Cystectomy, nephrectomy (simple), nephrostomy, orchiectomy, orchiopexy, pyelolithotomy, transurethral resection of bladder tumor or prostate, urethral reimplantation, ureterolithotomy

nor crossmatch was of historic interest only.

THE ABBREVIATED CROSSMATCH

Abbreviated crossmatching (ABO grouping and Rh typing, patient alloantibody screen, and an immediate-spin major crossmatch) is permitted for unimmunized patients, but is not widely practiced. Implementation of a type and screen protocol and an abbreviated crossmatch procedure in cases of massive transfusion have proven that the risk associated with transfusing uncrossmatched blood to a patient with no demonstrable clinically significant unexpected antibodies is minimal. The 11th edition of the AABB Standards specifies that the methods used for crossmatching must include those methods that demonstrate ABO incompatibility. If no clinically significant alloantibodies are detected by the antibody screen and there is no history of prior detection of an alloantibody, the AHG crossmatch is optional.

The abbreviated crossmatch is a very controversial topic. Proponents believe that an emphasis on careful clerical checking combined with the immediate-spin crossmatch is safe and cost-effective. When a carefully performed screening test for alloantibodies is included in the pretransfusion testing procedure, the primary purposes of the major crossmatch are to avoid inadvertent transfusion of ABO-incompatible blood and to recognize previously undetected clinically significant antibodies that react with antigens on the donor's red blood cells. Proper donor unit identification and the comparison of donor and recipient blood types is essential to guarantee that incompatible blood is not inadvertently selected and then issued for transfusion. In actual laboratory practice, donor units are selected because they are believed to be ABO-compatible. The incidence of error in identifying the ABO group of a donor is estimated to be less than 1 in 2,000,000 units. This frequency is insignificant when compared to the frequency of ABO-incompatible transfusions resulting from clerical errors, such as misidentification of patients or blood samples, which is reported to be about 1 in 10,000 units.

It has been suggested that the ABO group of all transfusion recipients be verified by retesting the blood prior to transfusion. This retesting should take the form of the immediate-spin crossmatch rather than repeating the ABO grouping of donor and recipient. In the opinion of some, the AHG major crossmatch provides minimal additional safety.

Opponents, however, believe that the immediate spin crossmatch is not sufficient. Studies have demonstrated that incompatibilities were undetected in 29 to 38% of crossmatches between type B patients and type A_2B donors with immediate spin after a 5-minute, room-temperature, incubation, but ABO incompatibilities were detected in the AHG phase of testing.

Other reasons for not adopting the abbreviated crossmatch have been cited. These reasons include the discovery of antibodies to low-incidence antigens present on donor red cells, which are not on reagent red cells but are in the recipient's serum. Unexpected ABO antibodies, maternal anti-A or anti-B in neonatal serum, and anti-A_1, have been detected by the AHG phase of the crossmatch. Because AHG detects most ABO and other blood group compatibilities, including donors with weak subgroups of A who have been mistyped as group O, many practitioners believe that it should remain an integral part of compatibility testing.

CURRENT MANDATED TESTS FOR PRETRANSFUSION SAMPLES

Testing of patient blood for transfusion must currently include the following:

1. ABO Grouping
   A. Anti-A and -B
   B. A_1 and B cells
2. Rh Typing
   A. Anti-D by direct agglutination
   B. Rh control, if required by reagent manufacturer
3. Alloantibody screen (indirect antiglobulin test)
   A. Methods demonstrating clinically significant antibodies
      (1.) 37° C incubation
      (2.) Antiglobulin test (AHG)

B. IgG-coated cells to confirm AHG reaction (Coombs' control or check cells)
4. Major Crossmatch
   A. Methods that demonstrate ABO incompatibility
   B. Methods that demonstrate clinically significant antibodies; can be eliminated in patients with the following:
      (1.) No history of significant antibodies
      (2.) A negative alloantibody screen

OPTIONAL PRETRANSFUSION TESTING

Testing of patient blood for transfusion may optionally include the following:

1. ABO Grouping
   A. Red cells with anti-A,B
   B. Serum/plasma with A_2 cells
2. Rh Typing
   A. D^u tests on patients
   B. Rh control with chemically modified reagents
3. Antibody screening (indirect antiglobulin test)
   A. Room temperature incubation
   B. Additives, such as albumin, low ionic strength salt solution, (LISS)
   C. Enzymes
   D. Polyspecific AHG in indirect antiglobulin testing
   E. Autocontrol or DAT
   F. Microscopic reading of tests (only for D^u and mixed field. A magnifier viewing lamp is adequate.)
4. Crossmatch
   A. 37° C and AHG testing when antibody screen is negative, with no previous record of clinically significant alloantibodies.

B. Room temperature incubation
C. Enzyme tests
D. AHG with polyspecific AHG
E. Minor crossmatch

ANTIBODY SCREENING (INDIRECT ANTIGLOBULIN TESTING)

As the preceding sections have elucidated, screening for alloantibodies is essential to the safety of blood transfusion. The screening test may be conducted in lieu of an AHG crossmatch but is usually conducted in conjunction with either the crossmatch or type and screen protocols.

Basic Screening for Antibodies

The most common technique for screening the serum of potential transfusion recipients is a two-cell procedure. Several commercial manufacturers market the erythrocytes of group O donors in two- or three-vial sets, as well as panels of 10 to 18 vials. These red cell suspensions contain a preservative and expire within a few weeks of preparation. With each set of screening cells (Table 6-6) or panel cells (Table 6-7), an analysis of the antigens present (antigen profile) is included. The lot number on the profile should correspond with the lot number on the vials.

The Two-Cell Screening Procedure

The basic procedure for testing the patient's serum for alloantibodies (see Chapter 14) is identical in principle to the major crossmatch procedure. The patient's

Table 6-6. Two Cell Reagent Erythrocyte Screening Set
Partial Listing of Antigens Present

Cell No.	Rh-hr					Kell		Duffy		Kidd		Lewis		MNS				P
	D	C	E	c	e	K	k	Fy^a	Fy^b	Jk^a	Jk^b	Le^a	Le^b	S	s	M	N	P_1
I	+	+	+	+	+	0	+	+	0	+	+	+	0	+	+	+	0	+
II	+	0	0	+	0	+	+	0	+	+	0	0	+	0	+	+	0	+

Table 6-7. Panel of Reagent Erythrocyte Cells

Cell No.	Rh-Hr								Kell						Duffy		Kidd	
	C	D	E	c	e	C^w	f	V	K	k	Kp^a	Kp^b	Js^a	Js^b	Fy^a	Fy^b	Jk^a	Jk^b
1	+	+	+	0	+	0	0	0	+	+	0	+	+	+	0	+	0	+
2	+	+	0	0	+	+	+	0	0	+	0	+	0	+	+	+	+	+
3	0	+	+	+	0	0	0	0	0	+	0	+	0	+	+	+	+	+
4	+	0	0	+	+	0	+	0	0	+	0	+	0	+	0	+	+	0
5	0	0	+	+	+	0	+	0	0	+	0	+	0	+	+	+	+	0
6	0	0	0	+	+	0	+	0	0	+	+	+	0	+	0	+	0	0
7	0	0	0	+	+	0	+	0	0	+	0	+	0	+	+	0	0	0
8	0	+	0	+	+	0	+	0	0	+	0	+	0	+	+	+	+	0
9	0	0	0	+	+	0	+	0	0	+	0	+	0	+	0	0	+	0
10	0	0	0	+	+	0	+	0	0	+	0	+	0	+	+	+	0	0

	Lewis		P	MNS				Lutheran		Sex-Linked	Additional
Antigens	Le^a	Le^b	P^1	M	N	S	s	Lu^a	Lu^b	Xg^a	
1	0	+	+	0	+	+	+	0	+	0 M	
2	+	0	+	+	+	0	+	0	+	+ F	
3	0	+	+	0	+	0	+	0	+	+ M	
4	0	+	+	+	0	+	0	+	+	+ F	Co (b+)
5	0	+	0	+	+	+	+	0	+	+ M	
6	0	+	0	+	+	0	+	0	+	0 M	
7	0	+	+	+	0	+	+	0	+	0 M	Co(b+)
8	+	0	+	+	+	+	0	0	+	0 M	
9	0	0	+	+	+	+	0	0	+	+ F	
10	0	+	0	0	0	0	+	0	+	+ F	
11	—	—	—	—	—	—	—	—	—	—	I (neg)

serum is combined with red cells and these combinations undergo the same phases as a crossmatch: immediate spin (room temperature) and 37° C, followed by the addition of AHG (Table 6-8).

Table 6-8. Two Cell Screening Procedure

		Erythrocytes		
		I	II	Auto
Substance	Patient's serum	X	X	X
	Patient's cells			X
	Reagent cell I	X		
	Reagent cell II		X	
Tests or Examination Phase	Immediate spin			
	22% Albumin (optional)	X	X	
	37 °C Incubation			
	Saline Wash 3X			
	AHG			
	Control cells (if no agglutination in previous steps)			

Preliminary Antibody Identification

If agglutination is observed in the screening cells, the temperature and mode of reactivity suggest which blood group systems are the most likely to be involved. It is important to remember that the cells are group O; hence, antibodies such as anti-A_1 will not be detected by this method of screening.

If the following reactions are observed, preliminary identification of an antibody or antibodies can be made.

Patient Results

Cell No.	Room Temperature	37° C	AHG	Control Cells
I	Neg	1+	3+	
II	Neg	2+	2+	
Auto	Neg	Neg	Neg	2+

Using the two-cell screen antigen profile (Table 6-6), a list of possible antibodies should be developed. In this case, the temperature and mode of reactivity are characteristic of Rh antibodies. Both the D and c antigens are present on both of the reagent cells. Although these reactions could represent a mixture of two antibodies, such as anti-D and anti-c or anti-C and anti-Kell, anti-D or anti-c are the most likely choices.

Panel Cell Identification

After agglutination has been observed in screening cells, it is necessary to test the patient's serum with more reagent cells to have a large enough variety of antigen arrangements to establish the identity of the antibody. The panel of reagent cells is treated in the same manner as the screening cells. The results of the patient's serum that was previously screened follow:

Patient Results

Cell No.	R.T.	37°C	AHG	Control Cells
1	Neg	1+	3+	
2	Neg	1+	3+	
3	Neg	1+	3+	
4	Neg	Neg	Neg	2+
5	Neg	Neg	Neg	2+
6	Neg	Neg	Neg	2+
7	Neg	Neg	Neg	2+
8	Neg	1+	3+	
9	Neg	Neg	Neg	2+
10	Neg	Neg	Neg	2+
11	Neg	Neg	Neg	2+
Auto	Neg	Neg	Neg	

If the pattern of reactivity is matched against the antigens in the erythrocytes of the panel of cells (Table 6-7), the identity of the antibody or antibodies can be tentatively established. To conclusively identify an antibody, other factors, such as the absence of the antigen on the patient's erythrocytes to the probable alloantibody, need to be investigated.

SOLVING ANTIBODY PROBLEMS

Most antibody-associated problems encountered in the blood bank can be re-

solved using a systematic approach. Problems associated with alloantibodies or autoantibodies can be encountered in a variety of areas, including the following:

1. ABO discrepancies, such as missing or additional antibodies or antigens (refer to Chapter 4 for additional information)
2. Rh grouping, for example in the presence of a positive DAT or serum protein abnormality
3. Positive alloantibody screening
4. Incompatible crossmatches
5. Transfusion reactions (refer to Chapter 11)
6. Jaundice in the newborn (Refer to Chapter 10)
7. Positive DAT, such as AIHA, HDN, transfusion reactions, drugs

To investigate a blood bank problem, it is important to categorize information in the areas discussed in the following sections.

First Step—Patient History

Age, Sex, and Race. The race of a patient may offer a clue as to antibody specificity because specific antigens are more often lacking in individuals of certain races. For example, the Fy (a−b−) phenotype is found in 68% of the Black population and in less than 1% of the White population. By comparison, the U negative phenotype is primarily found in Blacks and the K (Cellano) negative phenotype is more prevalent in Whites.

Blood Bank Records. Records should be checked to confirm that the current ABO group and Rh type of the patient match the previous typing, and to alert the technologist to problems that may have been detected previously. Past records, however, only provide clues and should *not* be relied on exclusively.

Transfusion History. It is important to document any history of transfusion, such as the number of transfused units, the dates of transfusion, and why the units were transfused. The transfusion history should also include all blood products received in the past 3 months, such as Rh$_o$ immune globulin, plasma products, factor VIII concentrates, gamma globulin, nongroup-specific platelets, or cryoprecipitate, because a plasma product may contain an alloantibody of sufficient concentration to be detected in the alloantibody screen. A history of recent infusion with volume expanders, such as dextran, may explain the presence of marked rouleaux.

Obstetric History. A complete history should include the number of pregnancies, any stillbirths, abortions, or infants affected with hemolytic disease of the newborn or jaundice. If the patient is pregnant or postpartum, the administration of antenatal or postnatal Rh$_o$ immune globulin should be included with the transfusion history.

Drug History. Medications in current and long-term use by the patient should be recorded. Prescription drugs and over-the-counter medications taken presently and within the past year must be noted. Long-term effects have been noticed with some drug therapy, even after completion of treatment. Many drugs have been associated with a positive DAT and some with autoimmune hemolytic anemia. A listing of drugs that have been cited as the cause of a possible DAT is presented in Tables 6-9 and 6-10.

Admitting Diagnosis. The current diagnosis should include the primary diagnosis as well as a complete medical history of any other conditions that could be expected to be associated with abnormal serologic findings. Examples of serologic conditions and related disorders are presented in Table 6-11.

Table 6-9. Substances Reported to Cause a Positive DAT

Acetaminophen*
Aminopyrine
Amphotericin B
Antihistamines
Carbromal
Cephalosporins
Chlorinated hydrocarbon insecticides
Chlorpropamide
Chlorpromazine
Cloxacillin
Cyclophosphamide
Dexchlorpheniramine maleate
Dipyrone
Erythromycin
Ethosuximide
Fenfluramine hydrochloride
Furosemide
Hydralazine hydrochloride
Hydrochlorothiazide
Ibuprofen**
Indomethacin
Insulin
Isoniazid
Levodopa
Mefenamic acid
Melphalan
Mephenytoin
Methadone hydrochloride
Methotrexate
Methyldopa
Methysergide maleate
Penicillin G
Phenacetin†
Phenylbutazone
Phenytoin sodium
Probenecid
Procainamide
Quinidine
Quinine sulfate
Rifampin
Streptomycin sulfate
Sulphonamides
Tetracycline hydrochloride
Tolbutamide
Triamterene

*Available in over-the-counter medications.
**Available in over-the-counter medications in concentrations under 200 mg.
†Phenacetin-containing medications have been temporarily withdrawn from distribution by most manufacturers pending FDA action.

Second Step—Preliminary Serologic Testing

1. Obtain fresh clotted and anticoagulated specimens from the patient.
2. Centrifuge and examine the serum of the clotted specimen for hemolysis and icteric appearance.
3. Wash red blood cells from the anticoagulated specimen four times and repeat ABO grouping.
4. Perform a direct antiglobulin test (DAT) from the anticoagulated sample. If a broad-spectrum (polyspecific) AHG antiserum is used initially, additional information can be gained by repeating the DAT with anti-IgG and anticomplement antisera.
5. If the patient has a positive DAT or if

Table 6-10. Trade Names* of Medications Containing Substances Reported to Cause a Positive DAT

Achromycin (Tetracycline hydrochloride)	Maxzide (Triamterene)
Advil (Ibuprofen)	Mesantoin (Acetylsalicylic acid)
Aldoclor (Methyldopa)	Momentum (Ibuprofen)
Aldomet (Methyldopa)	Motrin (Ibuprofen)
Aldoril (Hydrochlorothiazide)	Mysteclin (Tetracycline hydrochloride)
Aldoril (Methyldopa)	Nuprin (Ibuprofen)
Alkeran (Melphalan)	Orinase (Tolbutamide)
Antazole (Antihistamine)	Polaramine (Dexchlorpheniramine maleate)
Antistin (Antihistamine)	Polycillin-PRB (Probenecid)
APC with codeine (Phenacetin)**	Ponderax (Fenfluramine hydrochloride)
Apresazide (Hydrochlorothiazide)	Pondimin (Fenfluramine hydrochloride)
Apresoline HCl (Hydralazine hydrochloride)	Ponstel (Mefenamic acid)
Azolid (Phenylbutazone)	Procan SR (Procainamide)
Benemid (Probenecid)	Pronestyl (Procainamide)
Butazolidin (Phenylbutazone)	Propoxyphene (Benzenethanol)
Carbropent (Carbromal)	Pyradone (Aminopyrin)
Cephalexin (Cephalosporin)	Quinidine
Cloxapen (Cloxacillin)	Quinine
Cytoxan (Cyclophosphamide)	Rifadin (Rifampin)
Diabinese (Chlorpropamide)	Rifamate (Rifampin, isoniazid)
Dieldrin (Chlorinated hydrocarbon insecticide)	Rimactane (Rifampin)
Dilantin (Phenytoin sodium)	Sansert (Methysergide maleate)
Dolophine (Methadone)	Serpasil-Apresoline (Hydralazine hydrochloride)
Dyazide (Triamterene)	Sinemet (Levodopa)
Dyrenium (Triamterene)	Sub-Quin (Procainamide)
Fungizone (Amphotericin B)	Sumycin (Tetracycline hydrochloride)
Heptachlor (Chlorinated hydrocarbon insecticide)	Tegopen (Cloxacillin)
Indocin (Indomethacin)	Thorazine (Chlorpromzine)
INH (Isoniazid)	Topicycline (Tetracycline hydrochloride)
Insulin	Toxaphene (Chlorinated hydrocarbon insecticide)
Keflex (Cephalexin)	Tylenol (Acetaminophen)
Keflin (Cephalothin sodium)	Unipres (Hydralazine hydrochloride)
Larodopa (Levodopa)	Zarontin (Ethosuximide)
Lasix (Furosemide)	

*The trade names cited are examples. It is impractical to list the names of all products containing each drug. If any questions exist about the composition of a drug, the latest edition of a pharmaceutical index should be consulted.

**Temporarily withdrawn from the market

References

Billups, N. F.: American Drug Index, 30th Ed. Philadelphia, J. B. Lippincott, 1986.
Fischbach, F. T.: A Manual of Laboratory Diagnostic Tests, 2nd Ed. Philadelphia, J. B. Lippincott Co., 1984.
Hansten, P. D.: Drug Interactions, 3rd Ed. Philadelphia, Lea & Febiger, 1975.
Kastrup, E. K. (Ed): Facts and Comparisons. Philadelphia, J. B. Lippincott, 1986.
Petz, L. D. and S. N. Swisher: Clinical Practice of Blood Transfusion. NY, Churchill Livingstone, 1981, p. 655.
Widmann, F. K. (Ed): Technical Manual, 9th Ed. Arlington, VA, Am. Assoc. of Blood Banks. 1985, p. 261.

the control performed with Rh modified tube and slide typing is positive, the Rh test must be repeated using saline or chemically modified anti-Rh$_o$ (D) antisera. If the DAT and autocontrol are negative, repeat the test with modified tube and slide anti-Rh$_o$ (D) antisera; the manufacturer's directions, however, must state that saline-suspended cells can be used.

6. Repeat the alloantibody screen. An autocontrol must be included. Two screening sets should be set up. One set should be incubated at room temperature 15° C and 4° C. The other set should be incubated at 37° C (with or without albumin) and carried through to the AHG phase. If results are positive with either or both of these screening procedures, a panel of reagent red cells can be set up and treated in the same manner as the screening sets. Note: Always grade reactions and observe for hemolysis.

Table 6-11. Serologic Conditions Associated with Representative Diseases or Clinical Conditions

Serologic Problem	Clinical Disorder
Cold autoantibody	Autoimmune disorders (e.g., cold agglutinin disease)
Warm autoantibody	Hemolytic anemia, carcinoma, lymphoma, systemic lupus erythematosus
Anti-P	PCH, childhood viral infections
Anti-I, anti-IH	Pneumonia, lymphoma, viral infections
Anti-i	Infectious mononucleosis, cirrhosis

Third Step—Evaluation and Identification of an Antibody

Antibodies are often classified as "warm" or "cold," indicating the temperature at which the antibody reacts best. Another classification is IgM or IgG. IgM antibodies react best at room temperature or colder; IgG antibodies react best at 37° C and in the AHG phase.

INVESTIGATION OF ANTIBODIES THAT REACT BEST AT ROOM TEMPERATURE

Antibodies that are representative of this category include anti-A, anti-B, anti-A,B and anti-A_1. Other examples include anti-Le^a and anti-Le^b, anti-P_1, anti-M, and anti-N. The auto-control (patient's serum and erythrocytes) may be positive or negative and except for unusual situations, the DAT will be negative. Problems related to this category can be divided into three types:

1. ABO discrepancy or incompatible crossmatch with both a negative antibody screen and auto control
2. Positive alloantibody screen with a negative auto control
3. Positive alloantibody screen with a positive or variable auto control

ABO Discrepancy or Incompatible Crossmatch with Both a Negative Antibody Screen and Auto-Control. Problems related to an ABO discrepancy are usually caused by anti-A_1 in an A_2 or A_2B person. Resolve this problem by testing the patient's cells with anti-A_1 and testing the serum with A_1 and A_2 cells.

If an ABO discrepancy is not detected, other reasons for this type of problem include the presence of a weak antibody or an antibody to a low-incidence antigen. The presence of a weak antibody that reacts only with homozygous cells, such as anti-M, can create a problem. If the screening cells are MN but the reverse grouping or donor cells are MM, the antibody will not be detected with the screening cells but will react with the donor or reverse grouping cells. In other cases, such as anti-P_1, Lewis $^{a+b}$, or anti-H, the antibody may react only with those cells that have the most antigen. The presence of an antibody in the patient's serum reacting with a low incidence antigen on donor or reverse grouping cells can also create problems. In this situation, red cells from another donor or another set of reagent red cells will undoubtedly be nonreactive.

Positive Alloantibody Screen with a Negative Auto-Control. If the alloantibody screening cell reactions strengthen with colder temperatures and the autocontrol remains negative, the pattern of reactivity should be examined using two reagent screening cells followed by a panel of reagent red cells. It is important to note if the reactivity in a single test phase is variable in strength and inconsistent with a single antibody specificity. This may indicate the following:

1. A dosing antibody that may react better with cells homozygous for the antigen.
2. An antibody directed toward an antigen that has variable strength among donors, such as P_1, Lewis, Sd^a.
3. Multiple antibodies.

When examining the reagent cell antigen profile for alloantibodies present in the patient's serum, the temperature and mode of reactivity suggest which blood group systems are the most likely to be involved. An example follows.

Reagent Red Blood Cell Screening Cells
Partial Listing of Antigens Present

Cell No.	Rh-hr					Kell		Duffy		Kidd		Lewis		MNS				P
	D	C	E	c	e	K	k	Fy^a	Fy^b	Jk^a	Jk^b	Le^a	Le^b	S	s	M	N	P_1
I	+	+	0	+	+	+	0	0	+	+	+	0	+	+	+	+	+	+
II	+	0	+	+	0	0	+	+	0	+	0	0	+	0	+	+	0	+

Patient Results

Cell No.	4° C	15° C	Room Temperature
I	3+	3+	±
II	3+	3+	±
Auto	Neg	Neg	Neg

Patient Results

Cell No.	Room Temperature	37° C	AHG	Control Cells
I	±	Neg	±	2+
II	±	Neg	±	2+
Auto	Neg	Neg	Neg	2+

Based on the results obtained with the patient's sera, a list of possible antibodies should be developed. In this case, reactions in both red cells that were enhanced by cold incubation suggest an anti-M, anti-P_1, or anti-Le^b. The reaction noted in the AHG phase is suggestive of the fixation of complement at room temperature rather than a IgG type antibody. Further testing demonstrated the following results.

Reagent Red Blood Cell Panel Antigen Profile
Partial Listing of Antigens Present

Cell No.	Rh-hr					Kell		Duffy		Kidd		Lewis		MNS				P
	D	C	E	c	e	K	k	Fy^a	Fy^b	Jk^a	Jk^b	Le^a	Le^b	S	s	M	N	P_1
1	+	0	0	+	+	+	0	+	+	+	0	0	0	+	0	+	+	+
2	+	0	0	+	+	0	+	0	+	+	+	0	+	+	+	+	0	0
3	+	+	+	+	+	0	+	0	+	+	+	0	+	+	+	+	0	+
4	0	0	0	+	0	0	+	+	+	+	0	0	+	0	+	+	0	+
5	0	0	+	+	0	+	+	+	+	0	+	0	+	0	+	+	+	+
6	0	+	0	0	+	+	+	+	+	+	0	0	+	+	+	+	+	+
7	0	+	+	0	+	0	+	0	+	+	+	0	+	0	+	+	+	+
8	0	+	0	0	+	0	+	+	+	0	+	+	0	0	+	+	0	0
9	0	+	+	+	+	0	+	+	+	+	+	+	0	+	0	0	+	+
10	0	+	0	0	+	0	+	0	+	+	+	0	+	0	+	+	+	+
11	0	0	0	+	+	+	+	0	+	+	+	+	0	0	0	0	+	+

Patient Results

Cell No.	4°C	15°C	Room Temperature
1	3+	3+	±
2	Neg	Neg	Neg
3	3+	3+	±
4	3+	3+	±
5	3+	3+	±
6	3+	3+	±
7	3+	3+	±
8	Neg	Neg	Neg
9	3+	3+	±
10	3+	3+	±
11	3+	3+	±
Auto	Neg	Neg	Neg

The pattern of reactivity excludes anti-M and anti-Le^b as possibilities but fits the pattern and mode of reactivity of anti-P$_1$. The autocontrol must remain negative.

MULTIPLE ANTIBODIES. In some cases, more than one antibody may be formed. Cold-reacting antibodies that may be found singly or in combination include anti-Le^a, anti-Le^b, anti-M, anti-N, and anti-P$_1$. The configuration of most panel cells is designed to provide at least one cell that is antigen-negative for similarly acting antibodies. In the preceding anti-P$_1$ example, the possibilities of anti-M and anti-Le^b could be excluded because of the differential reactivity of specific cells. Cells No. 2 and 8 are positive for M antigen but negative for P$_1$ antigen. Cell No. 2 is positive for Le^b antigen but negative for the P$_1$ antigen. The patient's sera did not react with

cells No. 2 and 8; therefore, anti-M and anti-Le^b could be excluded.

If anti-M and anti-Le^b were the two possibilities, the reactivity of cells No. 1 and 8 would be important in distinguishing anti-M from anti-Le^b.

Cell	Lewis			MNS			P
No.	Le^a	Le^b	S	s	M	N	P$_1$
1	0	0	+	0	+	+	+
2	0	+	+	+	+	0	0
3	0	+	+	+	+	0	+
4	0	+	0	+	+	0	+
5	0	+	0	+	+	+	+
6	0	+	+	+	+	+	+
7	0	+	0	+	+	+	+
8	+	0	0	+	+	0	0
9	+	0	+	0	0	+	+
10	0	+	0	+	+	+	+
11	+	0	0	0	0	+	+

FOLLOW-UP. If a patient has an antibody that reacts at room temperature and the ABO grouping does not give the expected results, repeat the ABO grouping using reverse grouping cells that lack the antigen to the corresponding alloantibody. For example, if the patient has anti-M and the initial ABO grouping was as follows:

	Antisera		Forward Typing	Reagent Cells		Reverse Grouping
Anti-A	Anti-B	Anti-A,B		A$_1$	B	
Pos	Neg	Pos	A	Pos	Pos	O

The correct ABO grouping would be demonstrated by using M antigen negative reagent red cells for the reverse grouping.

	Antisera		Forward Typing	Reagent Cells		Reverse Grouping
Anti-A	Anti-B	Anti-A,B		A$_1$ (M neg)	B (M neg)	
Pos	Neg	Pos	A	Neg	Pos	A

Positive Alloantibody Screen with a Positive or Variable Autocontrol. Antibodies that react at room temperature or colder temperatures are referred to as *cold agglutinins.* Because nonspecific autoantibodies as well as specific cold antibodies can agglutinate a patient's own red cells as well as the reagent screening or panel cells, they may mask alloantibodies. When a positive DAT is found and the autoantibody is of a high titer and high thermal range, a pathologic condition such as cold-type hemolytic anemia (discussed in detail in the

following section) may be present. In paroxysmal cold hemoglobinuria (PCH), the patient's serum contains a cold, complement-fixing "Donath-Landsteiner" antibody that produces both in vivo and in vitro hemolysis.

The characteristics of cold agglutinins that can be encountered in normal serum versus cold agglutinins associated with pathologic conditions are listed in Table 6-12.

LABORATORY INVESTIGATION. Several techniques can be used to differentiate

Table 6-12. Characteristics of Cold Agglutinins

Normal Serum	Pathologic Cold Agglutinins
Not associated with in vivo hemolysis or occlusion	Associated with hemolytic anemia or vascular occlusion on exposure to the cold, particularly the extremities
Titer no greater than 1:64	High titer, above 1:1000
Thermal range (10 to 15° C)	Active in vitro up to 30° C
Example: Anti-H	Examples: Anti-I

harmless from pathologic cold-reacting antibodies. It is current practice to omit extensive testing (Table 6-13) to differentiate nonhemolytic, cold autoantibodies but alloantibodies with anti-M, anti-N, anti-P, and anti-Lewis specificity are identified.

Basic testing includes the following:

1. Determining the thermal range of the antibody by testing the patient's serum versus reagent red cells (Group O adult) at 4° C, room temperature, and 37° C.
2. Performing a DAT on the patient's red cells using polyspecific, IgG, and anti-C3 antiglobulin antisera. The IgG reaction should be negative and anti-C3 should be positive.
3. Titrating the serum (optional).

TESTING IN THE PRESENCE OF COLD AUTOAGGLUTININS. Autoantibodies can coat erythrocytes and cause spontaneous agglutination, leading to false positive results in the ABO and Rh groupings. In collecting the patient sample, a prewarmed technique can be used.

Anticoagulated red cells should be collected, kept at 37° C, and washed with 37° C saline to remove autoantibody. These cells can be used for reliable forward cell typing and DAT testing. Specimens without anticoagulant are immediately placed in warm water, while transporting, incubated at 37° C for 10 to 15 minutes before testing,

and washed with prewarmed saline before alloantibody testing. Autocontrols must be performed simultaneously at each phase of testing. If the autocontrol is positive, it may be due to nondispersed agglutination caused by cancer or spontaneous agglutination produced by IgG sensitized red cells.

Autoabsorption, or absorbing the patient's serum onto his own red cells, is an alternate technique. After autoabsorption, the usual compatibility testing using the patients auto-absorbed serum can be performed. In cases of recent transfusion, prewarmed testing techniques should be used for compatibility and antibody detection. Autoabsorption is *not* recommended.

An antibody screen with an autocontrol must be done on the absorbed serum. If the alloantibody screen is still positive, a panel must be run with the auto-absorbed serum to determine antibody specificity. If the autoantibody is very potent, the autoabsorption may have to be repeated several times before all the autoantibody is removed and the serum is used for reverse grouping, alloantibodies screening, or compatibility testing.

COMPATIBILITY TESTING. Transfusion of a patient with an urgent need for blood should not be withheld if a documented nonpathologic cold agglutinin is present and the compatibility tests are negative at 37° C. Antibodies that react optimumly at room temperature and are nonreactive when the prewarmed technique is used are

Table 6-13. Agglutination Patterns of Typical Cold Agglutinins

Antibody	I	i	H	IH
A$_1$	4+	0–1+	0–1+	0–2+
A$_2$	4+	0–1+	2–3+	4+
B	4+	0–1+	2–3+	4+
O (adult)	4+	0–1+	4+	4+
O (cord)	0–2+	4+	3–4+	0–2+
Auto	0–4+	0–1+	0–2+	0–2+

usually considered clinically insignificant antibodies (anti-Le[a], anti-Le[b], anti-I, anti-IH, anti-P[1], anti-A[1], anti-M, and anti-N). Units that are crossmatch-compatible are considered suitable for transfusion, but in actual practice, antigen-negative blood is ideally chosen.

INVESTIGATION OF ANTIBODIES THAT REACT BEST AT 37° C OR IN THE AHG PHASE OF TESTING

The types of antibodies that are representative of this category include Anti-Fy[a], anti-Fy[b], anti-S, anti-s, anti-Jk[a], anti-Jk[b], anti-K, anti-k and all of the Rh antibodies. Such antibodies are found in approximately 0.3 to 2% of the population, depending on the incidence of previous transfusions or pregnancies.

Although some of these antibodies, such as high-titered Rh antibodies, occasionally react in saline at room temperature or at 37° C, they usually react in the AGH phase. Antibodies commonly found individually or in combination are Rh, Kell, and Duffy antibodies.

After testing both reagent screening cells and a panel of reagent red cells, the probable antibody specificity can be determined (as previously described). The final step is to test the patient's pretransfusion specimen to be certain that it lacks the corresponding antigen or antigens.

In compatibility testing, donors whose red cells have the antigen against the patient's alloantibody may demonstrate major side incompatibility. Compatible donors should *not* be selected on the basis of compatibility results alone. If the antibody is of a low titer, it may react with some but not all red cells that are antigen-positive.

If a specific antibody is present, the patient's erythrocytes should be typed for the corresponding antigen. The patient should lack the antigen that corresponds to the alloantibody. Red blood cell typing may not be accurate if the patient has been recently transfused. In such cases, mixed-field agglutination may be observed. The reticulocyte-rich top layer of cells can be harvested for cell typings if the patient has been transfused within the last 3 months.

PROBLEMS IN SEROLOGIC TESTING

Alloantibody Problems

A variety of situations or conditions can present problems in antibody identification or produce pseudo-alloantibody reactions. These situations include the following:

Low-titer antibodies
High titer-low avidity antibodies
Antibodies to low-incidence antigens
Passively acquired ABO antibodies
Polyagglutination
Panagglutination
Albumin-agglutinating phenomenon
Antibody to the red cell preservative
LISS autoagglutinin
Rouleaux formation

LOW-TITER ANTIBODIES

Low-titer antibodies can present a problem because they are difficult to detect in vitro. Certain IgG antibodies, such as anti-Kidd, anti-Duffy, and anti-Dombrock, rarely exhibit titers greater than 1:4. Antibodies to antigens of the Kidd system (anti-Jk[a], anti-Jk[b], and anti-Jk[ab]) are notorious for their rapid disappearance from the blood soon after the last immunizing dose.

If weak agglutination reactions are observed, an antibody of low titer should be suspected. To investigate this type of situation, the following techniques can be used.

1. Lengthen the incubation time
2. Alter the serum/cell ratio by adding 1 or 2 extra drops of serum
3. Try different enhancement media such as enzymes, polybrene, or LISS
4. Repeat testing with a fresher specimen

HIGH-TITER, LOW-AVIDITY ANTIBODIES

High-titer, low-avidity (HTLA) antibodies are antibodies with similar serologic characteristics that have a low antigen-binding capacity and a high titration value. Examples of HTLA antibodies include the following: Anti-Chido, anti-Rodgers, anti-Yk[A], anti-Cs[A], anti-Kn[A], anti-McC[A] and anti-SD[A].

The HLTA antibodies produce weak reactions with most red cells in AHG; agglutination is not enhanced by using enzymes. To establish the presence of an HTLA antibody, the following procedures should be performed:

1. Titrate to establish "high titer"
2. Test with red cells that lack high frequency factors
3. Test with cord red blood cells
4. Test with C4-coated red cells
5. Perform neutralization studies Anti-Chido and anti-Rodgers can be neutralized with plasma or serum from donors positive for the corresponding antigen. Anti-Sd(a) (Sid) can be neutralized with urine from most Sda+ humans and from guinea pigs.

ANTIBODIES TO LOW INCIDENCE ANTIGENS

Antibodies to low-incidence antigens may not be detected with reagent screening cells. However, they can become apparent because of an incompatibility with a DAT negative donor unit. The specificity of the antibody is of purely academic interest. Only the nature of the problem, which is the presence of an antibody to an occasional donor unit, should be determined.

PASSIVELY ACQUIRED ABO ANTIBODIES

Passively acquired ABO antibodies can be detected after massive transfusion with blood products that are not ABO group-specific. This type of situation may manifest itself as a mixed-field reaction in forward typing or an ABO discrepancy.

Reactions are usually strongest at room temperature. A positive autocontrol or DAT may be evident, depending on the amount of transfused plasma and the patient's total blood volume.

POLYAGGLUTINATION

Polyagglutination is a condition in which erythrocytes are agglutinated by all or nearly all human sera. In testing patients or donors, a useful clue is the fact that the auto-control is usually negative.

If polybrene enhancement is used, erythrocytes displaying polyagglutination will not agglutinate. Normal erythrocytes carry a negative charge at and near the surface, when cells are mixed with positively charged polybrene, the negative charge is overcome and the erythrocytes aggregate. In contrast, most polyagglutinable erythrocytes carry less of a negative charge because of the reduction of sialic acid at the membrane and thus fail to aggregate in polybrene.

PANAGGLUTINATION

Panagglutination is caused by an antibody that is capable of agglutinating all erythrocytes tested, including the patient's own red cells. The pattern of reactivity is nonspecific.

ALBUMIN AGGLUTINATING PHENOMENON

This rare phenomenon is caused by an antibody in the patient's serum that is reactive with sodium caprylate, a stabilizer, used in many commercial albumin preparations.

Initially, the serum may appear to contain an autoantibody, but further testing reveals that these reactions occur only when albumin is used. Most albumin-agglutinating phenomenon reactions are generally observed after immediate spin or 37° C incubation, although some examples have been found to be detectable only after the AHG phase. In these cases, an autocontrol in albumin is positive but the DAT is negative.

ANTIBODY TO THE RED CELL PRESERVATIVE

Occasionally, a patient's serum may contain antibodies directed against a specific chemical or antibiotic in a preservative solution. Reactions with reagent erythrocytes from different diagnostic companies may vary because the compositions of the preservatives are dissimilar.

A typical example of this condition produces agglutination of reagent red cells but compatible crossmatches with all donor units. The serum usually reacts at room temperature on immediate spin with all red cells suspended in the preservative. The problem can be resolved by washing the reagent red cells to remove the preservative and retesting the serum in saline suspended cells.

LISS AUTOAGGLUTININ

Occasionally, a patient's serum appears to contain a panagglutinin when a low ionic strength salt solution (LISS) is included as an enhancement. The phase of reactivity can be varied, but agglutination has been observed at room temperature-immediate spin and/or the AHG phase. Because it is important to rule out the possibility of a specific clinically significant antibody, testing with other enhancement media should be conducted.

ROULEAUX FORMATION

Rouleaux formation represents a type of pseudo-agglutination in which all erythrocytes are aggregated because of a property of the serum being tested. The appearance of the red cells, resembling stacks of coins, is often more translucent and refractile than in true agglutination.

Rouleaux produce a change in the surface charge of the red cell membrane because of an alteration in the serum or plasma. Serum alterations are caused by exogenous administration of solutions such as dextran, fibrinogen, or polyvinyl pyrolidone (PVP) or by intrinsic protein abnormalities related to a disease.

When washed cells are used for testing, no discrepancy should be noted in forward ABO grouping or Rh testing. Occasionally, rouleaux formation causes a problem in AHG testing even with washed erythrocytes. In this situation, addition of 2 drops of saline and 2 drops of albumin before addition of the patient's serum should correct the problem. Albumin corrects the abnormal albumin/globulin reaction, and saline disperses rouleaux formation.

Problems in Compatibility Testing

Problems with incompatible crossmatches parallel most of the conditions previously discussed in solving antibody problems. The principal types of problems that can produce agglutination/incompatibility in the major crossmatch are the following:

1. Incorrect ABO grouping of patient or donor
2. An alloantibody in the patient's serum reacting with the corresponding antigen on the donor's erythrocytes
3. An autoantibody in the patient's serum reacting with the corresponding antigen on the donor's erythrocytes
4. Prior coating of the donor's erythrocytes, which produces a positive DAT
5. Abnormalities in the patient's serum
6. Contaminants in the test system (such as bacterial contamination of reagents)

Combining information from both the crossmatching observations (such as how many donor units are incompatible) and antibody screening results allows efficient resolution of many problems (Tables 6-14 and 6-15). If the crossmatch is incompatible but the reagent screening red cells are nonreactive, this may indicate one of the following:

1. Incorrect ABO grouping
2. An anti-A_1 in the serum of A_2 patient
3. An antibody against a low frequency antigen
4. A positive direct AHG test on donor red cells

The status of the patient's auto-control is also useful to know. If a patient has a positive autocontrol, it is important to check his/her transfusion history. If the patient has been transfused within the last 3 months, alloantibody may be attached to any remaining transfused erythrocytes. In these cases, antibody elution studies on the patient's erythrocytes may be helpful in resolving the problem. If the autocontrol agglutination results are combined with the antibody screening reactions and crossmatching results, a systematic approach to problem solving can be followed.

THE DIRECT ANTIGLOBULIN TEST (DAT)

The direct antiglobulin test (DAT) is used to detect erythrocyte sensitization with im-

Table 6-14. Problem-Solving Incompatible Crossmatches (Negative Autocontrol)

If a patient has a *negative* autocontrol, this information will aid in proceeding to the appropriate technique to solve the problem.

Temperature of Reactivity: Room Temperature—Immediate Spin

Antibody Screen	Crossmatch	Possible Causes	Resolution
Positive	Compatible or incompatible	IgM alloantibody	Refer to section entitled investigation of antibodies that react best at room temperature
	Compatible or incompatible	IgM autoantibody	Refer to section entitled investigation of antibodies that react best at room temperature
	Compatible	Antibody to red cell preservative in screening cells	Refer to section entitled problems in serologic testing
Positive	All units incompatible	Passively acquired ABO antibody	
	One or a few units incompatible	Anti A₁	Type patient with anti-A₁ lectin
		Mistyped unit of donor blood	Quarantine unit—return to blood supplier or reprocess if an in-house unit
		Dosage or variable reactivity	Test using a prewarming technique or absorbed serum
			Test with homozygous and heterozygous RBCs
		Antibody to low-frequency antigen	

Temperature of Reactivity: After Incubation at 37° C or in the AHG Phase

Positive	Compatible or incompatible	IgG alloantibody	Refer to section entitled Investigation of Antibodies that React Best at 37° C or in the AHG Phase of testing
Negative	All units incompatible	Passively acquired ABO antibody	
	One / few units incompatible	Donor has positive DAT	Return unit to blood supplier or discard
		Dosage or variable reactivity	Increase ratio of serum to cells
			Use enhancement technique (eg., enzymes)
			Retest with homozygous and heterozygous red cells
		Antibody to low-frequency antigen	

munoglobulins and / or complement in vivo (refer to Chapters 3 and 13 for a full discussion of the principle of the test). If in vivo sensitization or coating of red cells does take place, a positive DAT should be detected.

The most frequent source of a false positive result is the use of refrigerated, clotted blood samples in which complement components coat erythrocytes in vitro. Any positive DAT results obtained from a clotted blood sample should be confirmed using a freshly collected EDTA anticoagulated specimen. In vitro coating of erythrocytes and other sources of error should be excluded before further investigation of the

Table 6-15. Problem-Solving Incompatible Crossmatches (Positive Autocontrol)*

If a patient has a positive autocontrol, the information will aid in proceeding to the appropriate technique to solve the problem.

Temperature of Reactivity: Room temperature—immediate spin

Antibody Screen	Crossmatch	Possible Causes	Resolution
Positive	Compatible or Incompatible	IgM autoantibody	Refer to section entitled investigation of antibodies that react best at room temperature
	Incompatible	Rouleaux	Refer to problems in antibody identification
	Compatible	Preservative in screening red cells	
	Compatible	Panagglutination caused by LISS	
Negative	All incompatible	Passively acquired ABO antibody	

Temperature of Reactivity: After incubation at 37° C or in the AHG phase

Positive	All or most compatible	Rouleaux	Refer to section entitled problems in serologic testing
	Incompatible	Panagglutination caused by LISS Albumin agglutinating phenomenon	
Positive or Negative	Variable	Hemolytic disease of the newborn (HDN) Transfusion reaction Autoimmune disorder Drug-induced condition	

*Check patient's transfusion history. If patient has received a recent transfusion (within 3 months), alloantibody may be attached to transfused cells. Antibody elution studies from the patient's red cells may be useful.

potential causes of a positive DAT (Table 6-16). It is equally important to rule out the possibility of false negative results (Table 6-17).

Table 6-16. Potential Sources of Error: False Positive Direct Antiglobulin Test

1. Improperly collected specimens, for example blood collected into tubes containing silicone gel or from an intravenous line containing 5% or 10% dextrose rather than dextrose with lactated Ringer's solution, using a large bore rather than a small bore needle, or drawing too small a volume of blood into anticoagulant.
2. Use of refrigerated clotted whole blood samples
3. Bacterial contamination due to storage of a specimen or from a septic patient
4. Contaminated saline due to leaching of colloidal silica particles from glass or metallic ions from metal containers
5. Dirty glassware, i.e., contamination with dust or detergent
6. Incomplete dispersion of red blood cells produced by overcentrifugation

Immune Hemolysis and the DAT

Positive DAT results with polyspecific or monospecific AHG antisera (anti-IgG or anti-C3d) may be encountered in a variety of clinical conditions (Table 6-18) associated with immune hemolysis. A positive

Table 6-17. Potential Sources of Error: False Negative Direct Antiglobulin Test

1. Loss of AHG antisera potency due to factors such as bacterial contamination or improper storage
2. Inadequate or improper technique when washing red cells, which produces residual proteins, for example unbound globulins, that neutralize the AHG antisera
3. Incorrect RBC suspensions
4. Improper time or speed of centrifugation
5. Omitting AHG antisera from the test
6. Interruptions or delays in the testing process
7. Use of a saline wash solution with too low pH (less than 6.0)
8. Use of saline that has been autoclaved and stored in plastic containers.

Table 6-18. Direct Antiglobulin Test Results Using an EDTA Specimen

| Type of AHG Sera | | | Cells Probably | Possible |
Polyspecific	Anti-IgG	Anti-C3d	Sensitized With	Explanation
Positive	Positive	Positive	IgG and C3d	Warm antibody autoimmune hemolytic anemia, including drug-induced AIHA
				Post-transfusion of incompatible blood
Positive	Positive	Negative	IgG and C4	Warm antibody autoimmune hemolytic anemia, including drug-induced AIHA
				Post-transfusion of incompatible blood
Positive	Negative	Positive	C3d and/or C4	Warm antibody autoimmune hemolytic anemia, including drug-induced AIHA
				Cold agglutinin disease
				Post-transfusion of incompatible blood
Positive	Positive	Negative	IgG	Warm antibody autoimmune hemolytic anemia, including drug-induced AIHA
				Post-transfusion of incompatible blood
				Drug-induced cell sensitization (Without *in vivo* hemolysis)

DAT, however, does *not* always indicate that the erythrocytes have a shortened survival. A small percentage of healthy donors as well as about 10% of hospital patients can have a positive DAT without clinical signs of immune hemolysis.

Conditions associated with immune hemolysis, such as HDN and delayed transfusion reactions, can be caused by alloantibodies. Conditions, such as autoimmune hemolytic anemias or drug-induced antibodies can be caused by autoantibodies. Immune hemolysis is the manifestation of an antigen-antibody reaction, which results in shortened red cell survival. Serologic findings do not determine whether or not a patient has hemolytic anemia, but they are important in establishing the immune origin and type of hemolytic anemia. This is important because each type of hemolytic anemia is treated differently.

The diagnosis of immune hemolysis depends on clinical findings and laboratory data, for example a decreased or decreasing hemoglobin and hematocrit or an increased reticulocyte count. It is important to note that immune hemolysis may *not* result in anemia if the bone marrow is able to compensate for the loss of erythrocytes from the circulation.

Evaluations of elution studies (see Chapter 14) have demonstrated that routine studies are nonproductive. Because most patients have serum antibody of the same specificity, it has been suggested that elutions be restricted to cases in which immune hemolysis is clinically suspected and when elutions may add clinically useful information or improve transfusion safety, such as in delayed transfusion reactions. An algorithm has recently been developed (Table 6-19) that outlines the rapid systematic evaluation of all positive direct antiglobulin tests.

Alloantibodies as the Cause of Immune Hemolysis

The detection of alloantibodies has been previously discussed in this chapter. A full discussion of the mechanism and symptoms of immune hemolysis in hemolytic disease of the newborn (HDN) or transfusion reactions is presented in Chapters 10 and 11, respectively. Most patients with immune hemolysis demonstrate alloantibodies. In rare cases such as HDN or transfusion reactions, a positive DAT may be observed in the absence of demonstrable alloantibodies.

Autoimmune Hemolytic Anemia

Autoimmune hemolytic anemia can be classified into 4 groups:

Table 6-19. Preparation of an Eluate in Cases of a Positive Direct Antiglobulin Test*
Polyspecific Antiglobulin Test Positive

Anti-IgG	Anti-C3d	Recently Pregnant or Transfused	Negative Pretransfusion DAT	Hematology	Jkᵃ antigen	Action
+	±	Yes	Yes			Eluate
+	±	Yes	No			Consult medical director
+	±	No		Abnormal		Consult medical director
+	±	No		Normal		No eluate
−	−	No				No eluate
−	−	Yes				Eluate
−	+	No				No eluate
−	+	Yes			+	No eluate
−	+	Yes			−	Eluate

NA = not applicable

* Johnston, M. F., and Belota, M. K.: Determination of the need for elution studies for positive direct antiglobulin tests in pretransfusion testing, Am. J. Clin. Pathol. 90 (1): p. 58-62, 1988.

1. Warm-reactive autoantibodies—the most common
2. Cold-reactive autoantibodies—less than 20% of cases
3. Paroxysmal cold hemoglobinuria (PCH)—rare
4. Drug-induced hemolysis—less than 20% of cases

Warm Autoimmune Hemolytic Anemia (WAIHA)

WAIHA is associated with antibodies reactive at warm temperatures, 37° C. In more than three fourths of cases, the red cells are coated with both IgG and complement, although some may demonstrate coating with IgG alone or more infrequently complement coating. In WAIHA, there is very little serum autoantibody because the antibody reacts optimally at 37° C and is being continuously adsorbed by erythrocytes in vivo. An elution should demonstrate an autoantibody, but testing for specificity is not routinely necessary. Serologic characteristics of WAIHA are presented in Table 6-20.

Cold Autoimmune Hemagglutinin Disease (CHAD)

Cold autoimmune hemagglutinin disease (CHAD), in either the acute or chronic form, is the most common type of hemolytic anemia associated with cold-reactive autoantibodies. The acute form is often secondary to *Mycoplasma pneumoniae* infection or lymphoproliferative disorders, such as lymphoma. The chronic form is seen in older patients and produces a mild to moderate degree of hemolysis, with Raynaud's phenomena and hemoglobinuria occurring in cold weather.

In CHAD, a cold-reactive IgM autoantibody that reacts with erythrocytes in the peripheral circulation when the body temperature falls to 32° C or below, binds complement to red cells. Hence, complement is the only globulin detected on erythrocytes. Eluates prepared from red cells collected at 37° C will not demonstrate antibody reactivity in the eluate.

Paroxysmal Cold Hemoglobinuria (PCH)

Paroxysmal cold hemoglobinuria (PCH) was previously associated with syphilis but is now more commonly seen as an acute transient condition secondary to viral infections, particularly in young children. PCH may also occur as an idiopathic chronic disease in older people.

The responsible autoantibody is an IgG protein that reacts with erythrocytes in colder parts of the body, causing the irreversible binding of complement components C3 and C4, to red cells. At warmer

Table 6-20. Serologic Characteristics in WAIHA (Patient not transfused in the last 120 days)

Component	Reagent Screening	Panel of Reagent RBCs	Possible Resolution	
Patient Serum Antibody Screen	Positive	Specific reactions	Identify auto or alloantibody	
		Nonspecific reactions	Autoabsorption	Screen and identify underlying allo-antibody If serum is neg. use for X-match
Patient red cells	Negative Rh typing	No free antibody Positive control	Saline or chemically reduced antisera	
	Positive DAT (IgG) Elution (optional) specificity	Pos: identify antibody; Neg: Drug + RBCs		

temperatures, red cells are hemolyzed and the antibody elutes from the cells. Eluates are also nonreactive. This IgG autoantibody, a biphasic hemolysin, can be demonstrated through the Donath-Landsteiner test (see Chapter 14). The autoantibody has anti-P specificity and reacts with all except the rare p or p^K phenotypes. Examples of these exceptions have been described as having anti-IH specificity.

Drug-Induced Positive DATs and Hemolysis

Positive DAT results may be drug-induced (Table 6-21) and may or may not be accompanied by hemolysis. The modes of reactivity have been described as being the result of four basic mechanisms (Table 6-22):

1. Drug adsorption
2. Immune complex
3. Membrane modification
4. Autoantibody formation

DRUG ADSORPTION

Penicillin is a representative example of a drug that displays drug adsorption. In this type of mechanism, the drug strongly binds to any protein, including red cell membrane proteins. This binding produces a drug-red cell-hapten complex that can stimulate antibody formation. The antibody is specific for this complex, and no reactions will take place unless the drug is adsorbed onto the erythrocytes. Massive doses of IV penicillin are needed to coat the red cells sufficiently for antibody attachment to occur.

Table 6-21. Interpretation of Direct Antiglobin Test (DAT)

Result	Interpretation	Cause
Negative	Clinically established hemolysis	Poor technique
		IgA or IgM coating patient's red cells
		Patient antibody has increased dissociation constant
		IgG concentration on red cells too low to be detected
Positive	IgG positive clinical and transfusion history	
	Eluate positive	Transfusion reaction
		Warm: AIHA
		HDN
		Unknown
	Eluate negative	ABO HDN
		Drug Antibody
		Unknown
	C3d positive recently transfused elute positive	Transfusion Reaction
	C3d positive recently transfused elute negative	Cold AIHA
		Drug mechanism
		Unknown
	No transfusion	Cold AIHA
		Drug mechanism
		Unknown

Table 6-22. Drug-Induced Positive DAT

	Drug Adsorption	Immune Complex	Membrane Modification	Autoantibody Formation
Common cause	IgG	Complement	Nonserologic	IgG
Antibody Screening	Negative*	Positive†	Negative	Variable‡
Eluate reactivity with reagent RBCs	Nonreactive	Nonreactive	Nonreactive	Reactive§
Penicillin treated RBCs	Reactive with patient's serum and eluate	Nonreactive	Nonreactive	Nonreactive
Drug needed in the test system	Yes	Yes	No	No

* Unless alloantibodies are present in the sample.
† If the drug and complement are present in the test system.
‡ If the autoantibody is high enough in titer, screening tests may be positive with all cells tested.
§ Reacts with all normal cells tested, occasionally showing Rh-like specificity.

Approximately 3% of affected patients demonstrate a positive DAT, and less than 5% of them develop hemolytic anemia because of the drug. The hemolysis of erythrocytes is usually extravascular and occurs slowly. It is not life-threatening and will abate when penicillin is withdrawn. There appears to be no connection between this type of antibody production and allergic penicillin sensitivity caused by IgE production.

Other drugs that display drug absorption are cephalothin derivatives such as cefalothin sodium and quinidine.

IMMUNE COMPLEX

The mechanism of immune complexing is displayed by a variety of drugs, including phenacetin, quinine, rifampin, and stibophen. In this interaction, the drug and antibody form a complex in the serum and attach nonspecifically to the erythrocytes. Once attached, this complex initiates the complement cascade, which culminates in intravascular hemolysis. The immune complex may dissociate from the red cell membrane after complement activation and attach to another red cell. This action allows a small amount of drug to produce a severe anemia. When the offending drug is discontinued, the hemolytic process disappears quickly.

MEMBRANE MODIFICATION

Drugs of the cephalosporin type, such as Keflin, occasionally cause a positive DAT with polyspecific and monospecific AHG antisera by membrane modification. In this type of mechanism, the drug alters the membrane so that there is a nonspecific adsorption of globulins, including IgG, IgM, IgA, and complement. Hemolysis is not a frequent complication in this type of membrane augmentation.

AUTOANTIBODY FORMATION

Drugs such as methyldopa (Aldomet), L-dopa, and mefanamic acid (Ponstel) have been implicated in positive DATs because of autoantibody formation. The autoantibody formed recognizes a part of the red cell and therefore reacts with most normal erythrocytes. Some drug-induced autoantibodies have been shown to have specificities that appear to be of the RH type, but most have no apparent specificity. Antibody production ceases with withdrawal of the drug.

Problem-Solving in DAT Testing

Weak AHG reactions frequently cause concern in blood banking. Various conditions (summarized in Table 6-23) can produce weak reactions.

Table 6-23. Investigation of Weak Antiglobulin Reactions

Condition	Cause
Mixed-field agglutination*	Mixture of patient and donor antigens posttransfusion Interdonor incompatibility Fetomaternal hemorrhage Chimerism caused by intrauterine transfusion, dispermy, or bone marrow grafts Polyagglutination caused by Tn-activation, CAD, and some acquired B-like antigens
Low titer antibodies	Certain IgG antibodies rarely have titers greater than 1:4. Examples: Kidd, Duffy, Dombrock
HTLA antibodies	Antibodies with low binding capacity and high titration values. Examples: Anti-Chido, anti-Rodgers, anti-Yk^a, anti-Cs^a, anti-Kn^a, and anti-McC^a Similar serologic characteristics
Complement fixation—cold agglutination	During incubation at room temperature or lower, red cells adsorb various complement components (e.g., C4 and C3; from fresh serum containing cold agglutinins. Adsorbed components are reactive at the AHG phase with corresponding anti-complement fragments, if present, in AHG. Positive autocontrol if cold auto antibody. Negative autocontrol if anti-A$_1$ and anti-H

* Mixed-field agglutination appears as agglutinated erythrocytes uniformly dispersed in a background of nonagglutinated erythrocytes when viewing a microscopic field using low (10×) power.

CHAPTER SUMMARY

Historical Development of Crossmatching

Although the transfusion of blood has been practiced since the nineteenth century, it was not until 1907 that the crossmatching of blood was first described. The major milestones in compatibility testing include the demonstration of the relative importance of red blood cell typing and the matching test, the development of rapid techniques for crossmatching, and the advent of high protein, antiglobulin, and enzyme techniques. Many scientists have contributed to the basic theories and practice of blood transfusion.

The Classic Crossmatch: Procedure and Rationale

Although the classic crossmatch has been modified, the same basic principles are fundamental to contemporary testing. The classic crossmatch consists of a major and a minor crossmatch. The major side of the crossmatch contains patient serum and donor's erythrocytes; the minor crossmatch consists of the reverse combination, patient erythrocytes and donor plasma. A high-protein substance, usually 22% albumin, is added to one tube of the major and minor side as an enhancement agent. Testing at different temperatures and the addition of other agents assists in the detection of various types of antibodies.

Modern Developments in Pretransfusion Testing

Although the terms crossmatch and compatibility test are sometimes used synonymously, the crossmatch is presently only part of compatibility testing in the United States. Compatibility testing now includes ABO and Rh typing of the donor and patient, screening of the donor's and patient's serum for alloantibodies, and crossmatching. Since 1980, there has been a change in attitude about pretransfusion testing because of a more restrictive economic climate. New protocols have been developed based on a balance among patient safety; elimination of the number of unwanted transfusion reactions; the simplicity, sensitivity, and specificity of selected methods; and the speed with which test procedures can be performed.

The type and screen procedure has emerged as an acceptable alternative to crossmatching blood in many cases of elective surgery. This protocol consists of performing an ABO grouping and Rh typing, and performing an indirect antiglobulin test for alloantibodies.

During the 1980s, other practices such as the use of anti-A,B antisera and A$_2$ erythrocytes in ABO grouping, D^u testing, and the appropriate use of antiglobulin (AHG) testing began to be eliminated or modified. These changes include deletion of the AHG phase of the crossmatch if the antibody screen was negative, and deletion of the direct antiglobulin test (DAT) or the commonly used autocontrol as part of pretransfusion testing. The minor crossmatch became of historic interest only.

Abbreviated crossmatching (ABO grouping and Rh typing, patient alloantibody screen, and an immediate-spin major crossmatch) is now permitted for unimmunized patients but is not widely practiced. Implementation of a type and screen protocol and an abbreviated crossmatch procedure in cases of massive transfusion has proven that the risk associated with transfusing uncrossmatched blood to a patient with no demonstrable clinically significant unexpected antibodies is minimal.

Testing of patient blood for transfusion must currently include ABO grouping, Rh typing, alloantibody screening, and the major crossmatch. Optional pretransfusion testing, such as ABO grouping with anti-A,B, and D^u testing on patients, may be included.

Antibody Screening (Indirect Antiglobulin Testing)

Screening for alloantibodies is essential to the safety of blood transfusion. The screening test may be conducted in lieu of an AHG crossmatch; however, it is usually conducted in conjunction with the crossmatch, or type and screen protocol. The most common technique for screening the serum of patients is a two-cell procedure that consists of using the erythrocytes of group O donors in two separate vials. If agglutination is observed in the screening cells, the temperature and mode of reactivity suggest which blood group system antibodies are the most likely to be involved. It is important to remember that the cells are group O; hence, antibodies such as anti-A_1 are not detected by this method of screening. If agglutination is observed in either of the screening cells, testing the patient's serum with more reagent red cells

is necessary to have a variety of antigen arrangements to establish the identity of the antibody. If the pattern of agglutination is matched against the antigens in the erythrocytes of the panel of cells, the identity of the antibody or antibodies can be tentatively established. To conclusively identify an antibody, other factors such as the absence of the antigen on the patient's erythrocytes to the probable alloantibody should be investigated.

Solving Antibody Problems

Most antibody-associated problems encountered in the blood bank can be resolved using a systematic approach. Problems associated with alloantibodies or autoantibodies can be encountered in situations such as ABO discrepancies, Rh typing, positive alloantibody screening, incompatible crossmatches, transfusion reactions, hemolytic disease of the newborn (HDN), and positive direct antiglobulin tests (DATs). To initiate investigation of a problem, it is important to obtain a thorough patient history and check blood bank records and the patient's history of transfusion, pregnancy, and drugs. The admitting diagnosis of the patient may also be helpful because some diseases or clinical conditions are characterized by specific serologic problems.

Preliminary serologic testing should consist of examining a fresh blood specimen from the patient for hemolysis and icteric appearance. Other testing should include repeating the ABO grouping and DAT. If the patient's DAT or autocontrol are positive, the Rh typing should be repeated with an appropriate antisera. If the patient's alloantibody screening results are positive, the serum should be additionally tested with a panel of reagent red cells.

Difficulties can be encountered involving antibodies that react best at room temperature, such as anti-A_1 or anti-M. Problems of this type may be demonstrated by an ABO discrepancy or incompatible crossmatch with both a negative antibody screen and autocontrol, a positive alloantibody screen and negative autocontrol, or a positive alloantibody screen with a positive or variable autocontrol. Other types of problems may involve antibodies that react best at 37° C or in the AHG phase of testing. Antibodies representative of this category include anti-Fy^a, anti-Fy^b, and anti-Kell.

Problems in Serologic Testing

Various situations or conditions can present problems in serologic testing. These include low-titer antibodies, high-titer, low-avidity antibodies, antibodies to low-incidence antigens, passively acquired ABO antibodies, polyagglutination, panagglutination, albumin-agglutinating phenomenon, antibody to red cell preservative, LISS autoagglutination, and rouleaux formation.

Low-titer antibodies can be difficult to detect in vitro. If weak agglutination reactions are observed, an antibody of low titer should be suspected. To investigate a problem of this type, the incubation time can be lengthened, the serum:cell ratio can be altered, different enhancement media can be used, or testing can be repeated with a fresh specimen. High titer, low-avidity (HTLA) antibodies have a low antigen-binding capacity and a high titration value. To establish the presence of an HTLA antibody, the patient's serum can be titrated to establish "high titer," or be tested with erythrocytes that lack high frequency factors, cord blood cells, and C4-coated red cells. Neutralization studies can also be performed. Antibodies to low-incidence antigens may not be detected with reagent screening cells but may demonstrate their presence through incompatibility with a DAT-negative donor unit. Passively acquired ABO antibodies may manifest themselves as mixed-field reactions in forward typing or an ABO discrepancy.

Polyagglutination is a condition in which the patient's erythrocytes are agglutinated by all or nearly all human sera but the autocontrol is usually negative. Panagglutination is caused by an antibody that is capable of agglutinating all erythrocytes tested, including the patient's own cells. The pattern of reactivity is nonspecific. The albumin agglutinating phenomenon is a rare condition caused by an antibody in the patient's serum that is reactive with sodium caprylate, a stabilizer used in many commercial albumin preparations. Occasionally, a patient's serum may contain antibodies directed against a specific chemical or antibiotic in a preservative solution. When this condition is present, the patient's serum agglutinates reagent screening red cells but is compatible with all donor units. LISS autoagglutinin can also produce serologic problems. In this type of reaction, the patient's serum appears to contain a panagglutinin when low ionic strength salt solution (LISS) is included as an enhancement medium. Rouleaux formation represents a type of pseudo-agglutination in which all erythrocytes are aggregated because of a property of the serum being tested.

The principal types of problems that can produce agglutination or incompatibility in the major crossmatch are incorrect ABO grouping of patient or donor, an alloantibody in the patient's serum that reacts with the corresponding antigen on the donor's red cells, an autoantibody in the patient's serum reacting with the corresponding antigen on the donor's red cells, prior coating of the donor's red cells which produces a positive DAT, abnormalities in the patient's serum, or contaminants in the test system.

Combining information from both the crossmatching observations and alloantibody screening results allows efficient resolution of many problems. If the crossmatch is incompatible but the reagent screening cells are nonreactive, it may indicate incorrect ABO grouping, an anti-A$_1$ in the serum of an A$_2$ patient, an antibody against a low frequency antigen, or a donor with a positive DAT. Knowledge of the status of the patient's autocontrol is also useful. When the autocontrol agglutination results are combined with the alloantibody screening reactions and crossmatching results, a systematic approach to problem solving can be followed.

The Direct Antiglobulin Test (DAT)

The direct antiglobulin test (DAT) is used to detect erythrocyte sensitization with immunoglobulins and/or complement in vivo.

The most frequent source of a false positive result is the use of refrigerated, clotted blood samples in which complement components coat erythrocytes in vitro. It is equally important to rule out the possibility of false negative results.

Positive DAT results with polyspecific or monospecific AHG antisera (Anti-IgG or Anti-C3d) may be encountered in a variety of clinical conditions associated with immune hemolysis, but a positive DAT does *not* always indicate shortened erythrocyte survival. The diagnosis of immune hemolysis depends on clinical findings as well as laboratory data. Elution studies are of limited value in establishing the presence of an antibody.

Autoimmune hemolytic anemia can be classified into four groups: warm-reactive autoantibodies, cold-reactive autoantibodies, paroxysmal cold hemoglobinuria (PCH), and drug-induced hemolysis. Warm autoimmune hemolytic anemia (WAIHA) is associated with antibodies reactive at warm temperatures. Cold hemagglutinin disease (CHAD), in either the acute or chronic form, is the most common type of hemolytic anemia associated with cold reactive autoantibodies. Paroxysmal cold hemoglobinuria (PCH) is commonly seen as an acute transient condition secondary to viral infections, particularly in young children, or may occur as an idiopathic chronic disease in older people. The causative IgG autoantibody, a biphasic hemolysin, can be demonstrated by the Donath-Landsteiner test. Positive DAT results may be drug-induced and may or may not be accompanied by hemolysis. The mechanisms of drug induced positive DATs have been described as being caused by four basic mechanisms: drug absorption, immune complexes, membrane modification, and autoantibody formation. Penicillin is a representative example of a drug that displays drug adsorption. The mechanism of immune complexing is displayed by a variety of drugs, including phenacetin, quinine, rifampin, and stibophen. Drugs of the cephalosporin type, such as Keflin, occasionally cause a positive DAT with polyspecific and monospecific AHG antisera by membrane modification. Drugs such as methyldopa (Aldomet), L-dopa, and mefanamic acid

(Ponstel) have been implicated in positive DATs due to autoantibody formation.

Weak DAT reactions can be caused by situations such as a mixture of patient and donor antigens post-transfusion, interdonor incompatibility, low titer or HTLA antibodies, or complement fixation by cold agglutinins.

REVIEW QUESTIONS

1. Ottenberg was credited with:
   A. Encouraging the mixing of patient and donor sera and erythrocytes
   B. Performing ABO testing before transfusion
   C. A 48-hour "in vitro" hemolysis test
   D. Condoning the use of group O blood without crossmatching
   E. Performing crossmatching at 37° C

2. The first blood bank for the storage of donor units was established at Cook County Hospital in Chicago in:
   A. 1906
   B. 1915
   C. 1921
   D. 1937
   E. 1945

3. Agglutination "in vitro" may express itself as ____ "in vivo."
   A. Clumping of erythrocytes
   B. No reaction because of dilution
   C. Hemolysis
   D. Hives
   E. An elevated body temperature

4. The major crossmatch consists of a mixture of:
   A. Donor serum and patient erythrocytes
   B. Donor serum and donor erythrocytes
   C. Patient serum and donor erythrocytes
   D. Patient serum and patient erythrocytes
   E. Either A or D

5–7. Select the correct answers for the crossmatch results of the following cases in questions 5, 6, and 7.
   A. Major side compatible
   B. Major side incompatible
   C. Minor side incompatible
   D. Major and minor sides compatible

5. If an A_2 Rh+ patient with anti-A_1 were crossmatched with an A_1 donor, the results would be:

6. If an O Rh+ patient with an anti-Kell were crossmatched with an O Rh− (Kell negative) donor with anti-D, the results would be:

7. If an O Rh− patient were crossmatched with an O Rh+ donor, the results would be:

8. The type and screen protocol consists of:
   1. ABO grouping
   2. Rh typing
   3. Alloantibody screening
   4. HIV screening
   5. HBsAg screening
   A. 1 only
   B. 1 and 2
   C. 1, 2, and 3
   D. 1, 4, and 5
   E. All of the above

9. The major reason for performing a pretransfusion or autocontrol is to:
   A. Confirm ABO grouping
   B. Detect an alloantibody that is sensitizing transfused erythrocytes
   C. Detect an antibody that is not detectable in the patient's serum
   D. Confirm the presence of a cold antibody
   E. Both B and C

10. An abbreviated crossmatch consists of:
    A. ABO grouping
    B. Rh typing
    C. Alloantibody screening
    D. An immediate spin crossmatch
    E. All of the above

11. The primary purpose(s) of the major crossmatch is (are) to:
    1. Avoid inadvertent transfusion of ABO-incompatible blood
    2. Avoid inadvertent transfusion of Rh positive blood to an Rh negative person
    3. Demonstrate previously undetected alloantibodies
    4. Demonstrate previously undetected autoantibodies
    5. Detect a drug-induced hemolytic anemia
    A. 1 only
    B. 1 and 2
    C. 1 and 3

D. 4 only
E. 4 and 5

12. Screening cells for the detection of alloantibodies will not detect:
    A. Anti-M
    B. Anti-N
    C. Anti-A_1
    D. Anti-K
    E. Anti-c

13. Problems associated with alloantibodies or autoantibodies can be encountered in all of the following clinical conditions except:
    A. ABO discrepancies
    B. Donor reactions
    C. Transfusion reactions
    D. Hemolytic disease of the newborn
    E. Positive direct antiglobulin test

14. All of the following factors are important patient history considerations in the investigation of a blood bank problem, except:
    A. Transfusion history
    B. Obstetric history
    C. Recent history of prescriptive medications
    D. Recent history of nonprescriptive medications
    E. Dietary history

15–19. Arrange the steps in the preliminary serologic testing of an antibody problem in the correct sequence of performance:
    A. Perform a direct antiglobulin test
    B. Obtain a fresh specimen from the patient
    C. Repeat the alloantibody screen
    D. Wash the patient's erythrocytes and repeat the ABO grouping
    E. Perform a panel examination for antibody identification

15. _____
16. _____
17. _____
18. _____
19. _____

20–25. Match the following alloantibodies with their usual optimum temperature or mode of reactivity.
    A. Room temperature or colder
    B. 37° C or antiglobulin testing

20. Anti-A
21. Anti-Le[b]
22. Anti-K

23. Anti-S
24. Anti-Fy^a
25. Anti-M
20. ____
21. ____
22. ____
23. ____
24. ____
25. ____
26. If a major crossmatch is incompatible at room temperature but the alloantibody screen and autocontrol are both negative, the problem can be the result of:
   A. Anti-A$_1$ in an A$_2$ or A$_2$B patient
   B. A donor with a positive direct antiglobulin test
   C. An antibody in the patient's serum reacting with a low incidence antigen on the donor's erythrocytes
   D. An antibody in the donor's serum
   E. All of the above, except D

27. If an antibody panel displays variable strength reactions, which of the following should be considered?
   1. Multiple antibodies
   2. Dosage effect
   3. An antibody directed toward an antigen that has variable strength among donors (e.g., P$_1$)
   4. A drug-related antibody
   5. A typical cold-reacting antibody
   A. only 1
   B. 1 and 2
   C. 1, 2, and 3
   D. 2, 3, and 4
   E. only 5

28. If a patient's serum produces the following reactions with screening cells, what are the most probable antibodies?
   A. Anti-D or anti-c
   B. Anti-K and anti-k
   C. Anti-Le^b or anti-s
   D. Anti-M or anti-P$_1$
   E. None of the above

Reagent Red Blood Cell Screening Cells
Partial Listing of Antigens Present

Cell No.	Rh-hr					Kell		Duffy		Kidd		Lewis		MNS				P
	D	C	E	c	e	K	k	Fy^a	Fy^b	Jk^a	Jk^b	Le^a	Le^b	S	s	M	N	P$_1$
I	+	+	0	+	+	+	0	0	+	+	+	0	+	+	+	+	+	+
II	+	0	+	+	0	0	+	+	0	+	0	0	+	0	+	+	0	+

Patient Results

Cell No.	Room Temp.	37°C	AHG	Coombs Check Cells
I	2+	Neg	±	2+
II	2+	Neg	±	2+
Auto	Neg	Neg	Neg	2+

29. Pathologic conditions can stimulate the production of cold agglutinins with the following characteristics:
   A. A high titer and a thermal range of 10–15° C
   B. Associated with hemolytic anemia and a titer no greater than 1:64
   C. A high titer and associated with anti-H

   D. A high titer and active in vitro up to 30° C
   E. Not associated with in vivo hemolysis and having a thermal range of 10–15° C

30. If a patient's serum produces the following reactions, what is the most probable antibody?

Reagent Red Blood Cell Screening Cells
Partial Listing of Antigens Present

Cell No.	Rh-hr					Kell		Duffy		Kidd		Lewis		MNS				P
	D	C	E	c	e	K	k	Fy^a	Fy^b	Jk^a	Jk^b	Le^a	Le^b	S	s	M	N	P$_1$
I	+	+	0	+	+	+	0	0	+	+	+	0	+	+	+	+	+	+
II	+	0	+	+	0	0	+	+	0	+	0	0	+	0	+	+	0	+

Patient Results

	RT	37 °C	AHG	CC
I	Neg	±	1+	2+
II	Neg	±	1+	2+

Red Blood Cell Panel Antigen Profile
Partial Listing of Antigens Present

Cell No.	Rh-hr					Kell		Duffy		Kidd		Lewis		MNS				P
	D	C	E	c	e	K	k	Fy^a	Fy^b	Jk^a	Jk^b	Le^a	Le^b	S	s	M	N	P$_1$
1	+	0	0	+	+	+	0	+	+	+	0	0	0	+	0	+	+	+
2	+	0	0	+	+	0	+	0	+	+	+	0	+	+	+	+	0	0
3	+	+	+	+	+	0	+	0	+	+	+	0	+	+	+	+	0	+
4	0	0	0	+	0	0	+	+	0	+	0	0	+	0	+	+	0	+
5	0	0	+	+	0	+	+	+	+	0	+	0	+	0	+	+	+	+
6	0	+	0	0	+	+	+	+	+	+	+	0	+	0	+	+	+	+
7	0	+	0	0	+	0	+	0	+	+	+	0	+	0	+	+	0	0
8	0	+	0	0	+	0	+	+	0	0	+	+	0	0	+	+	0	0
9	0	+	+	+	+	0	+	+	+	+	+	+	0	+	0	0	+	+
10	0	+	0	0	+	0	+	0	+	+	+	0	+	0	+	+	+	+
11	0	0	0	+	+	+	+	0	+	+	+	+	0	0	0	0	+	+

Patient Results

Cell No.	37 °C	AHG*	Enzyme Enhancement
1	Neg	1+	3+
2	Neg	1+	3+
3	Neg	1+	3+
4	Neg	1+	3+
5	Neg	1+	3+
6	Neg	Neg	Neg
7	Neg	Neg	Neg
8	Neg	Neg	Neg
9	Neg	1+	3+
10	Neg	Neg	Neg
11	Neg	1+	3+
Auto	Neg	Neg	Neg

* All negative AHG results had 2+ positive check cells

A. Anti-D

B. Anti-c

C. Anti-Fy^a and Fy^b

D. Anti-Le^b

E. Anti-M

31. If a weakly reacting antibody is encountered in the AHG phase of testing, what can be done to potentially enhance the reaction?

A. Extend the incubation time at 4° C

B. Alter the serum:cell ratio by adding 1 or 2 additional drops of serum

C. Titrate the serum to establish the titer

D. Add enzymes to the system

E. Both B and D

32. The term "high-titer–low-avidity" (HTLA) antibodies refers to:

A. High-titer cold agglutinins
B. Antibodies that produce strong AHG reactions
C. Antibodies that react at 37° C
D. Antibodies that have low antigen binding capacity
E. Antibodies that are enhanced by enzymes

33. A mixed-field agglutination pattern of patient's serum and donor's cells can be due to:
   A. Cold agglutinins
   B. Passively acquired antibodies
   C. HTLA antibodies
   D. A type A patient crossmatched with a type B donor
   E. All of the above

34. Polybrene does *not* enhance the agglutination of
   A. IgG type antibodies
   B. Polyagglutinated erythrocytes
   C. Anti-D
   D. Anti-K
   E. All of the above, except **B**

35–39. Match the following terms with their respective descriptions:
35. Panagglutination
36. Polyagglutination
37. Albumin agglutinating phenomenon
38. Antibody to a preservative
39. Rouleaux formation
A. RBCs agglutinated by all or nearly all human sera; autocontrol is usually negative
B. Agglutination caused by sodium caprylate

C. Pseudo-agglutination caused by a serum property
D. Antibody capable of agglutinating all RBCs tested, including the autocontrol
E. Agglutination of reagent RBCs but compatible crossmatches

40. If a patient has a negative alloantibody screen but one or a few units are incompatible, the reason that would *not* be a possibility is:
   A. Anti-A_1
   B. Antibody to preservative
   C. Mistyped unit of blood
   D. Dosage effect
   E. Antibody to a low frequency antigen

41. Which of the following is *not* a potential cause of a false positive direct antiglobulin test?
   A. Use of EDTA anticoagulated blood
   B. Use of refrigerated clotted whole blood
   C. Bacterial contamination
   D. Dirty glassware
   E. Overcentrifugation of erythrocytes

42. Which of the following is *not* a potential cause of a false negative direct antiglobulin test?
   A. Incorrect red cell suspension
   B. Contaminated saline
   C. Bacterial contamination
   D. Delays in the testing process
   E. Omitting AHG from the test

43–45. Fill in the correct answers in the following table.

Direct Antiglobulin Test Results				
Polyspecific AHG	Anti-IgG	Anti-C3d	Cells Probably Sensitized with	Possible Explanation
Positive	Negative	Positive	43	Cold agglutinin disease
Positive	44	45	IgG	Post-transfusion of incompatible blood

43.
   A. IgM
   B. IgG
   C. C3d
   D. C4
   E. Both C and D
44.
   A. Positive
   B. Negative

45.
   A. Positive
   B. Negative

46. Autoimmune hemolytic anemia can be due to:
   A. Warm-reactive autoantibodies
   B. Cold-reactive autoantibodies
   C. Drugs

D. Alloantibodies of the warm type

E. All of the above, except D

47. A positive direct antiglobulin test (DAT) result brought about by drugs can be caused by a (an) _____ mechanism.

    A. Drug adsorption

    B. Immune complex

    C. Membrane modification

    D. Autoantibody formation

    E. All of the above

48. One of the most common drugs that can produce an IgG type of positive DAT is:

    A. Aldomet

    B. Salicylate

    C. Vitamin B$_6$

    D. Valium

    E. Paraaminobenzoic acid (PABA)

49. Which of the following is *not* a cause of mixed-field agglutination?

    A. Interdonor incompatibility

    B. Fetal-maternal hemorrhage

    C. Weak IgM antibodies

    D. Chimerism

    E. Polyagglutinins

50. What can cause a negative direct antiglobulin test (DAT) in the presence of clinically established hemolysis?

    A. An increased antibody dissociation constant

    B. Poor technique

    C. Low IgG levels on erythrocytes

    D. IgM or IgA coating of erythrocytes

    E. All of the above

33. B	42. B
34. B	43. E
35. D	44. A
36. A	45. B
37. B	46. E
38. E	47. E
39. C	48. A
40. B	49. C
41. A	50. E

BIBLIOGRAPHY

Beck, M.L. Hicklin, B., and Pierce, S.R.: Unexpected limitations in the use of commercial antiglobulin reagents. Transfusion, *16*:71-75, 1976.

Boral, L.I., and Henry, J.B.: The Type and Screen: A safe alternative and supplement in selected surgical procedures. Transfusion, *17*:163-168, 1977.

Bruce, M., Watt, A.H., Hare, W., Blue, A., and Mitchell, R.: A serious source of error in antiglobulin testing. Transfusion, *26*(2):177-181, 1986.

Chaplin, H.: Clinical usefulness of specific antiglobulin reagents in autoimmune hemolytic anemia. Prog. Hematol., *8*25-49, 1973.

Cordle, D., et al.: Safety and cost containment data advocate abbreviated crossmatching. Abstract of paper at 39th Annual Meeting of the American Association of Blood Banks, Transfusion, *26*(6): 1986.

Dzik, W.H., and Darling, C.A.: Positive Direct antiglobulin Test (DAT) due to anti-formaldehyde antibodies. Transfusion, *26*(6):578, 1986.

Freedman, J., Wright., J., Lim, F.C., and Garvey, M.B.: Hemolytic warm IgM autoagglutinins in autoimmune hemolytic anemia. Transfusion, *27*(6):464-467, 1987.

Garratty, G., and Petz, L.D.: The significance of red cell bond complement components in the development of standards and quality control for the anticomplement, components of antiglobulin sera. Transfusion, *16*:297-306, 1976.

Garratty, G.: Abbreviated pretransfusion testing. Transfusion *26*(3):217-219, 1986.

Geisland, J.R., Milam, J.D.: Spuriously positive direct antiglobulin tests caused by silicone gel. Transfusion, *20*:711-713, 1980.

Giblett, E.R.: Blood group alloantibodies: An assessment of some laboratory practices. Transfusion, Vol. *17*:299-307, 1977.

Gilliland, B.C., Leddy, J.P. and Baughn, J.H.: The detection of cell-bound antibody on complement coated human red cells. J. Clin. Invest. *49*:898-906, 1970.

Grindon, A.J., and Wilson, M.J.: False-Positive DAT caused by variables in sample procurement. Transfusion *21*:313-314, 1981.

Issitt, P.D.: Applied Blood Group Serology. 3rd Ed. Miami, Montgomery Scientific, 1985. pp. 478-495.

Judd, W.J.: Streamlining Serological Testing: Scientific Considerations. Blood Banking in a Changing Environment. Edited by D.M. Smith Arlington, Va.,

ANSWERS

1. B	17. A
2. D	18. C
3. C	19. E
4. C	20. A
5. B	21. A
6. C	22. B
7. D	23. B
8. C	24. B
9. E	25. A
10. E	26. E
11. C	27. C
12. C	28. D
13. B	29. D
14. E	30. B
15. B	31. E
16. D	32. D

American Association of Blood Banking, 1984, pp. 15-40.

Kim, B., and Anderson, H.: Correspondence from American Red Cross, Blood Services, Rochester, New York, December, 1985.

Moscow, J.A., Casper, A.J., Kodis, C., and Fricke, W.A.: Positive direct antiglobulin test results after intravenous immune globulin administration. Transfusion, 27(3):248-249, 1987.

Noto, T.A.: How to interpret a positive DAT. Diagn. Med. Sept/Oct.: 59-61, 64-67, 70, 1982.

Ortho Diagnostics Product Brochure, Results of Parallel Tests Using an EDTA Specimen, Raritan, NJ, Ortho Diagnostics, Inc., 1977.

Oberman, H.A.: The crossmatch-A brief historical perspective. Transfusion, 21(6):645-651, 1981.

Oberman, H.A., et al.: Role of the crossmatch in testing for serologic incompatibility. Transfusion. 22:12-16, 1982.

Park, H.: Limitations of the immediate-spin crossmatch. Transfusion, 25(6):588, 1985.

Pliska, C.: Low ionic strength solution (LISS). Lab. Med. 11(3):159-164, 1980.

Pohl, B.A.: Immediate-spin crossmatch: How serious are the problems? Transfusion, 25(6):589, 1985.

Proujan, B. (Ed.): Changes to 12th edition of Standards Announced—Testing of Recipient Blood. AABB News Briefs. 11(6):3, 1988.

Robertson, V. M., Dickson, L. G., Romond, E. H., and Ash, R.C.: Positive antiglobulin tests due to intravenous immunoglobulin in patients who received bone marrow transplant. Transfusion 27(1):28-31, 1987.

Salama, A., Gottsche, B., Schleiffer, T., and Mueller-Eckhardt, C.: Immune complex mediated intravascular hemolysis due to IgM cephalosporin-dependent antibody. Transfusion 27(6):460-463, 1987.

Schmidt, P. J., Samia, C. T., Gregory, K. R., and Leparc, G. F.: Rational reduction in pretransfusion testing. Lab. Med. 17(8):467-470, 1986.

Sererat, Surapong, et al.: Why not antiglobulin compatibility testing? Transfusion, 25(6):589, 1985.

Shirley, R.S., et al.: The efficacy of performing red cell elutions in pretransfusion testing of patients with positive antiglobulin tests. Transfusion, 24:417, 1984.

Shulman, I.A., et al.: Unreliability of the immediate-spin crossmatch to detect ABO incompatibility. Transfusion. 25(6):589, 1985.

Standards for Blood Banks and Transfusion Services, Arlington, VA, 11th Ed. 1984, pp. 24-26.

Steane, E.A., et al.: A proposal for compatibility testing incorporating the manual hexadimethrine bromide (Polybrene) Test. Transfusion, 25(6):540-544, 1975.

Steane, S.: Drug-Induced Red Blood Cell Sensitization and Destruction. In Pittiglio, D.H. (Ed.): Modern Blood Banking and Transfusion Practices. Philadelphia, F.A. Davis, p. 447-458, 1985.

7

Clinical Problems in Blood Banking

> At the conclusion of this chapter, the reader will be able to:
> • Analyze and solve serologic problems related to blood group systems, drugs, and hemolytic disease of the newborn.

Chapter Outline

In this chapter, typical examples of serologic problems encountered in the blood bank are presented. The first seven groups of case studies integrate the concepts and practices presented in preceding chapters. The last group of case studies represent specific antibody problems that can be encountered in obstetric and neonatal situations. Additional information related to the last group of cases can be found in Chapter 10, Hemolytic Disease of the Newborn.

ABO DISCREPANCY

Case 1

Submitted by Polly F. Kay, MT(ASCP), MHS
School of Medical Technology
Anderson Memorial Hospital
Anderson, South Carolina

HISTORY AND LABORATORY DATA

A unit of blood from a healthy homologous donor yielded the following results on processing:

	Anti-A	Anti-B	Anti-A, B	Anti-D	Rh control	A₁ cells	B cells
Forward RBC typing	1+	3+	3+	3+	Neg		
Serum reverse typing						3+	Neg

QUESTIONS

1. What blood type does the forward typing indicate?

2. What blood type does the reverse serum typing indicate?
3. What additional tests should be done to confirm this donor's phenotype?

DISCUSSION

1. The forward typing indicates group AB.
2. The reverse serum grouping indicates group B.
3. To resolve this discrepancy, the donor's serum was tested with three A_1 cells, three A_2 cells, and three O cells. The donor's red cells were additionally tested with anti-A_1 lectin, and no agglutination was observed. The following reactions were observed with the donor's serum and the panel of known cells.

Laboratory Data (Case 1)

Patient Results

Reagent Cell No. and Type	Reaction
1 A_1	3+
2 A_1	3+
3 A_1	3+
4 A_2	Neg
5 A_2	Neg
6 A_2	Neg
7 O	Neg
8 O	Neg
9 O	Neg

The serum antibody was identified as anti-A_1. Because the donor's cells failed to agglutinate the anti-A_1 lectin, the cells were classified as A_2. Other subgroups of A were excluded because of the original reaction observed with the anti-A reagent. Anti-A reagent agglutinates A_1 and A_2 red cells. Refer to Chapter 4 for a full discussion of discrepancies in the ABO system.

CONCLUSION

This donor is of the A_2B phenotype with an anti-A_1 antibody.

Rh ANTIBODIES

Case 2

HISTORY AND LABORATORY DATA

A 24-year-old White woman, group AB Rh negative, D^u positive, phenotype cde/cde, received 2 units of AB positive blood when her first child was delivered. Three years later, she received another 2 units of AB positive (RH_o) blood at the same hospital. This patient's husband is Rh negative as were her first two children. She never received antenatal or postpartum immune globulin D. One year later, she had the following test results when a prenatal screen was performed during her third pregnancy.

Laboratory Data (Case 2)

Reagent Red Blood Cell Screening Cells
Partial Listing of Antigens Present

Cell No.	Rh-hr					Kell		Duffy		Kidd		Lewis		MNS				P
	D	C	E	c	e	K	k	Fy^a	Fy^b	Jk^a	Jk^b	Le^a	Le^b	S	s	M	N	P_1
I	+	0	+	+	+	0	+	+	0	+	+	0	+	+	+	+	0	+
II	0	+	0	+	0	0	+	0	+	+	0	0	+	0	+	+	0	+

Patient Results

Cell No.	Immediate Spin	37° C	AHG	Coombs Control
I	Neg	Neg	2+	
II	Neg	Neg	Neg	2+

Reagent Red Blood Cell Panel Antigen Profile
Partial Listing of Antigens Present

Cell No.	Rh-hr					Kell		Duffy		Kidd		Lewis		MNS				P
	D	C	E	c	e	K	k	Fy^a	Fy^b	Jk^a	Jk^b	Le^a	Le^b	S	s	M	N	P$_1$
1	0	0	0	+	+	0	+	+	+	+	0	0	0	+	0	+	+	+
2	0	0	0	+	+	0	+	0	+	+	+	0	+	+	+	+	0	0
3	0	+	+	+	+	0	+	0	+	+	+	0	+	+	+	+	0	+
4	+	0	+	+	0	0	+	+	0	+	0	0	+	0	+	+	0	+
5	+	0	+	+	0	0	+	+	+	0	+	0	+	0	+	+	+	+
6	+	+	0	0	+	+	+	+	+	+	0	0	+	0	+	+	+	+
7	+	+	0	0	+	0	+	0	+	+	+	0	+	0	+	+	0	0
8	+	+	+	0	+	0	+	+	0	0	+	+	0	0	+	+	0	+
9	+	+	0	+	+	0	+	+	+	+	+	+	0	+	0	0	+	+
10	+	+	0	0	+	+	0	0	+	+	+	0	+	0	+	+	+	+
11	+	0	0	+	+	0	+	0	+	+	+	+	0	0	0	0	+	+

Patient Results

Cell No.	Immediate Spin	37° C	AHG	Coombs Control
1	Neg	Neg	Neg	2+
2	Neg	Neg	Neg	2+
3	Neg	Neg	Neg	2+
4	Neg	Neg	2+	
5	Neg	Neg	2+	
6	Neg	Neg	2+	
7	Neg	Neg	3+	
8	Neg	Neg	2+	
9	Neg	Neg	1+	
10	Neg	Neg	1+	
11	Neg	Neg	2+	

QUESTIONS

1. Based on the antigen profile of the two screening cells and the phase of reactivity, name all the possible alloantibodies that could be present in this patient's serum.

2. Based on the possible alloantibodies identified in answer No. 1 and the antigen profile of the panel of reagent red cells, what is the identity of the alloantibody?

3. Could other techniques be used to enhance the reactivity of this antibody?

4. Why would a D^u positive person develop an alloantibody to a related Rh antigen?

5. What type of blood should this patient have received in the past and what type must she receive if future transfusions are necessary?

DISCUSSION

1. Reactivity in the AHG phase suggests either an Rh antibody or an AHG reactive antibody. Based on the major antigens cited in two cell antigen profiles, several alloantibodies are possible: anti-D, anti-E, anti-e, anti-Fy^a, anti-Jk^b, and anti-S.

2. The patient's antibody-containing serum does not react with any of the red cell antigens expressed on panel cells 1, 2, or 3. She is also known to be e antigen-positive. Therefore, the pattern and mode of reactivity of the antibody or antibodies exclude all the possible antibodies cited in Answer 1, but are consistent with anti-D.

3. Yes, enzyme treatment of reagent screening and/or panel cells is an excellent method of strengthening the reactivity of Rh antibodies. Such treatment usually produces reactions at 37° C.

4. The expression of a positive test for D^u when the results of D antigen testing are negative may be caused by either a mosaic or suppression of the D antigen. Refer to Chapter 5 for a full discussion of D^u. In this case, the patient was a true D^u (not a suppressed D antigen) and the introduction of D antigen by transfusion was recognized by her immune system as foreign. A secondary anamnestic response occurred when the D antigen was reintroduced following the delivery of her second child.

5. This patient should have received D (Rh$_o$) and D^u negative blood. She *must* receive D and D^u negative blood if future transfusions are needed.

Conclusion

Transfusion-induced anti-D alloantibody.

Case 3

History and Laboratory Data

A 43-year-old Black woman was admitted for a cholecystectomy. The patient had 4 living children; the youngest was 15 years old. She had no history of prior transfusions. An alloantibody was discovered on the routine preoperative blood bank work-up.

Laboratory Data (Case 3)

Blood grouping	B Positive
Indirect antiglobulin test (Coombs')	Positive
Reactive phases	AHG and 37° C with ficin-treated reagent cells
DAT	Negative

The results of the two-cell screening and the panel of reagent red cells follow:

Reagent Red Blood Cell Screening Cells
Partial Listing of Antigens Present

Cell No.	Rh-hr					Kell		Duffy		Kidd		Lewis		MNS				P
	D	C	E	c	e	K	k	Fy^a	Fy^b	Jk^a	Jk^b	Le^a	Le^b	S	s	M	N	P$_1$
I	0	+	0	+	+	0	+	0	+	+	+	0	+	+	+	+	0	+
II	+	0	+	+	0	0	+	+	0	+	0	0	+	0	+	+	0	+

Patient Results

Cell No.	Immediate Spin	37° C	AHG	Coombs Control	37° C Enzyme-Treated
I	Neg	Neg	Neg	2+	Neg
II	Neg	Neg	2+		3+
Auto	Neg	Neg	Neg	2+	Neg

Reagent Red Blood Cell Panel Antigen Profile
Partial Listing of Antigens Present

Cell No.	Rh-hr					Kell		Duffy		Kidd		Lewis		MNS				P
	D	C	E	c	e	K	k	Fy^a	Fy^b	Jk^a	Jk^b	Le^a	Le^b	S	s	M	N	P$_1$
1	0	0	0	+	+	0	+	+	+	+	0	0	0	+	0	+	+	+
2	0	0	0	+	+	0	+	0	+	+	+	0	+	+	+	+	0	0
3	0	+	0	+	+	0	+	0	+	+	+	0	+	+	+	+	0	+
4	+	0	+	+	0	0	+	+	0	+	0	0	+	0	+	+	0	+
5	+	0	+	+	0	0	+	+	+	0	+	0	+	0	+	+	+	+
6	+	+	0	0	+	+	+	+	+	+	0	0	+	+	+	+	+	+
7	+	+	0	0	+	0	+	+	0	+	+	0	+	0	+	+	+	+
8	+	+	+	0	+	0	+	0	0	0	+	+	0	+	+	0	0	0
9	+	+	0	+	+	0	+	+	+	+	+	+	0	+	0	0	+	+
10	+	+	0	0	+	+	0	0	+	+	+	0	+	0	+	+	+	+
11	+	0	0	+	+	0	+	0	+	+	+	+	0	0	0	0	+	+

Patient Results

Cell No.	Immediate Spin	37° C	AHG	Coombs Control
1	Neg	Neg	Neg	2+
2	Neg	Neg	Neg	2+
3	Neg	Neg	Neg	2+
4	Neg	Neg	2+	
5	Neg	Neg	2+	
6	Neg	Neg	Neg	2+
7	Neg	Neg	Neg	3+
8	Neg	Neg	2+	
9	Neg	Neg	Neg	1+
10	Neg	Neg	Neg	1+
11	Neg	Neg	Neg	2+

QUESTIONS

1. Based on the antigen profile of the two screening cells and the phase of reactivity, name all the possible alloantibodies that could be present in this patient's serum.

2. Based on the possible alloantibodies identified in answer No. 1 and the antigen profile of the panel of reagent red cells, what is the identity of this alloantibody?

3. What additional testing should be conducted to confirm the identity of the antibody?

4. Briefly describe some of the characteristics of the antigen-antibody system to which this alloantibody belongs.

5. What was the source of this patient's antigen exposure?

DISCUSSION

1. Reactivity in the AHG phase suggests either an Rh antibody or an AHG reactive antibody. The major antigens reacting in the two-cell antigen screening test suggest the presence of one or more of several alloantibodies: anti-D, anti-E, anti-Fy^a, and anti-Jk^a. The known presence of the D (Rh$_o$) antigen, however, excludes the possibility of anti-D.

2. The pattern of reactivity in AHG distinguishes the alloantibody as anti-E.

3. If possible, the patient's red cells should be tested for the presence of the corresponding antigen. In this case, it was possible to test the patient's red cells accurately because she had not been transfused within the last 3 months. Her red cells were E Negative.

4. The E antigen is part of the Rhesus (Rh) blood group system described in Chapter 5. Anti-E is usually an IgG (sometimes IgM) antibody and does not bind complement. Seventy percent of White persons are E negative. This antibody has been implicated in hemolytic reactions and HDN.

5. Most cases of anti-E represent alloantibodies formed in response to E positive erythrocyte transfusions or pregnancies, although a few are believed to be secondary to naturally occurring antigens. In this case, the patient had had four pregnancies, which were probably the source of the antigenic exposure.

CONCLUSION

Anti-E alloantibody, probably resulting from previous pregnancies.

Case 4

HISTORY AND LABORATORY DATA

A 20-year-old woman was a prenatal outpatient (8 weeks gestation). She had no history of prior transfusions but had had one previous pregnancy. The patient was group A Rh positive and demonstrated a positive alloantibody screening test. During the patient's last pregnancy, another blood bank had identified the alloantibody Fy^a in the patient's serum. Her past records did not include any additional antigen testing.

Laboratory Data (Case 4)

Reagent Red Blood Cell Screening Cells
Partial Listing of Antigens Present

Cell No.	Rh-hr					Kell		Duffy		Kidd		Lewis		MNS				P
	D	C	E	c	e	K	k	Fy^a	Fy^b	Jk^a	Jk^b	Le^a	Le^b	S	s	M	N	P$_1$
I	+	0	+	+	+	0	+	+	0	+	+	0	+	+	+	+	0	+
II	0	+	0	+	0	+	0	0	+	+	0	0	+	0	+	+	+	+

Patient Results

Cell No.	Immediate Spin	37° C	AHG
I	3+	1+	+
II	±	Neg	±

Reagent Red Blood Cell Panel Antigen Profile
Partial Listing of Antigens Present

Cell No.	Rh-hr					Kell		Duffy		Kidd		Lewis		MNS				P
	D	C	E	c	e	K	k	Fy^a	Fy^b	Jk^a	Jk^b	Le^a	Le^b	S	s	M	N	P$_1$
1	0	0	0	+	+	0	+	+	+	+	0	0	0	+	0	+	+	+
2	0	+	0	+	+	0	+	0	+	+	+	0	+	+	+	+	+	0
3	0	+	0	+	+	0	+	+	+	+	+	0	+	+	+	0	+	+
4	+	+	+	+	0	0	+	+	0	+	0	0	+	0	+	+	+	+
5	+	0	+	+	0	0	+	+	+	0	+	0	+	0	+	+	0	+
6	+	+	0	0	+	+	+	+	+	+	0	0	+	+	+	+	0	+
7	0	+	0	0	+	0	+	0	+	+	+	0	+	0	+	+	0	+
8	0	0	+	+	+	0	+	+	0	0	+	+	0	0	+	+	0	0
9	0	0	0	+	+	0	+	0	+	+	+	+	0	+	0	+	0	+
10	0	+	0	0	+	+	0	+	+	+	+	0	+	0	+	0	+	+

Patient Results

Cell No.	Immediate Spin	37° C	AHG	Coombs Control
1	±	Neg	± micro	
2	±	Neg	± micro	
3	Neg	Neg	Neg	2+
4	±	Neg	± micro	
5	2+	1+	± micro	
6	2+	1+	± micro	
7	2+	1+	± micro	
8	2+	1+	± micro	
9	2+	1+	1+	
10	Neg	Neg	Neg	2+
Auto	Neg	Neg	Neg	2+

QUESTIONS

1. Based on the pattern of reactivity, does this patient have only the previously identified anti-Fy^a?
2. What antibody (antibodies) is (are) suggested by the screening and panel cells?
3. Why are the reactions of the I screening cell as well as the panel cells No. 5 through No. 9 stronger than those of the other reactive cells?
4. Would additional tests be of value?
5. Was this patient immunized as the result of her previous pregnancy?

DISCUSSION

1. No. The pattern of reactivity and the specific cells demonstrating agglutination in both the screening cells and panel of cells do *not* suggest the presence of a Fy^a alloantibody. The screening cells suggest an antibody that has an optimal thermal range of 4 to 20° C. The specific blood group antigens present on the group O reagent cells that exhibit this behavior are Lewis, MNS, and P.
2. The agglutination pattern, graded by strength as well as specificity, is typical of the reactivity demonstrated by anti-M. Most examples of anti-M have a definite affinity for cooler temperatures. Anti-M is usually an IgM antibody, although it may occasionally be an IgG antibody, and it usually does not bind complement. It typically reacts in the saline phase, but it may occasionally react in the AHG phase. Refer to Chapter 5 for a full discussion of the MNS system.
3. Examination of the MN phenotypes of the reagent cells demonstrates that the stronger-reacting cells are homozygous MM cells rather than heterozygous MN cells. The difference in strength of agglutination is caused by the "dosage effect."
   Almost all anti-M antibodies show

some dosage effect. Anti-M displays dosage at 4 to 20° C. This means that it reacts more strongly with MM cells than with MN cells. Additionally, if an anti-M reacts at 37° C, it generally will do so only with type MM cells.

4. In this case, it was important to exclude an underlying anti-Fy^a because of the previously identified alloantibody in the patient's history. The patient's red cells were typed for Fy^a antigen and found to be positive. Therefore, the previous identification of the alloantibody as anti-Fy^a, was an error. The patient's red cells were also typed for the M and N antigen. She was found to be M (negative) and N (positive).

5. No. Testing of both the patient's husband and their first baby revealed that both were M (negative) and N (positive). Anti-M is a fairly frequent environmentally stimulated antibody. The usual mode of stimulation is through exposure to antigenically similar, naturally occurring substances by either ingestion or inhalation.

CONCLUSION

Anti-M.

COLD-REACTING ANTIBODIES

Case 5

HISTORY AND LABORATORY DATA

A 6-year-old Black boy had a diagnosis of congenital spherocytosis with acute hemolytic anemia. On admission, his hematocrit was 16% and one unit of packed red cells was ordered for transfusion. According to the patient's pediatrician, the child had never been transfused. The patient was group A Rh positive. All units crossmatched were weakly incompatible at room temperature, 37° C and AHG.

The patient's DAT was negative with polyspecific, IgG, and C3d antisera. Although the DAT was negative, an elution technique was performed. The elution studies, however, failed to demonstrate a specific antibody. The results of his two-cell reagent screening cells and an accompanying panel of reagent red cells follows.

Laboratory Data (Case 5)

Reagent Red Blood Cell Screening Cells
Partial Listing of Antigens Present

Cell No.	Rh-hr					Kell		Duffy		Kidd		Lewis		MNS				P
	D	C	E	c	e	K	k	Fy^a	Fy^b	Jk^a	Jk^b	Le^a	Le^b	S	s	M	N	P$_1$
I	+	0	+	+	+	0	+	+	0	+	+	0	+	+	+	+	0	+
II	0	+	0	+	0	+	0	0	+	+	0	0	+	0	+	+	0	+

Patient Results

Cell No.	Immediate Spin	37° C	AHG
I	±	±	±
II	±	1+	±

Reagent Red Blood Cell Panel Antigen Profile
Partial Listing of Antigens Present

Cell No.	Rh-hr					Kell		Duffy		Kidd		Lewis		MNS				P
	D	C	E	c	e	K	k	Fy^a	Fy^b	Jk^a	Jk^b	Le^a	Le^b	S	s	M	N	P_1
1	0	0	0	+	+	0	+	+	+	+	0	0	0	+	0	+	+	+
2	0	+	0	+	+	0	+	0	+	+	+	0	+	+	+	+	0	0
3	0	+	0	+	+	0	+	0	+	+	+	0	+	+	+	+	0	+
4	+	+	+	+	0	0	+	+	0	+	0	0	+	0	+	+	0	+
5	+	0	+	+	0	0	+	+	+	0	+	0	+	0	+	+	+	+
6	+	+	0	0	+	+	+	+	+	+	0	0	+	0	+	+	+	+
7	+	+	0	0	+	0	+	0	+	+	+	0	+	0	+	+	+	+
8	+	0	+	+	+	0	+	+	0	0	+	+	0	0	+	+	0	0
9	+	0	0	+	+	0	+	+	+	+	+	+	0	+	0	0	+	+
10	+	+	0	0	+	+	0	0	+	+	+	0	+	0	+	+	+	+
11	+	0	0	+	+	0	+	0	+	+	+	+	0	0	0	0	+	+

Patient Results

Cell No.	Immediate Spin	37° C	AHG
1	±	±	±
2	±	±	±
3	±	±	±
4	±	±	±
5	±	±	±
6	±	±	±
7	±	±	±
8	±	±	±
9	±	±	±
10	±	±	±
11	±	±	±
Auto	±	±	±

QUESTIONS

1. What is the cause of the positive DAT?
2. What does the reactivity pattern of the Group O reagent red cells indicate?
3. What technique can be used to cross-match units for transfusion?

DISCUSSION

1. With a negative DAT, the cause of the hemolysis is more likely to be related to the spherocytosis and a superimposed infection than a cold autoagglutinin.
2. The reactivity observed in the screening and panel cells, and the autocontrol is typical of a nonspecific cold agglutinin. Because the patient had no history of transfusion, it is unlikely that he has an alloantibody.

3. Compatible blood should not be difficult to find, especially if a pre-warmed crossmatch is performed.

CONCLUSION

Nonspecific cold autoagglutinin.

AHG-REACTING ANTIBODIES

Case 6

HISTORY AND LABORATORY DATA

A 90-year-old White woman with chronic renal failure was admitted to the hospital to be transfused with 3 units of packed red cells. Her hemoglobin was 6.0 dL. She had received numerous past transfusions, but had not been transfused for the past 3 months. Her history also included one pregnancy.

She was group O Rh positive, and one of the 3 units crossmatched was incompatible. Her alloantibody screen was also positive. However, her DAT was negative. Results of the screening and a panel of reagent red cells are presented below. Investigation of her past medical records indicated that anti-Kell had been identified in her serum at another hospital 14 months earlier and anti-S had been eluted from her red cells during the same hospitalization.

Laboratory Data (Case 6)

Reagent Red Blood Cell Screening Cells
Partial Listing of Antigens Present

Cell No.	Rh-hr					Kell		Duffy		Kidd		Lewis		MNS				P
	D	C	E	c	e	K	k	Fy^a	Fy^b	Jk^a	Jk^b	Le^a	Le^b	S	s	M	N	P_1
I	+	0	+	+	+	0	+	+	0	+	+	0	+	+	+	+	0	+
II	0	+	0	+	0	+	0	0	+	+	0	0	+	0	+	+	0	+

Patient Results

Cell No.	Immediate Spin	37° C	AHG	Coombs Control Cells
I	Neg	Neg	Neg	2+
II	Neg	Neg	2+	

Reagent Red Blood Cell Panel Antigen Profile
Listing of Antigens Present

Cell No.	Rh-Hr								Kell						Duffy		Kidd	
	C	D	E	c	e	C^w	f	V	K	k	Kp^a	Kp^b	Js^a	Js^b	Fy^a	Fy^b	Jk^a	Jk^b
1	+	+	+	0	+	0	0	0	+	+	0	+	0	+	0	+	0	+
2	+	+	0	0	+	+	0	0	0	+	0	+	0	+	+	+	+	0
3	0	+	+	+	0	0	0	0	0	+	0	+	0	+	+	+	+	0
4	+	0	0	+	+	0	+	0	0	+	0	+	0	+	0	+	+	+
5	0	0	+	+	+	0	+	0	0	+	0	+	0	+	+	+	+	0
6	0	0	0	+	+	0	+	0	0	+	0	+	0	+	0	+	0	+
7	0	0	0	+	+	0	+	0	0	+	0	+	0	+	+	0	0	+
8	0	+	0	+	+	0	+	0	0	+	0	+	0	+	0	0	+	0
9	0	0	0	+	+	0	+	0	0	+	0	+	0	+	+	+	+	+
10	0	0	0	+	+	0	+	0	0	+	0	+	0	+	+	+	+	+

Antigens Present (continued)

Cell No.	Lewis		P	MNS				Lutheran		Sex-Linked		Additional
	Le^a	Le^b	P_1	M	N	S	s	Lu^a	Lu^b	Xg^a		
1	0	+	+	0	+	+	+	0	+	0	M	
2	+	0	+	+	+	0	+	0	+	+	M	Co (b+)
3	0	+	+	0	+	0	+	0	+	+	M	
4	0	+	+	+	0	+	0	+	+	+	F	Co (b+)
5	0	+	0	+	+	+	+	0	+	+	M	
6	0	+	0	+	+	0	+	0	+	0	M	
7	0	+	+	+	0	+	+	0	+	0	M	Co (b+)
8	+	0	+	+	+	+	0	0	+	0	M	
9	0	0	+	+	+	+	0	0	+	+	F	
10	0	+	0	0	0	0	+	0	+	+	F	
11												I (neg)

Patient Results

Cell No.	Immediate Spin	37° C	AHG	Coombs Control Cells
1	Neg	1+	2+	
2	Neg	Neg	Neg	2+
3	Neg	Neg	Neg	2+
4	Neg	Neg	Neg	2+
5	Neg	Neg	Neg	2+
6	Neg	Neg	Neg	2+
7	Neg	Neg	Neg	1+
8	Neg	Neg	Neg	2+
9	Neg	Neg	Neg	1+
10	Neg	Neg	Neg	2+
11	Neg	Neg	Neg	2+
Auto	Neg	Neg	Neg	2+

QUESTIONS

1. Based on the reactions of the two screening cells and the panel of reagent red cells, what antibody (antibodies) is (are) present?
2. What antibody is producing the incompatible crossmatch?
3. Why was a second antibody not demonstrated?
4. Briefly describe some of the characteristics of the undetectable antibody.
5. What type blood should this woman receive?

DISCUSSION

1. The pattern of reactivity is consistent only with anti-K.
2. The anti-K was reacting with one of the crossmatched units, which was found to be K (positive).
3. The titer of the anti-S was undoubtedly too low to be clinically detectable.
4. Anti-S usually occurs as an immune antibody in the sera of multiparous women or multitransfused patients. Rare examples of environmentally stimulated anti-S which react best in saline at room temperature have been observed. This antibody is capable of causing HDN. He-molytic transfusion reactions attributable to it have also occurred. The antibody is most often found in conjunction with other antibodies, except anti-A and anti-B.

Anti-S is not a commonly detected alloantibody despite the frequency of the S antigen in the general population. This suggests that the S antigen is capable of initiating an immune response only in very susceptible individuals. A full discussion of the MNS system is presented in Chapter 5.
5. Because anti-S was reported from a previous eluate, this patient should be transfused only with K-neg, S-neg units even though the anti-S is not demonstrable at present.

CONCLUSION

Anti-K with a history of anti-S.

Case 7

HISTORY AND LABORATORY DATA

A 70-year-old White woman was hospitalized for a below-the-knee amputation. She had received 3 units of packed red cells during a surgical procedure 7 months earlier. She had also received 2 units of packed red cells to correct a mild anemia one week earlier. Her obstetrical history included two living children and one miscarriage.

Her blood type was group B Rh negative. She had had a negative alloantibody screen one week earlier. A repeat alloantibody screen performed while cross-matching the preoperative units of blood revealed a positive alloantibody screen. She also exhibited a positive DAT. An eluate of the patient's red cells and serum revealed the following pattern of reactivity using two screening cells and a red cell reagent panel.

Laboratory Data (Case 7)

Direct Antiglobulin Profile

	Polyspecific Anti-Human Serum (Rabbit)	Control Pts Washed RBCs + Normal Saline	Anti-Human Serum Anti-IgG (Rabbit)	Anti-Human Serum Anti-C3d Serum (Rabbit)
Red cell test results	1+ micro	Negative	1+ micro	Negative

Reagent Red Blood Cell Screening Cells (Using an eluate from the patient's red cells)

Cell No.	Rh-hr					Kell		Duffy		Kidd		Lewis		MNS				P
	D	C	E	c	e	K	k	Fy^a	Fy^b	Jk^a	Jk^b	Le^a	Le^b	S	s	M	N	P$_1$
I	+	0	+	+	+	0	+	+	0	+	+	0	+	+	+	+	0	+
II	0	+	0	+	0	0	+	0	+	+	0	0	+	0	+	+	0	+

Patient Results

Cell No.	Immediate Spin	37° C	AHG	Coombs Control Cells
I	Neg	Neg	1+	
II	Neg	Neg	Neg	2+

Reagent Red Blood Cell Panel Antigen Profile
Partial Listing of Antigens Present

Cell No.	Rh-hr					Kell		Duffy		Kidd		Lewis		MNS				P
	D	C	E	c	E	K	k	Fy^a	Fy^b	Jk^a	Jk^b	Le^a	Le^b	S	s	M	N	P$_1$
1	0	0	0	+	+	0	+	+	+	+	0	0	0	+	0	+	+	+
2	0	0	0	+	+	0	+	0	+	+	+	0	+	+	+	+	0	0
3	0	+	0	+	+	0	+	0	+	+	+	0	+	+	+	+	0	+
4	+	0	+	+	0	0	+	+	0	+	0	0	+	0	+	+	0	+
5	+	0	+	+	0	0	+	+	+	0	+	0	+	0	+	+	+	+
6	+	+	0	0	+	+	+	+	+	+	0	0	+	+	+	+	+	+
7	+	+	0	0	+	0	+	0	+	+	+	0	+	0	+	+	+	+
8	+	+	+	0	+	0	+	+	0	0	+	+	0	0	+	+	0	0
9	+	+	0	+	+	0	+	+	+	+	+	+	0	+	0	0	+	+
10	+	+	0	0	+	+	0	0	+	+	+	0	+	0	+	+	+	+
11	+	0	0	+	+	0	+	0	+	+	+	+	0	0	0	0	+	+

Patient Results

Cell No.	Immediate Spin	37° C	AHG
1	Neg	2+	
2	Neg	Neg	2+
3	Neg	Neg	2+
4	Neg	2+	
5	Neg	2+	
6	Neg	2+	
7	Neg	Neg	1+
8	Neg	2+	
9	Neg	1+	
10	Neg	Neg	1+

QUESTIONS

1. What is the identity of the alloantibody?

2. Why was the patient's alloantibody screen negative before and positive at the time of this crossmatch?

3. Should additional tests be performed?

4. Why was the DAT positive?

5. Briefly discuss the characteristics of the blood group system involved in this case.

DISCUSSION

1. The patient's serum and elution both demonstrated anti-Fy^a reactivity.

2. Post-transfusion sensitization against Fy^a antigen, consistent with a delayed hemolytic transfusion reaction, caused the differences in the test observations. The original antigenic exposure probably

occurred as the result of the pregnancy or the packed red cells administered 7 months previously. The anti-Fy^a was not detected on the alloantibody screen one week earlier or when the specimen was retested. However, the most recent transfusion undoubtedly produced a secondary anamnestic response.

3. Yes. When the two units transfused one week earlier were typed for the Fy^a antigen, both were found to be Fy^a positive.

4. The positive DAT resulted rom the transfused Fy^a positive red cells being coated with the patient's Fy^a alloantibody.

5. The Fy^a antigen belongs to the Duffy blood group system. Anti-Fy^a is usually an IgG antibody, sometimes capable of binding complement. This antibody has been implicated in hemolytic transfusion reactions and HDN. It usually develops in response to antigenic exposure through transfusion or pregnancy to Fy^a positive red cells. A complete discussion of this blood group system can be found in Chapter 5.

CONCLUSION

Anti-Fy^a associated with delayed hemolytic transfusion reaction.

Case 8

HISTORY AND LABORATORY DATA

A 33-year-old man was admitted for a perforated ulcer. He had a history of multiple transfusions. A stat crossmatch for 8 units of packed cells was ordered while the patient was in surgery.

The man was group A Rh positive. He had a positive alloantibody screen and negative DAT. The results of the two cell screening and subsequent reagent red cell panel follow.

Laboratory Data (Case 8)

Reagent Red Blood Cell Screening Cells
Partial Listing of Antigens Present

Cell No.	Rh-hr					Kell		Duffy		Kidd		Lewis		MNS				P
	D	C	E	c	e	K	k	Fy^a	Fy^b	Jk^a	Jk^b	Le^a	Le^b	S	s	M	N	P$_1$
I	+	+	0	+	+	+	0	0	+	+	+	0	+	+	+	+	0	+
II	+	0	+	+	0	0	+	+	0	+	0	0	+	0	+	+	0	+

Patient Results

Cell No.	Immediate Spin	37° C	AHG	Coombs Control
I	Neg	Neg	2+	
II	Neg	Neg	Neg	2+

Reagent Red Blood Cell Panel Antigen Profile
Partial Listing of Antigens Present

Cell No.	Rh-hr					Kell		Duffy		Kidd		Lewis		MNS				P
	D	C	E	c	e	K	k	Fy^a	Fy^b	Jk^a	Jk^b	Le^a	Le^b	S	s	M	N	P$_1$
1	+	0	0	+	+	+	0	+	+	+	0	0	0	+	0	+	+	+
2	+	0	0	+	+	0	+	0	+	+	+	0	+	+	+	+	0	0
3	+	+	+	+	+	0	+	0	+	+	+	0	+	+	+	+	0	+
4	0	0	0	+	0	0	+	+	0	+	0	0	+	0	+	+	0	+
5	0	0	+	+	0	+	+	+	+	0	+	0	+	0	+	+	+	+
6	0	+	0	0	+	+	+	+	+	+	0	0	+	+	+	+	+	+
7	0	+	+	0	+	0	+	0	+	+	+	0	+	0	+	+	0	0
8	0	+	0	0	+	0	+	+	0	0	+	+	0	0	+	+	0	0
9	0	+	+	+	+	0	+	+	+	+	+	+	0	+	0	0	+	+
10	0	+	0	0	+	0	+	0	+	+	+	0	+	0	+	+	+	+
11	0	0	0	+	+	+	+	0	+	+	+	+	0	0	0	0	+	+

Patient Results

Cell No.	Immediate Spin	37° C	AHG	Coombs Control
1	Neg	Neg	2+	
2	Neg	Neg	Neg	2+
3	Neg	Neg	Neg	1+
4	Neg	Neg	Neg	2+
5	Neg	Neg	2+	
6	Neg	Neg	2+	
7	Neg	Neg	Neg	2+
8	Neg	Neg	Neg	3+
9	Neg	Neg	Neg	2+
10	Neg	Neg	Neg	2+
11	Neg	Neg	1+	
Auto	Neg	Neg	Neg	2+

QUESTIONS

1. Based on the two-cell screening, what are the possible alloantibodies in this patient's serum?
2. What is the identity of the alloantibody or antibodies?
3. Briefly discuss the characteristics of the blood group system involved in this case.
4. How is the antibody formed?

DISCUSSION

1. The results of the two-cell screening suggest the presence of either an Rh or AHG reactive alloantibody. The antigens present in the I cell but not in the II cell are C, K, Fy^b, Jk^b, and S.
2. The reaction in the AHG phase of the 1, 5, 6, and 11 cell indicates that one alloantibody is present: Anti-K.
3. The K antigen is part of the Kell system and is present in 9% of the White population. Anti-K is usually an IgG antibody but may rarely be observed as an IgM antibody. Typically, it reacts in the antiglobulin phase, although it may be observed at 37° C in albumin. It may bind complement. This antibody has been implicated in HDN and hemolytic transfusion reactions. A complete discussion of this blood group system can be found in Chapter 5.
4. Antibody formation usually results from erythrocyte antigen exposure, either during pregnancy or through transfusions. In this case, prior blood transfusions had exposed the patient to the Kell antigen.

CONCLUSION

Anti-Kell induced through prior blood transfusions.

Case 9

HISTORY AND LABORATORY DATA

An 18-year-old White woman (group O Rh positive) was 24 hours post-partum. Because of a low hematocrit, 2 units of packed red cells were ordered. The patient had no known history of pregnancy or prior transfusions.

Two of 4 units crossmatched produced incompatible results. The patient's indirect antiglobulin alloantibody screening test was also positive. The results of these tests follow.

Laboratory Data (Case 9)

Reagent Red Blood Cell Screening Cells
Partial Listing of Antigens Present

Cell No.	Rh-hr					Kell		Duffy		Kidd		Lewis		MNS				P
	D	C	E	c	e	K	k	Fy^a	Fy^b	Jk^a	Jk^b	Le^a	Le^b	S	s	M	N	P_1
I	+	0	+	+	+	0	+	+	0	+	+	0	+	+	+	+	0	+
II	0	+	0	+	0	0	+	0	+	+	0	+	+	0	+	+	0	+

Patient Results

Cell No.	Immediate Spin	37° C	AHG	Coombs Control Cells
I	Neg	Neg	Neg	2+
II	±	±	1+	2+

Reagent Red Blood Cell Panel Antigen Profile
Partial Listing of Antigens Present

Cell No.	Rh-hr					Kell		Duffy		Kidd		Lewis		MNS				P
	D	C	E	c	e	K	k	Fy^a	Fy^b	Jk^a	Jk^b	Le^a	Le^b	S	s	M	N	P$_1$
1	+	0	0	+	+	+	0	+	+	+	0	0	0	+	0	+	+	+
2	+	0	0	+	+	0	+	0	+	+	+	0	+	+	+	+	0	0
3	+	+	+	+	+	0	+	0	+	+	+	0	+	+	+	+	0	+
4	0	0	0	+	0	0	+	+	0	+	0	0	+	0	+	+	0	+
5	0	0	+	+	0	+	+	+	+	0	+	0	+	0	+	+	+	+
6	0	+	0	0	+	+	+	+	+	+	0	0	+	+	+	+	+	+
7	0	+	+	0	+	0	+	0	+	+	+	0	+	0	+	+	+	+
8	0	+	0	0	+	0	+	+	0	0	+	+	0	0	+	+	0	0
9	0	+	+	+	+	0	+	+	+	+	+	+	0	+	0	0	+	+
10	0	+	0	0	+	0	+	0	+	+	+	0	+	0	+	+	+	+
11	0	0	0	+	+	+	+	0	+	+	+	+	0	0	0	0	+	+

Patient Results

Cell No.	Immediate Spin	37° C	AHG	Coombs Control Cells
1	Neg	Neg	Neg	2+
2	Neg	Neg	Neg	2+
3	Neg	Neg	Neg	2+
4	Neg	Neg	Neg	2+
5	Neg	Neg	Neg	2+
6	Neg	Neg	Neg	2+
7	Neg	Neg	Neg	1+
8	1+	±	2+	
9	1+	±	2+	
10	Neg	Neg	Neg	1+
11	±	Neg	1+	

QUESTIONS

1. Based on the reactions in the two-cell screening panel, what antibodies are probably in this serum?
2. What is the identity of the alloantibody or antibodies?
3. Briefly discuss the characteristics of the blood group system involved in this case.
4. How is the antibody formed?

DISCUSSION

1. The II cell of the screening cells was the only reactive cell. The following antigens are present on this cell but not on the I cell: C, Fy^b, and Le^a.
2. The pattern of reactivity of the panel of reagent red cells is consistent with the pattern and type or reactivity seen with anti-Le^a.

3. The Le (a) antigen is part of the Lewis blood group system. Anti-Le^a is an IgM antibody, known to fix complement, and is capable of producing hemolytic transfusion reactions. HDN has not been reported due to anti-Le^a. A full discussion of the Lewis blood group system is presented in Chapter 5.
4. Patients develop anti-Le^a through inhalation or ingestion of Le^a-like antigenic determinants. Transient anti-Le^a is not uncommon during pregnancy.

CONCLUSION

Anti-Le^a related to pregnancy.

Case 10

HISTORY AND LABORATORY DATA

A 76-year-old Black man was admitted for sepsis and kidney failure. He was group AB Rh negative. His history included receiving two units of packed cells 5 years before. The patient had also been recently transfused; therefore, mixed field agglutination patterns were observed when other Rh antigens were tested.

Rh$_o$(D) Neg; D^u neg; rH′ (C) 1+MF; rh″(E) 1+MF; hr′(c)2+MF; hr″(e) 2+MF

During the preparation of several units of packed red cells for transfusion, a negative alloantibody screen was observed and a weakly positive DAT was detected. No alloantibodies were detected using multiple testing techniques.

Laboratory Data (Case 10)

Direct Antiglobulin Profile

	Polyspecific Anti-human serum (Rabbit)	Control Pts washed RBCs + Normal Saline	Anti-Human Serum Anti-IgG (Rabbit)	Anti-Human Serum Anti-C3d serum (rabbit)
Red cell test results	Positive ± weak microscopic	Negative	Positive ± strong microscopic	Negative

Heat ether eluate of the patient's red cells revealed the following pattern of reactivity using two screening cells and a red cell reagent panel.

Reagent Red Blood Cell Screening Cells
Antigens Present

Cell No.	Rh-hr					Kell						Duffy	
	D	C	E	c	e	K	k	Kp^a	Kp^b	Js^a	Js^b	Fy^a	Fy^b
I	+	0	+	+	+	+	+	0	+	0	+	0	+
II	0	+	0	+	0	0	+	0	+	0	+	0	+

Antigens Present (continued)

Cell No.	Kidd		Lewis		MNS				P
	Jk^a	Jk^b	Le^a	Le^b	S	s	M	N	P$_1$
I	+	+	0	+	+	+	+	0	+
II	+	+	+	0	+	0	+	+	0

Patient Results

Cell No.	Immediate Spin	37° C	AHG	Coombs Control Cells
I	Neg	Neg	Neg	2+
II	Neg	Neg	Neg	2+

Reagent Red Blood Cell Panel Antigen Profile
Antigens Present

Cell No.	Rh-Hr								Kell						Duffy		Kidd	
	C	D	E	c	e	C^w	f	V	K	k	Kp^a	Kp^b	Js^a	Js^b	Fy^a	Fy^b	Jk^a	Jk^b
1	+	+	+	0	+	0	0	0	+	+	0	+	+	+	0	+	0	+
2	+	+	0	0	+	+	0	0	0	+	0	+	0	+	+	+	+	0
3	0	+	+	+	0	0	0	0	0	+	0	+	0	+	+	+	+	0
4	+	0	0	+	+	0	+	0	0	+	0	+	0	+	0	+	+	+
5	0	0	+	+	+	0	+	0	0	+	0	+	0	+	+	+	+	0
6	0	0	0	+	+	0	+	0	0	+	+	+	0	+	0	+	0	+
7	0	0	0	+	+	0	+	0	0	+	0	+	0	+	+	0	0	+
8	0	+	0	+	+	0	+	0	0	+	0	+	0	+	+	+	+	0
9	0	0	0	+	+	0	+	0	0	+	0	+	0	+	0	+	+	+
10	0	0	0	+	+	0	+	0	0	+	0	+	0	+	+	+	0	+

Antigens Present (continued)

Cell No.	Lewis		P	MNS				Lutheran		Sex-Linked		Additional
	Le^a	Le^b	P$_1$	M	N	S	s	Lu^a	Lu^b	Xg^a		
1	0	+	+	0	+	+	+	0	+	0	M	
2	+	0	+	+	+	0	+	0	+	+	F	
3	0	+	+	0	+	0	+	0	+	+	M	
4	0	+	+	+	0	+	0	+	+	+	F	Co (b+)
5	0	+	0	+	+	+	+	0	+	+	M	
6	0	+	0	+	+	0	+	0	+	0	M	
7	0	+	+	+	0	+	+	0	+	0	M	Co (b+)
8	+	0	+	+	+	+	0	0	+	0	M	
9	0	0	+	+	+	+	0	0	+	+	F	
10	0	+	0	0	0	0	+	0	+	+	F	
11	—	—	—	—	—	—	—	—	—	—		I (neg)

Patient Results

Cell No.	Immediate Spin	37° C	AHG	Coombs Control
1	Neg	Neg	2+	
2	Neg	Neg	Neg	2+
3	Neg	Neg	Neg	2+
4	Neg	Neg	Neg	2+
5	Neg	Neg	Neg	2+
6	Neg	Neg	Neg	2+
7	Neg	Neg	Neg	2+
8	Neg	Neg	Neg	2+
9	Neg	Neg	Neg	2+
10	Neg	Neg	Neg	2+
11	Neg	Neg	Neg	2+
Auto	Neg	Neg	Neg	2+

QUESTIONS

1. Based on the results of the screening and reagent panel cells, what is the identity of the antibody in the eluate?
2. Why was the patient's serum alloantibody screen negative?
3. What further tests should be done?
4. Briefly describe the blood group system involved in this case.

DISCUSSION

1. The heat ether eluate prepared from the patient's red cells was positive with one cell tested. This cell is positive for Js^a antigen.
2. The patient had an extremely low titer of alloantibody. The presence of Js^a antibody, however, was enough to coat the Js^a positive transfused cells. It was suspected that the patient had an anti-Js^a, but samples of the previously transfused units were unavailable to confirm whether or not a positive Js^a unit of blood was transfused.
3. The patient's DAT should be monitored to detect increases in its strength.
4. The Js^a antigen is one of the Kell blood group antigens. Anti-Js^a was discovered in 1958 during routine compatibility tests in the serum of a previously transfused White man. The Js^a (Sutter) antibody is typically an AHG reacting antibody. The Js^a antigen is present in about 20% of Blacks but is apparently absent in Whites. The Kell blood group system is fully described in Chapter 5.

CONCLUSION

Anti-Js^a.

MULTIPLE ANTIBODIES

Case 11

HISTORY AND LABORATORY DATA

A 72-year-old White woman with degenerative osteoarthritis was admitted for elective total knee replacement surgery. She was group O Rh negative. Her transfusion and obstetric histories were unavailable. In preparation of the two units of packed red cells preoperatively, both units were incompatible; however, the autocontrol was negative. The two-cell screening test was also positive. The results of the two-cell screening procedure and a reagent panel of red cells follow.

Laboratory Data (Case 11)

Reagent Red Blood Cell Screening Cells
Partial Listing of Antigens Present

Cell No.	Rh-hr					Kell		Duffy		Kidd		Lewis		MNS				P
	D	C	E	c	e	K	k	Fy^a	Fy^b	Jk^a	Jk^b	Le^a	Le^b	S	s	M	N	P_1
I	0	+	0	0	+	0	+	0	+	+	+	0	+	+	+	+	0	+
II	+	0	+	+	0	+	0	+	0	+	0	0	+	0	+	+	0	+

Patient Results

Cell No.	Immediate Spin	37° C	AHG
I	Neg	Neg	2+
II	Neg	1+	3+

Reagent Red Blood Cell Panel Antigen Profile
Partial Listing of Antigens Present

Cell No.	Rh-hr					Kell		Duffy		Kidd		Lewis		MNS				P
	D	C	E	c	e	K	k	Fy^a	Fy^b	Jk^a	Jk^b	Le^a	Le^b	S	s	M	N	P_1
1	0	0	0	+	+	0	+	+	+	+	0	0	0	+	0	+	+	+
2	0	0	0	+	+	0	+	0	+	+	+	0	+	+	+	+	0	0
3	0	+	0	+	+	0	+	0	+	+	+	0	+	+	+	+	0	+
4	+	0	+	+	0	0	+	+	0	+	0	0	+	0	+	+	0	+
5	+	0	+	+	0	0	+	+	+	0	+	0	+	0	+	+	+	+
6	+	+	0	0	+	+	+	+	+	+	0	0	+	0	+	+	+	+
7	+	+	0	0	+	0	+	0	+	+	+	0	+	0	+	+	0	0
8	+	+	+	0	+	0	+	+	0	0	+	+	0	0	+	+	0	0
9	+	+	0	+	+	0	+	+	+	+	+	+	0	+	0	0	+	+
10	+	+	0	0	+	+	0	0	+	+	+	0	+	0	+	+	+	+
11	+	0	0	+	+	0	+	0	+	+	+	+	0	0	0	0	+	+

Patient Results

Cell No.	Immediate Spin	37° C	AHG	Control Check Cells
1	Neg	Neg	Neg	2+
2	Neg	Neg	Neg	2+
3	Neg	Neg	1+	
4	Neg	1+	2+	
5	Neg	1+	2+	
6	Neg	1+	2+	
7	Neg	1+	2+	
8	Neg	1+	2+	
9	Neg	1+	2+	
10	Neg	1+	2+	
11	Neg	1+	2+	

QUESTIONS

1. Based on the two cell screening test, what is (are) the possible alloantibody or antibodies?
2. Is the pattern of cell reactivity in the panel of reagent red cells consistent with any specific alloantibody?
3. What other tests would support the agglutination results?
4. Briefly discuss the antigen-antibody systems involved in this case.

DISCUSSION

1. The reaction with screening cell I in only the antiglobulin phase implies either a low titer Rh antibody or an AHG reactive antibody. Possible antigens present on the I cell that would fit into one of these categories include: C, e, k, Fy^b, or Jk^b.

The reaction of the II cell with albumin at 37° C suggests the presence of high-titered Rh antibody (the D, E and c antigens are present on this cell) or a high titered anti-K which can exhibit reactivity at 37° C in albumin.

2. The patient's serum demonstrated agglutination in cells 3 through 11. The AHG pattern of the panel cells excludes most of the antibodies identified as possibilities for the I screening cell (Anti-e, anti-k, anti-Fy^b, and anti-Jk^b). The pattern of anti-C, however, would not be excluded if a second antibody existed in the serum.

Cells 4 through 11 exhibited agglutination at the 37° C phase, which is similar to the activity displayed in screening cell II. This pattern of reactivity excludes the other probable antibodies (anti-E, anti-c, or anti-K) identified in question 2 but is consistent with the presence of the alloantibody, anti-D.

3. Testing of the patient's red cells for the absence of D and C antigens would confirm the patient's ability to produce corresponding antibodies, if she had been antigenically stimulated by antigenic exposure and had the capability of mounting an immune response.

The patient is already known to lack the D antigen; therefore, anti-D is one of the probable alloantibodies. Results of additional antigen testing of her red cells were C–Negative, E–Positive, e–Positive, K–Positive, k–Positive, Fy^b–Negative, JK^b–Negative.

4. The D and C antigens belong to the Rhesus (Rh) blood group system. Most anti-D and anti-C antibodies are of the IgG type, although anti-D is occasionally demonstrated in the IgM form and rarely as IgA. The formation of anti-D is usually stimulated by antigenic exposure during pregnancy or through transfusion to D

(Rh$_o$) positive RBCs. Anti-C is produced in response to the transfusion of C positive erythrocytes.

Anti-D is a well-known cause of HDN and can produce a hemolytic transfusion reaction, if the corresponding D antigen is introduced into the circulation of a patient with the alloantibody. Anti-C has also been implicated in hemolytic transfusion reactions, if the antigen and corresponding antibody are united.

Anti-C is a rare antibody in Rh positive persons, and is rarely the only alloantibody, if it occurs, in Rh negative subjects. The combination of anti-D and anti-C in Rh negative subjects is more common.

CONCLUSION

Anti-D and anti-C alloantibodies, cause unknown.

Case 12

HISTORY AND LABORATORY DATA

An 83-year-old White man was suffering from anemia (hematocrit 22%) and congestive heart failure. He was receiving two types of medication, Bumex and Demerol. He was group O Rh positive (most probable genotype R$_2$r) and had been transfused with 6 units of packed cells over the last 2½ to 4½ months.

A weakly positive DAT and positive alloantibody screen were discovered on the pretransfusion workup. An initial serum antibody panel and elution studies using conventional techniques were nonspecific. The specimen was referred to a reference laboratory for further studies. His phenotype was performed using autologous red cells obtained by using simplified reticulocyte-rich cell separation techniques. Additional antigen typings: M+N+S−s+; P1+; Le(a−b+); K−; Fy(a+b−); Jk(a−b+). DAT: IgG−1+, C3−neg.

Laboratory Data (Case 12)

Direct Antiglobulin Profile

	Polyspecific AHG (Rabbit)	Control (Pts Washed Red Cells + Normal Saline)	AHG Anti-IgG (Rabbit)	AHG Anti-C3d (Rabbit)
Red cell negative results	Positive ± Micro	Negative	Positive 1+	Negative

Enzyme-Treated Reagent Red Blood Cell Screening Cells
Partial Listing of Antigens Present

Cell No.	Rh-hr					Kell		Duffy		Kidd		Lewis		MNS				P
	D	C	E	c	e	K	k	Fy^a	Fy^b	Jk^a	Jk^b	Le^a	Le^b	S	s	M	N	P$_1$
I	0	+	+	+	+	0	+	+	0	+	0	0	+	0	+	+	0	+
II	+	0	+	+	0	0	+	0	+	+	+	0	+	+	+	+	0	+

Patient's Serum Results

Cell No.	Immediate Spin	37° C	AHG	Coombs Control
I	Neg	±	1+	
II	Neg	Neg	Neg	2+

Enzyme-Treated Red Blood Cell Panel Antigen Profile
Partial Listing of Antigens Present

Cell No.	Rh-hr					Kell		Duffy		Kidd		Lewis		MNS				P
	D	C	E	c	e	K	k	Fy^a	Fy^b	Jk^a	Jk^b	Le^a	Le^b	S	s	M	N	P$_1$
1	0	0	0	+	+	0	+	+	+	+	0	0	0	+	0	+	+	+
2	0	0	0	+	+	0	+	0	+	+	+	0	+	+	+	+	0	0
3	0	+	+	+	+	0	+	0	+	+	+	0	+	+	+	+	0	+
4	+	0	0	+	0	0	+	+	0	+	0	+	+	0	+	+	0	+
5	+	0	+	+	0	0	+	+	+	0	+	0	+	+	+	+	+	+
6	+	+	0	0	+	+	+	+	+	+	0	0	+	0	+	+	+	+
7	+	+	+	0	+	0	+	0	+	+	+	0	+	0	+	+	+	+
8	+	+	0	0	+	0	+	+	0	0	+	+	0	0	+	+	0	0
9	+	+	+	+	+	0	+	+	+	+	+	+	0	+	0	0	+	+
10	+	+	0	0	+	+	0	0	+	+	+	0	+	0	+	+	+	+
11	+	0	0	+	+	0	+	0	+	+	+	+	0	0	0	0	+	+

Patient's Serum Results

Cell No.	Immediate Spin	37° C	AHG	Coombs Control
1	Neg	Neg	1+	
2	Neg	Neg	1+	
3	Neg	±	2+	
4	Neg	Neg	Neg	2+
5	Neg	Neg	Neg	2+
6	Neg	±	2+	
7	Neg	±	2+	
8	Neg	±	2+	
9	Neg	±	2+	
10	Neg	±	2+	
11	Neg	±	1+	
Auto	Neg	Neg	Neg	2+

Questions

1. What does the positive DAT profile suggest?
2. Why was an enhancement technique used to further study the patient's serum?
3. What antibody (antibodies) does (do) the results of the two enzyme-treated screening cells suggest?
4. Can this patient have an antibody to a self-antigen?
5. Would an elution prepared from the patient's positive DAT cells be of value?

DISCUSSION

1. Positive reactions with both polyspecific and IgG AHG suggest the presence of an IgG type antibody. Refer to Chapter 6 for a full discussion of the causes of a positive DAT.

2. Enhancement techniques such as enzyme treatment or polybrene frequently strengthen the reactions of certain antigen-antibody systems, e.g., Rh. Techniques such as enzyme treatment, however, can also destroy antigen receptor sites. For example, the treatment of Fy^a positive cells with trypsin or papain makes them nonreactive with anti-Fy^a sera.*

3. The antigens present on the I screening cell but not on the II cell are C, e, and Fy^a. The enzyme-treated panel reactions at 37° C are consistent with anti-C activity. The additional reactions in the AHG phase suggest the presence of another alloantibody.

A negative autocontrol excludes the possibility that a nonspecific autoantibody is clouding the picture. Enzyme treatment should have destroyed the Fy^a receptor sites; therefore, anti-Fy^a should be excluded for this reason and also because the patient is Fy^a Positive. The only other possibility based upon the reagent screening cell reactivity is anti-e. The patient, however, is also positive for the e antigen.

4. Yes. The detection of a possible anti-e in this patient's serum is somewhat unexpected because the patient's own reticulocyte-rich red cells are e positive. However, an adsorption using R2R2 red

*Zmijewski, Fletcher: *Immunohematology* (2nd ed.), New York, Appleton Century Crofts, 1972, p. 166.

cells on the serum was performed and there was no significant reduction in the strength of this antibody after adsorption.

Like the D antigen, the e antigen is a structure with many different components. It is probable that this patient is an e "mosaic." In this mosaic, the e antigen lacks one or more of the normal components. Just like individuals with the D^u mosaic, these individuals can produce antibodies to that portion of the antigen which they lack. In this case, the patient was undoubtedly transfused with normal e positive red cells, which elicited the observed antibody response. Refer to Chapter 5 for a full discussion of the Rh blood group system.

5. In this case, elution of the red cells and analysis of the eluate did not yield any specific reactions.

CONCLUSION

Anti-C and Anti-e.

Case 13

HISTORY AND LABORATORY DATA

A 94-year-old White woman was admitted to the hospital because of gastrointestinal (GI) hemorrhage. She was group A Rh positive. Her transfusion history included 4 units of packed red cells 1 month prior to admission and another 4 units of packed red cells 10 days previously. Her medications included alpha-methyldopa, cephalothin, penicillin, Persantine, Feosol, and Lasix. In preparing 4 units for transfusion, a positive alloantibody screen and a weakly positive DAT were detected.

Laboratory Data (Case 13)

	Direct Antiglobulin Profile			
	Polyspecific Anti-Human Serum (Rabbit)	Control Pts Washed RBCs + Normal Saline	Anti-Human Serum Anti-IgG (Rabbit)	Anti-Human Serum Anti-C3d Serum (rabbit)
Red cell test results	Positive ± micro	Negative	Positive ± micro	Negative

Reagent Red Blood Cell Screening Cells
Partial Listing of Antigens Present

Cell No.	D	C	E	c	e	K	k	Fy^a	Fy^b	Jk^a	Jk^b	Le^a	Le^b	S	s	M	N	P$_1$
I	+	0	+	+	+	0	+	+	0	+	+	0	+	+	+	+	0	+
II	0	+	0	+	0	+	0	0	+	+	0	0	+	0	+	+	0	+

Patient Results

Cell No.	Immediate Spin	37° C	AHG	Coombs Control Cells
I	Neg	1+	2+	
II	Neg	Neg	Neg	3+

Reagent Red Blood Cell Panel Antigen Profile
Partial Listing of Antigens Present

Cell No.	D	C	E	c	e	K	k	Fy^a	Fy^b	Jk^a	Jk^b	Le^a	Le^b	S	s	M	N	P$_1$
1	0	0	0	+	+	0	+	+	+	+	0	0	0	+	0	+	+	+
2	0	+	0	+	+	0	+	0	+	+	+	0	+	+	+	+	0	0
3	0	+	0	+	+	0	+	0	+	+	+	0	+	+	+	+	0	+
4	+	+	+	+	0	0	+	+	0	+	0	0	+	0	+	+	0	+
5	+	0	+	0	0	0	+	+	+	0	+	0	+	0	+	+	+	+
6	+	+	0	0	+	+	+	+	+	+	0	0	+	+	+	+	+	+
7	+	+	0	0	+	0	+	0	+	+	+	0	+	0	+	+	+	+
8	+	0	+	+	+	0	+	+	0	0	+	+	0	0	+	+	0	0
9	+	0	0	+	+	0	+	+	+	+	+	+	0	+	0	0	+	+
10	+	+	0	0	+	+	0	0	+	+	+	0	+	0	+	+	+	+
11	+	0	0	+	+	0	+	0	+	+	+	+	0	0	0	0	+	+

Patient Results

Cell No.	Immediate Spin	37° C	AHG	Coombs Control Cells
1	Neg	Neg	Neg	2+
2	Neg	Neg	Neg	2+
3	Neg	Neg	Neg	3+
4	Neg	2+	3+	
5	Neg	Neg	Neg	2+
6	Neg	Neg	Neg	2+
7	Neg	Neg	Neg	1+
8	Neg	2+	3+	
9	Neg	Neg	Neg	1+
10	Neg	Neg	Neg	2+
11	Neg	Neg	Neg	2+
Auto	Neg	Neg	Neg	2+

Reagent Red Blood Cell Screening Cells
Partial Listing of Antigens Present

Cell No.	Rh-hr					Kell		Duffy		Kidd		Lewis		MNS				P
	D	C	E	c	e	K	k	Fy^a	Fy^b	Jk^a	Jk^b	Le^a	Le^b	S	s	M	N	P_1
I	+	0	+	+	+	0	+	+	0	+	+	0	+	+	+	+	0	+
II	0	+	0	+	0	+	0	0	+	+	0	0	+	0	+	+	0	+

Patient Results
Using an Eluate from the Patient's Red Cells

Cell No.	Immediate Spin	37° C	AHG	Coombs Control Cells
I	Neg	Neg	Neg	2+
II	Neg	Neg	2+	

Reagent Red Blood Cell Panel Antigen Profile
Partial Listing of Antigens Present

Cell No.	Rh-hr					Kell		Duffy		Kidd		Lewis		MNS				P
	D	C	E	c	e	K	k	Fy^a	Fy^b	Jk^a	Jk^b	Le^a	Le^b	S	s	M	N	P_1
1	0	0	0	+	+	0	+	+	+	+	0	0	0	+	0	+	+	+
2	0	+	0	+	+	0	+	0	+	+	+	0	+	+	+	+	0	0
3	0	+	0	+	+	0	+	0	+	+	+	0	+	+	+	+	0	+
4	+	+	+	+	0	0	+	+	0	+	0	0	+	0	+	+	0	+
5	+	0	+	+	0	0	+	+	+	0	+	0	+	0	+	+	+	+
6	+	+	0	0	+	+	+	+	+	+	0	0	+	+	+	+	+	+
7	+	+	0	0	+	0	+	0	+	+	+	0	+	0	+	+	+	+
8	+	0	+	+	+	0	+	+	0	0	+	+	0	0	+	+	0	0
9	+	0	0	+	+	0	+	+	+	+	+	+	0	+	0	0	+	+
10	+	+	0	0	+	+	0	0	+	+	+	0	+	0	+	+	+	+
11	+	0	0	+	+	0	+	0	+	+	+	+	0	0	0	0	+	+

Patient Results
Using an Eluate from the Patient's Red Cells

Cell No.	Immediate Spin	37° C	AHG	Coombs Control Cells
1	Neg	Neg	2+	2+
2	Neg	Neg	Neg	2+
3	Neg	Neg	Neg	3+
4	Neg	Neg	2+	
5	Neg	Neg	2+	
6	Neg	Neg	2+	
7	Neg	Neg	Neg	1+
8	Neg	Neg	2+	
9	Neg	Neg	1+	
10	Neg	Neg	Neg	2+
11	Neg	Neg	Neg	2+
Auto	Neg	Neg	Neg	2+

QUESTIONS

1. What is the identity of the antibody or antibodies in the patient's serum?
2. What is the identity of the antibody or antibodies from the eluate?
3. Explain the inconsistency between the serum and eluate.
4. What further tests should be conducted?
5. Explain the mechanism of the involved reaction.

Discussion

1. The pattern of reactivity of the patient's serum is consistent with the reactions of an anti-E.

2. The elution from the patient's red cells produced the reactivity pattern of an anti-Fy^a.

3. The inconsistency between the serum and elution alloantibodies may be related to recent transfusions of Fy^a positive blood. A delayed hemolytic transfusion reaction cannot be excluded with the available data.

The absence of anti-Fy^a in the serum may be explained by its adsorption onto transfused Fy^a positive cells. Alternatively, passive infusion of anti-Fy^a in donor blood plasma could explain this set of circumstances if the patient received whole blood. In units of packed cells, the little donor plasma that remains is unlikely to be detectable.

4. The patient's E and Fy^a antigen status should be determined. If possible, the antigen status of the transfused units should also be determined. In this case, the patient was both E and Fy^a antigen negative. Several of the previously transfused units of blood were either E or Fy^a antigen-positive.

5. Based on the positive DAT, the eluate specificity, and the patient's and donor's phenotype, there is serologic evidence of a transfusion reaction. This type of reaction can occur when the patient has produced an antibody through previous exposure to a blood group antigen but has no demonstrable level of antibody at the time of transfusion.

The transfused red cells act as a secondary antigenic stimulus. The corresponding antibody is produced while the transfused red cells are still circulating, thus resulting in a positive DAT. When a previously negative DAT becomes positive or a positive DAT increases in strength after transfusion, this type of reaction should be investigated and further transfusions delayed until an eluate prepared from the patient's red cells can be tested.

In this case, if additional units are required for transfusion therapy, they should be negative for both the E and Fy^a antigens. Approximately 25% of A Rh positive units should be E neg and Fy^a neg.

Conclusion

Anti-E and anti-Fy^a.

Case 14

History and Laboratory Data

An 85-year-old Black woman had a history of chronic GI bleeding. She had received multiple transfusions over the last decade. Her last transfusion of 2 units of packed red cells had been 6 months previously. She was admitted to the hospital for anemia, and 4 units of packed red cells were ordered for administration. Her blood type was group A Rh positive.

A weakly reacting alloantibody, anti-Fy^a, had been demonstrated in her serum 6 months previously. Her alloantibody screen was positive again on this admission. The results of the two-cell screening procedure and reagent cell panel follow.

Laboratory Data (Case 14)

Reagent Red Blood Cell Screening Cells
Partial Listing of Antigens Present

Cell No.	Rh-hr					Kell		Duffy		Kidd		Lewis		MNS				P
	D	C	E	c	e	K	k	Fy^a	Fy^b	Jk^a	Jk^b	Le^a	Le^b	S	s	M	N	P$_1$
I	+	0	+	+	+	0	+	+	0	+	0	0	+	0	+	+	0	+
II	0	+	0	+	0	0	+	0	+	0	+	0	+	+	+	+	0	+

Patient Results

Cell No.	Immediate Spin	37° C	AHG	AHG Check Cells
I	Neg	Neg	±	2+
II	Neg	Neg	Neg	2+

Reagent Red Blood Cell Panel Antigen Profile
Partial Listing of Antigens Present

Cell No.	Rh-hr					Kell		Duffy		Kidd		Lewis		MNS				P
	D	C	E	c	e	K	k	Fy^a	Fy^b	Jk^a	Jk^b	Le^a	Le^b	S	s	M	N	P$_1$
1	+	0	0	+	+	0	+	+	+	+	0	0	0	+	0	+	+	+
2	+	0	0	+	+	0	+	0	+	+	+	0	+	+	+	+	0	0
3	+	+	0	+	+	0	+	0	+	+	+	0	+	+	+	+	0	+
4	0	0	+	+	0	0	+	+	0	+	0	0	+	0	+	+	0	+
5	0	0	+	+	0	0	+	+	+	0	+	0	+	0	+	+	+	+
6	0	+	0	0	+	+	+	+	+	+	0	0	+	+	+	+	+	+
7	0	+	0	0	+	0	+	0	+	+	+	0	+	0	+	+	+	+
8	0	+	+	0	+	0	+	0	0	0	+	+	0	0	+	+	0	0
9	0	+	0	+	+	0	+	+	+	+	+	+	0	+	0	0	+	+
10	0	+	0	0	+	+	0	0	+	+	+	0	+	0	+	+	+	+

Patient Results

Cell No.	Immediate Spin	37° C	AHG	AHG Check Cells
1	Neg	Neg	±	
2	Neg	Neg	±	
3	Neg	Neg	±	
4	Neg	Neg	±	
5	Neg	Neg	±	
6	Neg	Neg	±	
7	Neg	Neg	±	
8	Neg	Neg	Neg	2+
9	Neg	Neg	±	
10	Neg	Neg	±	
Auto	Neg	Neg	Neg	2+

QUESTIONS

1. Based on the reactions of the I screening cell, what is (are) the possible alloantibody or alloantibodies?
2. Is anti-Fy^a the only alloantibody present?
3. What additional testing could confirm the identity of the alloantibody or antibodies exhibited by the reagent red cells?

4. What type blood should this patient receive?
5. What percentage of blood would be appropriate for this patient?

DISCUSSION

1. The antigens that are present only in the I screening cell are: D, E, e, Fy^a, and Jk^a.
2. No. The reactions in cells 1, 4, 5, 6, and 9 are consistent with the pattern of anti-Fy^a; however, additional reactions in cells 2, 3, 7, and 10 suggest the presence of another alloantibody. Anti-D is excluded because the patient is known to be Rh$_o$ positive. Both anti-E and anti-e can be excluded because the No. 8 cell did not react; it has both the E and e antigens. All the reactive cells, however, possess either the Fy^a antigen and/or the Jk^a antigen. Therefore, anti-Jk^a is the second alloantibody present in this serum.
3. Additional antigens can be tested for on the patient's red blood cells. In this case, an antigen profile was performed. It demonstrated the following:

Additional Patient Antigens

Rh$_o$ (D) 4+; rh′ (C) neg; rh″ (E) 3+; hr′ (c) 3+; hr″ (e) 3+; Rh cont neg.

Le^a	Le^b	M	N	S	s	Fy^a	Fy^b	Jk^a	Jk^b	K	k
0	+	+	+	+	+	0	+	0	+	0	+

4. Obviously, this patient should receive ABO-compatible blood. Because anti-Jk^a and anti-Fy^a often cause shortened red cell survival, she should receive only blood typed as negative for Jk^a and Fy^a antigens.

5. Approximately 8% of A positive units should be suitable for this patient. The Duffy and Kidd blood group systems are fully discussed in Chapter 5.

CONCLUSION

Anti-Fy^a and anti-Jk^a, probably transfusion-induced.

Case 15

HISTORY AND LABORATORY DATA

A 22-year-old Black woman with polycystic ovaries was admitted for bilateral ovarian wedge resections. She had no history of prior transfusion or pregnancy. Her preoperative crossmatch for 2 units of packed red cells demonstrated incompatibilities with both units and a positive alloantibody screen. Reactions were at both 37° C and AHG. Her blood type was group A Rh positive and her DAT was negative. The results of her serum tested with two screening cells and a panel of reagent red cells follow.

Laboratory Data (Case 15)

Reagent Red Blood Cell Screening Cells
Partial Listing of Antigens Present

Cell No.	Rh-hr					Kell		Duffy		Kidd		Lewis		MNS				P
	D	C	E	c	e	K	k	Fy^a	Fy^b	Jk^a	Jk^b	Le^a	Le^b	S	s	M	N	P$_1$
I	+	+	+	+	+	0	+	+	0	+	+	+	0	+	+	+	0	+
II	0	0	0	+	0	+	+	0	+	+	0	0	+	0	+	+	0	+

Patient Results

Cell No.	Immediate Spin	37° C	AHG
I	1+	±	2+
II	1+	±	2+

Reagent Red Blood Cell Panel Antigen Profile
Antigens Present

Cell No.	Rh-Hr								Kell						Duffy		Kidd	
	C	D	E	c	e	C^w	f	V	K	k	Kp^a	Kp^b	Js^a	Js^b	Fy^a	Fy^b	Jk^a	Jk^b
1	+	+	+	0	+	0	0	0	+	+	0	+	+	+	0	+	0	+
2	+	+	0	0	+	+	0	0	0	+	0	+	0	+	+	+	+	0
3	0	+	+	+	0	0	0	0	0	+	0	+	0	+	+	+	+	0
4	+	0	0	+	+	0	+	0	0	+	0	+	0	+	0	+	+	+
5	0	0	+	+	+	0	+	0	0	+	0	+	0	+	+	+	+	0
6	0	0	0	+	+	0	+	0	0	+	+	+	0	+	0	+	0	+
7	0	0	0	+	+	0	+	0	0	+	0	+	0	+	+	0	0	+
8	0	+	0	+	+	0	+	0	0	+	0	+	0	+	+	+	+	0
9	0	0	0	+	+	0	+	0	0	+	0	+	0	+	0	0	+	+
10	0	0	0	+	+	0	+	0	0	+	0	+	0	+	+	+	0	0

Antigens Present (continued)

Cell No.	Lewis		P	MNS				Lutheran		Sex-Linked	Additional
	Le^a	Le^b	P$_1$	M	N	S	s	Lu^a	Lu^b	Xg^a	
1	0	+	+	0	+	+	+	0	+	0 M	
2	+	0	+	+	+	0	+	0	+	+ F	
3	0	+	+	0	+	0	+	0	+	+ M	
4	0	+	+	+	0	+	0	+	+	+ F	Co (b+)
5	0	+	0	+	+	+	+	0	+	+ M	
6	0	+	0	+	+	0	+	0	+	0 M	
7	0	+	+	+	0	+	+	0	+	0 M	Co (b+)
8	+	0	+	+	+	+	0	0	+	0 M	
9	0	0	+	+	+	+	0	0	+	+ F	
10	0	+	0	0	0	0	+	0	+	+ F	
11											I (neg)

Patient Results

Cell No.	Immediate Spin	37° C	AHG	Coombs Control Cells
1	1+	±	2+	
2	1+	±	2+	
3	1+	±	2+	
4	1+	±	2+	
5	1+	±	2+	
6	1+	±	3+	
7	1+	±	1+	
8	1+	±	2+	
9	Neg	Neg	Neg	2+
10	1+	±	2+	
11	1+	±	2+	
Auto	Neg	Neg	Neg	2+

Questions

1. Based on the reactions of the screening cells, what is (are) the possible alloantibody (alloantibodies)?

2. Based on the reactions of the screening cells combined with the panel cell reactions, what is (are) the possible alloantibody (alloantibodies)?

3. What additional testing could confirm the identity of the suspected alloantibody or antibodies?

4. Briefly discuss the characteristics of this woman's genotype.

5. What type blood should this patient receive?

Discussion

1. The type of reaction exhibited by the screening cells is typical of Lewis antibodies. Reactions at room temperature with the fixation of complement becoming apparent during the AHG phase of testing are a common observation.

2. Each of the two screening cells is positive for one of the Lewis antigens. The panel cell reactions also display reactivity with cells that are positive for either the Le^a or Le^b antigens.

3. Testing the patient's RBCs for the presence of Le^a and Le^b antigens would validate the possibility of the suspected alloantibodies. If the patients lacks the Le^a and Le^b antigens, she could theoretically form antibodies to these nonself-antigens. This patient was subsequently typed and found to be Le^a Negative and Le^b Negative.

4. The genotype Le (a–b–) occurs in 22% of Blacks and 6% of Whites. Persons with this genotype may produce anti-Le^a and/or anti-Le^b. Development of Le^a and/or Le^b antibodies is usually due to exposure to some agent other than red blood cells.

5. It is the usual practice to select Le^a and Le^b negative blood if the corresponding alloantibodies are identified in the patient's circulation. However, Mollison[*] believes that transfusing across the anti-Le^a, Le^b barrier can be done without any serious reactions.

Conclusion

Anti-Le^a and anti-Le^b.

*Mollison, P.L.: Blood Transfusion in Clinical Medicine, 5th ed., pp. 489 and 512-514.

POSITIVE DIRECT ANTIGLOBULIN TESTS

Case 16

HISTORY AND LABORATORY DATA

A 65-year-old White woman had carcinoma of the breast and was currently receiving chemotherapy. She was group A, Rh negative (rr). Her medications included Nitro-Dur, Lasix, Solu-Medrol, cefoxitin, and Zantac. She had received two units of packed red cells three days before. The patient had no other history of transfusion, but was the mother of three children.

Two units of packed red cells were ordered to correct her anemia. As a result of crossmatching, a weakly positive autocontrol was demonstrated. A direct antiglobulin profile was performed on the current specimen and on a specimen that had been used for crossmatching 3 days earlier. The results of these tests follow. Further tests of the patient's serum and an eluate, all prepared from the patient's red cells with reagent red cells, were nonreactive.

Laboratory Data (Case 16)

	Direct Antiglobulin Profile			
	Polyspecific Anti-Human Serum (Rabbit)	Control Pts Washed RBCs + Normal Saline	Anti-Human Serum Anti-IgG (Rabbit)	Anti-Human Serum Anti-C3d Serum (Rabbit)
Red cell test results				
Fresh specimen	Positive 1+ micro	Negative	Positive 1+ micro	Negative
72-hr-old specimen	Negative	Negative	Negative	Negative

QUESTIONS

1. What is the most probable cause of this patient's positive DAT?
2. What medications could be responsible for this positive DAT?
3. Are the laboratory findings clinically significant?

DISCUSSION

1. Reactivity to IgG antisera suggests the possibility of allo-immunization; however, only a short interval has elapsed since any known red cell antigenic exposure. Therefore, the possibility of a drug-related cause of the positive AHG is more likely.
2. This patient's positive AHG may be associated with cefoxitin and/or Lasix therapy. This drug has been reported to cause a positive DAT with a nonreactive eluate in 3% or less of patients receiving this medication.
3. No. If this patient is not hemolyzing her erythrocytes, the DAT findings are clinically insignificant.

CONCLUSION

Positive DAT, probably drug-induced.

Case 17

HISTORY AND LABORATORY DATA

A 71-year-old White man was admitted to the hospital because of fatigue. He had an established diagnosis of lymphoma and was presently receiving five different medications: prednisone, Leukovorin, Lasix, Clotrimasol, and Allopurinol. He had received several units of packed red cells over the last 3 months.

Because his hematocrit was low, 4 units of packed red cells were ordered. A positive autocontrol was demonstrated during the crossmatch procedure. He had a weakly positive DAT, but no alloantibodies were detected in his serum.

Laboratory Data (Case 17)

Direct Antiglobulin Profile

	Polyspecific Anti-Human Serum (Rabbit)	Control Pts Washed RBCs + Normal Saline	Anti-Human Serum Anti-IgG (Rabbit)	Anti-Human Serum Anti-C3d Serum (Rabbit)
Red cell test results	Positive 1+ micro	Positive 1+ micro	Positive 1+ micro	Positive 1+ micro

QUESTIONS

1. Do the DAT reactions suggest the possible cause of the positive DAT?
2. What procedure or procedures should be performed next?
3. Can the causative agent be identified?

DISCUSSION

1. No. The cause of the positive DAT is difficult to identify specifically from the DAT reactions. The control test is positive, which demonstrates that an autoantibody is present; however, another underlying reaction could also be present.
2. In the case of a positive DAT, an elution should be prepared from the patient's red cells. The eluate and a serum sample should be tested simultaneously. In this case, an eluate was prepared from the patient's red cells. The eluate and serum were tested, but no reactions were demonstrated with the reagent red cells.
3. In this case, the agent responsible for the positive DAT was considered to be a nonspecific weak autoantibody, possibly related to the patient's lymphoproliferative disorder.

CONCLUSION

Positive DAT, possibly related to the patient's lymphoproliferative disorder.

Case 18

HISTORY AND LABORATORY DATA

A 52-year-old Black woman was admitted to the hospital following a motor vehicle accident. She was started on penicillin intravenously upon admission. She had no previous history of transfusion or pregnancy.

Laboratory tests performed several days after admission revealed evidence of hemolytic anemia (slightly elevated bilirubin, increased reticulocyte count, and decreased hemoglobin and hematocrit). A DAT profile was ordered. The results follow.

Laboratory Data (Case 18)

Direct Antiglobulin Test Profile

	Polyspecific Anti-Human Serum (Rabbit)	Control Pts Washed RBCs + Normal Saline	Anti-Human Serum Anti-IgG (Rabbit)	Anti-Human Serum Anti-C3d Serum (Rabbit)
Cell test results	1+	Negative	Negative	±
Repeat testing (2 days later)	1+	Negative	Negative	±

QUESTIONS

1. What do the results of the DAT suggest?

2. Should the patient's alloantibody screen be positive?
3. What is the most probable reason for this patient's positive DAT?

4. Can drugs, such as the one the patient is receiving, produce a positive DAT?
5. What additional tests should be performed?

DISCUSSION

1. A positive DAT with polyspecific and anti-C3d antisera suggests the possibility of a drug-related reaction. A full discussion of drug-induced positive DATs is presented in Chapter 6.
2. No. If the positive DAT were related only to drug therapy, the alloantibody screening test would be negative.
3. Several significant facts suggest the cause of the positive DAT. The patient has no history of prior transfusions or pregnancy. Additionally, the DAT did not react with IgG sera and the alloantibody screen was negative. Because the patient was receiving intravenous penicillin, the positive DAT is probably related to this therapy.
4. Yes. Penicillin has been reported to cause a positive DAT in 3% of patients receiving large doses of the drug intravenously. However, hemolytic anemia associated with penicillin therapy is rare. If the patient is hemolyzing his or her own red cells, penicillin-induced immune hemolysis should be suspected.
5. The patient's serum and an eluate prepared from the DAT-positive RBCs should be tested against penicillin-treated red cells (see Chapter 14). In this case, the serum and eluate reacted strongly against penicillin-treated red cells. However, the serum and eluate continued to be negative, with red cells not treated with the drug.

CONCLUSION

Drug-induced positive DAT due to penicillin antibodies.

Case 19

HISTORY AND LABORATORY DATA

An 84-year-old Black man was admitted to the hospital because of a seizure disorder and gastrointestinal (GI) bleeding. The patient had no history of prior transfusions. He was receiving several medications: Dilantin, Cimetidine, and alpha-methyldopa (Aldomet). The Aldomet had been administered for the last 24 hours. He had no evidence, either clinically or by laboratory studies, of hemolysis.

Because of the GI bleeding, a type and crossmatch for 6 units of packed cells was ordered. The patient was group B, Rh positive and demonstrated a positive autocontrol during the crossmatch procedure. His serum alloantibody screening cells were nonreactive. Subsequent testing revealed the following DAT profile.

Laboratory Data (Case 19)

	Direct Antiglobulin Profile			
	Polyspecific Anti-Human Serum (Rabbit)	Control Pts Washed RBCs + Normal Saline	Anti-Human Serum Anti-IgG (Rabbit)	Anti-Human Serum Anti-C3d Serum (Rabbit)
Red cell test results	1+	Negative	1+	Negative

QUESTIONS

1. What is the most probable reason for the patient's positive DAT?
2. Should an elution of the positive DAT red cells be performed?
3. What conclusions can be drawn from the laboratory data?
4. Discuss the consequences of the observed reaction "in vivo."

DISCUSSION

1. Because the patient had no history of prior transfusions, it is unlikely that the positive DAT is due to a specific blood group system antibody. However, the accuracy of a patient's history may be questionable, particularly with elderly or disoriented patients.

2. Yes, an elution of the DAT positive red cells should be performed. In this case, elution of the patient's red cells revealed the presence of non-specific reactivity against all panel cells. The results of this procedure follow.

Reagent Red Blood Cell Screening Cells
Partial Listing of Antigens Present

Cell No.	Rh-hr					Kell		Duffy		Kidd		Lewis		MNS				P
	D	C	E	c	e	K	k	Fy^a	Fy^b	Jk^a	Jk^b	Le^a	Le^b	S	s	M	N	P$_1$
I	+	+	0	0	+	+	0	0	+	0	+	+	0	+	+	0	+	+
II	+	0	+	+	0	0	+	+	0	+	0	0	+	0	+	+	0	+

Patient Results (using an elution from patient's RBCs)

Cell No.	Immediate Spin	37° C	AHG
I	Neg	Neg	1+
II	Neg	Neg	±

Reagent Red Blood Cell Panel Antigen Profile
Partial Listing of Antigens Present

Cell No.	Rh-hr					Kell		Duffy		Kidd		Lewis		MNS				P
	D	C	E	c	e	K	k	Fy^a	Fy^b	Jk^a	Jk^b	Le^a	Le^b	S	s	M	N	P$_1$
1	+	0	0	+	+	0	+	+	+	+	0	0	0	+	0	+	+	0
2	+	0	0	+	+	0	+	0	+	+	+	0	+	+	+	+	0	+
3	+	+	+	+	+	0	+	0	+	+	+	0	+	+	+	+	0	+
4	0	0	0	+	0	0	+	+	0	+	0	0	+	0	+	+	0	0
5	0	0	+	+	0	+	+	+	+	0	+	0	+	0	+	+	+	+
6	0	+	0	0	+	0	+	+	+	+	0	0	+	+	+	+	+	+
7	0	+	+	0	+	0	+	0	+	+	+	0	+	0	+	+	+	+
8	0	+	0	0	+	0	+	+	0	0	+	+	0	0	+	+	0	0
9	0	+	+	+	+	0	+	+	+	+	+	+	0	+	0	0	+	+
10	0	+	0	0	+	+	0	0	+	+	+	0	+	0	+	+	+	+
11	0	0	0	+	+	0	+	0	+	+	+	+	0	0	0	0	+	+

Patient Results

Cell No.	Immediate Spin	37° C	AHG
1	Neg	Neg	±
2	Neg	Neg	1+
3	Neg	Neg	1+
4	Neg	Neg	2+
5	Neg	Neg	±
6	Neg	Neg	2+
7	Neg	Neg	2+
8	Neg	Neg	1+
9	Neg	Neg	±
10	Neg	Neg	2+
11	Neg	Neg	1+
Auto	Neg	Neg	±

3. The pattern of reactivity observed in the DAT and reagent red cells is consistent with an alpha-methyldopa-induced autoantibody. The eluate prepared from red cells of patients taking this drug usually reacts with all cells without the presence of the drug in the test system, indicating the development of a warm-reactive autoantibody. The in vitro tests for compatibility cannot be used to predict the cell survival of transfused red cells because all units may appear incompatible when unadsorbed serum is used.

A full discussion of drug-induced positive DATs is presented in Chapter 6.

4. Approximately 10 to 30% of patients taking Aldomet have a positive DAT while less than 1% develop hemolytic anemia. Because the treatments of AIHA and drug-induced anemia are different, it is important that the cause of the anemia be determined. In patients who do experience a hemolytic anemia caused by the drug therapy, the hemolysis usually regresses within a few weeks after cessation of the drug.

Transfusion may be of some benefit to patients showing signs of erythrocyte hemolysis, but the benefit is usually only temporary. The transfused red cells are eliminated at the same accelerated rate as the patient's own red cells. If the patient is not hemolyzing, the autoantibody is probably not clinically significant.

CONCLUSION

Drug-induced positive DAT caused by antibody to Alpha-methyldopa (Aldomet).

Case 20

HISTORY AND LABORATORY DATA

A 75-year-old White man was diagnosed as having idiopathic (autoimmune) thrombocytopenia. He also had concurrent anemia and was admitted for transfusion therapy. Two years previously, the patient had exhibited a strongly positive DAT (IgG and C3d). Nonspecific warm and cold autoantibodies were also reported at that time, but no alloantibodies were detected.

On this admission, this group A, Rh positive patient had both a positive DAT and a positive indirect antiglobulin reaction in the AHG phase. Reactions were also observed at 5° C. He had not received any transfusions within the last 3 months and was not receiving any medications.

Laboratory Data (Case 20)

Direct Antiglobulin Profile

	Polyspecific Anti-Human Serum (Rabbit)	Control Pts Washed RBCs + Normal Saline	Anti-Human Serum Anti-IgG (Rabbit)	Anti-Human Serum Anti-C3d Serum (Rabbit)
Red cell test results	Positive 4+	Negative	Positive 3+	Negative

Reagent Red Blood Cell Screening Cells
Partial Listing of Antigens Present

Cell No.	Rh-hr					Kell		Duffy		Kidd		Lewis		MNS				P
	D	C	E	c	e	K	k	Fy^a	Fy^b	Jk^a	Jk^b	Le^a	Le^b	S	s	M	N	P$_1$
I	+	0	+	+	+	0	+	+	0	+	+	0	+	+	+	+	0	+
II	0	+	0	+	0	0	+	0	+	+	0	0	+	0	+	+	0	+

Patient Results

Cell No.	Immediate Spin	37° C	AHG
I	±	Neg	4+
II	±	Neg	3+

Reagent Red Blood Cell Panel Antigen Profile
Partial Listing of Antigens Present

Cell No.	Rh-hr					Kell		Duffy		Kidd		Lewis		MNS				P
	D	C	E	c	e	K	k	Fy^a	Fy^b	Jk^a	Jk^b	Le^a	Le^b	S	s	M	N	P_1
1	0	0	0	+	+	0	+	+	+	+	0	0	0	+	0	+	+	+
2	0	0	0	+	+	0	+	0	+	+	+	0	+	+	+	+	0	0
3	0	+	0	+	+	0	+	0	+	+	+	0	+	+	+	+	0	+
4	+	0	+	+	0	0	+	+	0	+	0	0	+	0	+	+	0	+
5	+	0	+	+	0	0	+	+	+	0	+	0	+	0	+	+	+	+
6	+	+	0	0	+	+	+	+	+	+	0	0	+	+	+	+	+	+
7	+	+	0	0	+	0	+	0	+	+	+	0	+	0	+	+	+	+
8	+	+	+	0	+	0	+	+	0	0	+	+	0	0	+	+	0	0
9	+	+	0	+	+	0	+	+	+	+	+	+	0	+	0	0	+	+
10	+	+	0	0	+	+	0	0	+	+	+	0	+	0	+	+	+	+
11	+	0	0	+	+	0	+	0	+	+	+	+	0	0	0	0	+	+

Patient Results

Cell No.	Immediate Spin	37° C	AHG	5° C
1	±	Neg	4+	4+
2	±	Neg	3+	4+
3	±	Neg	3+	4+
4	±	Neg	3+	4+
5	±	Neg	4+	4+
6	±	Neg	4+	4+
7	±	Neg	4+	4+
8	±	Neg	4+	4+
9	±	Neg	4+	4+
10	±	Neg	3+	4+
Auto	±	Neg	4+	4+

QUESTIONS

1. What does the reactivity pattern suggest?
2. What additional tests can be performed?
3. Should any precautions be taken when transfusing this patient?

DISCUSSION

1. The serum demonstrates a nonspecific cold autoantibody strongly reactive in the AHG phase and at 5° C.
2. In this case, an autoabsorption with formaldehyde-treated rabbit red cell eliminated the antibody reactions. This confirmed the presence of a nonspecific cold agglutinin. No alloantibody was detected.
3. A warming coil is suggested for future transfusions.

CONCLUSION

Persistently strong positive DAT, idiopathic nonspecific cold agglutinin.

ADVANCED-LEVEL CASE STUDIES

Case 21

HISTORY AND LABORATORY DATA

A 20-year-old Black man with a known diagnosis of mild hemophilia was admitted to the hospital because of injuries sustained in a motor vehicle accident. A crossmatch for 6 units of blood was ordered. The patient was currently receiving AHF and had been transfused with packed red cells within the last 3 months. He was also receiving Colace medication.

At the time of crossmatching the currently requested units of blood, both a positive alloantibody screen and a weakly positive DAT were discovered. All of the crossmatches were incompatible. The patient was group A Rh positive with the most probable genotype R_2R_2. The results of the DAT profile and patient's serum with a two-cell screening set and a panel of reagent red cells follow. An eluate prepared from the DAT positive cells was negative with the two screening cells (I and II) and the panel of reagent red cells.

Laboratory Data (Case 21)

Direct Antiglobulin Profile

	Polyspecific Anti-Human Serum (Rabbit)	Control Pts Washed RBCs + Normal Saline	Anti-Human Serum Anti-IgG (Rabbit)	Anti-Human Serum Anti-C3d Serum (Rabbit)
Red cell test results	Positive 1+ weak	Negative	Positive ±	Negative

Reagent Red Blood Cell Screening Cells
Partial Listing of Antigens Present

Cell No.	Rh-hr					Kell		Duffy		Kidd		Lewis		MNS				P
	D	C	E	c	e	K	k	Fy^a	Fy^b	Jk^a	Jk^b	Le^a	Le^b	S	s	M	N	P$_1$
I	+	0	+	+	+	0	+	+	0	+	+	0	+	+	+	+	0	+
II	0	+	0	+	0	+	0	0	+	+	0	0	+	0	+	+	0	+

Patient Results

Cell No.	Immediate Spin	37° C	AHG	Coombs Control Cells
I	Neg	±	1+	
II	Neg	Neg	Neg	2+

Reagent Red Blood Cell Panel Antigen Profile
Antigens Present

Cell No.	Rh-Hr								Kell						Duffy		Kidd	
	C	D	E	c	e	C^w	f	V	K	k	Kp^a	Kp^b	Js^a	Js^b	Fy^a	Fy^b	Jk^a	Jk^b
1	+	+	+	0	+	0	0	0	+	+	0	+	0	+	0	+	0	+
2	+	+	0	0	+	+	0	0	0	+	0	+	0	+	+	+	+	0
3	0	+	+	+	0	0	0	0	0	+	0	+	0	+	+	+	+	0
4	+	0	0	+	+	0	+	0	0	+	0	+	0	+	0	+	+	+
5	0	0	+	+	+	0	+	0	0	+	0	+	0	+	+	+	+	0
6	0	0	0	+	+	0	+	0	0	+	0	+	0	+	0	+	0	+
7	0	0	0	+	+	0	+	0	0	+	0	+	0	+	+	0	0	+
8	0	+	0	+	+	0	+	0	0	+	0	+	0	+	0	0	+	0
9	0	0	0	+	+	0	+	0	0	+	0	+	0	+	+	+	+	+
10	0	0	0	+	+	0	+	0	0	+	0	+	0	+	+	+	+	+

Antigens Present (continued)

Cell No.	Lewis		P	MNS				Lutheran		Sex-Linked		Additional
	Le^a	Le^b	P$_1$	M	N	S	s	Lu^a	Lu^b	Xg^a		
1	0	+	+	0	+	+	+	0	+	0	M	
2	+	0	+	+	+	0	+	0	+	+	M	Co (b+)
3	0	+	+	0	+	0	+	0	+	+	M	
4	0	+	+	+	0	+	0	+	+	+	F	Co (b+)
5	0	+	0	+	+	+	+	0	+	+	M	
6	0	+	0	+	+	0	+	0	+	0	M	Co (b+)
7	0	+	+	+	0	+	+	0	+	0	M	
8	+	0	+	+	+	+	0	0	+	0	M	
9	0	0	+	+	+	+	0	0	+	+	F	
10	0	+	0	0	0	0	+	0	+	+	F	
11												I (neg)

Patient Results

Cell No.	Immediate Spin	37° C	AHG	Coombs Control Cells
1	Neg	±	1+ weak	
2	Neg	±	1+ weak	
3	Neg	Neg	Neg	2+
4	Neg	±	1+ weak	
5	Neg	±	1+ weak	
6	Neg	±	1+ weak	
7	Neg	±	1+ weak	
8	Neg	±	1+ weak	
9	Neg	±	1+ weak	
10	Neg	±	1+ weak	
11	Neg	±	1+ weak	
Auto	Neg	Neg	Neg	2+

Enzyme-Enhanced Reagent Red Blood Cells + Patient's Serum

Cell No.	37° C
1	2+
2	2+
3	Neg
4	2+
5	2+
6	2+
7	2+
8	2+
9	2+
10	2+
11	2+
Auto	Neg

QUESTIONS

1. What antibody or antibodies are present in the patient's serum?
2. Why was the eluate negative? What further tests can be performed?
3. Would crossmatching only units negative for the antigen(s) to the corresponding antibody (antibodies) identified in questions No. 1 and 2 yield compatible results.
4. What further steps should be taken?
5. Briefly discuss the characteristics of the last antibody identified.

DISCUSSION

1. The weak pattern of AHG reactivity was further enhanced with enzymes, and both patterns were consistent with anti-e.

2. The eluate did not contain an antibody to any of the antigens present on the screening or panel cells. Medications could be ruled out as the source of a drug-induced DAT because the patient was receiving no medications implicated in producing a positive DAT. The patient, however, had been and was receiving AHF.

The eluate was tested against three A_1 and three A_2 cells. Although the eluate was nonreactive with group O cells, agglutination was observed with A_1 reagent cells. Demonstration of the presence of anti-A is consistent with passive acquisition of anti-A by way of AHF concentrate.

3. No. In this case, when the patient was crossmatched with six units of O Positive, e-negative packed red cells, one unit was incompatible.

4. In this case, the hospital blood bank was unable to identify any additional alloantibodies and sent a specimen of the patient's blood as well as segments from the incompatible unit to a reference laboratory. The reference laboratory identified another alloantibody, anti-Kp^a. Additional antigen typings were also performed: M−N+S−s+; P_1−; Le(a−b+); K−k+; Fy(a−b+); Jk(a−b+); Kp^a−.

5. Anti-Kp^a is an antibody to a low-frequency antigen. This antibody has been implicated in HDN. It has also been implicated in transfusion reactions and often causes shortened red cell survival. The frequency of the antigen in the random population is 2%. For a full discussion of the Kell blood group system, refer to Chapter 5.

CONCLUSION

Anti-e, anti-A_1, and anti-Kp^a.

Case 22

HISTORY AND LABORATORY DATA

A 71-year-old White woman is group A_2 Rh positive (R_1R_1). She has an established diagnosis of multiple myeloma and has received numerous transfusions over the last 10 years. Her most recent transfusion was 4 months ago. She was admitted for anemia and fatigue secondary to multiple myeloma. She has been receiving two medications, Keflex and Tolinase.

Four units of packed cells were ordered for transfusion. All of the 4 units cross-matched were incompatible microscopically. Her alloantibody screen was weakly positive, as was the autocontrol. A DAT profile was also performed.

Laboratory Data (Case 22)

Direct Antiglobulin Profile

	Polyspecific Anti-Human Serum (Rabbit)	Control Pts Washed RBCs + Normal Saline	Anti-Human Serum Anti-IgG (Rabbit)	Anti-Human Serum Anti-C3d Serum (Rabbit)
Red cell test results	Positive ± weak	Negative	Positive ± weak	Negative

Reagent Red Blood Cell Screening Cells
Partial Listing of Antigens Present

Cell No.	Rh-hr					Kell		Duffy		Kidd		Lewis		MNS				P
	D	C	E	c	e	K	k	Fy^a	Fy^b	Jk^a	Jk^b	Le^a	Le^b	S	s	M	N	P$_1$
I	+	0	+	+	+	+	+	+	0	+	0	0	+	+	+	+	0	+
II	0	+	0	+	0	0	+	0	+	0	+	0	+	0	+	+	0	+

Patient Results

Cell No.	Immediate Spin	37° C	AHG	Coombs Control Cells
I	Neg	Neg	±	3+
II	Neg	Neg	±	3+

Reagent Red Blood Cell Panel Antigen Profile
Partial Listing of Antigens Present

Cell No.	Rh-hr					Kell		Duffy		Kidd		Lewis		MNS				P
	D	C	E	c	e	K	k	Fy^a	Fy^b	Jk^a	Jk^b	Le^a	Le^b	S	s	M	N	P$_1$
1	0	0	0	+	+	0	+	+	+	+	0	0	0	+	0	+	+	+
2	0	0	0	+	+	0	+	0	+	+	+	0	+	+	0	+	0	0
3	0	0	+	0	+	0	+	0	+	+	+	0	+	0	+	+	0	+
4	+	0	+	+	0	0	+	+	0	+	0	0	+	+	0	+	+	+
5	+	0	+	+	0	0	+	+	+	0	+	0	+	+	+	+	+	+
6	+	+	0	0	+	+	+	+	+	+	+	0	+	0	+	+	+	+
7	+	+	0	0	+	0	+	0	+	0	0	+	0	0	+	+	0	0
8	+	+	+	0	+	0	+	0	+	+	+	+	0	+	0	0	+	+
9	+	+	0	+	+	+	0	+	0	+	+	0	+	0	+	+	+	+
10	+	+	0	0	+	+	0	0	+	+	+	0	+	0	+	+	+	+

Patient Results
Elution of DAT Positive Cells

Cell No.	Immediate Spin	37° C	AHG	Coombs Control
1	Neg	Neg	±	2+
2	Neg	Neg	±	2+
3	Neg	Neg	±	2+
4	Neg	Neg	±	2+
5	Neg	Neg	±	2+
6	Neg	Neg	±	2+
7	Neg	Neg	±	2+
8	Neg	Neg	±	2+
9	Neg	Neg	±	2+
10	Neg	Neg	±	2+
Auto Control	Neg	Neg	±	2+

Patient Results
Serum (Using Prewarming Technique)

Cell No.	Immediate Spin	37° C	AHG	Coombs Control
1	Neg	±	1+	
2	Neg	±	1+	
3	Neg	±	1+	
4	Neg	±	1+	
5	Neg	±	1+	
6	Neg	Neg	±	2+
7	Neg	Neg	±	2+
8	Neg	Neg	±	2+
9	Neg	±	1+	
10	Neg	Neg	±	2+
Auto Control	Neg	Neg	Neg	2+

QUESTIONS

1. What is the cause of the positive DAT?
2. Can other crossmatch techniques be attempted?
3. What do the results of the serum alloantibody tests suggest?
4. What is the explanation for the weakly reacting reagent cells and the continuing incompatible units?

DISCUSSION

1. A heat ether eluate prepared from the patient's red cells was inconclusive because it reacted with all panel cells tested (panagglutinin). Two of the medications presently being given to the patient (Keflex and Tolinase) have been implicated in producing a positive DAT. Screening the eluate for cephalosporin antibodies (Chapter 14) could rule out Keflex as the source of the positive DAT. If this procedure yields negative results, the patient's disorder or her medication, Tolinase, may be the cause.

2. Yes. Consistent with the diagnosis of multiple myeloma, the patient's serum and cells are exhibiting very strong rouleaux formation. The rouleaux seem only to interfere with testing at extended incubations at room temperature and below. Saline replacement technique did produce a negative autocontrol; however, the crossmatched units continued to be incompatible.

3. The prewarmed serum reactivity was consistent with the activity of anti-c. The patient's genotype would also support the possibility of this alloantibody. The weak reactions in the c negative cells could not be explained. When c negative units were crossmatched using a prewarming technique, 3 out of 4 units continued to be incompatible.

4. This patient's specimen and segments from the c (negative)-incompatible units were forwarded to a reference laboratory for further study. The reference laboratory confirmed the findings of the blood bank and identified the cause of the weakly reacting cells and incompatible crossmatches.

The report stated that this specimen exhibited a high-titer low avidity (HTLA) antibody, anti-York. These antibodies generally cause agglutination reactions at the AHG phase. Reactions range from weakly macroscopic to microscopic positives. The corresponding Yk^a antigen is present on 92 to 98% of the red cells of the random population; therefore, the major problem this antibody causes is the incompatibility of nearly all donor units when crossmatching. Anti-Yk^a has not been implicated in hemolytic transfusion reactions or in increased red cell destruction: Anti-Yk^a is often found in the presence of other alloantibodies. If transfusions are needed, this patient should receive c negative crossmatch-compatible units.

CONCLUSION

Cold autoagglutinin, anti-York, and anti-c.

Case 23

An 86-year-old White woman was admitted for a fractured hip and anemia. She had received 13 units of packed red cells over the last 4 months. Her blood type was group O Rh positive (genotype R²r, cDE/cde).

During the preparation of 2 units of packed cells preoperatively, one of the units was weakly incompatible. The alloantibody screening cells were very weakly positive (microscopically). The DAT was positive.

Laboratory Data (Case 23)

Direct Antiglobulin Profile

	Polyspecific Anti-Human Serum (Rabbit)	Control Pts Washed RBCs + Normal Saline	Anti-Human Serum Anti-IgG (Rabbit)	Anti-Human Serum Anti-C3d Serum (Rabbit)
Red cell test results	Positive 1+	Negative	Positive 1+	Negative

Reagent Red Blood Cell Screening Cells
Partial Listing of Antigens Present

Cell No.	Rh-hr					Kell		Duffy		Kidd		Lewis		MNS				P
	D	C	E	c	e	K	k	Fyᵃ	Fyᵇ	Jkᵃ	Jkᵇ	Leᵃ	Leᵇ	S	s	M	N	P₁
I	+	0	+	+	+	0	+	+	0	+	+	0	+	+	+	+	0	+
II	0	+	0	+	0	+	0	0	+	+	0	0	+	0	+	+	0	+

Patient Results
Using an Eluate from the DAT Positive RBCs

Cell No.	Immediate Spin	37° C	AHG	Coombs Control Cells
I	Neg	Neg	Neg	2+
II	Neg	Neg	2+	

Reagent Red Blood Cell Panel Antigen Profile
Partial Listing of Antigens Present

Cell No.	Rh-hr					Kell		Duffy		Kidd		Lewis		MNS				P
	D	C	E	c	e	K	k	Fyᵃ	Fyᵇ	Jkᵃ	Jkᵇ	Leᵃ	Leᵇ	S	s	M	N	P₁
1	0	0	0	+	+	0	+	+	+	+	0	0	0	+	0	+	+	+
2	0	+	0	+	+	0	+	0	+	+	+	0	+	+	+	+	0	0
3	0	+	0	+	+	0	+	0	+	+	+	0	+	+	+	+	0	+
4	+	+	+	+	0	0	+	+	0	+	0	0	+	0	+	+	0	+
5	+	0	+	+	0	0	+	+	+	0	+	0	+	0	+	+	+	+
6	+	+	0	0	+	+	+	+	+	+	0	0	+	+	+	+	+	+
7	+	+	0	0	+	0	+	0	+	+	+	0	+	0	+	+	+	+
8	+	0	+	+	+	0	+	+	0	0	+	+	0	0	+	0	+	0
9	+	0	0	+	+	0	+	+	+	+	+	+	0	+	0	0	+	+
10	+	+	0	0	+	+	0	0	+	+	+	0	+	0	+	+	+	+
11	+	0	0	+	+	0	+	0	+	+	+	+	0	0	0	0	+	+

Patient Results
Using an Eluate from the DAT Positive RBCs

Cell No.	Immediate Spin	37° C	AHG
1	Neg	Neg	1+
2	Neg	Neg	2+
3	Neg	Neg	2+
4	Neg	Neg	3+
5	Neg	Neg	2+
6	Neg	Neg	2+
7	Neg	Neg	1+
8	Neg	Neg	2+
9	Neg	Neg	2+
10	Neg	Neg	1+
11	Neg	Neg	2+
Auto	Neg	Neg	±

Adsorbed Eluate

Cell No.	Immediate Spin	37° C	AHG	Coombs Control Cells
I	Neg	Neg	Neg	2+
II	Neg	Neg	2+	

Adsorbed Eluate

Cell No.	Immediate Spin	37° C	AHG	Coombs Control
1	Neg	Neg	± micro	2+
2	Neg	Neg	Neg	2+
3	Neg	Neg	Neg	3+
4	Neg	Neg	Neg	2+
5	Neg	Neg	Neg	2+
6	Neg	Neg	2+	
7	Neg	Neg	Neg	1+
8	Neg	Neg	Neg	2+
9	Neg	Neg	Neg	1+
10	Neg	Neg	2+	
11	Neg	Neg	Neg	2+
Auto	Neg	Neg	Neg	2+

Patient Results
Enzyme-Treated RBCs + Patient Serum

Cell No.	Immediate Spin	37° C
I	Neg	± micro
II	Neg	2+

Enzyme Treated RBCs + Patient Serum

Cell No.	Immediate Spin	37° C
1	Neg	±
2	Neg	2+
3	Neg	2+
4	Neg	3+
5	Neg	± micro
6	Neg	2+
7	Neg	2+
8	Neg	± micro
9	Neg	± micro
10	Neg	2+
11	Neg	± micro
Auto	Neg	Neg

QUESTIONS

1. What is the most probable cause of the positive DAT?
2. What procedure should be done next?
3. What is the significance of the positive DAT reaction?
4. If the alloantibody screening cells are negative or weakly nonspecific, does this indicate that no alloantibodies are present in the patient's serum?
5. What is the cause of the persistent weakly positive reactions?

DISCUSSION

1. The reactivity with both polyspecific and IgG antisera suggests a warm antibody.
2. An elution of the positive DAT cells was prepared. Although it demonstrated warm autoantibody activity, it was reactive with all cells (1+ to 3+). An adsorbed eluate was subsequently prepared to remove autoantibody reactivity. When testing the adsorbed eluate. an underlying anti-K was demonstrated.

Additional antigens were tested. A phenotype was performed on the top layer harvested from simplified cell separation. These results are as follows:

Antigen Profile

	Le^a	Le^b	M	N	S*	s*	P$_1$	Fy^{a*}	Fy^{b*}	Jk^{a*}	Jk^{b*}	K*	k*
Patient's Cells	0	+	+	+	+	+	+	+	0	0	+	0	+

* Chloroquine-treated cells

3. Based on the positive DAT, the eluate specificity, and the patient's phenotype, there is serologic evidence of a delayed transfusion reaction because of anti-K. This type of reaction can occur when the patient has been previously exposed to a blood group antigen but has no demonstrable level of antibody at the time of transfusion and compatible cross-matches. If the transfused cells are positive for the antigen, in this case Kell, the transfused red cells act as a secondary antigenic stimulus and the antibody is produced while the transfused red cells are still in the circulation.

4. No. A negative alloantibody screen does not unequivocally mean that alloantibodies are absent in the patient's serum. Antibodies may be present that are not represented on the group O screening cells, such as, low frequency antigens or immune anti-A. Low-titer alloantibodies can also be missed.

In this case, the weakly reactive nonspecific cell reactions with screening cells needed to be explained. An enzyme-enhanced technique was tried. The reactions using this technique demonstrated another antibody, anti-C. However, some of the cells continued to be weakly reactive. Additional cross-matches with K (neg) and C (neg) demonstrated weakly incompatible (microscopic) agglutination. The specimen was sent to a reference laboratory for further study.

5. In the hands of the reference laboratory, weak, nonspecific reactions were observed at the indirect antiglobulin phase with 75% of K and C negative red cells tested. HLA antibodies were suspected because of the weak, nonspecific, and stringy agglutination observed in this multiply transfused patient.

In an attempt to determine if these reactions were due to HLA antibodies, the patient's serum was adsorbed with pooled platelets. Platelets have white cell (HLA) antigens as well as ABO and unique platelet antigens and can be used to adsorb HLA antibodies.

After adsorption, the patient's serum was nonreactive with the previously positive red cells. Thus, it appears likely that the nonspecific reactivity at the AHG phase is caused by HLA antibody production.

CONCLUSION

Anti-K, anti-C, and HLA antibodies.

Case 24

HISTORY AND LABORATORY DATA

A 78-year-old White woman was diagnosed as having an evolving myeloproliferative disorder. Her blood type was group A Rh positive. She had been receiving folic acid, potassium, and Apresoline. She had received 5 units of packed RBCs one month before the detection and identification of an anti-Kell alloantibody in her serum. She also had a positive DAT with K specificity demonstrated from an eluate. The anti-C3d results were unexplained.

Direct Antiglobulin Profile

	Polyspecific Anti-Human Serum (Rabbit)	Control Pts Washed RBCs + Normal Saline	Anti-Human Serum Anti-IgG (Rabbit)	Anti-Human Serum Anti-C3d Serum (Rabbit)
Red cell test results	Positive 1+	Negative	Positive 1+	Positive ± micro

During the next 3-month period, she received an additional 4 units of Kell negative packed red cells. At the time of her next admission, a positive DAT was observed. The results of these tests follow.

Laboratory Data (Case 24)

Reagent Red Blood Cell Screening Cells
Partial Listing of Antigens Present

Cell No.	Rh-hr					Kell		Duffy		Kidd		Lewis		MNS				P
	D	C	E	c	e	K	k	Fy^a	Fy^b	Jk^a	Jk^b	Le^a	Le^b	S	s	M	N	P$_1$
I	+	0	+	+	+	0	+	+	0	+	+	0	+	+	+	+	0	+
II	0	+	0	+	0	+	0	0	+	+	0	0	+	0	+	+	0	+

Patient Results
Eluate of DAT Positive RBCs

Cell No.	Immediate Spin	37° C	AHG	Coombs Control Cells
I	Neg	Neg	±	1+
II	Neg	1+	2+	

Reagent Red Blood Cell Panel Antigen Profile
Antigens Present

Cell No.	Rh-Hr								Kell						Duffy		Kidd	
	C	D	E	c	e	C^w	f	V	K	k	Kp^a	Kp^b	Js^a	Js^b	Fy^a	Fy^b	Jk^a	Jk^b
1	+	+	+	0	+	0	0	0	+	+	0	+	0	+	0	+	0	+
2	+	+	0	0	+	+	0	0	0	+	0	+	0	+	+	+	+	0
3	0	+	+	+	0	0	0	0	0	+	0	+	0	+	+	+	+	0
4	+	0	0	+	+	0	+	0	0	+	0	+	0	+	0	+	+	+
5	0	0	+	+	+	0	+	0	0	+	0	+	0	+	+	+	+	0
6	0	0	0	+	+	0	+	0	0	+	0	+	0	+	0	+	0	+
7	0	0	0	+	+	0	+	0	0	+	0	+	0	+	+	0	0	+
8	0	+	0	+	+	0	+	0	0	+	0	+	0	+	0	0	+	0
9	0	0	0	+	+	0	+	0	0	+	0	+	0	+	+	+	+	+
10	0	0	0	+	+	0	+	0	0	+	0	+	0	+	+	+	+	+

Antigens Present (continued)

Cell No.	Lewis		P	MNS				Lutheran		Sex-Linked		Additional Antigen
	Le^a	Le^b	P$_1$	M	N	S	s	Lu^a	Lu^b	Xg^a		
1	0	+	+	0	+	+	+	0	+	0	M	
2	+	0	+	+	+	0	+	0	+	+	M	Co (b+)
3	0	+	+	0	+	0	+	0	+	+	M	
4	0	+	+	+	0	+	0	+	+	+	F	Co (b+)
5	0	+	0	+	+	+	+	0	+	+	M	
6	0	+	0	+	+	0	+	0	+	0	M	
7	0	+	+	+	0	+	+	0	+	0	M	Co (b+)
8	+	0	+	+	+	+	0	0	+	0	M	
9	0	0	+	+	+	+	0	0	+	+	F	
10	0	+	0	0	0	0	+	0	+	+	F	
11												I (neg)

Patient Results
Eluate of DAT Positive RBCs

Cell No.	Immediate Spin	37° C	AHG	Coombs Control Cells
1	Neg	1+	2+	
2	Neg	Neg	±	2+
3	Neg	Neg	±	2+
4	Neg	Neg	±	2+
5	Neg	Neg	±	2+
6	Neg	Neg	±	2+
7	Neg	Neg	±	2+
8	Neg	Neg	±	2+
9	Neg	Neg	±	2+
10	Neg	Neg	±	2+
11	Neg	Neg	Neg	2+
Auto	Neg	Neg	Neg	2+

Patient Results—Serum

Cell No.	Immediate Spin	37° C	AHG	Coombs Control Cells
I	Neg	Neg	±	1+
II	Neg	1+	2+	

Patient Results—Serum

Cell No.	Immediate Spin	37° C	AHG	Coombs Control Cells
1	Neg	1+	2+	
2	Neg	Neg	2+	
3	Neg	Neg	±	2+
4	Neg	Neg	±	2+
5	Neg	Neg	±	2+
6	Neg	Neg	±	2+
7	Neg	Neg	±	2+
8	Neg	Neg	±	2+
9	Neg	Neg	±	2+
10	Neg	Neg	±	2+
11	Neg	Neg	Neg	2+
Auto	Neg	Neg	Neg	2+

QUESTIONS

1. What is the identity of the antibody in the eluate?
2. What is the explanation for the weakly reactive agglutination pattern in the reagent cells with the patient's serum?
3. Does the reaction pattern of the reagent cells suggest the presence of any other alloantibodies?
4. Briefly describe the characteristics of the most recently discovered antibody in this patient's serum.

DISCUSSION

1. The patient's heat eluate was weakly reactive with all panel cells tested. She is not receiving any medications known to cause a positive DAT. Anti-K specificity was demonstrated in the eluate. Because this patient has been recently transfused, with K negative units only, the presence of anti-K in her eluate is probably caused by the Matuhasi-Ogato Phenomenon. This phenomenon occurs when a specific antigen-antibody complex forms and another antibody that is not directed against an antigen on the red cells involved in the specific complex is unable to bind to the complex and can be recovered in eluates subsequently made.
2. Weak, nonspecific reactions were observed at the AHG phase with most of the K negative red cells tested. In an attempt to determine if these reactions were caused by HLA antibodies, the patient's serum was adsorbed with pooled platelets. After adsorption, the patient's serum was nonreactive with the previously positive (K negative) red cells. Thus, it appears likely that the nonspecific reactivity at the AHG phase was due to HLA antibody production.
3. Yes. The strongly reacting No. 2 cell is consistent with anti-C^w reactivity.
4. The C^w antigen is part of the Rhesus blood group system. It is present in about 1% of the population. Anti-C^w is formed either through previous transfusions or pregnancies, or more rarely through inhalation or ingestion of similar antigens. Anti-C^w has been implicated in hemolytic transfusion reactions and HDN.

CONCLUSION

Anti-K, anti-C^w, and HLA antibodies.

*Issit, P. D.: *Spectra Biological Applied Blood Group Serology*, ed.2, p. 346.

Case 25

HISTORY AND LABORATORY DATA

A 67-year-old White woman received 1 unit of fresh frozen plasma and 6 units of packed RBCs 1 month earlier for injuries sustained in a motor vehicle accident. Four units of packed red cells were ordered preoperatively for orthopedic repair of injuries sustained in that accident. She was the mother of eight children and reported that all pregnancies had been normal and all of her children were healthy at birth. Her blood type was group O Rh positive.

All of the crossmatches were incompatible and the alloantibody screen was also positive. Agglutination occurred in all phases of the crossmatches and antibody screening (RT, 37° C, AHG). Additionally, the patient's auto control was positive.

Laboratory Data (Case 25)

Reagent Red Blood Cell Screening Cells
Partial Listing of Antigens Present

Cell No.	Rh-hr					Kell		Duffy		Kidd		Lewis		MNS				P
	D	C	E	c	e	K	k	Fy^a	Fy^b	Jk^a	Jk^b	Le^a	Le^b	S	s	M	N	P$_1$
I	+	0	+	+	+	+	+	+	0	+	0	0	+	+	+	+	0	+
II	0	+	0	+	0	0	+	0	+	0	+	0	+	0	+	+	0	+

Reagent Red Blood Cell Panel Antigen Profile
Partial Listing of Antigens Present

Cell No.	Rh-hr					Kell		Duffy		Kidd		Lewis		MNS				P
	D	C	E	c	e	K	k	Fy^a	Fy^b	Jk^a	Jk^b	Le^a	Le^b	S	s	M	N	P$_1$
1	0	0	0	+	+	0	+	+	+	+	0	0	0	+	0	+	+	+
2	0	0	0	+	+	0	+	0	+	+	+	0	+	+	+	+	0	0
3	0	+	0	+	+	0	+	0	+	+	+	0	+	+	+	+	0	+
4	+	0	+	+	0	0	+	+	0	+	0	0	+	0	+	+	0	+
5	+	0	+	+	0	0	+	+	+	0	+	0	+	0	+	+	+	+
6	+	+	0	0	+	+	+	+	+	+	0	0	+	+	+	+	+	+
7	+	+	0	0	+	0	+	0	+	+	+	0	+	0	+	+	+	+
8	+	+	+	0	+	0	+	0	0	0	+	+	0	0	+	+	0	0
9	+	+	0	+	+	0	+	+	+	+	+	+	0	+	0	0	+	+
10	+	+	0	0	+	+	0	0	+	+	+	0	+	0	+	+	+	+

Initial Patient Results

Cell No.	Immediate Spin	37° C	AHG
I	2+	2+	3+
II	1+	±	4+

Initial Patient Results

Cell No.	Immediate Spin	37° C	AHG
1	±	Neg	3+
2	1+	±	4+
3	1+	1+	4+
4	2+	3+	3+
5	2+	3+	3+
6	2+	3+	3+
7	1+	1+	2+
8	2+	3+	3+
9	2+	3+	±
10	2+	3+	3+
Auto Control	1+	3+	4+

QUESTIONS

1. What is the most probable explanation for the reactions observed in the initial reagent red cell screening?
2. What procedures can be performed to investigate the presence of any other antibodies?
3. Are any additional alloantibodies present in the patient's serum?
4. Can all of the weakly reactive agglutinations be attributed to the presence of the cold antibody?

5. What is the appropriate type of blood for transfusing this patient?

DISCUSSION

1. The initial reagent red cell panel demonstrated agglutination of all cells (pan-agglutination) and a positive (4+) autocontrol. This is the type of pattern that is typical of a cold autoagglutinin.

2. Because of the strong cold autoagglutinin, the patient's serum was subjected to a double autoabsorption of the patient's papain-treated cells. The strength of the auto control decreased to ±.

Repeat testing was conducted with absorbed serum. The results of this testing follow.

Patient Results—Absorbed Patient's Serum

Cell No.	Immediate Spin	37° C	AHG
I	Neg	2+	3+
II	Neg	Neg	±

Patient Results—Absorbed Patient's Serum

Cell No.	Immediate Spin	37° C	AHG	Coombs Control
1	Neg	Neg	±	2+
2	Neg	Neg	±	2+
3	Neg	Neg	±	2+
4	Neg	1+	3+	
5	Neg	±	3+	
6	Neg	Neg	3+	
7	Neg	Neg	±	2+
8	Neg	±	3+	
9	Neg	Neg	±	
10	Neg	Neg	3+	
Auto Control	±	±	±	2+

3. Yes. Removal of the strong reactivity due to the cold agglutinin unmasked a pattern of reactivity that was consistent with other alloantibodies. The I screening cell suggests antibodies to any of the following antigens: E, K, Fy^a, Jk^a, and S. However, the panel of reagent cell agglutination excludes Anti-Fy^a, -Jk^a, and -S. It is consistent with anti-E and anti-K in addition to the cold autoagglutinin.

The patient's red cells were phenotyped and found to be negative for both the E and K antigens.

4. No. subsequent testing by a reference laboratory disclosed that the patient also had a high-titer low-avidity (HTLA) antibody. These antibodies generally cause weak reactions ranging from weakly macroscopic to microscopic reactions in the AHG phase of testing. The Knopps (Kn^a) and McCoy (McC^a) antigens are of high frequency and are present on more than 98% of the red cells of the random population. These antigens have often been found to be phenotypically related. Neither anti-Kn^a or anti-McC^a is known to cause reduced red cell survival following transfusion of antigen positive units.

5. The patient should receive O positive, E negative, Kell negative crossmatch-compatible (or least incompatible) donor units for transfusion. Prewarming or cold autoabsorption should be considered if the cold agglutinin causes crossmatching difficulties.

CONCLUSION

Anti-E, anti-K, anti-Kn^a/McC^a, and a cold agglutinin.

Case 26

Submitted by Polly F. Kay, MT(ASCP), MHS, and Marion Hursey
School of Medical Technology
Anderson Memorial Hospital
Anderson, South Carolina

HISTORY AND LABORATORY DATA

A 62-year-old Black man was admitted to the hospital with a 5.6 dL hemoglobin. He had a long history of atherosclerotic coronary heart disease and severe end-stage renal disease. The patient was on maintenance chronic hemodialysis and had a history of previous transfusions 1 and 5 years before admission.

On an earlier admission the same year, this serum demonstrated an antibody (or antibodies) which reacted with all cells of a reagent panel. Randomly crossmatched blood was incompatible with 72 units of blood in the blood bank. A specimen was submitted to a reference laboratory for antibody identification. The results indicated that the serum contained an Rh alloantibody of "broad specificity" and that his red cells lacked one or more high frequency Rh antigens; the serum was compatible only with Rh Null cells.

Additional samples were referred to an AABB reference laboratory for confirmation of the antibody identification and help in obtaining blood for transfusion. The only positive reactions during Rh phenotyping were with anti-D (Rh$_o$) and anti-c (hr') antisera. Exact specificity of the antibody could not be confirmed as either anti-hr^s or anti-hr^B.

Family members were located and their samples were also sent to the AABB reference laboratory for testing. Three children were incompatible with the patient's serum. A sister was compatible and appeared to have the same Rh phenotype as the patient. The sister donated blood, three times to date. These units were frozen until transfused. One other rare donor, who is hr^s (−), hr^B (−), Hr$_o$ (−), was located. This donor is participating in an autologous frozen blood program for herself; however, she released two of her frozen units for this patient. These units were stored frozen until needed.

On admission in June of that year, the patient was admitted to Coronary Care with a 6.1 g/dL hemoglobin and a possible myocardial infarction. Two units of the frozen blood were successfully crossmatched and transfused. The patient left the hospital against medical advice. In August, he was again admitted with severe anemia. Another frozen unit was crossmatched and transfused. Colonic polyps were discovered at this time, but surgery was postponed until more compatible blood could be located.

Blood samples were sent to the National Red Cross Rare Donor Center in Washington, D.C. and to the Atlanta Red Cross for mass random crossmatching by capillary technique with predominantly Black donors. To date, approximately 3000 donors have been tested. One additional donor appears to be compatible and three are microscopically incompatible. The Rh phenotypes of these donors have not yet been determined. All 4 units have been frozen and are available for an emergency.

The patient later underwent surgery, successfully, for the colonic polyps after receiving the last two originally identified compatible units from his sister and the rare donor. A system has evolved in which his sister will continue to donate blood on a periodic basis. These units will be frozen for future use. In the meantime, the Red Cross continues to screen donors for other sources of blood for this patient.

QUESTIONS

1. When a patient's alloantibody screen is positive and an extraordinary number of donors is incompatible, what could some of the reasons be?
2. Why would a patient develop alloantibodies of this type?
3. Is it harmful to transfuse a patient with this type of problem?
4. Why was it important to locate suitable donors in this situation?

DISCUSSION

1. It is important in cases of positive alloantibody screens and panagglutination that the pattern of reactivity be investigated. If activity is strong at room temperature or colder, a cold agglutinin must be excluded. Assuming that the patient's DAT and autocontrol are negative, other facts can be excluded. In this case, significant reactivity of the patient's serum in the AHG phase with all donors tested suggests an alloantibody to a high-incidence antigen.
2. Alloantibodies to high incidence antigens occur because the patient lacks the corresponding antigen. Hence, transfusion of almost all units of donor blood could stimulate antibody production against the corresponding antigen.
3. Not always. Transfusion of antigen-positive blood that is not known to reduce red survival, such as Knopps/McCoy, presented in the previous case, can generally be given without a transfusion reaction. However, the attending physician

should decide if transfusing least incompatible blood is in the best interest of the patient.

4. Antibodies of the Rh system are known to cause hemolytic transfusion reactions when antigen-positive blood is transfused to a patient with the corresponding antibody. In this case, the exact specificity of the antibody could not be confirmed as either anti-hr^s or anti-hr^B. Therefore, it was important that hr^s (−), hr^B (−), and Hr$_o$ (−) donors be located. Refer to Chapter 5 for a full discussion of the Rh system.

CONCLUSION

Probable anti-hr^s or anti-hr^B.

MATERNAL AND RELATED CASE STUDIES OF HEMOLYTIC DISEASE OF THE NEWBORN

Case 27

HISTORY AND LABORATORY DATA

A well-hydrated White baby boy was 1 day old when the neonatologist observed that he was beginning to appear jaundiced. This baby was the first child of a 28-year-old computer analyst who had no previous obstetric history or history of prior blood transfusion. The pregnancy had been normal.

Stat total bilirubin, hemoglobin and hematocrit, blood type and Rh, and direct antiglobulin tests were ordered on the baby. A cord blood sample had not been collected at delivery. A blood grouping and Rh testing and a screening test for alloantibodies were requested on the mother.

Laboratory Data. The baby's laboratory results:

Total bilirubin	10.8 mg/dL
Hemoglobin	16.9 g/dL
Hematocrit	0.52
Blood group and Rh	A$_1$, Rh Positive
Direct antiglobulin test	Negative

The mother's laboratory results:

Blood group and Rh	O, Rh Negative
Alloantibody screen	Negative

TREATMENT

The baby was immediately started on phototherapy. Subsequent total bilirubin tests were no higher than the 24-hour value and continued to decrease over the next 48 hours. At the time of discharge, the total bilirubin was 6.9 mg/dL.

QUESTIONS

1. What was the most probable cause of this infant's jaundice?
2. What additional laboratory tests could have been of value?
3. Why was phototherapy the treatment of choice?

DISCUSSION

1. Although the mother was Rh negative and the baby was Rh positive, the absence of prior exposure to red cell antigens through pregnancy, miscarriage, abortion, or blood transfusion makes the presence of anti-D antibody highly unlikely even if fetal maternal hemorrhage had occurred during the pregnancy. The fact that the mother is Group O and the baby Group A, suggests an ABO incompatibility, which is particularly common between Group O mothers and Group A babies.

Clinical signs and symptoms are usually mild if the HDN is associated with ABO incompatibility. The laboratory data further suggest that the baby's jaundice was the result of anti-A antibodies. The laboratory results of normal hemoglobin and hematocrit, moderately elevated total bilirubin, and a negative direct antiglobulin test are typical in cases such as this.

2. An elution procedure on the infant's erythrocytes may have demonstrated the presence of anti-A.

3. Phototherapy is a commonly used noninvasive method of treatment in cases of jaundice. The ultraviolet light increases the breakdown of bilirubin pigment that has accumulated in the skin. This treatment is effective in mild cases of jaundice.

CONCLUSION

Hemolytic disease of the newborn caused by ABO incompatibility.

Case 28

HISTORY AND LABORATORY DATA

A 34-year-old geologist was initially seen by her obstetrician at 10 weeks gestation. This was her first pregnancy. She had no previous history of miscarriage, abortion, or prior blood transfusion. A routine prenatal laboratory workup included blood group and Rh type, and alloantibody screening.

Laboratory Data. Blood Group A, Rh(D) negative, D^u negative
Alloantibody Screen Negative

Supplementary Clinical Data. At 22 weeks gestation, the patient fell down a steep embankment while on a geologic field survey for her company. She was taken to the emergency room of a nearby hospital because she sustained some minor cuts. No vaginal bleeding, uterine tenderness, or abdominal pain were noted by the emergency room physician. A subsequent visit to her obstetrician a week later also revealed no abnormalities.

The remainder of this woman's pregnancy proceeded normally. She went into spontaneous labor at 40 weeks (full term) of gestation. A normally developed baby girl was subsequently delivered. The baby had no signs of pallor or jaundice.

The following routine laboratory tests were ordered on the cord blood: blood grouping, total bilirubin, hemoglobin, hematocrit, and direct antiglobulin test. Immune globulin (Rh₀ IgG) was ordered for the mother.

Supplementary Laboratory Data. The baby's cord blood test results are:

Blood group and Rh	A, Rh(D) Positive
Total bilirubin	2.4 mg/dL
Hemoglobin	19.8 g/dL
Hematocrit	0.58
Direct antiglobulin test (DAT)	Positive (3+)

A postpartum blood specimen from the mother revealed that she was Group A, Rh(D) negative and D^u negative with a positive alloantibody screen. The antibody was identified as anti-D, present in a titer of 1:64. A subsequent elution of the baby's red blood cells also revealed the presence of anti-D.

Follow-Up Data. At 24 hours of age, the baby began to develop jaundice. A blood sample from the baby's heel for total bilirubin was 4.3 mg/dL. Phototherapy was begun immediately. On day 2, the baby's bilirubin rose to its maximum value of 9.8 mg/dL. Both the mother and baby were discharged on the third day postpartum.

QUESTIONS

1. Is this patient a candidate for immune globulin (Rh₀) D?
2. What is the possible cause of the anti-D antibody in this case?
3. Could this situation have been averted or anticipated?

DISCUSSION

1. The three *exclusionary* criteria for Rh immune globulin (RhIg) are:

A. If the mother is Rh₀(D) positive or D^u positive. In mothers with the D^u phenotype, however, the situation is controversial. If these women are also C+, the D^u phenotype is the result of gene suppression caused by the presence of the C gene in a "trans" position. Mothers with this type of D^u *cannot* be immunized to D or produce anti-D antibodies. Other D^u phenotypes, which are rare, can produce anti-D but are not usually given Rh immune globulin prophylactically.

B. If both mother and baby are Rh(D) Negative.

C. Rh(D) negative mothers who demonstrate anti-D antibody due to active immunization are not candidates for RhIg prophylaxis. However, the sole presence of anti-D, is *not* definitive proof that active immunization has occurred. Administration of antenatal Rh immune globulin could contribute to a positive test for alloantibodies and must be ruled out through either documentation of the patient's obstetric history or laboratory testing. Anti-D antibody that has been passively acquired is usually weakly reactive. However, anti-D that results from active antibody production is generally high-titered and can be inactivated by treating the serum with substances such as 2-mercaptoethanol. Mothers who received antenatal Rh immune globulin should also receive postpartum RhIg.

2. Because this patient had no prior history of miscarriage, abortion, or previous pregnancies, it must be assumed that feto-maternal hemorrhage occurred after the trauma of falling.

3. Rh immune globulin is a concentrated solution of IgG anti-D antibody. A normal dose contains 300 μg, which is sufficient to counteract the immunizing effects of 15 mL of Rh Positive fetal erythrocytes or 30 mL of whole blood.

The Kleihauer-Betke test is helpful in identifying and determining a semi-quantitative estimate of the amount of fetal erythrocytes in the maternal circulation. This allows calculation of the total dose of Rh-immune globulin required.

Conclusion

Hemolytic disease of the newborn caused by Rh_o (D) incompatibility.

Case 29

HISTORY AND LABORATORY DATA

A 23-year-old pregnant woman was admitted for delivery. She had no history of prior transfusions; however, a previous pregnancy 5 years earlier had resulted in a stillborn infant. Because the patient was group O Rh negative, she had received antenatal Rh immune globulin three months before admission.

Following this delivery, postpartum Rh immune globulin was ordered. The results of the type and screen procedure revealed a positive alloantibody in her serum. The baby's cord blood DAT was also positive. The mother's serum and an eluate of the baby's red cells were tested. The results were similar.

Laboratory Data (Case 29)

Reagent Red Blood Cell Screening Cells
Partial Listing of Antigens Present

Cell No.	Rh-hr					Kell		Duffy		Kidd		Lewis		MNS				P
	D	C	E	c	e	K	k	Fy^a	Fy^b	Jk^a	Jk^b	Le^a	Le^b	S	s	M	N	P$_1$
I	+	0	+	+	+	0	+	+	0	+	+	0	+	+	+	+	0	+
II	0	+	0	+	0	0	+	0	+	+	0	0	+	0	+	+	0	+

Patient Results

Cell No.	Immediate Spin	37° C	AHG	Coombs Control
I	Neg	Neg	2+	
II	Neg	Neg	Neg	2+

Reagent Red Blood Cell Panel Antigen Profile
Partial Listing of Antigens Present

Cell No.	Rh-hr					Kell		Duffy		Kidd		Lewis		MNS				P
	D	C	E	c	e	K	k	Fy^a	Fy^b	Jk^a	Jk^b	Le^a	Le^b	S	s	M	N	P$_1$
1	0	0	0	+	+	0	+	+	+	+	0	0	0	+	0	+	+	+
2	0	0	0	+	+	0	+	0	+	+	+	0	+	+	+	+	0	0
3	0	+	0	+	+	0	+	0	+	+	+	0	+	+	+	+	0	+
4	+	0	+	+	0	0	+	+	0	+	0	0	+	0	+	+	0	+
5	+	0	+	+	0	0	+	+	+	0	+	0	+	0	+	+	+	+
6	+	+	0	0	+	+	+	+	+	+	0	0	+	+	+	+	+	+
7	+	+	0	0	+	0	+	0	+	+	+	0	+	0	+	+	+	+
8	+	+	+	0	+	0	+	+	0	0	+	+	0	0	+	+	0	0
9	+	+	0	+	+	0	+	+	+	+	+	+	0	+	0	0	+	+
10	+	+	0	0	+	+	0	0	+	+	+	0	+	0	+	+	+	+
11	+	0	0	+	+	0	+	0	+	+	+	+	0	0	0	0	+	+

Patient Results

Cell No.	Immediate Spin	37° C	AHG	Coombs Control
1	Neg	Neg	Neg	2+
2	Neg	Neg	Neg	2+
3	Neg	Neg	Neg	2+
4	Neg	1+	2+	
5	Neg	Neg	2+	
6	Neg	Neg	2+	
7	Neg	1+	3+	
8	Neg	±	2+	
9	Neg	±	1+	
10	Neg	Neg	1+	
11	Neg	Neg	2+	

QUESTIONS

1. What is the identity of the alloantibody in the patient's serum and the eluate of the baby's erythrocytes?
2. What is the most probable explanation for the presence of this antibody?
3. What further tests should be considered?
4. Is this situation common?
5. Is antenatal Rh immune globulin administration an effective method of prevention of HDN due to anti-D?

DISCUSSION

1. Although both anti-D and anti-E are the most probable alloantibodies in this case, the alloantibody was anti-D.
2. Occasionally strong reactions (2 to 3+), including reactions in the albumin 37° C phase, may be seen 3 months after administration of Rh immune globulin. A positive cord blood DAT with anti-D demonstrated by elution may also be expected.
3. It is suggested that the patient be rechecked in 6 months to totally exclude the possibility of an additional actively acquired alloantibody.
4. According to Bowman,* 28% of ABO-compatible babies born to mothers who have received antenatal RhIg will have a positive DAT (weak). One-fourth of women receiving RhIg at 28 weeks, 34 weeks, and delivery will have residual passively acquired anti-D at 6 to 9 months postpartum. Another poorly referenced "rule of thumb" is that the anti-D titer at 8 to 12 weeks after the administration of IgG should be 1:4 or less if caused by passively acquired antibody and greater than 1:4 if caused by immunization.
5. Rh immunization may be prevented in at least 94% of instances by antenatal prophylaxis at 28 weeks' gestation.

CONCLUSION

Anti-D (Probably passively acquired antenatal immune globulin).

*Bowman, John M.: *Eradication of Rh Hemolytic Disease of the Fetus and Newborn*, presented at the Harvard Medical School Course in Eradication of Rh Hemolytic Disease of the Fetus and Newborn, May 21-22, 1981.

Case 30

HISTORY AND LABORATORY DATA

A 38-year-old woman was 4 months pregnant (gravida 3, para 2). Her husband is homozygous for the D antigen. She was being followed for anti-D sensitization and possible HDN because she is group O Rh negative with a positive indirect antiglobulin test at room temperature, 37° C, and AHG phases. The alloantibody had been previously identified as anti-D. Anti-D was again the only alloantibody recognized in the patient's serum. Her anti-D titers follow.

One Month Ago

Dilution	IS	37° C	AHG
1:1	3+	4+	3+
1:2	3+	3+	3+
1:4	3+	3+	3+
1:8	±	3+	3+
1:16	Neg	2+	3+
1:32	±	2+	2+
1:64	Neg	1+	1+
1:128	Neg	Neg	1+
1:256	Neg	Neg	Neg
1:512	Neg	Neg	Neg
1:1024	Neg	Neg	Neg

Present

Dilution	IS	37° C	AHG
1:1	4+	3+	3+
1:2	3+	3+	3+
1:4	3+	3+	3+
1:8	2+	3+	3+
1:16	1+	2+	2+
1:32	±	2+	2+
1:64	Neg	1+	2+
1:128	Neg	1+	1+
1:256	Neg	1+	1+
1:512	Neg	±	±
1:1024	Neg	Neg	Neg

QUESTIONS

1. Based on the previous and current agglutination results, what are the patient's anti-D titers?
2. Comment on the observations in question 1.
3. What is the significance of the results of the present titer?

4. What is the probable Rh$_o$ phenotype of the fetus?
5. Will interventions be necessary before delivery of this infant?

DISCUSSION

1. The patient's previous anti-D titer was 1:64 (albumin) and 1:128 (AHG). The present titer is 1:512 (Albumin and AHG).
2. There was a fourfold increase in strength of the anti-D in the mother's serum since the previous study one month before.
3. A rising titer indicates antigenic stimulation that is encouraging antibody production. Another method of assessing antibody avidity is to score the titer. The scoring of this titer follows:

One Month Previously

Dilution	AHG	Score
1:1	3+	10
1:2	3+	10
1:4	3+	10
1:8	3+	10
1:16	3+	10
1:32	2+	8
1:64	1+	5
1:128	1+	5
1:256	Neg	0
1:512	Neg	0
1:1024	Neg	0
		68 Total

Present

Dilution	AHG	Score
1:1	3+	10
1:2	3+	10
1:4	3+	10
1:8	3+	10
1:16	2+	8
1:32	2+	8
1:64	2+	8
1:128	1+	5
1:256	1+	5
1:512	±	2
1:1024	Neg	0
		76 Total

4. The fetus is probably Rh$_o$ (D) positive.
5. An assortment of diagnostic and therapeutic interventions may be necessary

in this case. Various procedures are discussed in Chapter 10; intrauterine transfusion may be necessary.

CONCLUSION

Hemolytic disease of the newborn caused by anti-D.

Case 31

HISTORY AND LABORATORY DATA

A 40-year-old Black lawyer was referred to a medical center obstetrician by her family physician after she was diagnosed as pregnant (approximately 8 weeks gestation). Her medical history indicated that she had received 2 units of Group O, Rh negative packed red cells during the delivery of her first child. Rh immune globulin was administered postnatally because she was a suitable candidate. Routine prenatal laboratory testing was ordered.

Laboratory Data

Blood group and Rh	O, Rh (D) and D^u negative
Alloantibody screen	Positive
Antibody identification	Anti-Kell antibody, titer 1:32

Supplementary Testing

A *repeat* titer of anti-Kell was performed at 28 weeks gestation; this titer was 1:128.

QUESTIONS

1. What tests should be performed routinely at delivery?
2. Would prophylactic treatment with immune globulin D have protected the mother against development of this antibody?
3. What is the significance of a rising titer?

DISCUSSION

1. Current standards do not require that Rh(D) Negative mothers be tested at delivery for alloantibodies or have a repeat Rh(D) and D^u test performed. If, however, the Rh(D) and D^u tests have not been previously determined in prenatal cases or in patients admitted for abortion or amniocentesis, they must be performed on delivery or hospital admission.

The cord blood from newborn infants of Rh(D) and D^u negative mothers should be tested for D antigen. The presence of alloantibodies in the mother's serum and the infant's clinical condition determine whether or not a DAT should be done. Routine protocols differ from one hospital to another.

2. No. Immune globulin (IgG) anti-D is effective *only* against the D antigen. It would not protect the mother against immunization to any other foreign antigen.

3. A fourfold or greater increase in alloantibody titer suggests an active immunologic response. In this case, the increase of the anti-Kell titer suggests that fetal erythrocytes bearing the Kell antigen have entered the maternal circulation and are stimulating alloantibody production. The performance of alloantibody titers is presented in Chapter 14. Although the numeric value of an alloantibody titer is not positively correlated to the severity of HDN, the patient should be closely monitored. Tests such as paternal Kell antigen typing or amniocentesis would be of value.

CONCLUSION

Hemolytic disease of the newborn caused by anti-Kell.

8

Transfusion Policies and Practices

At the conclusion of this chapter, the reader will be able to:
- Describe the requirements for the selection of blood for transfusion to a patient.
- Discuss the risk of immunization when transfusing a patient.
- Name at least six common surgical procedures for which the type and screen protocol is appropriate.
- Explain the steps that must be followed in transfusion emergency situations.
- Name the first sign of immunization in a patient who has received blood possessing a foreign antigen.
- Define the term "massive transfusion."

- List the clinical priorities in massive transfusion situations.
- Name and describe six adverse conditions associated with the rapid infusion of massive amounts of blood.
- Explain the purpose of an exchange transfusion of a newborn infant.
- Discuss the selection of donor blood for exchange transfusion of a newborn infant.
- Describe the special blood requirements of patients with cold-reacting alloantibodies or a warm autoantibody.

Chapter Outline

ROUTINE TRANSFUSION REQUESTS

Most of the blood provided by a blood bank is used by patients undergoing surgical procedures or with acute unexpected blood loss. The balance is used for correction of chronic anemias not treatable by surgery or other means and for patients with special needs, such as oncology or dialysis patients.

In the early 1980s, the need to eliminate the time and expense of unnecessary crossmatching was recognized. Based on the established prospective need for blood in specific surgical procedures, the type and screen protocol (discussed in Chapter 6) was developed. Blood banks have now established what types of cases are most likely to use blood and the average number of units of blood usually required. The prospective use of blood varies from one hospital to another, depending on factors such as the patient's presurgical condition and age, and the type of surgical technique used. Table 8-1 presents a summary of a typical blood order schedule.

Selection of Blood for Crossmatching

The *first requirement* for blood selection is the ABO group of the patient (Table 8-2). Whenever possible, blood of the same group should be given (see discussion of the universal donor and the universal recipient). This requirement is absolute in the case of group O recipients. The use of group O whole blood for other ABO groups is not acceptable except for a group O recipient. If volume replacement is needed, red blood cells can be resuspended in saline or volume expanders can be infused. The subgroups A and AB are unimportant unless the patient has potent anti-A_1 or anti-H, in which case donor blood group A_2 or A_2B, or A_1 or A_1B, respectively, would be selected.

When blood of the same ABO group is not available, the next choice is red blood cells of a group that are compatible by major crossmatch. The most important consideration is that the donor red blood cells must be compatible with both the recipient's anti-A or anti-B and any other clinically significant antibody the prospective recipient may have. This is because every foreign red blood cell transfused becomes instantly and totally surrounded by the recipient's plasma, which provides complete contact between antigens on the donor's red blood cells and the patient's plasma antibodies. If the patient's plasma contains an antibody to the corresponding antigen on the foreign red blood cells the two will combine and a serious reaction may take place. The reverse situation, in which the donor's plasma has the antibody and the recipient's red blood cells have the antigen, is not as dangerous. The incoming donor antibody is instantly diluted by the recipient's much larger volume of plasma before the antibody has an opportunity to interact with the recipient's red blood cells.

THE UNIVERSAL DONOR

The term "universal donor" often has been applied to group O, Rh negative blood products. There is no such thing as a universal donor! The use of this term for group O individuals is based on the lack of A, B, and D antigen on the red blood cells. The plasma of group O persons, however, does contain anti-A and anti-B, which is able to react with recipient red blood cells of other blood groups. The extraction of plasma from whole blood units removes about 80% of the antibody from the unit. If the residual antibody is high in titer, a considerable amount of activity remains. If a significant amount of anti-A and anti-B accumulates in the patient's circulation, it prevents reverting to transfusing blood of the patient's own blood type. Washed or deglycerolized red blood cells contain little or no residual plasma with accompanying antibodies.

The use of group O blood does not prevent sensitization of the patient to other blood group antigens that may be missing from their own red blood cells. Indiscriminate use of group O Rh negative blood may also produce a shortage of this type and could have serious consequences if a group O Rh negative person needed to be transfused.

THE UNIVERSAL RECIPIENT

A group AB recipient lacks both anti-A and anti-B and may safely receive red blood cells from donors of other blood groups. Group O, however, is the poorest choice because it contains some anti-A, anti-B, and cross-reacting anti-A,B.

Other Requirements

The *second requirement* in the selection of blood is the Rh group of the patient. Testing for $RH_o(D)$ is considered sufficient. The risk of immunization depends on factors such as the immunogenicity of a specific antigen, the frequency of the antigen in the donor population, and an individual's capacity to form antibodies.

Table 8-1. Surgical Blood Order Schedule

Type of Surgery	Maximum Standard Crossmatch Order (Units)	Type of Surgery	Maximum Standard Crossmatch Order (Units)
Dental Surgery		Meniscectomy	0
Full mouth extraction	0	Minor hand or foot surgery	0
Extraction, impacted molars	0	Open reduction	T&S
		Osteotomy	1 PC
General Surgery		Removal of hip pin	T&S
Abdominal-perineal resection	4PC	Shoulder reconstruction	T&S
Amputation	T&S	Spinal fusion	2 PC
Anal fistula excision	T&S	Synovectomy	0
Appendectomy	T&S	Total hip replacement	4 PC
Breast biopsy	T&S	Total knee replacement	T&S
Cholecystectomy	T&S		
Colon resection	2 PC	*Plastic Surgery*	
Colostomy or closure	T&S	Augmentation mammoplasty	T&S
Esophageal resection	4 PC	Facelift	0
Excision of anal fissure or fistula/		Reduction mammoplasty	T&S
sphincterotomy	0	Rhinoplasty	0
Excision of skin lesions	0	Skin flap	T&S
Exploratory laparotomy	T&S	Skin graft, minor	T&S
Gastrectomy	4 PC	Skin graft, major (severe burns)	T&S
Gastroscopy	0		
Hemicolectomy	2 PC	*Pulmonary and Vascular Surgery*	
Hemorrhoidectomy	0	Abdominal aortic aneurysm	
Hernia repair, hiatal	2 PC	resection	4 WB and 2 PC
Hernia repair, inguinal or femoral	0	Aortofemoral bypass graft	4 WB and 2 PC
Hernia repair, ventral	T&S	Aortoiliac bypass graft	4 WB and 2 PC
Lymph node biopsy	0	Bronchoscopy	0
Mastectomy, modified radical	2 PC	Endarterectomy: femoral or carotid	2 PC
Mastectomy, simple	T&S	Femoral–femoral bypass graft	2 PC
Parathyroidectomy	T&S	Femoral–popliteal bypass graft	2 PC
Sigmoidectomy	2 PC	Thoracotomy	4 PC
Splenectomy	T&S		
Thyroid lobectomy	T&S	*Gynecologic and Obstetric Surgery*	
Vagotomy and antrectomy	T&S	Cesarean section	T&S
Vein stripping	T&S	Dilatation, curettage, and	
		conization	0
Ear, Nose, and Throat		Hysterectomy, radical and pelvic	
Caldwell-LUC	T&S	lymphadenectomy	4 PC
Excision of submandibular gland	0	Hysterectomy, simple (including	
Myringotomy	0	TAH/BSO)	T&S
Laryngectomy	1 PC	Hysterectomy and anterior-	
Mastoidectomy	0	posterior repair	1 PC
Neck dissection (radical)	4 PC	Laparoscopic tubal ligation	T&S
Parotidectomy	0	Marshall-Marchetti procedure	0
Septoplasty	0	Ovarian wedge resection, ovarian	
Tonsillectomy and adenoidectomy	T&S	cystectomy	T&S
Transantral ethmoidectomy	T&S	Stamey procedure	T&S
Tympanoplasty	0	Tuboplasty	T&S
		Uterine suspension, fulguration of	
Orthopedic Surgery		endometrial implants	T&S
Amputation, toe	0	Vaginal plastic procedures	T&S
Arthroscopy	0		
Arthrotomy–removal of loose body	0	*Neurosurgery*	
Carpal tunnel repair	0	Carpal tunnel release	T&S
Excision, Morton's neuroma	0	Craniotomy for aneurysm	T&S
Fracture, closed reduction	0	Craniotomy for tumor	T&S
Fracture, open reduction, internal		Craniotomy for traumatic	
fixation	2 PC	hematoma (acute)	T&S
Hip nailing/hip screw	3 PC	Craniotomy for chronic subdural	
Leg amputation	0	hematoma	T&S

Table 8-1. (continued)

Type of Surgery	Maximum Standard Crossmatch Order (Units)
Craniotomy for AVM	T&S
Craniotomy for rhizotomy	T&S
Craniotomy for EC-IC	T&S
Depressive laminectomy (cervical, thoracic, or lumbar)	T&S
Laminectomy for disc removal (lumbar)	T&S
Laminectomy for rhizotomy	2 WB + 2 PC
Bilateral T_{2-3} sympathectomy	0
Laminectomy for spinal tumor	2 WB + 2 PC
Shunts, VP and VA, (if an alloantibody is detected 2 WB should be available)	T&S
Laminectomy for chordotomy	2 WB + 2 PC
Percutaneous chordotomy	T&S
Craniotomy for excision of abscess	2 WB
Burr hole for tapping of cyst or abscess	T&S
Carotid endarterectomy	T&S
Ophthalmologic Surgery	
Cataract removal	0
Recession, eye	0
Entropion or extropion repair	0
Urologic Surgery	
Cystectomy, radical	4WB
Cystectomy, segmental	T&S
Cystoscopy	0
Cystourethropexy	0
Fulguration of bleeding bladder tumor	1 PC
Hydrocelectomy	0
Ileal conduit–colon conduit	1 PC
Needle biopsy, prostate	0
Nephrectomy, radical	4 WB
Nephrectomy, simple	T&S
Nephrostomy	T&S
Orchiectomy	T&S
Orchiopexy	T&S
Penile prosthesis	T&S
Perineal prostatectomy	2 PC
Prostate biopsy	0
Pyelolithotomy	T&S
Suprapubic prostatectomy	2 PC
Transurethral resection of bladder tumor	T&S
Transurethral resection of prostate	T&S
Ureteral dilatation	0
Ureteral reimplantation	T&S
Ureterolithotomy	T&S

Key: T&S = Type and Screen
         WB = Whole Blood
         PC = Packed Red Blood Cells

Table 8-2. Selection of Donor Blood According to ABO Group

Patient's Type	Donor Blood 1st choice	Donor Blood 2nd choice*	Donor Blood 3rd choice*
0	0	None	
A	A	O (RBCs)	
A_1 with anti-H	A_1	None	
A_2 with anti-A_1	A_2	O (RBCs)	
B	B	O (RBCs)	
AB	AB	A or B RBCs†	O RBCs
A_1B with anti-H	A_1B	A_1 or B RBCs†	
A_2B with anti-A_1	A_2B	A_2 or B RBC†	O RBC

* When donor blood of recipient's group is not available.

† It does not make much difference which of these is chosen. Because they are mutually incompatible, both must not be given concurrently. Type B has the advantage of avoiding possible complications due to the presence of anti-A_1 or anti-H in the recipient serum.

(From Huestis, D.W., Bove, J.R., and Busch, S.: Practical Blood Transfusion. (3rd ed.). Boston, Little, Brown and Co., 1982, p. 206.)

RH$_o$(D) is an important antigen because of its immunogenicity and the fact that a person has an 85% chance of receiving Rh positive blood. Although D^u is less immunogenic than D, D^u positive individuals can produce anti-D. Therefore, the D^u status of a recipient does not need to be determined; he/she should receive Rh negative blood. D^u positive donors are regarded as Rh positive donors. The comparative risk of immunization to antigens other than A, B, and Rh$_o$(D) based on the number of antibodies encountered and the frequencies of the antigens in the population, in descending order, is K, c, E, k, e, Fy^a, C, Jk^a, S, Jk^b, and s.

The *third requirement* is the use of antigen-negative blood in patients in whom an alloantibody is detected. An alloantibody should be identified before blood is selected for transfusion. If a situation is clinically urgent, it is sometimes necessary to issue blood which is crossmatch incompatible. The crossmatch technique by which the antibody reactivity is strongest should be used and recorded.

Blood Shortages

Inability of a blood bank to meet patient needs for blood and blood products may result from a shortage of blood within the regional system or depletion of certain types in the blood bank inventory because of massive transfusion needs.

A shortage of blood may be due to:

1. Increased general demand, e.g., major disaster.
2. Insufficient blood collections, e.g., seasonal variation.
3. Disproportionate collection and need of specific blood types, e.g., group O Rh negative, group B Rh positive.
4. Inability to provide antigen-negative blood for a patient with an antibody to a high incidence antigen or in cases of multiple alloantibodies.

In addition to increased donor recruitment efforts for all blood or specific types of blood, donation of autologous blood (see Chapter 2) may alleviate the problems.

EMERGENCY TRANSFUSION SITUATIONS

Orderly management of a patient requiring urgent blood transfusions requires communication of the severity of the need and the extent of the emergency to the blood bank by the attending physician. This allows a determination of the anticipated blood use and the extent of pretransfusion testing that can be completed before issuing the blood.

Emergency Processing and Issuing of Blood

When there is a desperate need for blood, uncrossmatched or partially crossmatched blood might be requested by a physician. When blood is released before the crossmatch is completed, an Emergency Release Form (Fig. 8-1 A, B) must be completed. This form, which must be signed by the ordering physician, indicates that the patient's life will be in jeopardy without an emergency transfusion. Such a statement does not absolve the blood bank from its responsibility to issue properly labelled donor blood or to complete typing and compatibility testing as soon as possible.

Steps To Follow in an Emergency

When an urgent request for blood is received:

1. Immediately obtain a blood specimen from the patient and attach a numbered bracelet on the patient's arm. Both the specimen and the patient should be minimally identifiable by number if time does not permit additional information or if other information about the patient, for example, name, is unknown. Blood specimens *must* be collected before any blood is administered.
2. Promptly determine the ABO group and Rh type of the patient, and begin compatibility testing. Determination of the group and Rh types should take less than 5 minutes. Most patients can receive volume support during this brief interval. Any blood that is released before pretransfusion testing is fully completed should be group and type compatible. The blood typing must be from the patient's current specimen. Previous blood bank records must *not* be used to determine the recipient's blood group and the blood group must not be taken from other records, e.g., driver's license. If group O blood is to be used in a patient of an unknown type, it should be in the form of packed red blood cells and the patient should be switched to his or her own type as soon as possible (see Table 8-3).
3. Indicate, in a conspicuous fashion on the tag or label attached to the donor units, that compatibility testing has not been completed at the time of issue.

I request the release of blood for _____,
                                         Patient's Name or Identification

_____ , _____ , _____ , _____ ,
Hospital ID Number   Location   Age   Sex
_____ , at _____ on _____ .
        Race   Time   Date

Nature of the Emergency: _____

I believe this patient's life will be in jeopardy *without* an emergency transfusion; therefore, I accept the responsibility for, and release the Blood Bank Medical Director and Blood Bank personnel of the responsibility for, any adverse patient reaction resulting from this transfusion, which might have been prevented if time had allowed for complete pretransfusion testing.

I further understand that the Blood Bank personnel will complete routine compatibility testing as soon as possible and that they will report the results immediately to me.

                         Signed: _____ , M.D.

A

FOR BLOOD BANK USE:

The patient's AB and RH groups (if known) are _____ .

Patient Alloantibody   A. Not performed
Screen   B. Immediate spin only
                            C. Centrifuged post-incubation
                            D. Completed

Donor Unit Number   Stage of crossmatch when released;
1. _____   A. No pretransfusion testing performed
                            B. Immediate spin only
                            C. Centrifuged post-incubation

2. _____   A. No pretransfusion testing performed
                            B. Immediate spin only
                            C. Centrifuged post-incubation

3. _____   A. No pretransfusion testing performed
                            B. Immediate spin only
                            C. Centrifuged post-incubation

_____   _____
      Blood Bank Technologist   Date
B

Fig 8-1. Example of an emergency release of blood form. A, Physician's release form; B, Form for blood bank use.

4. Complete compatibility tests promptly (stat), even though the transfusion has already been started. If an incompatibility is detected at any stage of testing, immediately notify the patient's physician and the blood bank medical director, and, if possible, retrieve the donor units at once.

5. Complete all records and forms as in a routine situation.

Table 8-3. Principles to be Followed When Switching Blood Types Because of Shortages

Patient's Blood Type and Rh Type	Principle
O negative	1. Use only group O, Rh negative blood if patient is sensitized to Rh_o (D). 2. Use group O, D, and D^u negative, C negative and/or E positive blood in preference to Rh_o (D) positive blood. 3. Avoid transfusing anything but group O, Rh negative blood to patients (especially women) under 45. 4. Restrict the use of group O, Rh positive blood for group O, Rh negative patients to acute emergency situations, and then use only if the patient either has a negative antibody screen for anti-D or definitely lacks Rh antibodies. 5. If massive volumes of blood are required and switching to Rh positive blood is inevitable, avoid wasting group O, Rh negative blood by switching as early as possible.
A negative or B negative	1. Use only Rh negative blood if patient is sensitized to Rh_o (D), i.e., group specific, Rh negative or group O, Rh negative packed RBCs. 2. Use D and D^u negative, C negative and/or E positive in preference to Rh_o (D) positive. 3. Avoid transfusing anything but Rh negative blood to patients (especially women) under 45. 4. Restrict use of Rh positive blood to acute emergency situations, and then use only if the patient has a negative alloantibody screen for anti-D or definitely lacks Rh antibodies. 5. If massive volumes of blood are required and switching to Rh positive blood is inevitable, avoid wasting Rh negative blood by switching as early as possible. 6. Conserve group O blood. Only group O blood can be given to a group O recipient.
AB negative	1. Use only Rh negative blood if the patient is sensitized to Rh_O (D). 2. Use D and D^u negative, C negative and/or E positive in preference to Rh_o (D) positive. 3. Group A blood may be used (as packed RBCs) unless the patient has anti-A_1. 4. The patient should initially be switched to group A blood and then, secondarily, may be switched to group O blood. Always do this before switching Rh types. 5. Avoid transfusing anything but Rh negative blood to patient (especially women) under age 45. 6. Restrict the use of Rh positive blood to acute emergency situations and then use only if the patient has a negative alloantibody screen or definitely lacks Rh antibodies. 7. If massive volumes of blood are required and switching to Rh positive blood is inevitable, avoid wasting Rh negative by switching as early as possible. 8. Conserve group O blood. Only group O blood can be given to a group O recipient.
O positive	1. A group O patient may receive only group O blood. 2. Rh negative blood may be used, but this should be avoided due to supply problems.
A positive or B positive	1. Group O blood may be given as packed red cells. 2. Rh negative blood may be used, but this should be avoided because of supply problems.
AB positive	1. Group A blood may be used (as packed red cells, unless the patient has anti-A_1). 2. Switch initially to group A blood and then, secondarily, to group O blood. 3. Conserve group O blood. Only group O blood can be given to a group O recipient. 4. Rh negative blood may be used, but this should be avoided because of supply problems.

Compatibility Testing in the Emergency Situation

The hazard of transfusing blood to a patient whose serum has not been screened for alloantibodies must balance the risk of an unfavorable outcome, such as a hemolytic transfusion reaction, against the danger to the patient of postponing transfusion. An increased possibility of error exists when the haste and disruption created by an emergency upset routine procedures.

The most important function of the major crossmatch is confirmation of ABO compatibility. In general, IgG antibodies causing incompatible crossmatches result in decreased red blood cell survival of transfused cells but usually do not cause life-threatening intravascular hemolysis.

Changing Blood Groups

The blood bank policy manual should

contain established guidelines for switching to a different blood group during an urgent situation, such as massive transfusion. At times of blood shortage, the medical director of the blood bank and the patient's physician should not feel constrained to transfuse only ABO and Rh specific blood. When deciding on the appropriateness of switching blood types, it is essential that the patient's clinical condition be assessed to anticipate the extent of the prospective blood requirement. A plan for switching blood types should maintain the greatest flexibility in meeting the patient's total requirements.

The age and sex of a patient are an important consideration in selecting and switching blood types. For example, it would be well to avoid transfusing Rh positive blood to an Rh negative woman of childbearing age. In such cases, it is usually preferable to switch ABO groups, if feasible, before switching from Rh negative to Rh positive blood.

If the estimated total transfusion requirements of an actively bleeding Rh negative patient (with anti-D) exceed the available amount of appropriate Rh negative blood, the change to Rh positive should be done immediately to conserve this relatively scarce blood type. In such situations, the blood bank medical director should be consulted. If Rh positive blood must be given to an Rh negative patient, Rh negative blood should be given as soon as possible if additional transfusions are needed because immunization to the D antigen is likely to occur. The first evidence of immunization is usually the development of a positive DAT preceding detectable antibody in the patient's serum.

The principles of switching blood (Table 8-3) detail the strategy to be used in overcoming a shortage. When this is done, the transfused red blood cells should *always* be in the form of packed red blood cells rather than whole blood.

MASSIVE TRANSFUSION

Massive transfusion is defined as the administration of enough blood or compo-

nents within less than 24 hours to constitute a complete volume replacement. In an infant, this would be slightly more than half a unit and in an adult it would be 8 to 10 or more units. Situations associated with massive transfusion include treatment of acute bleeding associated with traumatic injury or surgery, and exchange transfusion subsequent to hemolytic disease of the newborn (HDN).

Physiologic Results of Hemorrhage

The various changes brought about by acute hemorrhage, e.g., decreased blood pressure, rapid and thready pulse, increased respiratory rate, and constriction of the peripheral blood vessels which produces cold, clammy-feeling skin, can be referred to as hypovolemic shock syndrome. Many factors affect the amount of hemorrhage that will cause shock, but a rapid loss of 15 to 20% of blood volume leads to shock symptoms in most individuals. Almost all patients with hemorrhagic or hypovolemic shock have lost 35 to 40% of their blood volume; an average adult in severe hypovolemic shock has probably lost about 2 liters of blood. In many cases, for example, internal injuries and fractures, not all of the lost blood is visible.

One of the first responses to severe, acute bleeding is the body's physiologic attempt to restore the circulating blood volume to normal by shifting fluid from extravascular to intravascular spaces. Although this fluid does not have the oxygen-carrying capabilities of red blood cells nor the osmotic properties of plasma, it does stabilize the circulation. The effect of this shift in fluid to the intravascular spaces is that the remaining circulating red blood cells will be diluted and produce the characteristic drop in red blood cell parameters: hemoglobin, hematocrit, and red blood cell count. Dilution begins almost as soon as the onset of hemorrhage and continues for as long as 72 hours after all bleeding has stopped. During this 3-day period, the hemoglobin and hematocrit values are unreliable because they do not reflect the total amount of bleeding during this period. In the first few hours of active bleeding, hemoglobin and hematocrit values may be misleadingly high despite obvious and substantial amounts of blood loss.

Initial Treatment of a Hemorrhaging Patient

Problems associated with massive transfusion may arise from one or more conditions including:

1. The primary state for which the blood is administered
2. Complications of the initial malady
3. Underlying secondary disorders
4. Abnormalities in the transfused blood.

It is *vital* that a blood specimen for blood bank use be obtained before transfusion is initiated. Identification of the patient with a wristband is essential to the safety of the impending blood transfusion (see Fig. 2-1). Errors such as misidentification of either the patient or the specimen are more likely to occur in this type of nonroutine situation.

The first priority in the treatment of a patient for massive transfusion is the restoration of blood volume. This allows the body to regain an acceptable blood pressure to enable oxygen and nutrients to be delivered to essential organs and to prevent or halt disseminated intravascular coagulation (DIC). Blood volume can be expanded with electrolytes, plasma substitutes, blood, or blood components. Electrolytes, for example, normal saline, are usually the first solutions to be administered to the critically injured patient. Emergency volume replacement solutions, for example, normal saline or lactated Ringer's, do not replace the oxygen-carrying capacity of the blood. If the circulation is effective, an increased rate of blood flow delivers an adequate quantity of oxygen to the tissues that will compensate for the lower level of hemoglobin. Following expansion of volume, the next priority is the restoration of an adequate level of hemoglobin to ensure that the patient's oxygen-carrying capacity does not drop below the level at which compensation is possible and to remove the

strain on the heart caused by the increased demand for cardiac output.

Adverse Conditions Associated with Massive Transfusion

Many adverse situations have been associated with the rapid infusion of massive amounts of blood. These situations include:

1. Citrate toxicity
2. Hypocalcemia
3. Hypothermia
4. 2,3 DPG depletion
5. Depletion of coagulation factors and platelets
6. Accumulation of biochemicals and microaggregates

CITRATE TOXICITY

In most transfusion situations, the infusion of blood mixed with anticoagulant-preservative and changes associated with storage (see Chapter 2) can be corrected by the patient's physiology shortly after infusion. After the administration of blood under usual circumstances, the patient's pH may initially reflect excess acid, but the subsequent metabolism of citrate results in a net excess of base. In cases of massive transfusion where the volume of transfusion is high and the rate is rapid, the patient's ability to compensate cannot keep up. This produces a need to correct disturbances in acid-base balance.

HYPOCALCEMIA

Ionized calcium, the physiologically active form of calcium, has been demonstrated to be lowered because of the massive transfusion of citrated blood, but this is rarely of clinical importance. This depression of ionized calcium is because the citrate concentration in a donor unit is sufficient to bind with the ionized calcium of the unit itself, with excess citrate remaining available to complex with calcium in the recipient.

Hypocalcemia is almost never witnessed because the body is able to mobilize additional calcium from bones as needed. Additionally, body cells rapidly metabolize infused citrate. Citrate is first converted to bicarbonate and ultimately to carbon dioxide and water. The general attitude is that a warm adult with a normally functioning liver can tolerate a unit of blood every 5 minutes without needing supplemental calcium. If this rate is exceeded or if hypothermia or severe liver disease exists, calcium infusion may be indicated, but calcium-containing solutions should not be administered through the same infusion lines as the blood because clotting in the line can result.

HYPOTHERMIA

Hypothermia can result from the rapid (more than 100 mL/minute for 30 minutes) transfusion of refrigerated blood. Large volumes of rapidly infused cold blood can lower the temperature of the sino-atrial node to below 30° C, at which point ventricular arrhythmias occur.

Warming blood during massive transfusion can avoid the adverse effects of hypothermia, such as cardiac arrhythmia, and enhance the body's homeostatic mechanism, which is being stressed. Warming of blood must be carefully controlled and should not slow the rate of infusion significantly.

2,3 DPG DEPLETION

If the oxygen-carrying capacity of the blood does decrease as a result of DPG depletion, the recipient may compensate by increasing the rate of blood flow to the tissues. The patient will be able to restore DPG biochemically to normal levels within a few hours. In most cases of massive transfusion, the level of DPG in the transfused blood is of no significance. However, DPG depletion can be potentially dangerous under the following circumstances:

1. When the volume of transfused blood results in an almost complete exchange within a few hours.
2. When all or most of the transfused blood has been stored for more than 1 or 2 weeks.

3. When the recipient lacks the ability to increase his/her cardiac output.

DEPLETION OF COAGULATION FACTORS

Massive transfusion is sometimes associated with coagulation abnormalities that have been attributed to dilution or the "washout" of coagulation factors or platelets. It has been established that massive transfusion with stored blood or plasma will not by itself reduce the activity of any plasma coagulation factors to a level at which hemostasis is compromised.

The occurrence of abnormal bleeding during massive transfusion indicates that simple dilution is *not* the only problem. Large amounts of plasma substitutes may aggravate a bleeding tendency. The bleeding time of an adult can be prolonged if more than one liter of dextran is rapidly transfused, presumably because dextran coats the platelets and impairs their function; however, coagulation function is not impaired by albumin, plasma protein fractions, or electrolytes except for their dilutional effect.

Although the patient's plasma maintains adequate levels of coagulation factors in uncomplicated situations where there is no increased rate of consumption, the major complication impairing hemostasis during massive transfusion is disseminated intravascular coagulation (DIC). DIC is almost inevitable when extensive tissue damage is accompanied by prolonged shock and the resultant poor perfusion. It leads to the loss of platelets as well as the consumption of plasma coagulation factors V, VIII, II (prothrombin), and factor I (fibrinogen). Secondary fibrinolysis complicates the situation by releasing fibrin breakdown products which, in turn, inhibit coagulation and platelet plug formation. If the circulation is improved by restoring blood volume to normal, this enhances the removal of activated clotting factors by the mononuclear phagocytic system or neutralization by normal circulatory inhibitors. As the patient's blood volume is being restored, it may be necessary to replace coagulation factors and platelets. If fibrinogen is low, cryoprecipitate should be transfused. Cryoprecipitate contains 250 mg of fibrinogen and the transfusion of 16 bags should raise fibrinogen level of the average adult by more than 100 mg/dL (see Chapter 9 for a complete discussion of blood components).

Although abnormal test results do not always correlate with clinical problems, a massively transfused patient should be monitored after or during transfusion. A platelet count, prothrombin time, and activated partial thromboplastin time should be performed. If abnormal bleeding occurs, platelet concentrates or fresh frozen plasma should be administered based on the laboratory test results and the patient's clinical symptoms. Additional tests may be indicated to evaluate the possibility of DIC.

DEPLETION OF PLATELETS

Platelet counts do decline in massively transfused patients and can fall below 100 $\times$ 10^9/L after infusion of 15 to 20 units of whole blood. Dilution of the patient's circulating platelets occurs as soon as the splenic pool reserves have been exhausted. Once the platelet reserves are exhausted, it takes 4 to 5 days for the synthesis of new platelets to restore the normal quantity.

At 1 to 6° C the microtubules in the platelets are disrupted; therefore, the lifespan of platelets in donated blood is limited. Recovery of viable platelets in whole blood is about 20% of normal after 72 hours. Platelet concentrates are the most effective method of preventing or correcting the dilutional thrombocytopenia of uncomplicated massive blood transfusion as well as augmenting the thrombocytopenia caused by DIC. Because platelet concentrates stored at room temperature for 72 hours have substantial quantities of the labile coagulation factors, a pool of eight platelet concentrates, with a volume of about 400 mL, should be considered the therapeutic equivalent of 1 to 2 units of fresh frozen plasma. Therefore, platelet concentrates can help to correct coagulation factor deficiencies and thrombocytopenia.

ACCUMULATION OF BIOCHEMICALS AND MICROAGGREGATES

Plasma potassium which accumulates in stored blood is of no significance in the massive transfusion of adult patients. Ammonia is also not significant, except for patients with severe liver failure. There is also no evidence of plasticizers leaching from blood containers.

Microaggregates composed of platelets, granulocytes, and fibrin increase progressively in stored blood but these aggregates are larger if red cells have been prepared by centrifugation. Microaggregate filters have been suggested after more than 5 to 10 units of blood have been transfused in rapid succession.

Compatibility Testing in Cases of Massive Transfusion

Following the infusion of many units of blood over a short period, the composition of circulating blood changes and the proportion of the patient's own red blood cells and plasma to the total blood volume decreases. Consequently, the pretransfusion specimen ceases to represent the patient's current status, and crossmatches using the initial specimen have limited validity.

If the pretransfusion specimen contained no alloantibodies, a saline immediate-spin crossmatch is permissible for confirmation of ABO compatibility. This is particularly applicable if 10 or more units of blood have been transfused; nothing is gained by continued crossmatching because most of the circulating blood is donor blood. If alloantibodies, however, were initially present in the patient specimen, the same policy of confirmation of ABO compatibility is permissible, provided that the donor blood has been screened for the corresponding antigen. This policy must be set forth in the laboratory procedures manual.

Exchange Transfusion

Exchange transfusion of a newborn infant is used in the treatment of both the anemia and hyperbilirubinemia that characterize hemolytic disease of the newborn (HDN; refer to Chapter 10 for a full discussion of HDN). Small amounts of blood are removed from the baby and replaced with donor blood until a one or two total blood volume exchange is accomplished. It is necessary to both maintain blood volume and prevent circulatory overload during the procedure.

Exchange transfusion replaces the antibody-coated red blood cells with compatible donor cells and removes bilirubin and circulating maternal antibody from the baby's plasma. A two-volume exchange achieves an 80 to 90% removal of red blood cells and 25 to 35% removal of bilirubin. The small amount of bilirubin removed is due to *extravascular* bilirubin, which is not removed by the procedure and is released into the plasma following the exchange transfusion.

Criteria for performing an exchange include:

1. The degree of anemia
2. The cord blood and plasma bilirubin level
3. The rate of the rise of bilirubin
4. The maturity of the baby

Performing an initial exchange transfusion or subsequent exchanges is based on restoring an adequate red cell volume and removing the product of red blood cell hemolysis, bilirubin. Generally, a bilirubin increase greater than 0.5 mg/dL per hour or a rise of 10 mg/dL in the first 24 hours is an indication for an exchange transfusion. Accumulation of bilirubin in nervous tissue, i.e., the brain, can result in *kernicterus,* which may occur at bilirubin levels of 20 mg/dL or greater in a full-term infant and lower levels in a premature infant. A 3- or 4-day old baby may be able to tolerate much higher levels than a premature infant.

SELECTION OF BLOOD IN SPECIAL CASES

Blood Requirements for Exchange Transfusion

Blood for the exchange transfusion of a newborn infant must be negative for the red blood cell antigen to which the mother has the corresponding antibody. It must also be ABO and RH group compatible with the infant's blood group (Table 8-4). If the mother's specimen is not available, group

Table 8-4. Selection of ABO Group Compatible for Exchange Transfusion

Mother's Group	Infant's Group	Donor Group
O, A, or B	O	O
O or B	A	O
A or AB	A	A or O
O or A	B	O
B or AB	B	B or O
A	AB	A or O
B	AB	B or O
AB	AB	AB, A, B, or O

O red blood cells must be selected. Rh positive blood may be given to an Rh positive infant whenever the mother lacks anti-D. Donor blood should also be negative for hemoglobin S and cytomegalovirus (CMV).

Blood Needed for Intrauterine Transfusion

Blood for intrauterine transfusion must be as fresh as possible and group O Rh negative. In addition, the red blood cells must be compatible with the mother's specimen. Because viable lymphocytes in the donated blood are capable of causing graft-versus-host disease, irradiated blood should be used (see Chapter 9 for a full discussion of blood products).

Transfusion of Newborn Infants

Newborn infants, particularly premature babies, often present problems when transfusion is required. There are important physiologic differences between the newborn and older children or adults. In the newborn infant, it is reasonable, on an immunologic basis, to provide sequential transfusions from the same donor who is antigen-compatible for some of the most immunogenic factors. In general, repeating the crossmatch with the same donor blood is unnecessary for the first 6 weeks of life. Although fresh heparinized blood provides the benefits of high 2,3 DPG levels, clotting factors, platelets, and a more physiologic pH, conventional blood bank units that are less than 1 week old have adequate 2,3 DPG and clotting factors. Clotting and platelets are not needed unless the baby has a bleeding tendency, in which case they can be administered as blood component concentrates.

Blood Needs of Patients with Cold Antibodies

Antibodies that are inactive below 37° C are of little clinical significance. When the crossmatches are incubated at 37° C (using the prewarming technique), red blood cells containing the antigen will not be agglutinated. If the patient's cold antibody is of a specific type, such as anti-M, antigen negative blood may be selected but is not mandatory.

Blood Needs of Patients with Warm Autoantibodies

When a patient with a warm autoantibody has to be transfused, the attending physician and blood bank medical director must decide jointly to administer blood that is not truly compatible in vitro. If autoabsorption is used to decrease the degree of agglutination, the crossmatch report should include the techniques used and the observed results.

Blood Needs of Patients with a Positive DAT

If a patient has a positive DAT, the following protocol is suggested for deciding whether or not the patient can be transfused.

A patient *can* be transfused if:

1. The alloantibody screening test is negative *and*
2. The crossmatched units are compatible *and*
3. There is no history of whole blood or packed red blood cell transfusion in the last three months

Note: The attending physician should be notified. One lavender-top (EDTA) and one red-top tube should be stored in the refrigerator prior to transfusion.

A patient *cannot* be transfused without further consultation if:

1. There is a history of transfusion of whole blood or packed red cells within the last 3 months *or*
2. The alloantibody screen is positive *or*
3. The crossmatched units are incompatible

Further steps should be taken as follows:

1. Notify the attending physician to determine the need for transfusion.
   A. If the patient's physician determines that a transfusion is needed as soon as possible (urgently), use the following guidelines:

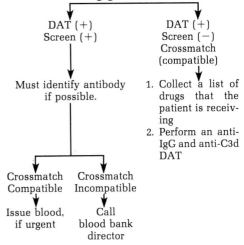

B. Perform an eluate if the patient is hemolyzing red cells and requires a transfusion. Signs of hemolysis include an elevated lactic dehydrogenase (LDH), an elevated bilirubin, and an increased reticulocyte count. Another sign of hemolysis is a decreasing hematocrit over a period of time without overt blood loss. Other guidelines for performing an elution procedure can be found in Table 6-19.

CHAPTER SUMMARY

Routine Transfusion Requests

Blood provided by a blood bank is for patients undergoing surgical procedures or for those with acute unexpected blood loss. Other patients may need transfusions to correct anemias. Because the need to eliminate unnecessary crossmatching has been recognized, the type and screen protocol has been developed for specific surgical procedures. Blood banks have now established the types of cases most likely to use blood and the average number of units of blood usually required. This prospective utilization of blood has been developed into an organized blood order schedule.

The first requirement for blood selection is the ABO group of the patient. Whenever possible, blood of the same group should be given; this requirement is absolute in the case of group O recipients. When blood of the same ABO group is not available, the next choice is packed red blood cells of a group that are compatible by major crossmatch. The term "universal donor" often has been applied to group O Rh negative blood products. There is no such thing as a universal donor. The use of this term for group O individuals is based on the lack of A, B, and D antigen on the erythrocytes. The use of group O does not prevent sensitization of the patient to other blood group antigens that may be missing from their own red cells. A group AB recipient lacks both anti-A and anti-B and may safely receive red cells from donors of other blood groups. However, group O is the poorest choice because it contains some anti-A, anti-B and cross-reacting anti-A,B. The second requirement in the selection of blood is the Rh type of the patient. $Rh_o(D)$ is an important antigen because of its immunogenicity and the fact that a person has an 85% chance of receiving Rh positive blood. Although D^u is less immunogenic than D, D^u positive individuals can produce anti-D. Therefore, the D^u status of a recipient does not need to be determined and he or she should receive Rh negative blood. The third requirement is the use of antigen-negative blood in patients in whom an alloantibody is detected. An alloantibody should be identified before blood is selected for transfusion. If a situation is clinically urgent, it is sometimes necessary to issue blood that is crossmatch-compatible.

Inability of a blood bank to meet patient needs for blood and blood products may result from a shortage of blood due to increased general demand, insufficient blood collections, disproportionate collection and need of specific blood types, or inability to provide antigen-negative blood for a patient with an antibody to a high-incidence antigen or in cases where multiple antibodies are present.

Emergency Transfusion Situations

Orderly management of a patient requiring urgent blood transfusion requires communication of the severity of the need and the extent of the emergency to the blood bank by the attending physician. When there is a desperate need for blood, uncrossmatched or partially crossmatched blood might be requested by a physician. In these situations, an emergency release form must be completed.

When an urgent request for blood is received, a blood specimen should be immediately obtained from the patient and a numbered bracelet attached on his or her arm. Other steps that must be followed include prompt determination of the group and type of the patient, beginning of compatibility testing, indication in a conspicuous fashion on the tag or label attached to the donor units that compatibility testing has not been completed at the time of issue, complete compatibility tests promptly, and completion of all records and forms as in a routine situation. The hazard of transfusing blood to a patient whose serum has not been screened for alloantibodies must balance the risk of an unfavorable outcome against the danger to the patient of postponing transfusion. An increased possibility of error exists when the haste and disruption created by an emergency upsets routine procedures.

The blood bank policy manual should contain established guidelines for switching to a different blood group during an urgent situation such as massive transfusion. It is essential that the patient's clinical condition be assessed to anticipate the extent of the prospective blood requirement. A plan for switching blood types should maintain the greatest flexibility in meeting the patient's total requirements.

Massive Transfusion

Massive transfusion is defined as the administration of enough blood or components within less than 24 hours to constitute a complete volume replacement. In an infant, this is slightly more than half a unit and in an adult 8 to 10 or more units.

Various changes such as decreased blood pressure, rapid and thready pulse, increased respiratory rate, and hypovolemic shock syndrome can be brought about by acute hemorrhage. Problems associated with massive transfusion may arise from one or more conditions, including the primary state for which the blood is administered, complications of the initial malady, underlying secondary disorders, or abnormalities in the transfused blood. Errors such as misidentification of either patient or specimen are more likely to occur in this type of nonroutine situation.

The first priority in the treatment of candidates for massive transfusion is restoration of blood volume to regain an acceptable blood pressure to enable oxygen and nutrients to be delivered to essential organs and to prevent or halt disseminated intravascular coagulation (DIC). Following expansion of volume, the next priority is the restoration of an adequate level of hemoglobin to ensure that the patient's oxygen-carrying capacity does not drop below the level at which compensation is possible and to remove the strain from the heart caused by the increased demand for cardiac output.

Various adverse situations have been associated with rapid infusion of massive amounts of blood. These include citrate toxicity, hypocalcemia, hypothermia, 2,3 DPG depletion, depletion of coagulation factors and platelets, and accumulation of biochemicals and microggregates. After infusion of many units of blood over a short period of time, the composition of circulating blood changes and the proportion of the patient's own red cells and plasma to the total blood volume decreases. Consequently, the pretransfusion specimen ceases to represent the patient's current status, and crossmatches using the initial specimen have limited validity.

Exchange transfusion of a newborn infant is used in treatment of both the anemia and hyperbilirubinemia that characterize hemolytic disease of the newborn. Exchange transfusion replaces the antibody-coated erythrocytes with compatible donor cells as well as removing bilirubin and circulating maternal antibody from the baby's plasma. Criteria for performing an exchange include degree of anemia, cord blood and plasma bilirubin level, rate of the rise of bilirubin, and the maturity of the baby.

Selection of Blood in Special Cases

Blood for exchange transfusion must be negative for the erythrocyte antigen to which the mother has the corresponding antibody. It must also be ABO and Rh compatible with the infant's blood group. If the mother's specimen is not available, group O erythrocytes must be selected.

Blood for intrauterine transfusion must be as fresh as possible; it must also be group O Rh negative. The donor unit must be compatible with the mother's specimen. Because viable lymphocytes in the donated blood are capable of causing graft-versus-host disease, irradiated blood should be used.

Newborn infants, particularly premature ones, often present problems when a transfusion is required. It is reasonable, on an immunologic basis, to provide sequential transfusions from the same donor who is antigen-compatible for some of the most immunogenic factors. Although fresh heparinized blood provides additional benefits, conventional blood bank units less than 1 week old can be used. Clotting and platelets are not needed unless the baby has a bleeding tendency, in which case, they can be administered as blood component concentrates.

Patients with cold-reacting alloantibodies may present special problems. Although this type of antibody is considered of no clinical significance, in vitro agglutination can be avoided when a prewarming technique is used. If the patient's cold antibody is a specific type such as anti-M, antigen-negative blood may be selected but is not mandatory.

When a patient with a warm autoantibody has to be transfused, the attending physician and blood bank medical director must jointly decide whether to administer blood that is not truly compatible in vitro. If autoabsorption is used to decrease the degree of agglutination, the crossmatch report should include the techniques used and the observed results.

REVIEW QUESTIONS

1-4. Arrange the following requirements in the correct sequence of priority for the selection of blood for a patient.
A. Rh (Rh$_o$) specific
B. ABO group specific
C. Antigen negative blood in patients with an alloantibody
D. Group O whole blood
E. Major crossmatch ABO-compatible erythrocytes

1. ____
2. ____
3. ____
4. ____

5. Group O Rh negative blood has several disadvantages when used as "universal donor" blood for a patient of a different blood type. Which of the following is *not* a disadvantage?
A. Anti-A and anti-B can react with the recipient's erythrocytes
B. It can prevent switching back to the patient's own blood type
C. It can provide for the immediate emergency needs of a patient until his/her ABO group is determined
D. It can produce a shortage of this type of blood
E. None of the above

6. The poorest ABO choice of blood for an AB recipient is:
A. Group A
B. Group B
C. Group AB
D. Group O
E. Both Group A and Group B

7. If a patient is group O and donor blood of the recipient's own type is not available, what other type (or types) can be used as packed erythrocytes?
A. Group A

B. Group B
C. Group AB
D. Either **A** or **B**
E. None of the above

8. If a patient is group A$_2$ with anti-A$_1$ and donor blood of the recipient's own group is not available, what other type (or types) can be used as packed erythrocytes?
A. A$_1$
B. B
C. A$_1$B
D. A$_2$B
E. O

9. If a patient is group A$_2$B with anti-A$_1$ and donor blood of the recipient's own group is not available, what other type (or types) can be used as packed erythrocytes?
A. A$_1$
B. A$_2$
C. B
D. A$_1$ or B
E. A$_2$ or B

10. The risk of immunization when transfusing a patient depends on all of the following factors except:
A. The patient's antigen status
B. The ABO group of the patient
C. The immunogenicity of the antigen
D. The frequency of the antigen in the donor population
E. The individual's capacity to form antibodies

11-15. When an urgent request for blood is received, certain procedural steps should be followed. Arrange the following procedural steps in their proper sequence.
A. Determine the patient's ABO and Rh group
B. Complete compatibility testing
C. Identify units of blood that have been partially crossmatched
D. Identify the patient and draw a blood specimen
E. Complete all records and forms

11. ____
12. ____
13. ____
14. ____
15. ____

16. The first evidence of immunization in a patient who has received blood possessing an antigen is:
    A. In vivo hemolysis
    B. Detectable antibody in the patient's serum
    C. A positive direct antiglobulin test
    D. Hemoglobinuria
    E. Increased blood pressure and respiration

17. If a group AB Rh Negative patient is admitted with massive bleeding, which of the following units of packed cells would be the *least* desirable to transfuse?
    A. Group O Rh Negative
    B. Group O (D Negative, C Negative, E Positive)
    C. Group O Rh Positive
    D. Group A Rh Negative
    E. Group A Rh Positive

18. In an adult, a massive transfusion is defined as the administration of more than ____ units of blood in less than 24 hours.
    A. 2–4
    B. 4–6
    C. 6–8
    D. 8–10
    E. 10–12

19. Hypovolemic shock can be caused by the rapid loss of ____% or more blood volume.
    A. 5–10
    B. 10–15
    C. 15–20
    D. 20–25
    E. over 25

20. From the list of adverse reactions associated with massive transfusion which of the following does *not* belong on the list?
    A. Citrate toxicity
    B. Permanent change in blood type
    C. Hypocalcemia
    D. Hypothermia
    E. Depletion of coagulation factors and platelets

21. The depletion of 2,3 DPG is usually *not* of concern unless one or more of the following is true:
    1. The volume of transfused blood results in an almost complete exchange within a few hours

2. All or most of the blood has been refrigerated for 1 or 2 weeks
    3. All of the units of blood are frozen deglycerolized RBCs
    4. The patient lacks the ability to increase cardiac output
    A. Only 1
    B. 1 and 2
    C. Only 3
    D. 1, 2 and 4
    E. All of the answers are correct

22. Bleeding due to impaired platelet function can occur in a massively transfused patient if _____ is rapidly administered.
    A. Albumin
    B. Whole blood
    C. Dextran
    D. Plasma protein fractions
    E. Electrolytes (e.g., normal saline)

23. The major complication that impairs hemostasis in an uncomplicated case of massive transfusion is:
    A. Thrombosis
    B. Primary fibrinolysis
    C. Accumulation of calcium
    D. Disseminated intravascular coagulation
    E. Loss of factor VIII

24. In an exchange transfusion of an infant, a one or two total blood volume exchange is accomplished. How much blood does this represent?
    A. 1/2 to 1 pint
    B. 1 to 2 pints
    C. 2 to 4 pints
    D. 4 to 8 pints
    E. 8 to 10 pints

25. The decision to perform an exchange transfusion in an infant is based on two or more of the following criteria:
    1. The degree of anemia
    2. The maturity of the baby
    3. The cord blood bilirubin level
    4. The infant's circulating plasma bilirubin level
    5. The rate of rise of the circulating plasma bilirubin
    A. 1 and 2
    B. 1, 2, and 3
    C. 3 and 4
    D. 3, 4 and 5
    E. All of the above

26. In the selection of blood for exchange transfusion, what characteristic or characteristics apply?
   - **A.** It must be negative for the RBC antigen to which the mother has the circulating antibody
   - **B.** It must be ABO and Rh compatible
   - **C.** It can be type O
   - **D.** It should be negative for cytomegalovirus (CMV)
   - **E.** All of the above

27. In the case of an exchange transfusion, if the mother is group O or A and the baby is group B, what donor type or types should be selected?
   - **A.** Group A
   - **B.** Group B
   - **C.** Group O
   - **D.** Group O or Group A
   - **E.** Group O or Group B

28. Blood selected for intrauterine transfusion should be two or more of the following:
   1. Compatible with the mother's blood
   2. As fresh as possible
   3. Group O Rh negative
   4. Irradiated
   5. Enriched with fresh frozen plasma
   - **A.** 1 and 2
   - **B.** 2 and 3
   - **C.** 3 and 4
   - **D.** 4 and 5
   - **E.** All of the above, except 5

29. If a newborn infant requires transfusions, which of the following factors is (are) important?
   1. Sequential transfusions from the same donor
   2. Repeating the crossmatch with each transfusion
   3. The use of fresh heparinized blood
   4. The use of bank blood that is less than 1 week old
   5. All of the above
   - **A.** 1 and 2
   - **B.** 1, 3 and 4
   - **C.** Only 3
   - **D.** 3 and 4
   - **E.** Only 5

30. If a patient has a cold antibody, what consideration or considerations is / are mandatory?
   - **A.** The antibody specificity should be determined
   - **B.** A prewarming technique should be used
   - **C.** The attending physician and blood bank director should decide to administer the blood
   - **D.** The patient's serum should be absorbed with group O cells
   - **E.** All of the above

ANSWERS

1.	B	**16.**	C
2.	E	**17.**	C
3.	C	**18.**	D
4.	A	**19.**	C
5.	C	**20.**	B
6.	D	**21.**	D
7.	E	**22.**	C
8.	E	**23.**	D
9.	E	**24.**	A
10.	B	**25.**	E
11.	D	**26.**	E
12.	A	**27.**	C
13.	C	**28.**	E
14.	B	**29.**	B
15.	E	**30.**	B

BIBLIOGRAPHY

Boyd, P. R., Sheedy, D. C., and Henry, J. B.: Type and screen: Use and effectiveness in elective surgery. Am. J. Clin. Pathol. *73*(5):694-699, 1980.

Dodsworth, H., and Dudley, H. A. F.: Increased efficiency of transfusion practice in routine surgery using pre-operative antibody screening and selective ordering with an abbreviated crossmatch. *Br. J. Surg.*, *72*:102-104, 1985.

Huestis, D. W., Bove, J. R., and Busch, S.: Practical Blood Transfusion. 3rd Ed. Boston; Little, Brown and Co.,

Heustis, D. W., Bove, J. R., and Case, J.: Practical Blood Transfusion, 4th ed. Boston, Little, Brown and Co., 1988, pp 169-210.

Insalaco, S. J., and Potter, A. R.: Neonatal transfusion therapy. Lab. Med., *16* (3): pp. 149-156, 1985.

Kuriyan, M., and Kim, D. U.: The maximum surgical blood order schedule: Choice of methods used in its development. Lab. Med. *19*(3):156-159, 1988.

McMican, A.: Neonatal transfusion therapy. Lab. Med., *19*:353-356, 1988.

Mollison, P.: Blood transfusion in Clinical Medicine 6th. Ed., Oxford, Blackwell Scientific, 1979.

Murphy, R. J. C., Malhotra, C., and Sweet, A. Y., Death following an exchange transfusion with hemoglobin SC blood. J. Pediatr. *96*:110, 1980.

Oberman, H. A.: Surgical Blood Ordering, Blood Shortage Situations, and Emergency Transfusion. In

Clinical Practice of Blood Transfusion. Edited by L. D. Petz and S. N. Swisher. New York, Churchill-Livingstone, 1981. pp. 393-404.

Perkins, H. A.: Strategies for massive transfusion. In Clinical Practice of Blood Transfusion. Edited by L. D. Petz, and S. N. Swisher. New York, Churchill-Livingstone, 1981. pp. 485-491.

Petz, L. and Swisher, S. N.: Blood transfusion in acquired hemolytic anemias. In Clin. Pract. Blood Transfusion. Edited by L. D. Petz and S. N. Swisher. New York, Churchill-Livingstone, 1981. pp. 623-661.

Schmidt, P. J., Samia, C. T. Gregory, K. R. and Leparc, G. F.: Rational reduction in pretransfusion testing, Lab. Med. 17(8):467-470, 1986.

Widmann, F.: Technical Manual (9th Ed.) Arlington, Va., American Association of Blood Banks, 1985. pp. 282-284.

9

Transfusion Therapy: Blood and Blood Components

At the conclusion of this chapter, the reader will be able to:

- List the components that can be prepared from one unit of whole blood.
- Explain the advantages of whole blood.
- List the advantages of packed red cells as compared to whole blood.
- Describe the most appropriate clinical applications for whole blood, packed red blood cells, washed red cells, and neocyte-enriched packed cells.
- State the currently approved FDA approved shelf-life of whole blood drawn into CPDA-1 anticoagulant.
- State the expiration time of packed red blood cells prepared in an open system.
- Compare and contrast the advantages and disadvantages of packed red blood cells.
- Discuss the purpose of red blood cell rejuvenation.
- Explain the advantages and disadvantages of neocytes.
- State the criteria for leukocyte-poor blood.
- Describe the clinical situation in which leukocyte-poor blood is most frequently indicated.
- List at least three techniques for preparing leukocyte-poor blood.
- Explain the process of freezing blood.
- Discuss the applications and advantages of deglycerolized red cells.
- State the proper storage conditions for platelet concentrates.
- State the maximum pH of stored platelet concentrates.
- State the required minimum percentage and concentration of platelets in random donor platelets.
- Describe the clinically appropriate condition or conditions for granulocyte transfusions.
- Define the term "graft-versus-host disease (GHVD)" and explain the mechanism of this disorder.
- Name at least three blood products that can cause GVHD.
- Describe how GVHD can be prevented.
- Compare the uses and differences between single-donor plasma and fresh-frozen single-donor plasma.
- Describe the characteristics and use of cryoprecipitate.
- Calculate the number of bags of cryoprecipitate needed, given the desired level of factor VIII activity and the patient's plasma volume.
- List the various blood anticoagulants.
- State the length of time in which a defrosted unit of cryoprecipitate must be given.
- Describe a method or methods for eliminating blood-borne viruses from cryoprecipitate.
- State the major disadvantage of Factor IX complex.
- Compare and contrast the synthetic red blood cell substitutes.
- Discuss the role of recombinant DNA technology in the production of blood components.

Chapter Outline

The collection and refrigerated preservation of whole human blood has been a well-established practice for more than 50 years in the United States. Although it was previously possible to enter glass bottles and remove the plasma from sedimented units, the introduction of plastic bags with attached multiple collection units and high speed temperature-controlled centrifuges made the current practice of blood component therapy a reality.

It is now possible to harvest a variety of blood components from a single unit of whole blood. The separation of a single unit of whole blood into multiple components has increased the effectiveness of blood utilization from each individual blood donation. The cellular components of whole blood are erythrocytes, leukocytes, and platelets (thrombocytes). The three major classes of whole blood plasma derivatives currently licensed in the United States are coagulation products, such as anti-hemophilic factor (AHF), immune globulins, and plasma volume expanders.

WHOLE BLOOD

The use of anticoagulated whole blood has been drastically reduced over the past two decades in favor of component therapy. In certain situations, however, all the constituents of whole blood are needed by a patient. Because of the extensive effort to utilize blood components, hospital blood banks may receive up to 99% of red cell units as packed cells rather than whole blood. Under these circumstances, whole blood is frequently not available when needed. Combining components to meet a patient's need for whole blood increases both the risk and cost of transfusion therapy to the patient.

Clinical Indications

Whole blood is appropriate for use if *both* enhanced oxygen-carrying capacity and blood volume replacement are needed. Whole blood is indicated for actively bleeding patients who have lost over 25% of their blood volume, i.e., acute massive blood loss. Fresh (less than 24-hour-old) whole blood is now considered unnecessary for the correction of coagulation deficiencies, and specific components are the appropriate and safer choice.

Methods

The collection of blood for use as whole blood or later separation into components is discussed in detail in Chapter 2. The quantity of anticoagulant (63 mL) such as citrate phosphate dextrose (CPD) is appropriate for 450 mL of whole blood. A 10% leeway is permitted in the volume of whole blood; therefore, a unit is considered satisfactory if it contains between 405 and 495 mL of whole blood. Less than 405 mL is unsatisfactory.

Storage Requirements

Whole blood must be refrigerated *as soon as possible* after collection. The temperature must be maintained at 1 to 6° C during storage and between 1 and 10° C if transported. The length of storage (shelf-life) varies with the type of anticoagulant used. Citrate phosphate dextrose (CPD) is currently approved by the FDA for storage for 21 days and citrate phosphate dextrose adenine-1 (CPDA-1) has an approved shelf-life of 35 days in most states.

Advantages

Whole blood carries less risk, particularly of blood-borne diseases, and is more cost-effective than combined component therapy if a bona fide need exists. The administration of packed red blood cells and fresh frozen plasma doubles the patient's risk of exposure to infectious agents and is more costly.

Disadvantages

Indiscriminate use of whole blood can reduce the availability of components to multiple patients. Additionally, congestive heart failure produced by hypervolemia can occur in patients who are not actively bleeding.

Special Notes

Whole blood (less than 4 or 5 days old) is the component of choice for exchange transfusion in newborn infants. This ensures plasma electrolyte concentrations that are tolerable for infants and also en-sures adequate levels of 2,3 diphosphogly-cerate (2,3 DPG).

RED BLOOD CELL PRODUCTS

Packed Red Blood Cells

In the interest of better patient care, the use of packed red cells has actively and effectively replaced whole blood for trans-fusion. Replacement of whole blood with packed red cells has been stimulated by the economic benefits of using blood products as components and has been successful.

CLINICAL INDICATIONS

Patients in need of the oxygen-carrying capabilities of the hemoglobin within red blood cells are candidates for packed red blood cells. Patients with chronic blood loss who cannot compensate for this loss through normal bone marrow replacement mechanisms and patients who lack normal bone marrow activity are examples of transfusion candidates.

METHODS

The desirable method of collection of blood for the preparation of packed red blood cells is to use blood collection units with an attached satellite bag. Collection of blood from the donor using this method is the same as collecting an individual unit of whole blood. The unit of whole blood may be allowed to sediment during refrigerated storage or centrifuged at any time up to the expiration date of the whole blood. The sep-aration of plasma from the unit is usually performed during initial processing of the donor unit and must be done within 6 hours of blood collection if fresh frozen plasma containing coagulation factors is desired.

Separation of plasma from the initial col-lection bag is performed by transferring the plasma from the top of the unit to a satellite bag with the aid of a plasma expressor or plasma separator. The amount of plasma transferred to the satellite bag can be weighed with a scale. Under most circum-stances, approximately 225 mL of plasma

are harvested. The red cells remaining in the original collection bag have a packed cell volume (hematocrit) of about 70%. The packed cell volume must *not* usually exceed 80%. Further processing of red cells to pro-duce washed red cells or frozen / deglycer-olized red cells may take place.

STORAGE REQUIREMENTS

After the plasma has been harvested, red cells must be stored and transported under the same conditions as whole blood. Red cells collected and separated in a closed system using integral tubing between the primary and satellite bag and properly re-frigerated have the same expiration date as the whole blood from which they were sep-arated, if the hematocrit does not exceed 80%. If the primary container is entered to remove the plasma or the sterility of the system is disrupted, the red cells have a 24-hour expiration. The new date and time of expiration must be noted on the label and in the records.

ADVANTAGES

Packed red cells minimize circulatory overload because of the reduced volume of the component compared to whole blood. Additionally, the volumes of anticoagulant and electrolytes, such as potassium, are re-duced.

DISADVANTAGES

The transfusion of red cells when whole blood is required necessitates additional transfusion of fresh-frozen plasma, result-ing in a doubled rate of exposure to blood-borne diseases, such as hepatitis, and for-eign antigens. The actual transfusion of packed red cells is slower than whole blood because of the increased viscosity of the component. Additionally, charges to the pa-tient are increased. In this situation, optimal medical care is compromised.

SPECIAL NOTES

Rejuvenating depleted 2,3 DPG and ATP to normal levels can be accomplished by incubating stored red cells with a rejuvenating solution. Several types of additive solutions are licensed for use with packed red cells. Some increase red cell levels of 2,3 DPG and/or ATP by adding substances such as adenine or pyruvate to red blood cells near the end of their shelf-life. To date, red cells stored in the anticoagulant preservative additive solutions Adsol (AS-1) or Nutricel (As-3) have not been studied or licensed for use with rejuvenation solutions. Rejuvenation may be performed up to 2 to 3 days after the red cells expire, provided they have been stored continuously at 1 to 6° C. One of the major advantages of rejuvenation is that it extends the use of outdated units of autologous blood which are still needed by their donors without incurring the additional cost associated with deglycerolization and freezing of red cells.

Rejuvenated red cells regain normal oxygen transport and delivery characteristics as well as improve post-transfusion survival. After rejuvenation, the red cells may be washed, reconcentrated, and transfused within 24 hours or glycerolized and frozen for later use.

Washed Red Blood Cells

The use of washed red blood cells has declined with the increased availability of deglycerolized red blood cells. This type of component, however, may be requested in special circumstances.

CLINICAL INDICATIONS

Disorders requiring saline-washed red blood cells are rare. Patients with paroxysmal nocturnal hemoglobinuria or hypersensitivity to plasma protein need red cells devoid of plasma protein. Emergency transfusion of group O red cells to a patient of another ABO type may also benefit from the removal of antibodies from the plasma.

METHODS

Packed red cells can be washed by multiple batch processing through centrifugation and decanting of the supernatant saline. It is generally more convenient to use equipment designed for deglycerolization of frozen red cells. The efficiency of washing depends on the amount of saline and the method used.

STORAGE REQUIREMENTS

Washed cells should be stored or transported in the same manner as whole blood. However, this type of red cell preparation must be used within 24 hours because it is prepared in an open system.

ADVANTAGES

Transfusing washed red cells reduces the incidence of febrile reactions due to leukocytes and platelets. The reduced number of microaggregates because of washing is advantageous to patients with pulmonary dysfunction, cardiopulmonary bypass patients, or recipients of massive transfusion.

Because of the trace amounts of residual protein in washed red cells, the product is almost devoid of plasma proteins, including regular and irregular antibodies. This may reduce the incidence of anaphylactic reactions due to plasma proteins or soluble substances in the plasma. Washing also eliminates anticoagulants, unwanted metabolites such as ammonia and accumulated lactic acid (lactate), and electrolytes such as potassium ion.

DISADVANTAGES

Preparation of washed red cells is a time-consuming and labor-intensive process. The additional cost to the patient may not be warranted. Although transfusion reactions associated with leukocytes and platelets may be reduced through the use of washed red cells, the use of this product is not the most efficient way to remove leukocytes. An expanded discussion of leukocyte-poor blood is presented later in this chapter.

Neocyte-Enriched Blood

In 1978, it was first demonstrated that young red blood cells (neocytes) had a longer in vivo survival than unfractionated cells from the same donor population. Neocytes have a significantly longer survival time than transfused mature red cells and pyruvate kinase, an age-dependent red cell enzyme activity that is 1.3 times greater than that of mature red cells. Separation of neocytes from more mature red cells is based upon on the age-dependent differences in density.

CLINICAL INDICATIONS

Because neocytes have an extended in vivo survival time, infusion of these red cells could theoretically reduce blood requirements in transfusion-dependent patients, such as those with thalassemia and chronic anemias.

METHODS

Neocytes can be prepared by apheresis or from an ordinary unit of blood. Techniques for isolating neocytes rely on the differences in density between neocytes and more mature red cells. Separation of neocytes with automated equipment from a unit of whole blood is based on the buoyant density of neocytes during centrifugation. When an automated cell processor is used, the larger, less dense red cells are expressed earlier than the older, heavier cells during deglycerolization and / or washing. The first half of the processed unit produces a uniformly younger cell population. The remaining half of the unit consists of older red cells. Units of anticoagulated whole blood must be processed within 24 hours of collection.

STORAGE REQUIREMENTS

Neocyte-rich units of red blood cells must be stored and transported in the same manner as whole blood. This type of product must be used within 24 hours if an open system is used in preparation.

ADVANTAGES

Each mL of erythrocytes theoretically deposits approximately 1 mg of iron in the tissue. A condition referred to as *hemochromatosis* is likely to develop in chronically transfused patients. Transfusion of

neocytes with a mean cell age of 30 days and a potential transfused survival of 90 days could reduce the needs of patients with chronic transfusion requirements, thereby reducing the subsequent deposition of iron in the tissues.

With some techniques it is possible to retain platelets, residual red cells, and plasma as transfusion products. This makes the processing of neocytes more economical. The residual fraction of older red cells may be transfused to patients for whom chronic red cell transfusion therapy is not indicated. If leukocytes are initially removed by sedimentation followed by filtration, the resulting product has $99.3 \pm 0.5\%$ of the leukocytes removed.

DISADVANTAGES

Some investigators suggest that neocyte transfusion does not significantly reduce transfusion requirements; however, considerable interest in this approach remains. Current techniques for neocyte preparation are technically difficult, time-consuming, and expensive. Automated techniques require costly equipment such as a continuous-flow cell separator or cell washer.

Leukocyte-Poor Blood

The standards for leukocyte reduction in leukocyte-poor blood have been based in the past on the percentage of reduction of leukocytes in a red cell product. From the standpoint of the recipient, the total number of leukocytes received is more significant than the percentage of reduction of the initial leukocyte count. Current AABB standards require removal of at least 70% of the leukocytes and retention of 70% of the original red cell mass.

The American Red Cross Blood Service standards have been revised on the basis of residual leukocyte count rather than percentage of reduction. These standards require red cells with leukocytes removed by centrifugation to contain no more than 1×10^9 leukocytes. Units that have leukocytes removed by washing should contain no more than 0.5×10^9 leukocytes. These standards reflect not what is desirable but what is actually achievable in practice.

CLINICAL INDICATIONS

The most frequent indication for leukocyte-poor blood is for use with patients who have suffered from febrile transfusion reactions due to leukocytes.

METHODS

Appraisal of available techniques for leukocyte removal suggests that a microaggregate filter should be used initially. The use of a filter at the bedside may be enough to prevent nonhemolytic febrile transfusion reactions in many patients. The major future role for microaggregate blood filters could well be in the prevention of febrile transfusion reactions. Laboratory processing of leukocyte-poor blood may be by two major techniques: open system procedures and closed system procedures:

Open System Procedures. Five different open systems have been described:

1. The IBM 2991 blood cell processor is an automated batch wash system. In this system, packed cells are introduced into the washing bag and the machine is programmed for a two-cycle saline wash with a 3-second override to remove the buffy coat, comprised mostly of leukocytes, at the end of each cycle.
2. The Haemonetics cell processor uses a continuous-flow system that is not efficient in removing leukocytes from red cells. To achieve satisfactory depletion of leukocytes, the buffy coat must be removed initially as a separate procedure.
3. Another method involves processing diluted upright packed red cells with saline followed by centrifugation. The buffy coat is manually removed with a conventional plasma extractor.
4. Filtration of packed red cells is another method of producing leukocyte-poor blood. Filters such as the Imugard IG500, the Erypur filter, and most recently the Sepaceel R-500A can be used. The Sepaceel filter allows hos-

pitals to prepare leukocyte-poor blood at the patient's bedside. This filter removes more than 99% of leukocytes with approximately 91% red cell recovery.
5. Frozen deglycerolized red cells, discussed in detail in the next section, are another leukocyte-poor blood product which involves the addition of glycerol to packed red cells frozen to $-60°$ C or below for storage. The process of glycerolization, freezing, and deglycerolization destroys leukocytes, particularly granulocytes.

Closed System Procedures Four different closed system techniques have been described.

1. In the upright spin technique, fresh whole blood is collected in a unit with a satellite pack unit. The entire unit is promptly centrifuged in an upright position. The plasma and buffy coat are manually expressed into a satellite pack using a plasma extractor. The red blood cells remain in the primary pack.
2. In the inverted spin technique, fresh whole blood is collected in a unit with a satellite pack unit. The entire unit is centrifuged upside down. With the unit in an inverted position, approximately 75 to 80% of the red cells are run into the satellite pack, leaving the majority of leukocytes in the primary collection unit.
3. The spin-filter method utilizes packed red cells that are at least 2 weeks old. The unit is centrifuged at $5000 \times g$ for 10 minutes at $4°$ C. Following centrifugation, the unit is transfused through a microaggregate filter.
4. Another closed method of leukocyte-poor blood preparation is the spin-cool-filter technique. Whole blood or packed red cells stored under refrigeration are centrifuged at $5000 \times g$ for 10 minutes in a refrigerated centrifuge. The unit is then stored at $4°$ C for a minimum of 3 hours before transfusion through a microaggregate filter.

STORAGE REQUIREMENTS

Leukocyte-poor red cells are stored and transported under the same conditions as whole blood except where the protocol specifies other conditions. An open system has a 24-hour shelf-life. A closed system retains the expiration date of original whole blood unit unless the procedure specifies otherwise.

ADVANTAGES

Leukocyte removal in the open systems discussed above is adequate for all but the most highly alloimmunized patients. It is estimated that units of blood containing less than 0.5×10^9/L leukocytes generally do not cause febrile reactions in alloimmunized patients, but a comparison of the total number of leukocytes remaining in red blood cell preparations processed by various methods can be misleading as an indication of effectiveness in preventing nonhemolytic, febrile transfusion reactions.

A retrospective study of transfusion reaction rates following the infusion of red cells to previously immunized patients processed by various techniques revealed the following rates:

1. Frozen deglycerolized blood was 1.9%
2. Spin-filter method was 3.6%
3. Inverted spin was 4.7%
4. Upright spin was 12%

A study of transfusion reaction rates in polytransfused patients with beta-thalassemia revealed the following nonhemolytic febrile transfusion rates: Imugard filter 1.4%, diluted upright spin 1.4%, spin-filter 16.2%, and packed red cells 25.9%.

Comparative evaluations of existing techniques concluded that the spin-cool-filter technique was the method of choice because of optimal residual leukocyte quantities and red cell recovery as well as simplicity, low cost, and retention of the original expiration date of the donor units. For highly alloimmunized patients requiring virtually total leukocyte removal, and where alloimmunization is to be avoided at any cost, deglycerolized red cells should be used.

DISADVANTAGES

The most commonly used methods for depleting red cells of leukocytes are the inverted spin procedure, which causes excessive red cell loss and poor leukocyte depletion, and the washing of red cells, which is expensive and produces a product with a 24-hour expiration date. The washing and buffy coat removal techniques remove a percentage of the total leukocytes; however, because granulocytes tend to be more dense than other leukocytes, these procedures may even leave a granulocyte-enriched leukocyte residual. With both the upright and the inverted spin techniques, leukocyte depletion is proportional to red cell loss, and the cut-off point for buffy coat removal is subjective. The effectiveness of the spin-filter procedure is related to the age of the blood. For this procedure to be clinically effective, the blood should be at least 15 days old.

In patients who have not previously experienced nonhemolytic febrile reactions due to leukocyte immunization, the cost of product processing is not warranted. Other reasons for using leukocyte-poor blood, such as the prevention of HLA immunization in renal allograft patients or possible reduction in leukocyte-transmitted diseases such as cytomegalovirus, are not warranted in most patients.

Frozen Deglycerolized Red Blood Cells

The science of cryobiology delves into the events which occur when cells are taken from their normal environmental temperature to temperatures below their freezing point. It is the phase transition of water to ice, when subfreezing temperatures are induced, possibly bringing death to cells. The relationship between low temperature and life remained largely unexplained until 1941, when Luyet and Gehenio published their classic, "Life and Death at Low Temperature." Since that time, great interest has flourished in preservation of cells by freezing. The major contribution brought on by this interest has been frozen red blood cells.

Glycerol, by virtue of its powerful water-binding properties, reduces the degree to which solvent water in biologic systems enters the nonsolvent crystalline ice phase. Glycerolization allows the preservation and extended storage of red cells. The in vivo survival and oxygen-carrying capabilities of the red cells are related to the length of time they are kept in the refrigerator between donation and freezing, not the length of storage at low temperatures. After thawing and deglycerolization, the end product results in the recovery of more than 85% of initial donor's red blood cells, which are largely free of the original plasma, leukocytes, and other formed elements.

CLINICAL INDICATIONS

Frozen / deglycerolized red cells are advocated in a variety of clinical situations, including:

1. Alloimmunized patients who have previously experienced nonhemolytic febrile transfusion reactions due to leukocytes or platelets.
2. Patients who are allergic to constituents of plasma proteins, such as those with IgA deficiencies.
3. Neonates or immunocompromised patients in whom the threat of exposure to cytomegalovirus exists.
4. Patients who need or desire autologous transfusions.

METHODS

While a protein solution such as plasma does not require control of the freezing rate or a cryoprotective additive, the cellular constituents of blood will not withstand the rigors of freezing and thawing unless a cryoprotective agent is added to the cells. Although many compounds have some cryoprotective capacity, only those which are nontoxic and biologically acceptable are used for the preservation of blood. Some typical cryoprotective additives are glycerol and dimethylsulfoxide (DMSO), which are intracellular additives that penetrate the cell, and glucose and polyvinylpyrrolidone (PVP), which function extracellularly.

The most popular method in current clinical use for freezing human red blood cells requires the intracellular additive glycerol in either high or low concentration. The high-concentration method uses a glycerol solution of approximately 45% with the slow freeze-thaw technique. The low-concentration method uses a glycerol solution of approximately 18% for the rapid freeze-thaw technique.

Freezing Technique. A unit of anticoagulated whole blood less than 5 days old is centrifuged at approximately 4400 rpm for 6 to 7 minutes. The supernatant plasma is removed with a plasma extractor and replaced with a solution of 45% glycerol. The thoroughly mixed, glycerolized red cells are then transferred to a suitable freezer-adapted plastic bag and a flat set of stainless steel canisters is placed around the plastic bag. The purpose of the canisters is to contain the blood in this specific geometric configuration to simplify storage and permit maximum surface area exposure during the freezing process. The entire unit is then placed in a $-80°$ C storage freezer, where cooling takes place over a period of several hours.

Thawing Technique. Frozen cells are thawed by agitation in a $35°$ C water bath for 10 minutes. The protocol for deglycerolization of high glycerol frozen blood is based on Dr. Meryman's concept of using diluent and wash solutions containing sodium chloride in successively decreasing concentrations to control the osmotic stress on the cells.

During the deglycerolization process, the red cells perform a series of gymnastics. In their transition from glycerol to the first saline solution, which is hypertonic, the red cells shrink into tight balls. The cells are then gradually expanded by the introduction of serially weaker salt solutions. The thawed glycerolized cells are continuously exposed to a decreasing gradient hypertonic wash of saline until isotonic conditions are reached using either a batch-wash technique or continuous-flow instrumentation. The end product will have a final intracellular glycerol concentration of less than 1% and a supernatant hemoglobin concentration within acceptable range. Thawed cells have a normal survival as determined by ^{51}Cr isotope technique and are sterile when tested in appropriate culture media.

STORAGE REQUIREMENTS

Following deglycerolization, the red cells can be stored and transported under the same conditions as whole blood, but a 24-hour dating restriction must be observed because the bag has been entered.

The expiration date for frozen red blood cells for routine transfusion is 10 years from the date of phlebotomy if stored at $-65°$ C or colder. Shipping frozen blood is possible with use of a suitable styrofoam container containing dry ice that will maintain the proper temperature.

Advantages

Reduction of Leukocytes and Platelets. Nonhemolytic febrile transfusion reactions are most frequently caused by leukocyte antibodies; hence, the administration of a product with a minimal number of leukocytes is the most common application of deglycerolized red cells. Leukocytes given to a sensitive recipient can produce diffuse capillary and endothelial damage, impair function of vital organs, and cause necrosis in tumors. These reactions can be prevented in a direct way by removing leukocytes from the blood to be transfused. The average total leukocyte count in a unit of frozen, deglycerolized red cells washed by continuous flow technique is $0.3 \times 10^9/L$, compared to batch-washed red blood cells with an average total leukocyte count of $8.8 \times 10^9/L$.

In addition to the prevention of nonhemolytic febrile transfusion reactions, the intentional transfusion of 5 units of deglycerolized red cells prior to cadaver renal allografting provides the optimum benefit for graft survival and renal function. Intentional transfusions of previously frozen cells are given, even if the hemoglobin level of the transplant candidate would not otherwise warrant transfusion in these cases at Massachusetts General Hospital, Boston. There is also a very low incidence of HLA antibody formation, a complication that could significantly reduce the number of potentially compatible kidney donors.

Because platelets are also reduced in deglycerolized red cells, the prevention of nonhemolytic febrile transfusion reactions in patients with platelet antibodies is another advantage of this blood product. Platelet antigen sensitization may also be decreased. Transfusing red cells that have a very low risk of subsequent HLA antibody formation is the optimum initial therapy for patients who need red cells early in their illness and who may later need platelets, for example, leukemia patients.

Plasma Protein Removal. The removal of plasma proteins is another one of the assets of deglycerolized red cells. The incidence of febrile transfusion reactions may be reduced or eliminated in patients who exhibit sensitivity to plasma proteins. Plasma removal is particularly important to IgA-deficient patients who have been previously immunized to IgA. In patients with classical hemophilia with anti-factor VIII antibodies, an anamnestic increase in antibody titers can occur if they are given whole blood or conventional red cells. Additionally, patients with paroxysmal nocturnal hemoglobinuria can experience hemolytic episodes if they are transfused with complement contained in the plasma of whole blood or packed cells.

Through the removal of plasma proteins which contain naturally occurring isoagglutinins and may include alloantibodies, a twofold benefit is gained. The passive transmission of antibodies is reduced by removing most of the plasma protein. In special circumstances, the transfusion of group O cells to patients of other ABO blood types is safer.

Reduction or Removal of Viruses. HEPATITIS. Although post-transfusion hepatitis has been reported following the transfusion of deglycerolized red cells, it appears that the rates of incidence and severity of post-transfusion hepatitis are considerably lower than the rates observed following the administration of conventional whole blood or red cells.

In one study of the incidence of post-transfusion hepatitis, no hepatitis occurred in a treatment group receiving 623 transfusions of frozen red blood cells resuspended in albumin. Albumin is heated to 60° C in preparation; hence it is considered hepatitis-free. A control group of 104 recipients receiving 441 units of frozen red cells resuspended in autologous plasma had an incidence of 9 cases per 1000. The same benefit can be anticipated with resuspension of red cells in hepatitis-free saline or other solutions.

The mechanism by which hepatitis virus is eluted or inactivated is unknown. It is presumed that the virus is physically displaced from within and without the red cell membrane through the washing process. Both detectable hepatitis associated antigen (HAA) and cytomegalovirus were eliminated from washed cells by both batch-washed and continuous flow techniques.

CYTOMEGALOVIRUS (CMV). CMV infections can be transmitted by blood transfusion. In one study, 52% of 72 patients with a history of multiple transfusions demonstrated CMV antibodies (sero-conversion) in an average of 8 weeks after transfusion. Attempts to grow CMV from deglycerolized red cells have been unsuccessful, presumably because leukocytes harboring the virus are destroyed during the addition and removal of glycerol.

A very low incidence of CMV infections has been observed in the newborn nursery among babies with respiratory distress syndrome who have been transfused with only deglycerolized group O, Rh-compatible red cells on a routine basis to prevent iatrogenic anemia. In evaluating the prevention of transfusion-acquired CMV and its severity in neonates, it was found that no infant in either group receiving seronegative (CMV antibody negative) blood developed a transfusion-acquired CMV infection. The incidence of transfusion-associated CMV infections among infants receiving CMV antibody positive blood was 32.4%. This data supports the concept that the use of deglycerolized red cells or CMV antibody negative blood prevents transfusion-acquired CMV infections. The use of deglycerolized red cells is preferred to screening donors for CMV antibody in an effort to prevent transfusion-acquired CMV infection.

Autologous Transfusion. Frozen red cells make autologous transfusion more practical. Receiving one's own blood is the only sure method of eliminating the possibility of antigenic exposure and acquisition of a blood-borne infectious disease, such as hepatitis or HIV.

Long-term preservation is useful for patients who have previously experienced major problems in crossmatching their blood, such as those with antibodies to high-incidence red cell antigens or those with extremely rare blood types. Storage of 5 units is generally recommended because the amount is great enough to be useful but not enough to occupy excessive freezer space. Frozen autologous blood storage is recommended for patients who are not expected to have crossmatching problems but who have an elective surgical procedure with predictable blood usage planned in the future. If a person's red cell status is normal, any amount of blood can be donated for frozen storage.

Autologous donation programs have been initiated for pregnant women, children, and adolescents but must be conducted with extreme care under a physician's supervision. The concept of autologous frozen blood has been applied to patients with sickle cell anemia. Long-term cryopreservation of sickle (HbSS) red cells opens the possibility of exploring autologous transfusion to treat sickle cell disease patients during anemic episodes that are not due to sickling. Cryopreserved hemoglobin SS-containing red cells retain their capacity to sickle and therefore are not expected to be of benefit in treating vascular complications of sickling. In vitro red cell losses due to freezing, thawing and deglycerolization are greater than in normal (HbAA) red cells; however, the remaining thawed red cells have metabolic characteristics and intravascular survival similar to those of fresh hemoglobin SS red cells. Because of the elimination to antigenic exposure and blood-borne infectious disease, deglycerolized red cells could prove useful for autologous transfusion of selected sickle cell anemia patients when they are severely anemic due to a complication not directly related to sickling.

Maintenance of 2,3 DPG and ATP levels. Freezing successfully prevents depletion of both the oxygen-carrying capabilities and energy levels of red cells, as demonstrated by the fact that 2,3 DPG and ATP levels in the red cells are not significantly lowered by freezer storage. The red cell survival in deglycerolized units stored for 48 hours was 87.8%, and at 72 hours it was 81.4%. Rejuvenated units had a survival of 82.5% at 72 hours. The average DPG at 72 hours was 7.2 μmol/g Hgb for nonrejuvenated blood and 13.7 μmol/g Hgb for rejuvenated blood. This characteristic is an advantage when considering long-term storage of rare types and surplus blood because of seasonal fluctuation in blood donations.

Elimination of Anticoagulants and Metabolites. Another benefit of frozen deglycerolized red cells is the elimination of anticoagulants and lactic acid. The potassium content of the resuspended cells is consistently low. These characteristics are helpful in the clinical care of patients with uremia, congestive heart failure, and the metabolic derangements that take place during multi-unit transfusions.

DISADVANTAGES

The high cost of a unit of deglycerolized red cells is the most frequently cited disadvantage; another is the limited 24-hour expiration time.

SPECIAL NOTES

It may be desirable to refreeze thawed units. The current AABB standard do not address refreezing thawed units because this should not be considered routinely desirable practice. However, if a high-priority blood unit is inadvertently thawed and/or deglycerolized, the physician responsible for the blood bank may sanction the refreezing of the unit. In cases of refreezing, documentation of the valuable nature of the unit and the reasons for refreezing must be recorded.

PLATELETS

Fresh Random Donor or Pooled Platelets

The introduction of blood platelets as a blood component became possible when plastic whole-blood donor collection bags with multiple satellite containers became available in the late 1960s. This technology permitted the separation, storage, and transport of platelet concentrates to be used as readily available blood bank components.

CLINICAL INDICATIONS

Patients with severe thrombocytopenia or platelet dysfunction with symptoms of bleeding are candidates for platelet concentrate transfusions to induce hemostasis or prevent intracranial bleeding and catastrophic hemorrhage in other organ systems. Severe thrombocytopenia is defined quantitatively as a platelet count less than 20×10^9/L. Conditions associated with severely decreased platelet counts include:

1. Bone marrow failure in conditions such as aplastic anemia.
2. Bone marrow suppression in patients receiving chemotherapy or radiation therapy.
3. Bone marrow replacement by malignant cells, as in acute leukemia or myeloid metaplasia.
4. Platelet consumption disorders.
5. Massive volume replacement for severe traumatic bleeding.
6. Abnormal platelet function.

Leukemia patients are frequent recipients of platelet concentrate transfusions. The Platelet Transfusion Subcommittee of the Acute Leukemia Task Force suggests platelet transfusion under the following circumstances:

1. Treatment of hemorrhage, including any overt bleeding such as epistaxis or hematuria.
2. Suspected or proven internal bleeding (intracranial, intracutaneous, or intramuscular).
3. If the risk of hemorrhage is high because the platelet counts falls below 10×10^9/L.

METHODS

Platelets survive poorly in stored refrigerated blood, therefore, whole blood is kept at room temperature (20 to 24° C) before separation. Platelets must be separated from whole blood promptly after collection in an anticoagulated primary donor unit with two satellite bags. Platelet-rich plasma (PRP) must be separated from whole blood by centrifugation within 6 hours after phlebotomy.

The unit of whole blood is first centrifuged at a low speed to separate PRP into the upper portion and red cells into the lower portion of the initial collection bag. The PRP is then expressed with a manual plasma extractor into an attached satellite bag, leaving the red cells in the original primary bag. This unit is usually separated from the satellite bags and labeled as packed red cells.

The remaining attached bags are recentrifuged at a high speed to produce an aggregated platelet button from the PRP. With a plasma extractor, approximately 200 mL of platelet-poor plasma is removed, leaving 50 mL of platelet-poor plasma with the platelet button. The 200 mL of plasma may be used as a single-donor unit of recovered plasma or fresh frozen plasma. The bag containing the platelet button and 50 mL of plasma is separated and allowed to rest undisturbed for an hour at room temperature to enhance platelet disaggregation. The platelets are then placed on a mechanical rotator to gently resuspend the platelet button. Most of the platelets from the whole blood unit are present in the platelet concentrate, which must be continuously agitated until used.

In addition to the labor-intensive process of recovering platelets from single units of anticoagulated blood, platelets may be collected by hemapheresis. Individual units of platelets from a unit of whole blood, also referred to as *random-donor platelets,* usually contain from 6 to 8×10^{10} platelets per bag. Federal regulations, however, require that only 75% of the sampled units contain a minimum of 5.5×10^{10} platelets per bag. Units of random-donor platelets are normally suspended in about 50 mL of plasma to maintain a pH of 6.0 or greater throughout the storage period. Platelets harvested from a single donor by pheresis usually contain 3 to 6×10^{11} platelets in about 200 mL of plasma per bag.

STORAGE REQUIREMENTS

Length of Time. The introduction of new types of plastic collection bags has produced extensive testing of platelet storage. Guidelines for testing platelets for transfusion indicate that platelets stored or processed with experimental techniques should be tested by a battery of laboratory procedures, observation of the hemostatic efficacy in patients, and determination of circulating survival time. These guidelines expedited approval by the FDA of second-generation platelet containers, which extended storage time from 3 to 5 days.

These new plastic bags permit increased gas exchange and can be stored for as long as 7 days. The most important concern is maintenance of the pH at greater than 6.0 to prevent loss of viability, which signals an irreversible change in the shape of platelets from a normal disc to spiny spheres. The pH at maximum platelet storage depends on many factors:

1. The anticoagulant in which the initial whole blood is collected.
2. The method of preparation.
3. The surface area and thickness of the storage container.
4. The type of plastic used.
5. The concentration of platelets and volume of plasma.
6. The adequacy of agitation.
7. The storage temperature.

It has become possible to lengthen platelet storage time from 3 to 5 days because the new blood bags are made of plastic films that optimize oxygen and carbon dioxide transfer. Increase of oxygen permeability by 25% was produced by decreasing the thickness of the plastic film or increasing the size of the bags. Second-generation storage bags designed to preserve platelets for 7 days prior to transfusion, with results comparable to those of platelets stored for 3 days in standard bags, are now available. However, if the platelets do not set enough oxygen, oxidative phosphorylation is blocked and the platelets accelerate their production of lactic acid threefold through glycolysis. Under low oxygen conditions, there is complete utilization of glucose, the pH is less than 6.0, and all the platelets assume the nonviable spiny sphere form. To keep the pH from falling below 6.0 when using the standard three day plastic bag, one must keep the maximum platelet count below 8×10^{10}. If the pH of the platelet concentrate rises above 7.3, there may be some loss of viability.

Temperature. Differences in pH, platelet count, morphology score, osmotic recovery, and release of lactic dehydrogenase (LDH) during storage have all been shown to be related to storage time, temperature, type of plastic storage bag, and type of agitation. Ideally, platelets should be stored at the lowest temperature compatible with normal survival to reduce metabolic requirements. Few studies of the viability of platelet concentrates stored at temperatures other than room temperature (20-24° C) and 4° C have been performed.

Present practice is to store platelet concentrates at room temperature with continuous gentle agitation. When platelet concentrates were stored for 3 days in conventional plastic bags, the difference in the mean life span after storage at 21° C was significantly different from that after storage at 18° C. Platelet viability is compromised after storage for 3 days at 18° C and possibly at 19.5° C, and this illustrates the need for quality control of temperature during short-term platelet storage. Reduction in viability after storage at lower temperature is correlated with a reduction in the number of normal discoid platelets. Cold-stored platelets (1 to 6° C) have been observed to provide immediate hemostasis, but after 48 hours they irreversibly lose their discoid shape and cannot reassemble their microtubules.

Because no studies have evaluated the effectiveness of platelet storage at temperatures other than room temperature in second-generation plastic bags, it would be prudent to store platelets collected in these containers at a temperature close to 22° C. This is particularly true for blood banks that store platelets in an open room where "room temperature" may be poorly controlled and exposure to temperatures below 20 or 21° C may occur.

The most desirable platelet storage temperature is 20 to 24° C, but core temperatures during shipping vary. Studies have demonstrated that single stryofoam containers with a coolant maintain the core temperature best.

Agitation. Agitation of cold-stored platelets causes clumping and rapid loss of cellular viability. The optimum method of storing platelet concentrates for transfusion is not known; therefore, they are stored in various types of plastic bags and on different types of agitators at 20 to 24° C. Although platelet storage requires some form of continuous gentle agitation, the best type of agitation is unknown. There is little in vivo data showing that a particular mode of agitation is better when used with one type of plastic bag than with another.

The storage of platelet concentrates for 5 days on a 6 rpm elliptical rotator is the least desirable method of storage; all other combinations gave acceptable and similar results. These modes of agitation were a 1 rpm elliptical rotator and 2 or 6 rpm circular rotators.

ADVANTAGES

A platelet concentrate prepared from a single unit of whole blood can elevate a patient's platelet count by 5 to 12×10^9 per L in 1 to 2 hours after infusion. The total dose of platelets required for a patient depends not only on the degree of thrombocytopenia but also on the patient's size and factors such as the presence of fever, sepsis, splenomegaly, and platelet antibodies.

A guideline for the effectiveness of the transfusion of platelets is to calculate a *corrected count increment* 1 to 2 hours after infusion. The following formula is used:

$$\text{Corrected count increment} = \frac{\left(\begin{array}{c} \text{Post-} \\ \text{transfusion} \\ \text{platelet count} \end{array} - \begin{array}{c} \text{Pretransfusion} \\ \text{platelet count} \end{array} \right) \times \begin{array}{c} \text{Body Surface} \\ \text{Area} \end{array}}{\text{Approximate total number of platelets infused}}$$

Another system for calculating transfusion effectiveness is the *percent recovery*. This formula, which takes splenic pooling into account by using the factor of $2/3$, is:

Percent recovery =

$$\frac{\text{Post-} \atop \text{transfusion} \atop \text{platelet count} - \text{Pretransfusion} \atop \text{platelet count} \times \text{Blood Volume}}{\text{Approximate total number of platelets infused} \times \frac{2}{3}}$$

The expected recovery of platelets is 60% at 1 hour and 40% at 24 hours. If a patient fails to demonstrate the expected platelet response, a refractory state should be suspected.

DISADVANTAGES

Various adverse reactions can result from the transfusion of platelet concentrates, including:

1. Bacterial contamination.
2. Transmission of viral blood-borne diseases such as hepatitis or AIDS.
3. Transmission of parasitic diseases, such as malaria, due to red blood cell contamination.
4. Pulmonary edema caused by plasma volume if more than 10 units are administered to a patient with poor cardiac status.
5. Febrile or allergic reactions caused by plasma proteins.
6. Anaphylaxis in IgA-deficient recipients.
7. Febrile reactions caused by leukocyte contamination.
8. Graft-versus-host disease in immunocompromised recipients if many viable lymphocytes are present in the concentrate.

SPECIAL NOTES

Platelet transfusions from donors mismatched for cross-reactive HLA antigens provide hemostasis and platelet survival equivalent to HLA-matched platelets in patients without platelet-specific antibodies. If HLA-matched platelets are unavailable from a family member, most hemapheresis programs choose donors for immunized patients with alloantibodies based on the recipient's HLA typing. However, even with fully HLA-matched platelets, 6 to 39% of platelet transfusions are unsuccessful. Patients negative for HLA-A2 antigens, however, have a better response

to single-donor platelets with major mismatches than those who possess the HLA-A2 antigen.

In addition to HLA typing, many programs include a screening test for lymphocytotoxicity (HLA) antibody to determine the degree of sensitization to the general population. Donor selection does not usually include a crossmatch, which uses patient serum against donor lymphocytes because the crossmatch procedure is believed to be a poor predictor of platelet survival giving high false positive and high false negative results (accuracy ranges from 30 to 75%).

Frozen Platelets

CLINICAL INDICATIONS

Patients with severe thrombocytopenia and bleeding or who are at a high risk of hemorrhage are candidates for platelet transfusions. Frozen units of platelets may be useful as autologous units or when fresh units are unavailable.

METHODS

Platelets have been frozen using the cryoprotective agent, DMSO, and stored in the vapor phase of liquid nitrogen ($-120°$ C) for as long as 3 years before inducing effective hemostasis. However, the freeze-thaw process causes a loss of 30 to 40% of the platelets, and about 50% of the platelets infused are in the nonviable form. Additionally, frozen platelets showed considerable structural damage, with 33% balloon forms counted after thawing as compared to less than 1% before freezing.

ADVANTAGES

Frozen autologous platelet concentrates have been used to support leukemic patients during thrombocytopenic periods, and in patients undergoing intensive chemotherapy for solid tumors. The use of frozen autologous platelets reduces alloimmunization and transfusion-related infections and provides platelets when needed. Frozen allogeneic platelets are also potentially useful. Freezing platelets from HLA-matched donors for alloimmunized patients would minimize the inconvenience to the donors, and frozen platelets from healthy donors could be used during emergencies.

DISADVANTAGES

Fresh platelets provide significantly better 1- and 24-hour corrected increments than frozen autologous platelets. To achieve the same effect as 1 unit of fresh, single-donor platelet pheresis product, 2 frozen units are necessary.

SPECIAL NOTES

Except in the case of alloimmunization, frozen autologous platelets are inferior to single-donor fresh platelets, and are significantly damaged in the freezing process.

GRANULOCYTES

Clinical Indications

Leukocyte concentrates, primarily neutrophils, may be of value to patients with severe neutropenia who have a life-threatening systemic infection uncontrolled by antibiotics. Patients who would most frequently be considered appropriate candidates are those with neutropenia induced by chemotherapy or radiation therapy.

Methods

Granulocyte concentrates are prepared by leukapheresis. Preparation of granulocyte concentrates from single units of whole blood does not produce a sufficient quantity to be of therapeutic value.

Storage Requirements

The present AABB standards specify that granulocytes be stored at 20 to 24° C without agitation for up to 24 hours. Although granulocytes may be stored for up to 24 hours, it is best to transfuse them as soon as possible after collection.

FACTORS RELATED TO THE STORAGE OF LEUKOCYTES

Recent studies have shown that after 8 hours of storage, granulocytes have a reduced ability to circulate, and migrate to a site of inflammation. When neutrophilic granulocytes (PMNs) are stored for 24 hours, several changes take place:

1. Decreased receptor affinity for chemotactic substances, associated with excessive hydrogen ion accumulation, particularly in units with a high concentration of leukocytes.
2. Decreased adherence properties.
3. Defective energy metabolism and glycogenolysis.

Storage of neutrophils produces a reduction in intracellular ATP levels, especially if the units are stored at 6° C. Because glycogen is the chief metabolic fuel source for phagocytosis and a facultative source for chemotaxis, alterations in the content or metabolism of glycogen in stored PMNs might cause impaired ATP maintenance and functional defects observed in the cells. Neutrophils (PMNs) stored at high concentration are particularly susceptible to depletion of ATP. Maintaining the intracellular ATP levels in stored leukocytes by adding bicarbonate buffer prevents reduction of ATP and aids maintenance of chemotactic function. Chemotactic impairment, observed in neutrophils stored for 24 hours in high concentrations, may be partially due to proteolytic autolysis.

PMNs stored for 48 hours, regardless of concentration, have defective degranulation of both primary and secondary granule contents. These cells have a defective capacity to degranulate in response to inflammatory stimuli.

Advantages

In patients at high risk of death due to an overwhelming bacterial infection that is uncontrollable through drug therapy, leukocyte transfusions may be of value.

Disadvantages

The major impediment to storage of granulocyte concentrates for transfusion is rapid impairment in the ability of the neutrophilic granulocytes to migrate toward inflammatory stimuli, both in vitro and in vivo. Although storage at room temperature is preferable to 6° C storage for the maintenance of chemotactic function, and maintaining pH may optimize chemotactic function, efforts to maintain chemotaxis of PMNs after storage have been largely unsuccessful. The major reason for impaired chemotaxis of stored granulocytes is still unknown and requires further investigation.

Special Notes

Although lymphocytes freeze well when glycerolized, granulocytes are extremely sensitive to the freezing/thawing process. This property of granulocytes restricts the freezing of these cells with present technologies. Only a few centers still advocate the therapeutic use of granulocyte concentrates obtained from patients with CML. All white cell units derived from CML donors should be irradiated to prevent GVHD. However, if the goal is transient myeloid engraftment, CML leukocytes that are *not* irradiated should be used.

IRRADIATED BLOOD AND BLOOD COMPONENTS

Since animal experiments in the mid-1950s, it has been known that the infusion of immunocompetent lymphocytes into animals with impaired immunity can lead to engraftment of donor cells, with an intense and frequently fatal immunologic reaction of engrafted cells against the host, or graft-versus-host disease. A similar graft-versus-host reaction was subsequently described in susceptible human recipients.

Graft-versus-host reactions are caused by the proliferation of mature donor-derived T lymphocytes in response to major and minor histocompatibility antigens in the host. The time needed for the disease to develop and the clinical manifestations of acute post-transfusion graft-versus-host disease are nearly identical to those of severe acute post-transplantation graft-versus-host disease, and their etiology has been assumed to be the same.

Graft-versus-host disease can occur after the transfusion of blood or various blood products, including:

1. Fresh and stored whole blood.
2. Packed red cells stored for as long as 12 days.
3. Buffy coat—poor or washed red cells.
4. Platelet concentrates.
5. Granulocyte concentrates.
6. Single units of fresh plasma.

Although graft-versus-host disease has not been reported after transfusion of frozen/deglycerolized red cells, a small number of viable lymphocytes may remain after deglycerolization and washing. Although processing frozen blood removes up to 95% of leukocytes, the remaining mononuclear cells can undergo normal blast transformation and mitotic activity in vitro.

The occurrence of graft-versus-host disease after transfusion of noncellular frozen blood products such as fresh frozen plasma (FFP) or cryoprecipitate has not been documented. Because no cryoprotective agent is used with these components, the final product is not expected to contain viable leukocytes; therefore, a graft-versus-host response is not expected in susceptible hosts.

The risk of graft-versus-host disease can be minimized, if not eliminated, by irradiating whole and various other components immediately before infusion. Studies are currently being conducted to evaluate the efficacy of irradiating blood and components before storage. Prophylactic irradiation of whole blood products and components before transfusion is presently the most efficient way to prevent post-transfusion graft-versus-host disease. In patients with post-transfusion graft-versus-host disease, approximately 90% die of acute complications of the disease, usually infection.

Clinical Indications

The infusion of lymphocyte-containing whole blood or blood components presents the risk of inducing graft-versus-host disease from the infused lymphocytes to patients who are immunosuppressed or have severe immunodeficiency disorders. Irradiation of these components can reduce this risk.

HIGH-RISK PATIENTS

Patients at the highest risk, with an absolute need for irradiated blood products, include:

1. Recipients of autologous or allogeneic bone marrow grafts. Recipients of autologous bone marrow may be expected to have the same risk of post-transfusion graft-versus-host disease as patients receiving allogeneic bone marrow.
2. Children with severe congenital immunodeficiency syndromes involving T lymphocytes. The degree of immunodeficiency in the host, rather than the number of transfused immunocompetent cells, determines whether graft-versus-host disease will occur.

INTERMEDIATE-RISK PATIENTS

Patients considered to be at less risk of developing graft-versus-host disease include:

1. Infants receiving intrauterine transfusions followed by exchange transfusions and possibly infants receiving only exchange transfusions. The immune mechanism of the fetus and newborn infant may not be sufficiently mature to reject foreign lymphocytes, and previous transfusions may induce a state of immune tolerance in the newborn. Transfused lymphocytes may continue to circulate for a prolonged time in some immunologically tolerant hosts without the development of graft-versus-host disease. There is insufficient evidence to rec-

ommend irradiation of transfused blood in all premature infants.
2. Patients receiving total body radiation or immunosuppressive therapy for disorders such as lymphoma and acute leukemia. Although routine irradiation of blood products given to these patients can be justified, it cannot be regarded as absolutely indicated because the risk of developing graft-versus-host disease is so small. However, blood product irradiation is advised for selected patients with hematologic malignancies, especially when transfusions are given at or near the time of sustained and severe therapy-induced immunosuppression.

LOWEST-RISK PATIENTS

Patients who are also at risk but are considered to be the least susceptible are:

1. Patients with solid tumors. The incidence of the development of graft-versus-host disease is difficult to determine. However, in nonhematologic malignancies such as neuroblastoma, the disease has developed. In one case, it developed after the infusion of a single unit of packed red cells.
2. Patients with aplastic anemia receiving anti-thymocyte globulin may theoretically be at increased risk of post-transfusion graft-versus-host disease during therapy-induced periods of lymphocytopenia.
3. AIDS patients. Although a theoretic risk of post-transfusion graft-versus-host disease may exist in patients with AIDS, the disease has not actually been observed in this disorder, and routine use of irradiated blood is not recommended.

Methods

A self-contained commercially available cesium[137] source is the most commonly used method of irradiating blood components. Quality control of irradiation equipment is essential to monitor the decay of the cesium source, which influences the length of time a unit is exposed to radiation. Once a unit has been exposed to a certain radiation dose and then removed from the source, it is not radioactive. Irradiated blood does not pose a threat of potential radiation exposure to staff members manipulating it or to patients to whom it is administered. If an irradiated unit is no longer needed for the intended recipient, it may be transfused safely to another patient who does not necessarily require such a special component.

No cases of post-transfusion graft-versus-host disease have been reported following administration of blood products irradiated with at least 1500 rad. A range from 1500 to 3000 rad is recommended as an effective and appropriate radiation dose. No obvious changes in clinical efficacy of products were reported from institutions that used as much as 5000 rad.

An alternate solution to providing quantities of irradiated blood is irradiating the units before storage. This requires packing red blood cells drawn into CPDA-1 to a hematocrit of $75 \pm 1\%$ and irradiating at 4000 rads on the day of donation. Analysis was conducted every 7 days. Irradiation caused a slight decrease in red cell ATP and 2,3 DPG and a slight increase in plasma hemoglobin compared to the controls. Methemoglobin, pH, and glucose consumption were identical to those of the nonirradiated controls. The evidence indicates that irradiation did not cause biochemical or metabolic changes in the red cells or differences between irradiated and nonirradiated stored red cells in function or viability.

Storage Requirements

Whole blood or blood components should be stored in the manner required for each specific component, whether or not the product is irradiated.

Effects of Radiation on Specific Cellular Components

LYMPHOCYTES

Ionizing radiation is known to inhibit lymphocyte mitotic activity and blast trans-

formation. Irradiation of normal donor lymphocytes with 1500 rad from a cesium[137] source causes a 90% reduction in mitogen-stimulated ^{14}C-thymidine incorporation. An 85% reduction in mitogen-induced blast transformation after exposure to 1500 rad and a 97 to 98.5% reduction in mitogenic response were noted after exposure to 5000 rads.

GRANULOCYTES

Ionizing radiation may impair granulocyte function, and this impairment is dose-dependent. The degree of actual damage to granulocytes is controversial. Chemotactic activity decreased linearly with increasing doses of irradiation, from 500 to 120,000 rads, but the reduction only reached statistical significance at 10,000 rad. A linear dose-response curve demonstrates that granulocyte locomotion is affected by very small doses of irradiation. A dose of 2000 rads is likely to eliminate lymphocytic mitotic activity and prevent graft-versus-host disease without causing significant damage to granulocytes or altering their chemotactic or bactericidal ability. Irradiation prior to transfusion has been demonstrated to contribute to defective oxidative metabolism, but this effect is highly variable.

MATURE RED BLOOD CELLS

Mature red cells appear to be highly resistant to radiation damage. After exposure to 10,000 rad, ^{52}Cr-labeled in vivo red cell survival was the same as that of untreated controls. In 1981, Button showed that stored red cells could be treated with up to 20,000 rads without changing their viability or in vitro properties, including ATP and 2,3 DPG levels, plasma hemoglobin, and potassium ions.

PLATELETS

Ionizing radiation may impair platelet function. Although this impairment is dose-dependent, the effect of irradiation on platelets has been difficult to characterize. Several studies have demonstrated unchanged in vivo platelet survival after exposure to 5000 to 75,000 rad. A 33% decrease in the expected platelet count increase was noted after transfusion of platelets exposed to 5000 rad, and similarly irradiated autologous platelets had a diminished ability to correct the bleeding times in a small number of volunteers who had consumed aspirin. In one study, platelet aggregation was not affected by exposure to 5000 rad, but an impaired response to collagen was noted.

Advantages

Blood product irradiation is believed to be the most efficient and probably the most economical method available to prevent post-transfusion graft-versus-host disease.

In addition, irradiation prior to storage may be of value in mass casualty situations in which a large number of patients may be suddenly immunosuppressed from inadvertent exposure to toxic chemical or nuclear radiation. In a disaster situation of this type, irradiation of blood immediately before transfusion may be impractical due to the lack of equipment or shortage of time.

Disadvantages

The cost of the equipment and additional labor requirements may be perceived as a disadvantage in a cost-benefit assessment.

PLASMA

Plasma is the noncellular, straw-colored fluid portion of anticoagulated whole blood that can be observed after whole blood is allowed to settle or is centrifuged. Chemically, plasma is comprised of water, electrolyte ions such as sodium (Na^+) and (K^+) potassium ions, and proteins. The soluble plasma proteins are primarily albumin, globulin, and coagulation factors.

At the present time, human donor plasma is the raw material for the production of more than 100 diagnostic and therapeutic products. The requirements for plasma cannot be met with the plasma byproducts of whole-blood collection; therefore, plasmapheresis techniques can be used to collect large quantities of donor plasma. Plasma can be separated from units of whole blood and stored as single-donor plasma or fresh-frozen plasma.

Plasma separated from outdated whole blood is somewhat different in chemical composition from plasma extracted from whole blood shortly after blood donation. The major change in plasma that has been in contact with red blood cells for an extended period of time is that it has higher levels of potassium ions and ammonia. Either form of plasma can be used for temporary volume replacement in patients who are depleted of whole blood or protein. Plasma may also be appropriate for coagulation factor replacement. However, when plasma which was immediately separated from whole blood originally collected in acid citrate dextrose (ACD) or citrate phosphate dextrose adenine (CPD) was stored at 6° C for 35 days, it was observed that activation of the coagulation, fibrinolytic, and kallikrein systems and decrease in coagulation inhibitors occurred. These conditions of storage had no significant effect on the levels of the main thrombin inhibitor, antithrombin III.

Components can be prepared from human plasma, such as cryoprecipitate or antihemophilic factor (AHF). Fractionation of human plasma can be into albumin or immune globulins. As the result of biotechnology, recombinant DNA-produced blood components such as albumin and factor VIII are anticipated in the near future.

Single-Donor Plasma

CLINICAL INDICATIONS

Patients with severe burns or hypovolemic shock are appropriate candidates for this blood component. Depending on the type of coagulation deficiency as well as the method of storage, patients with coagulation defects may also be suitable transfusion candidates.

METHODS

Single-donor plasma may be separated from a unit of whole blood using a plasma extractor. The original unit of whole blood should have been collected into an integral satellite bag system which allows for un-contaminated separation into the satellite bag. The separation must occur before the fifth day after the expiration date of the unit of whole blood.

STORAGE REQUIREMENTS

If the unit is *not* frozen, single-donor plasma must be stored at 1 to 6° C and may be kept for *no more* than 26 days from the date of whole blood collection if the anticoagulant CPD was used, or 40 days if CPDA-1 anticoagulant was used. When stored frozen at −18° C or lower, single-donor plasma has a shelf-life of up to 5 years.

ADVANTAGES

Specifically using plasma when colloid volume expansion or most coagulation factors are needed rather than whole blood reduces the risk of sensitization to cellular antigens and is cost-effective.

DISADVANTAGES

Single-donor plasma has the same risks of infectious disease due to blood-borne agents as a unit of whole blood. Transfusion reactions caused by plasma proteins and, to a lesser degree, cellular components are a possibility.

SPECIAL NOTES

Plasma from which cryoprecipitate has been removed must be so designated.

Fresh-Frozen Plasma

According to the National Institutes of Health (NIH), fresh-frozen plasma is defined as the fluid portion of 1 unit of human blood that has been centrifuged, separated, and frozen at 18° C or colder within 6 hours of collection. Fresh-frozen plasma contains:

1. Labile and stable components of the coagulation, fibrinolytic, and complement systems.

2. Proteins that maintain osmotic pressure and immunity.
3. Other proteins which have diverse activities.
4. Fats, carbohydrates, and minerals in concentrations similar to those in the circulation.

The use of fresh-frozen plasma has increased tenfold within the past 10 years and has reached almost 2 million units annually. Much of this increase over the last decade is related to decreases in whole blood availability rather than to use for labile coagulation factor replacement. Recent estimates are that fresh-frozen plasma is definitely or possibly indicated in 54% to 58% of patients. Educational efforts addressing the appropriate use of fresh-frozen plasma should be initiated.

CLINICAL INDICATIONS

Few specific indications for the use of fresh-frozen plasma exist. Indications are generally limited to the treatment of deficiencies of coagulation proteins for which specific factor concentrates are unavailable or undesirable. Appropriate use of fresh-frozen plasma belongs in the following categories according to the NIH:

1. Massive transfusion. Hemorrhage in patients receiving massive transfusions is caused more frequently by thrombocytopenia than by depletion of coagulation factors. Use of fresh-frozen plasma should be confined to patients in whom factor deficiencies are presumed to be the sole or primary problem. There is no evidence that the prophylactic administration of fresh-frozen plasma decreases transfusion requirements in patients receiving multiple transfusions who do not have documented coagulation defects.
2. Single or multiple coagulation protein deficiencies, either prophylactically or in the treatment of bleeding. Fresh-frozen plasma can be used to replace factor deficiencies of factors II, V, VII, IX, X, and XI if unacceptable or inappropriate specific component therapy is neither available nor appropriate.

3. Warfarin reversal. Patients who have been given the anticoagulant warfarin sodium are deficient in the functional vitamin K-dependent coagulation factors II, VII, IX and X, as well as proteins C and S. These functional deficiencies can be reversed by the administration of vitamin K. When such patients are actively bleeding or require emergency surgery, fresh-frozen plasma or single-donor plasma can be used to achieve immediate hemostasis.

4. Use in antithrombin III deficiency. Fresh-frozen plasma can be used as a source of antithrombin III in patients who are deficient in this inhibitor and are undergoing surgery, or who require heparin for treatment of thrombosis.

5. In conjunction with therapeutic plasma exchange for the treatment of thrombotic thrombocytopenic purpura.

6. Treatment of immunodeficiencies. Fresh-frozen plasma can serve as a source of immunoglobulin for children and adults with immunoglobulin deficiencies as an alternate to intravenous purified immune globulin. Fresh-frozen plasma is indicated in infants with secondary immunodeficiencies associated with severe protein loss caused by enteropathy and in patients in whom total parenteral nutrition is ineffective.

METHODS

After the collection of anticoagulated whole blood, fresh-frozen plasma can be prepared from a single heavy spin or from a double centrifugation to prepare a platelet concentrate at the same time. Each unit contains about 225 mL of plasma. The plasma should be frozen in a protective container within 6 hours after collection by placing it in a dry ice alcohol bath or in a freezer at $-30°$ C or below. The bag should be frozen in a horizontal position and stored in a vertical position so that inadvertent thawing will be noticed on visual inspection.

STORAGE REQUIREMENTS

Fresh-frozen plasma must be stored at $-18°$ C or below within 6 hours of collec-

tion. To maintain adequate levels of factors V and VIII, plasma must be stored frozen. The optimal storage is at $-30°$ C or colder with a dating period of 12 months after donation of the original unit of whole blood. If fresh-frozen plasma has not been used after 1 year of storage at $-18°$ C or colder, it may be relabeled and redesignated single-donor plasma. Thus redesignated, the plasma has 4 more years of shelf-life at $-18°$ C or colder.

When requested, the unit of fresh-frozen plasma must be thawed inside a clean plastic bag with agitation in a waterbath at temperatures between 30 and 37° C. It is important to prevent water contamination. If the intended use of the plasma is for the correction of labile coagulation factor deficiencies, it must be stored at 1 to 6° C after thawing. The FDA requires infusion within 6 hours after thawing if the plasma is intended for correcting coagulation deficiencies. A unit of fresh-frozen plasma thawed at 30 to 37° C and not transfused after storage at 1 to 6° C for 24 hours may be relabeled and redesignated single donor plasma. Records must include these changes.

Microwave thawing of fresh-frozen plasma is still considered an experimental technique. One of the major concerns of using this method of thawing is the leaching of plasticizer from the storage bag. Microwave-thawed plasma contains precipitated denatured protein (mainly albumin and fibrinogen), and a significant reduction of coagulation factors IX, X, XI and fibrinogen has been demonstrated with microwave-thawed plasma as compared to fresh plasma. A recent modification of the microwave-thawing method is the specially designed rotating temperature-controlled oven. With this equipment, no statistically significant differences in measured proteins compared with 37° C waterbath thawing were noted.

ADVANTAGES

The major advantage of fresh-frozen plasma is that, if appropriately used, it provides effective use of whole blood through component therapy. Through the use of plasma alone, the risk of alloimmunization to erythrocyte, leukocyte, and platelet antigens is reduced compared to the risk with use of whole blood.

The combined use of fresh-frozen plasma and packed red cells as a substitute for whole blood can have significant adverse effects in terms of the cost and safety of blood transfusion. The risks of fresh-frozen plasma include the same risks as whole blood: disease transmission, allergic and anaphylactoid reactions, and excessive intravascular volume. The incidence of non-icteric and icteric hepatitis following multiple transfusions of fresh-frozen plasma probably ranges between 3 and 10%. Although the risk is less than with whole blood or packed red cells, the potential for alloimmunization is present, as has been demonstrated by the infrequent formation of Rh antibodies.

Inappropriate use of fresh-frozen plasma could be avoided by the increased use of whole blood or safer, cheaper volume expanders. No justification exists for the use of fresh frozen plasma as a volume expander or as a nutritional source (NIH).

SPECIAL NOTES

Alternative therapies have been suggested (NIH):

1. Cryoprecipitate should be used when fibrinogen or von Willebrand factor is needed.
2. For treatment of hemophilia A, cryoprecipitate or factor VIII concentrates are available.
3. For the treatment of severe hemophilia B, factor IX complex is preferable. Both of these concentrates are prepared from pooled plasma, and the risk of virus transmission is high in untreated products. Factor IX concentrate carries the additional hazard of thrombogenicity.
4. Crystalloid, colloid solutions containing albumin or plasma protein fraction, hydroxyethyl starch, and dextran are preferred for volume replacement.
5. For nutritional support, amino acid solutions and dextrose are acceptable alternatives.

PLASMA COMPONENTS

Cryoprecipitated Antihemophilic Factor

Cryoprecipitated antihemophilic factor (AHF) is the cold insoluble precipitate of plasma remaining after fresh-frozen plasma obtained from whole blood or apheresis has been thawed between 1 and 6° C. Each bag of cryoprecipitated AHF contains an average of 80 or more factor VIII (FVIII:C) units, between 150 and 250 mg of fibrinogen, and fibronectin in less than 15 mL of plasma. Cryoprecipitate is the only concentrated fibrinogen product available. Fibrinogen preparations that were previously available are no longer prepared because of the high risk of infectious disease transmission.

CLINICAL INDICATIONS

Because cryoprecipitated AHF is a source of coagulation factor VIII, von Willebrand's factor (AHF-VWF), factor XIII, fibrinogen, and fibronectin, it is useful in the control of bleeding in a variety of clinical disorders. These conditions include factor VIII deficiency, von Willebrand's disease, factor XIII deficiency, and hypofibrinogenemia.

The National Hemophilia Foundation recommends that hemophiliacs, particularly children, receive cryoprecipitate. However, in mild or moderate cases, an attempt should be made to use desmopressin, an analog of the naturally occurring antidiuretic hormone, vasopressin, which has been shown to raise factor VIII levels in normal subjects and patients with mild to moderate hemophilia A and von Willebrand's disease.

For the treatment of bleeding in factor VIII-deficient patients, rapid infusion of cryoprecipitate (about 10 mL of diluted component per minute) of a loading dose is generally expected to produce the initial desired level of factor VIII:C with smaller maintenance doses every 8 to 12 hours. Patients should be monitored periodically by means of factor VIII plasma assays. A regimen of therapy for 10 or more days may be required to maintain hemostasis in afflicted patients after surgery.

The level of factor VIII needed for therapy or prophylaxis is not exactly predictable and varies with each clinical situation. A rule-of-thumb calculation of the number of bags of cryoprecipitate needed by factor VIII-deficient patients has been formulated. If a patient has antibodies to factor VIII, larger doses or more frequent doses may be needed to achieve hemostasis. The degree of factor VIII saturation of the extravascular space, which is equivalent to approximately 1.5 times the size of the intravascular space, can affect a patient's response to therapy. A lower dose response than expected can reflect the degree of extravascular space saturation.

Patients with von Willebrand's disease require smaller amounts of cryoprecipitate. Laboratory assays are helpful in monitoring patients with von Willebrand's disease as well as those suffering from hypofibrinogenemia.

Determination of Cryoprecipitate Quantity (Dosage) in Factor VIII Deficient Patients

Number of bags of cryoprecipitate required =

$$\frac{\text{Desired level of Factor VIII:C (\%)} \times \text{Patient's Plasma Volume (mL)}^*}{80^{**}}$$

* In lieu of an exact measure of plasma volume, 4% of the patient's body weight (Kg) $\times$ 1000 may be substitued.

** 80 represents the average number of units of factor VIII:C in a single unpooled bag of cryoprecipitate. If several bags of cryoprecipitate are pooled into one unit, the number of origional bags should be multiplied by 80 to obtain the number in the denominator.

EXAMPLE:
If the desired level of factor VIII:C activity is 70% and the patient's plasma volume is 2500 mL, the number of single bags of cryoprecipitate needed would be 22.

Number of bags required
$$= \frac{0.70 \times 2500 \text{ mL}}{80} = 22 \text{ bags}$$

METHODS

Plasma should be separated from erythrocytes within four hours of collection by heavy centrifugation. The plasma should be frozen within 2 hours of separation (or 6 hours of collection) in a freezer at 30° C or less. Frozen plasma should then be thawed at 1 to 6° C. The AHF-poor plasma is then separated from the cryoprecipitate after centrifugation, leaving about 15 mL of plasma with the cryoprecipitate. The precipitate should be frozen within 4 hours and stored at −18° C or below.

Units of cryoprecipitate can be pooled into groups of two to six units prior to freezing. They should be pooled promptly after preparation, using aseptic technique, and then refrozen immediately to prevent possible bacterial growth and loss of labile coagulation factors. These units must be labeled as pooled units.

STORAGE REQUIREMENTS

The shelf-life of cryoprecipitate when stored at −18° C or below is 12 months. On request, cryoprecipitate is thawed in a 30 to 37° C waterbath for up to 15 minutes. The cryoprecipitate should be resuspended in the residual 10 to 15 mL of plasma in the bag of wet cryoprecipitate or by adding 10 to 15 mL of sterile diluent (0.9% sodium chloride injection, USP, is preferred) and gently resuspending.

If several bags of cryoprecipitate are pooled, the precipitate in each concentrate should be mixed with 10 to 15 mL of sterile diluent (0.9% sodium chloride injection, USP) to ensure complete removal of all precipitate from the container. Cryoprecipitate that has been pooled prior to freezing usually requires no extra diluent.

Thawed units should be kept at room temperature and used as soon as possible. Storage in the refrigerator may cause reprecipitation of concentrated factor VIII. Cryoprecipitate must be administered within 6 hours of thawing and 4 hours of pooling. Thawed units may not be refrozen.

ADVANTAGES

Because of the small volume, cryoprecipitate is preferable to fresh-frozen plasma in the correction of bleeding conditions in certain disorders, for example, factor VIII deficiency. This component, however, should not be used unless a specific hemostatic defect for which this product is useful has been identified. Compatibility testing is not necessary. Although an ABO-compatibile product is preferred, it is not essential, nor is Rh status a consideration.

DISADVANTAGES

If cryoprecipitate is used for bleeding disorders other than those previously identified, it will be ineffective. Other disadvantages can include:

1. Febrile or allergic reactions
2. Bacterial contamination
3. Air embolism during administration
4. Hyperfibrinogenemia in massively transfused patients
5. Development of a positive direct antiglobulin test
6. Transmission of blood-borne diseases

SPECIAL NOTES

The transmission of blood-borne viruses in coagulation factor concentrates and other plasma products remains a serious health concern. Factor VIII and factor IX concentrates that have not been treated have been implicated in the transmission of a number of viral diseases, most notably hepatitis B, non-A, non-B hepatitis, and AIDS.

Approaches to virus inactivation in plasma products include:

1. Heating in the liquid state in the presence of low molecular weight stabilizers
2. Heating in the lyophilized state
3. Ultraviolet (UV) irradiation such as cobalt 60 exposure

The major problem with heat inactivation in achieving a balance between optimum viral destruction and retention of biologic activity of the heat-labile coagulation factors. To inactivate viruses with heat without a substantial loss of protein biologic activity in the liquid state requires the inclusion of high concentrations of stabilizers such as amino acids, sugars, and salts, or mixtures such as 2.75 M glycine and 50% sucrose. However, the inclusion of additives decreases the rate of virus inactivation at 60° C. An alternate approach is to remove excess water through lyophilization before heating. Heating at 60° C for 10 hours inactivates 104 infectious units of HBV virus, but increasing the temperature from 60 to 70 or 80° C causes a 90% or greater loss in AHF activity. An even greater decline in the rate of virus inactivation has been observed on heating AHF in the lypholized state at temperatures greater than 60° C, although no loss in AHF activity has been observed after 72 hours of heating at 60° C. Several proteins present in lyophilized AHF concentrates display an altered electrophoretic mobility as a result of exposure to 60° C for 24 hours.

Newer techniques to increase the yield and/or purity of AHF in concentrates include polyethylene glycol precipitation, solid- and liquid-phase chromatography with heparin, and polyelectrolytes. Direct adsorption of factor VIII:C from plasma by polyelectrolytes results in an overall yield of about 50% and a purity of approximately 1000-fold.

Monoclonal Absorption of Cryoprecipitate. The newest method of processing and purifying AHF concentrates is by monoclonal absorption. The purification of plasma proteins is achieved by using immunoaffinity chromatography.

With cryoprecipitate as the starting material, two methods of production are presently being used. These methods have some common characteristics, but differ in the specificity of the monoclonal antibody used for the purification of factor VIII:C and the method of viral inactivation. One product uses a monoclonal antibody directed toward the vWF portion of the factor VIII:C/vWF complex; the other product uses a monoclonal antibody specifically directed toward the factor VIII:C portion of the factor VIII:C/vWF complex. The other major processing difference is the method of virus inactivation. One method uses heat treatment of the product in a freeze-dried state at 60° C for 30 hours; the other uses a solvent/detergent treatment which is a chemical viral inactivation procedure.

Initial clinical trials have demonstrated no immediate adverse effects or symptoms of blood-borne diseases to date.

Factor IX Complex

Factor IX complex, Konyne[R], is a commercially prepared, heat-treated plasma product that contains coagulation factors II, IX, and X and low levels of factor VII. This product is approximately 50 times purified over whole plasma, and when reconstituted as directed, contains 25 times as much factor IX as an equal volume of fresh plasma.

CLINICAL INDICATIONS

The main indication for using factor IX complex is in the treatment of conditions caused by factor IX (hemophilia B or Christmas disease) deficiency. The use of factor IX complex for patients with factors II or X or mild cases of hemophilia B should be used if treatment with fresh-frozen plasma is not feasible or has proven ineffective. Other clinical indications include reversal of coumarin antigoagulant-induced hemorrhage as a secondary approach, if the risk of transmitting hepatitis is considered justifiable, and in the treatment of bleeding episodes in patients with hemophilia A (factor VIII deficiency) who have inhibitors to factor VIII.

METHODS

Reconstitute with Sterile Water for Injection, USP, and administer within 3 hours after reconstitution. Do not refrigerate after reconstitution. Administer by the intravenous route.

STORAGE REQUIREMENTS

Must be stored under refrigeration (2 to 8° C). Freezing should be avoided because breakage of the diluent bottle might occur. The product may be stored for a period of up to 1 month at a temperature not exceeding 25° C during travel.

ADVANTAGES

Factor IX complex is a rapid method of achieving and maintaining hemostasis in appropriate patients.

DISADVANTAGES

Factor IX complex is prepared from paid donors, in whom the risk of blood-borne disease is high. Heat treatment may not completely eliminate the risk of exposure to infectious agents. Cases of postoperative thrombosis have also been reported after the administration of this product.

SPECIAL NOTES

U.S. federal law prohibits dispensing factor IX complex without a prescription. In the treatment of specific coagulation disorders, deficiencies of factors II or X, and even cases of mild hemophilia B, the use of fresh-frozen plasma should be initially considered.

BLOOD SUBSTITUTES AND ALTERNATE SOURCES OF BLOOD COMPONENTS

Although saline solutions were used as early as 1833 for the treatment of cholera, the use of cystalloid solutions as substitutes for blood began around 1875. These solutions were developed because of the increasing incidence of complications associated with blood transfusion. The discovery of the ABO blood group system and the many scientific discoveries that followed led to the present era of blood transfusion.

While the use of human whole blood and blood components has many benefits, problems are also associated with it including the following:

1. An increasing demand for blood and blood products and a concomitant shortage of donors
2. The risk of transmitting blood-borne diseases
3. Cultural and religious objections to blood transfusion
4. Difficulty with collecting, storing, and transporting blood or blood components in underdeveloped countries or at disaster sites or in military situations
5. The time and cost factors associated with crossmatching

The traditional blood supply system is expected to continue to function for many years, but in the future the increasing demand may not be met. As an alternative to human-derived blood and blood components, substitutes and alternate sources are being developed. Substitutes must be nontoxic, nonpyrogenic, nonallergic, sterile, and easy to store at normal temperatures. These alternate blood replacement fluids must be equivalent to human blood in viscosity and osmotic pressure, and retained in the vascular system for a sufficient time to exert the required therapeutic effect. In addition, these substances must be eliminated by normal metabolism or excretion and must not affect normal hemostasis. They must also be relatively cheap to produce and easily administered. In the case of red cell substitutes, an additional requirement is that the substitute be able to give up oxygen to the tissues within the normal physiologic range of partial pressures.

Blood substitutes, whether they result from synthesis by organic chemistry procedures or from biologic processes through genetic engineering, are likely to make broad contributions to transfusion medicine. The future of hemoglobin-based blood substitutes may include obtaining the hemoglobin not from erythrocytes but by recombinant DNA technology. Recombinant DNA is already a reality in the production of some plasma protein products.

Red Cell Substitutes

Several types of synthetic red blood cell surrogates exist. These include the following:

1. Emulsions of perfluorocarbons
2. Stroma-free hemoglobin
3. Polymerized hemoglobin
4. Liposome-encapsulated hemoglobin

Perfluorocarbons

Perfluorochemicals (PFCs) are large organic compounds in which all the hydrogen atoms have been replaced by fluorine atoms. They are chemically inert, immiscible in water, and not metabolized. Oxygen transported by a PFC is carried in solution and has approximately 20 times the solubility for oxygen and carbon dioxide as does water, which is almost three times the oxygen-carrying capacity of blood. The PFC solution Fluosol-DA 20% was first administered to volunteers in 1979. American clinical trials were strictly limited to acutely anemic Jehovah's Witness patients who refused blood transfusion on religious grounds.

Experiments with Fluosol-DA have demonstrated a circulation half-life of about 13 hours and a tissue half-life of 9 days. These substances do not preferentially extract oxygen from the air. Because Fluosol-DA 20% does not contain sufficient PFC, only 10% by volume, the concurrent administration of 60 to 100% oxygen is required to dissolve a significant amount of oxygen, which can render the patient vulnerable to oxygen toxicity. The safety of PFCs has not yet been established, but pulmonary hypertension, bronchospasm, cytotoxicity, and retention by the liver and spleen have been reported. In addition, the emulsifying agent Pluronic F-68 may cause a clinical reaction involving the activation of complement. The stability of the current emulsion limits the shelf-life, even though it can be stored frozen for up to 1 year.

When PFC was assessed as a red cell substitute in acutely anemic patients, no adverse reactions were noted, but no significant beneficial effects were obvious because of the small increase in arterial oxygen content, brief half-life, and limited total dose. Further assessment of PFCs concluded that the solution was unnecessary in moderately anemic patients and ineffective in severely anemic patients. Although Fluosol-DA 20% was found ineffective as a blood substitute, it may be useful as an adjunct to radiation therapy in inoperable tumors and in angioplasty procedures.

Many of the limitations of PFCs will be lessened when a better biologically inert surfactant becomes available. New formulations of perfluorochemicals that correct the observed shortcomings of Fluosol-DA may be more effective.

Characteristics. The advantages of per-fluorocarbons are as follows:

1. Contain no antigens; no typing and crossmatching necessary
2. Easily synthesized from readily available materials
3. Free of infectious diseases
4. Do not carry carbon monoxide and could provide oxygen to a carbon monoxide victim until the patient replaces abnormal red cells
5. Small particle size enables the suspension to penetrate occluded vessels in conditions such as cerebral ischemia or myocardial infarction

The disadvantages of perfluorocarbons are as follows:

1. Potentially cause oxygen toxicity
2. Unstable in vitro—need to be frozen
3. Retention by liver and spleen and other adverse reactions
4. Have not been proven beneficial in severely anemic patients

HEMOGLOBIN SOLUTIONS

Hemoglobin solutions, such as stroma-free hemoglobin or polymerized hemoglobin, may be used as free solutions in the circulation, or may be encapsulated in a membrane.

Stroma-free hemoglobin. Stroma-free hemoglobin solution is another example of an oxygen-carrying blood substitute. In 1967, a major improvement was made in the preparation of free hemoglobin by removing the membrane fragments (stroma) from hemolyzed erythrocytes. Stroma-free hemoglobin is prepared by slowly lysing washed red cells with a buffered solution of water, followed by high-speed centrifugation and micropore filtration. This procedure separates the fragmented cell membrane into relatively large pieces that can be removed.

Removal of the stroma eliminated the earlier renal, cardiovascular, and coagulation problems, but free native tetrameric hemoglobin has an undesirably high oxygen affinity. To avoid excessively high colloid osmotic pressure, stroma-free hemoglobin is used at half the oxygen-carrying capacity of whole blood.

One of the disadvantages of free hemoglobin solutions as a blood substitute is the low circulation retention time, which is less than 8 hours. It is rapidly filtered by the kidneys, and may cause some nephrotoxicity. This can be improved by coupling the beta-chains of hemoglobin (cross-linked hemoglobin) through an organic phosphate compound.

CHARACTERISTICS. The advantages of stroma-free hemoglobin are as follows:

1. Excellent volume expanders
2. Potential candidate for an emergency resuscitative fluid

The disadvantages of stroma-free hemoglobin are as follows:

1. Toxicity
2. Can activate the complement system
3. Short half-life in the circulation
4. Significant oncotic effect and unacceptably high affinity for oxygen
5. Must be refrigerated or frozen

Polymerized Hemoglobin. The limitations of stroma-free hemoglobin (SFH) solutions have been partly removed by pyridoxylation (SFH-P) followed by polymerization (poly SFH-P) of hemoglobin. Polymerized pyridoxylated hemoglobin is currently the only modification of hemoglobin solution that approximates the oxygen-carrying capacity of whole blood and can be infused without altering the plasma oncotic pressure. It supports life in the absence of red cells while maintaining baseline hemodynamics and oxygen consumption. Poly SFH-P achieves a near-normal plasma hemoglobin and has a longer intravascular persistence than any unpolymerized product. These solutions have a normal oxygen-carrying capacity and a circulation half-life of 38 hours. The total hemoglobin concentration is 14 to 16 g/dL compared to the stroma-free hemoglobin concentration of 7 g/dL.

Poly SFH-P is an improved short-term red cell substitute. Because it is an effective oxygen carrier, it persists in the circulation much longer than SFH, and the tissue oxygenation effect is significantly improved. It has, however, a higher affinity for oxygen than for erythrocytes and a higher content of nonfunctional methemoglobin. Polymerization also causes a reduction in colloid osmotic pressure (COP) while maintaining a constant hemoglobin concentration.

Although nephrotoxicity is less likely with a polymer than with the hemoglobin tetramer, a major area of concern are toxicity problems associated with the administration of poly SFH-P. Nephrotoxicity is transient and is not believed to be associated with permanent renal damage. The cause of toxicity may be the presence of vasoactive substances in the hemoglobin solution, which affects renal blood flow. This belief is supported by the fact that the majority of recipients have developed transient bradycardia and mild hypertension during infusion. Another possibility is that the changes in renal function are related to the filtration of free hemoglobin through the kidneys because once hemoglobinemia disappears, renal function returns to normal.

An additional problem is that polymerized hemoglobin solutions may be immunogenic. Polymerized hemoglobin survives for a much longer time in the circulation than free hemoglobin, and these solutions retain a significant fraction of the tetramer. The question of the immunogenicity of the polymer is currently being investigated.

CHARACTERISTICS. The advantages of polymerized hemoglobin are as follows:

1. Relative simplicity of preparation
2. Approximates the oxygen carrying capacity of whole blood
3. Can be infused without altering the plasma oncotic pressure
4. Near-normal plasma hemoglobin
5. Longer intravascular persistence than any unpolymerized product
6. Tissue oxygenation effect is significantly improved in comparison to stroma-free hemoglobin

The disadvantages of polymerized hemoglobin are as follows:

1. A higher affinity for oxygen than erythrocytes
2. A higher content of nonfunctional methemoglobin
3. Nephrotoxicity
4. May be immunogenic

ENCAPSULATED HEMOGLOBIN

Another general approach for producing surrogate erythrocytes that seems to eliminate many of the problems plaguing SFH and poly SFH-P hemoglobin solutions is based on the concept of encapsulation of hemoglobin in membranes. The use of encapsulated hemoglobin as a red cell substitute has received relatively little attention in comparison to the research on PFCs and hemoglobin solutions.

Encapsulation dates back to 1964, when Chang first encapsulated hemoglobin in nylon membranes. Artificial cell membranes can now be formed using a variety of synthetic or biologic materials to produce desired variations in characteristics such as permeability and surface properties. Almost any substance, such as enzyme systems, cell extracts, or hormones, can be included in artificial cells.

The ideal biophysical criteria for artificial red cells include the following:

1. Adequate oxygen-carrying capacity and appropriate oxygen affinity
2. Rapid gas exchange
3. Satisfactory circulating half-life and thromboresistance
4. Chemical and physical stability
5. Biologic inertness (low pathogenic potential)
6. Satisfactory viscosity
7. Storage stability
8. Low immunogenicity

Encapsulation of hemoglobin in liposomes (hemosomes) is an alternative approach that minimizes many of the problems associated with the other methods of cell preparation. Liposomes can be prepared from a single phospholipid, a mixture of phospholipids, or mixtures of phospholipids and neutral lipids, for example phosphatidylcholine plus cholesterol. Hemosomes composed of polymeric phospholipids may offer specific advantages because of their reduced permeability and rate of aggregation, their increased resistance to hydrodynamic shear and chemical disruption, and their apparent thromboresistance. Because the toxicity, stability, and storage of these preparations still presents problems, recent research has been concerned with improving encapsulation techniques and producing nontoxic biodegradable membranes.

Hemoglobin has been successfully encapsulated in lipid vesicles at concentrations equal to that found in erythrocytes. A 10 g/dL quantity of hemoglobin encapsulated in an artificial cell results in an intracellular environment comparable to that of normal red blood cells. In this way, the enzymes enclosed in the artificial cells are stabilized by the high concentration of protein. Such vesicles can be stabilized by polymerization and have a half-life of several months.

A different approach to the preparation of vesicles is to encapsulate stroma-free hemoglobin in a polymerized hemoglobin membrane. The crosslinked membrane is permeable to oxygen and impermeable to hemoglobin in solution. These vesicles are capable of reversibly binding oxygen, are less than 4 μm in diameter, and have been reported to be stable under conditions of normal blood flow.

Liposome-embedded heme is also being investigated because oxygen binding is reversible and very rapid. In addition, oxygen volume dissolved in the solution is similar or superior to that of blood and the oxygen-binding affinity is close to that of blood. The particle is small in size and composed of bioacceptable heme and phospholipid. In vivo oxygenation of tissues, however, has not been extensively investigated.

A significant advance has been achieved by the development of neohemocytes, which are microcapsules containing purified human hemoglobin and 2,3-diphosphoglycerate. The microcapsule membrane is composed of phospholipids and cholesterol molecules that are biodegradable and biocompatible. Neohemocytes are substantially smaller than erythrocytes. The size range (0.1-1.0 μm) is small enough to allow free passage through capillaries.

Neohemocytes rather than hemosomes qualify as prototype artificial red cells because, in addition to having the general characteristics of hemosomes, they meet other essential specifications including lack of degradation of the encapsulated hemoglobin and a physiologically acceptable oxygen affinity. The six essential specifications for prototype cells include the following:

1. The microcapsule membrane must be biodegradable and physiologically compatible.
2. The encapsulation process must avoid significant hemoglobin degradation.
3. The oxygen affinity of hemoglobin must be reduced relative to that of free human hemoglobin.
4. The encapsulated hemoglobin must be sufficiently concentrated (more than 33% of that in erythrocytes).
5. There should be no evidence of overt intravascular coagulopathy.
6. The artificial cells must be small enough to pass unrestricted through normal capillaries.

For typical liposomes, emulsions, and microcapsules, the mononuclear phagocytic clearance process is dominant. Natural and synthetic glycolipids have been inserted into the liposomal membrane and tested for their ability to alter liposome clearance. Incorporation of these glycolipids did decrease uptake by the mononuclear phagocytic system, but many natural glycolipids are antigenic and thus would not be suitable for insertion. Inert carbohydrates attached to lipids may reduce clearance and binding of liposomes to tissues.

The overall clearance of neohemocytes consists of three processes: clearance resulting from irreversible binding to tissues followed by breakdown, clearance caused by rapid or early destruction or breakdown; and clearance from uptake by the mononuclear phagocytic system. The objective of neohemocytes is to have cells that do not result in blockage, that interact minimally with tissues, and that are relatively invisible to the mononuclear phagocytic system.

Encapsulation appears to be the approach most likely to lead to a blood substitute that has all the properties of erythrocytes, but major obstacles remain, including toxicity, stability, storage, and the question as to whether mass production can be cost-effective. Further studies are needed to resolve the problems of selecting an acceptable microencapsulating material, developing a microencapsulation process that yields the desired size range but avoids denaturation of hemoglobin and encapsulating a sufficient amount of hemoglobin while maintaining an acceptable final viscosity. Development of a nontoxic product that combines the functions of a plasma expander with the ability to carry and deliver oxygen to tissues could prove useful in the treatment of trauma, as a temporary substitute for red cells, and for the treatment of tissue ischemia.

Characteristics. The advantages of encapsulated hemoglobin are as follows:

1. Reduced permeability and rate of aggregation
2. Increased resistance to hydrodynamic shear and chemical disruption
3. Apparent thromboresistance
4. Substantially smaller than erythrocytes (neohemocytes)

The disadvantages of encapsulated hemoglobin are as follows:

1. Toxicity
2. Stability
3. Storage
4. Questionable cost-effectiveness

Alternate Cellular Technology

In Vitro Stem Cell Culturing

It is conceivable that pluripotent stem cells could be maintained in culture to replicate and differentiate into mature blood cells. Although it has been shown that cultures of human bone marrow cells may survive for several months, more basic information is needed about the processes that regulate the balance between self-renewal and differentiation of cells. Major problems associated with this technology include the production and harvesting of a sufficient number of functional cells (10^{10} to 10^{12}) for transfusion and the harvesting of mature functional cells free from microbial contamination.

Compatibility testing between donor and recipient will probably be necessary, thus negating the advantage of a universally compatible product. Questions remain as to whether in vitro stem cell culturing can be expanded to produce sufficient numbers of functional cells in a cost-effective way.

Artificial Platelets

Platelet substitute approaches have been similar to those of red cells. Although attempts to use phospholipids and the reconstitution of platelet membrane glycoproteins into lipid vesicles have been made, these experiments have failed to construct an artificial platelet that will mimic platelet function. Recent studies with liposomes as artificial red cells provide some encouragement, but researchers have been faced with the same problems. Another approach, the use of freeze-dried or fragmented platelets, has been unsuccessful in controlling bleeding.

Alternate Sources of Plasma Products

Recombinant DNA Technology

Recombinant DNA technology is believed to hold much promise as an alternate source of plasma proteins. Within the next decade, recombinant DNA products will probably replace at least several plasma derivatives, but each plasma protein will present its own collection of specific problems to the industry.

The major proteins currently recovered from human plasma fractionation are albumin, factor VIII, prothrombin complex, and immunoglobulins. Human plasma fractionation supplies the need for these products in the United States, but the world need is not being met. In addition, other plasma proteins cannot be recovered in high yield from plasma, or can be recovered only at the expense of another product. In 1982, 3.5 million liters of plasma were fractionated to meet American demands for plasma products. Large-scale production and purification capabilities must be available before genetic engineering can meet even the demand for plasma products in the United States.

Genetic engineering is a method by which proteins from sources such as human blood are produced. Bacteria, yeast, and, for very large molecules, mammalian cells are used because they replicate proteins more accurately. Because nonpathogenic microorganisms are used, the supply of protein becomes unlimited, is less expensive, and has a high degree of purity.

Recombininant DNA (rDNA) is a combination of gene identification and cloning techniques. A strand of DNA (gene) which codes for a specific product can be isolated, characterized, sequenced, and subjected to a series of chemical and enzymatic reactions. Genetic engineers identify the section of human DNA that governs the manufacture of a specific protein, enzymatically snip out that single gene, and then insert it into the DNA of a microorganism. The selected microorganism then reproduces it in sufficient quantities for collection and purification. A major challenge facing gene-cloning technology is expansion of production to meet the demand. In addition, although products produced by DNA technology would substantially eliminate the risk of blood-borne disease, care must be taken to avoid introducing new diseases from cell cultures.

SUBSTITUTES FOR PLASMA PRODUCTS

Plasma proteins can potentially be produced by microorganisms carrying the genetic code for these proteins. The first attempts at recombinant DNA technology have been successful in the cloning and expression of albumin, antithrombin III, urokinase, tissue plasminogen activator, alpha-1-antitrypsin, and factor IX; and recently factor VIII:C and von Willebrand factor.

The largest recombinant protein expressed to date is albumin. This required the ligation of separate DNA fragments to obtain the complete, circulating form of the molecule. Cloning, however, is not the most difficult aspect of producing factor IX and factor VIII. For example, factor VIII is believed to be large (molecular weight 100,000 and 300,000).

The number of DNA fragments required for a complete factor VIII molecule could

be a major complication, compounded by the fact that the messenger RNA for the protein is probably an extremely small trace. In fact, it is still not known in which organ the protein is synthesized. Factor VIII is extremely sensitive to proteases, and thus it is essential to ensure that organisms synthesizing the molecules have low endogenous levels of proteases. Because disrupting virtually any cell results in the release of proteases, it is desirable that a recombinant organism synthesizing factor VIII secrete the molecule into the medium. This puts severe limitations on purification procedures. In addition, factor IX is post-translationally modified by the action of liver enzymes dependent on vitamin K. Bacteria and yeast are not known to possess the vitamin K-dependent carboxylase system before it can deliver the functional factor IX zymogen. Therefore, a chemical modification procedure and/or expression in mammalian cells (resulting in the proper modification) is required to obtain a functioning protein.

The plasma fractionation industry currently isolates immunoglobulin fractions from plasma of donors hyperimmunized against known antigens. Production of immunoglobulin by methods other than plasma fractionation will probably be by cell fusion technique. Most companies are producing mouse-derived monoclonal antibodies. This experience should prove valuable for increased human antibody production, once the techniques for the routine production of human hybridomas have been developed. One major problem in the use of monoclonal antibodies as therapeutic agents will be proof that a product derived from a cancerous cell line is free of carcinogenic agents. This is particularly important because it has recently been shown that some types of human leukemia are caused by viral infections.

Albumin might be the first DNA recombinant transfusion product to be available in the field of transfusion. In 1985, several manufacturers announced that recombinant factor VIII will be available soon. These firms claim that the functional portion of the molecules has been cloned and synthesized by a recombinant mammalian cell line, but it is doubtful that recombinant factor VIII will be commercially available for several years. The predicted expression and actual commercial use and performance of DNA recombinant products have exceeded the projections:

Product	Expression		Commercialization	
	Predicted	Actual	Predicted	Actual
HB Vaccine	1982	1981	1990	1987
Factor VIII	1991	1984	1997	?
Albumin	1982	1981	1991	?

The ultimate success of recombinant DNA in producing plasma proteins will depend on the cost of these products compared to the cost of using human plasma fractions. The costs of these procedures differ for various products. It is crucial to take into account the interrelationships among demands for various plasma derivatives, some of which drive the plasma market. If albumin needs could be met by recombinant DNA but no hemophilia factors were produced, the cost of producing coagulation factors would be prohibitive. When large-scale production becomes a reality, the simultaneous manufacturing of a variety of derivatives must be guaranteed to have an adequate and continuous supply of products for patients who depend on these derivatives for survival. The biotechnology industry must be prepared to deal with changing economic patterns as recombinant DNA products affect traditional markets.

HEMAPHERESIS

Platelets, granulocytes, plasma, and plasma components such as factor VIII are frequently collected by the technique of hemapheresis. Using hemapheresis, the harvesting of blood components is efficient and the remaining constituents of whole blood can be immediately returned to the donor. This technique may also be used for the therapeutic withdrawal of unwanted or harmful components from a patient's blood.

Initial Development of Equipment

Early in the twentieth century, attempts were made to separate leukocytes from whole blood, but in the 1950s, the need to use blood and its derivatives efficiently produced the first actual equipment for separating blood continuously in a closed system. Prototype models of the present continuous flow blood cell separators were developed in the 1960s. The objective of the first equipment was to improve the efficiency of separating plasma and formed elements, but the modern continuous-flow blood cell separators were initially designed to harvest leukocytes.

Development of biomechanical equipment to fractionate whole blood was largely due to the influence of Dr. Edwin J. Cohn. During World War II, the need for plasma led Cohn to adapt De Laval's cream separator for separation of plasma from whole blood. The decade following the advent of the Cohn Fractionator was filled with experiments designed to separate leukocytes from whole blood by fractionation.

In 1961, Bierman reported the hematologic changes observed in donors after leukapheresis. Further studies of leukocyte depletion and replenishment led to improved designs of the separation bowls and equipment. Allen Latham, Jr. and the Arthur D. Little Company developed a discontinuous-flow set of bowls based on the basic principles of the Cohn Fractionator without its inherent cost and complexity. After the granting of the initial patent for this equipment, Latham supervised the first clinical trials of the equipment at the Boston Red Cross in 1973.

Later research was directed at refining the basic system and developing disposable equipment for the separation of blood into components. The results of these studies led to development of three separate pieces of equipment: one that automatically fractionated banked blood into plasma and packed red cells, a density-gradient centrifuge used to separate fractions of blood, a separator designed for use with healthy donors. The collaborative efforts of many scientists resulted in a reasonably effective, closed, continuous-flow centrifuge primarily designed to separate whole blood into individual cellular and plasma portions.

Continuous-flow Cell Separation

In response to the need for processing large volumes of blood from healthy donors to obtain an adequate collection, NCI and IBM announced the development of a continuous-flow blood cell separator. This was the first closed-centrifuge system in which it was possible to subject whole blood to an uninterrupted flow and a constant force field while collecting all of its components. Field testing of this equipment began in 1966, and it was manufactured to order through 1975.

In the early 1970s, a new automated continuous-flow system for granulocyte-only collection was developed and marketed. Rather than using a force field to separate individual components by densities, this system was based on the principle of filtration leukapheresis. This method had been used for 50 years to selectively remove granulocytes from whole blood. The principle of filtration leukapheresis relies on selective and reversible adherence of granulocytes to nylon wool fibers. The remaining components pass through the filter and are returned to the donor. This method produces the highest granulocyte yields per unit of donor time and minimizes unwanted cellular elements such as lymphocytes, platelets, and erythrocytes.

In 1978, another model that maintained the basic ideas of continuous flow centrifugation, selective separation by means of collection ports and concentric channels, and a rotating seal was introduced. The flexibility of this equipment was enhanced in 1980 by the addition of a variation to the separation channel. The dual-stage separation channel was introduced as a means of obtaining platelet concentrates with minimal leukocyte contamination.

Computer technology was applied to hemapheresis equipment in 1979. A microprocessor was introduced to control machine operation with a sealless system. Whole blood separation and component collection are performed in the centrifuge by means of specifically designed chambers that interconnect. This permits blood flow from the donor vein into the separation bag of the centrifuge, transfer of component-rich plasma within the centrifuge to the collection bag, and subsequent return of recombined fractions to the donor's vein. With this system, whole blood enters the chamber, the packed red cells are forced to the outside wall and extracted for return to the donor, and the plasma, rich in the desired cell fraction, is transferred to the collection bag, where the transferred component is concentrated along the periphery and cell-poor plasma is removed for reinfusion with the red cells. This entire sterile procedure is monitored continuously by the microprocessor.

Plasmapheresis

Automated devices for plasma procurement are also available. This equipment makes possible the on-line collection of approximately 500 mL of plasma from each donor without separating the donor from his/her own red cells. Automation of plasmapheresis improves on the time-consuming process of manual collection and eliminates the risk of returning the wrong red cells to a donor.

The use of automated equipment will alleviate some of the problems associated with obtaining a sufficient supply of normal human plasma. Plasmapheresis has been proposed and in some countries is actually used to supplement the plasma collected in other ways. Plasma and plasma components, such as cryoprecipitate for the initial isolation of factor VIII complex, can be obtained in greater quantity and more cost-effectively by automated plasmapheresis.

Therapeutic Hemapheresis

Therapeutic hemapheresis is the process of separating and removing a harmful constituent from a patient through the use of a blood cell separator. Plasma exchange is the most common form of therapeutic hemapheresis. In this procedure, aliquots of the patient's plasma are removed and replaced with either 5% albumin or normal plasma. The patient's red blood cells are returned with the replacement solution.

Removal of harmful substances in the plasma, such as antibodies or immune complexes, and concurrent administration of immunosuppressive or cytotoxic therapy are combined in most diseases treated by plasma exchange. Plasma exchange is believed to be generally effective in the treatment of the following diseases:

1. Hyperviscosity syndrome
2. Cryoglobulinemia
3. Myasthenia gravis
4. Goodpasture's syndrome
5. Thrombotic thrombocytopenia purpura
6. Guillain-Barré syndrome

The level of high-titer factor VIII inhibitor can be temporarily reduced by plasma exchange and may bring about some remission in post-transfusion purpura. Plasma exchange may be a useful adjunct to dietary treatment in reducing the circulating blood levels of phytanic acid in *Refsum's disease.* The efficacy of plasma exchange is less certain in conditions such as *systemic lupus erythematosus* and *rheumatoid arthritis.*

CHAPTER SUMMARY

Whole Blood

The use of anticoagulated whole blood has been drastically reduced over the past two decades in favor of component therapy. Whole blood is appropriate for use if enhanced oxygen-carrying capacity and blood volume replacement are needed, but indiscriminate use of whole blood can reduce the availability of components to multiple patients and produce hypervolemia in patients who are not actively bleeding.

Red Blood Cell Products

Patients in need of the oxygen-carrying capabilities of hemoglobin are candidates for packed red blood cells. The use of washed red blood cells has declined with increased availability of deglycerolized red blood cells, but this type of component may be requested in special circumstances. Pa-

tients with paroxysmal nocturnal hemoglobinuria (PNH) or hypersensitivity to plasma protein need red cells devoid of plasma protein and are appropriate candidates. Neocytes have a longer in vivo survival than unfractionated cells from the same donor population. Neocytes have a significantly longer survival time than transfused mature red cells, a higher reticulocyte count, and higher pyruvate kinase activity levels. Because neocytes have an extended in vivo survival time, infusion of these red cells can theoretically reduce blood requirements in transfusion-dependent patients. Leukocyte-poor blood is most frequently indicated for use in patients who have suffered from febrile transfusion reactions due to leukocytes. Frozen-deglycerolized red cells allow preservation and extended storage of erythrocytes. After thawing and deglycerolization, the end product results in the recovery of more than 85% of the initial donor's red blood cells, which are largely free of the original plasma, leukocytes, and other formed elements. The advantages of deglycerolized red cells include the reduction of leukocytes and platelets, plasma protein removal, reduction or removal of viruses such as hepatitis and cytomegalovirus, autologous blood storage for patients with antibodies to high-incidence antigens or those with extremely rare blood types, maintenance of 2,3 DPG and ATP levels, and elimination of anticoagulants and metabolites.

Platelets

The introduction of blood platelets as a blood component became possible when plastic whole blood donor collection bags with multiple satellite containers became readily available. This technology permitted the separation, storage, and transport of platelet concentrates to produce readily available blood bank components. Patients with severe thrombocytopenia or platelet dysfunction with symptoms of bleeding are candidates for platelet concentrate transfusions to induce hemostasis or for prophylactic use to prevent intracranial bleeding and catastrophic hemorrhage in other organ systems.

Granulocytes

Leukocyte concentrates, primarily neutrophils, may be of value to patients with severe neutropenia who have a life-threatening systemic infection uncontrolled by antibiotics. Patients who would most frequently be considered appropriate candidates are those with neutropenia induced by chemotherapy or radiation therapy. The major impediment to storage of granulocyte concentrates or transfusion is rapid impairment in the ability of the neutrophilic granulocytes to migrate toward inflammatory stimuli, both in vitro and in vivo.

Irradiated Blood and Blood Components

Graft-versus-host reactions are caused by proliferation of mature donor-derived T lymphocytes in response to major and minor histocompatibility antigens in the host. Graft-versus-host disease can occur after transfusion of blood or various blood products including fresh and stored whole blood, packed red cells stored for as long as 12 days, buffy coat-poor or washed red cells, platelet concentrates, granulocyte concentrates, or single units of fresh plasma. The risk of graft-versus-host disease can be minimized, if not eliminated, by irradiating whole and various other red cell components immediately before infusion.

The infusion of lymphocyte containing whole blood or blood components into patients who are immunosuppressed or have severe immunodeficiency disorders presents the risk of inducing graft-versus-host disease. Patients at the highest risk with an absolute need for irradiated blood products include recipients of autologous or allogeneic bone marrow grafts, and children with severe congenital immune deficiency syndromes involving T lymphocytes. Blood product irradiation is believed to be the most efficient and probably the most economical method available for prevention of post-transfusion graft-versus-host disease.

Plasma

Plasma can be separated from units of whole blood and stored as either single-donor plasma or fresh frozen plasma. Either form of plasma can be used for temporary volume replacement in patients who are depleted of whole blood or protein. Plasma may also be appropriate for coagulation factor replacement. Components such as cryoprecipitate are prepared from human plasma. Fractionation of human plasma can be into albumin or immune globulins.

Patients with severe burns or shock due to hypovolemia are appropriate candidates for single-donor plasma. Depending on the type of coagulation deficiency as well as the method of storage, patients with coagulation defects may also be suitable transfusion candidates. Using plasma rather than whole blood when colloid volume expansion or most coagulation factors are needed reduces the risk of sensitization to cellular antigens and is cost-effective, but single-donor plasma has the same risks of infectious disease due to blood-borne agents as a unit of blood. Transfusion reactions due to plasma proteins or cellular components are also a possibility.

Fresh-frozen plasma contains labile and stable components of the coagulation, fibrinolytic, and complement systems; proteins that maintain osmotic pressure and immunity; other proteins which have diverse activities; and fats, carbohydrates, and minerals in concentrations similar to those in the circulation. Few specific indications for the use of fresh frozen plasma exist. Indications are generally limited to the treatment of deficiencies of coagulation proteins for which specific factor concentrates are unavailable or undesirable. Use of fresh-frozen plasma is appropriate in patients who have received massive transfusions, in single or multiple coagulation deficiencies, for warfarin reversal, or in conjunction with therapeutic plasma exchange. The major advantage of fresh-frozen plasma is that if appropriately used, it provides effective use of whole blood through component therapy. With the use of plasma alone, the risk of alloimmunization to erythrocyte, leukocyte, and platelet antigens is lower than that with the use of whole blood.

Plasma Components

Cryoprecipitated antihemophilic factor (AHF) is the cold insoluble precipitate of plasma remaining after fresh-frozen plasma obtained from whole blood or apheresis has been thawed between 1 and 6° C. Because cryoprecipitated AHF is a source of coagulation factor VIII, von Willebrand's factor (AHF-VWF), factor XIII, fibrinogen, and fibronectin, it is useful in the control of bleeding in various clinical disorders including factor VIII deficiency, von Willebrand's disease, factor XIII deficiency, and hypofibrinogenemia.

The transmission of viral diseases by coagulation factor concentrates and other plasma products remains a serious health concern. Factor VIII and factor IX concentrates that have not been treated have been implicated in the transmission of several viral diseases, most notably hepatitis B, non-A, non-B hepatitis, and AIDS. Approaches to virus inactivation in plasma products include heating, ultraviolet radiation, and most recently monoclonal absorption of factor VIII (AHG).

Factor IX complex, Konyne[R], is a commercially prepared, heat-treated plasma product that contains coagulation factors II, IX, X, and low levels of factor VII. The main indication for factor IX complex is in the treatment of conditions caused by factor IX (hemophilia B or Christmas disease) deficiency. The use of factor IX complex for patients with factors II or X or mild cases of hemophilia B should be considered if treatment with fresh-frozen plasma is not feasible or has proven ineffective. Other clinical indications include reversal of coumarin anticoagulant-induced hemorrhage as a secondary approach if the risk of transmitting hepatitis is considered justifiable, and in the treatment of bleeding episodes in patients with hemophilia A (factor VIII deficiency) who have inhibitors to factor VIII. Factor IX complex is prepared from paid donors in whom the risk of bloodborne disease is high.

Blood Substitutes and Alternate Sources of Blood Components

While the use of human whole blood and blood components has many benefits, problems are associated with the use of these products. It is expected that the traditional blood supply system will continue to function for many years, but in the future the increasing demand may not be met. Substitutes and alternate sources are being developed as an alternative to human-derived blood or blood components.

Several types of synthetic red blood cell surrogates exist, including emulsions of perfluorocarbons, stroma-free hemoglobin, polymerized hemoglobin, and liposome-encapsulated hemoglobin.

It is conceivable that pluripotent stem cells could be maintained in culture to replicate and differentiate into mature blood cells. Major problems associated with this technology include the production and harvesting of a sufficient number of functional cells for transfusion and the harvesting of mature functional cells free from microbial contamination.

Although attempts to use phospholipids and the reconstitution of platelet membrane glycoproteins into lipid vesicles have been made, these experiments have failed to construct an artificial platelet that mimics platelet function.

Recombinant DNA technology is believed to hold much promise as an alternate source of plasma proteins. Within the next decade recombinant DNA products will probably replace at least several plasma derivatives. The major proteins currently recovered from human plasma fractionation are albumin, factor VIII, prothrombin complex, and immunoglobulins.

Hemapheresis

Platelets, granulocytes, plasma and plasma components such as factor VIII are frequently collected by the technique of hemapheresis. In the 1950s, the need to use blood and its derivatives efficiently produced the first equipment for separating blood continuously in a closed system. In 1978, another model that maintained the

basic ideas of continuous-flow centrifugation, selective separation by means of collection ports and concentric channels, and
a rotating seal was introduced. Computer
technology was applied to hemapheresis
equipment in 1979.

Automated devices for plasma procurement are also available. Automation of
plasmapheresis improves on the time-consuming process of manual collection and
eliminates the risk of returning the wrong
red cells to a donor. The use of this equipment will alleviate some of the problems
associated with obtaining a sufficient supply of normal human plasma.

Therapeutic hemapheresis is the process
of separating and removing a harmful constituent from a patient through the use of a
blood cell separator. Plasma exchange is
the most common form of therapeutic hemapheresis and is believed to be generally
effective in the treatment of hyperviscosity
syndrome, cryoglobulinemia, myasthenia
gravis, Goodpasture's syndrome, thrombotic thrombocytopenia purpura, and Guillain-Barré syndrome.

REVIEW QUESTIONS

1–4. Match the following blood products
with the most appropriate clinical application:
1. Whole blood (less than 4 or 5 days old)
2. Packed red blood cells
3. Washed red cells
4. Neocyte-enriched packed cells
   A. Exchange transfusion in newborn
      infants
   B. Patients with *paroxysmal nocturnal
      hemoglobinuria*
   C. If oxygen-carrying capacity and vol-
      ume replacement are needed
   D. Patients with thalassemia
   E. If the oxygen-carrying capabilities
      of hemoglobin are needed
5. The currently approved FDA approved
   shelf-life of whole blood drawn into
   CPDA-1 is _____ days.
   A. 18
   B. 21
   C. 28
   D. 32
   E. 35

6. Whole blood has the advantage of:
   A. Increasing the availability of com-
      ponents.
   B. Being less expensive than combined
      component therapy.
   C. Reducing the risks of combined
      component therapy.
   D. Reducing the risk of hypervolemia.
   E. Both B and C.
7. Packed red blood cells prepared in an
   open system have an expiration time of:
   A. 24 hours
   B. 48 hours
   C. 72 hours
   D. 21 days
   E. 28 days
8 and 9. Packed red blood cells have the
   advantage of 8. _____ but the dis-
   advantage of 9. _____.
8.
   A. Decreased exposure to infectious
      diseases
   B. Volume reduction
   C. Increased concentration of antico-
      agulant
   D. Increased K^+
   E. Increased viscosity
9.
   A. Increased cost
   B. Increased K^+
   C. Increased concentration of antico-
      agulant
   D. Increased viscosity
   E. No known disadvantages
10. The purpose of rejuvenation of packed
    red cells is:
    A. Depletion of 2,3 DPG
    B. Depletion of ATP
    C. Restoration of normal oxygen trans-
       port
    D. Reduction of the risk of hepatitis
       transmission
    E. Decrease of the antigenicity of
       erythrocyte antigens
11. A characteristic of neocytes is:
    A. A lower level of pyruvate kinase
       activity
    B. Longer transfusion survival time
    C. Greater density than mature eryth-
       rocytes
    D. Shorter transfusion survival time
    E. Higher hemoglobin content than ma-
       ture erythrocytes

12. Hemochromatosis may be reduced by transfusing:
   A. Packed red blood cells
   B. Whole Blood
   C. Washed red cells
   D. Neocytes
   E. Fresh whole blood

13 and 14

13. For blood to be considered to be leukocyte-poor by current standards and to be suitable for transfusion, the unit of blood must remove **13.** ___% of leukocytes and retain **14.** ___% of erythrocytes.

13.
   A. 30
   B. 50
   C. 70
   D. 90
   E. 100

14.
   A. 30
   B. 50
   C. 70
   D. 90
   E. 100

15. The ARC standards require that units having leukocytes removed by washing should contain *no more* than ___ leukocytes.
   A. 0.2×10^9
   B. 0.5×10^9
   C. 1.0×10^9
   D. 2.0×10^9
   E. 5.0×10^9

16. Leukocyte-poor blood is most frequently indicated clinically in patients who have:
   A. A high titer of alloantibodies to erythrocytes
   B. A high titer of alloantibodies to leukocytes
   C. Congestive heart failure
   D. Previously experienced febrile transfusion reactions
   E. High susceptibility to hepatitis

17. Of the available techniques used to prepare leukocyte-poor blood, the technique that has the greatest number of advantages for most alloimmunized patients is:
   A. Spin-cool-filter
   B. Upright spin
   C. Inverted spin
   D. Spin-filter

E. Deglycerolized red cells

18. The most commonly used methods for depleting red cells of leukocytes are:
   A. Washing and buffy-coat removal
   B. Inverted spin and washing
   C. Upright spin and inverted spin
   D. Spin-filter and washing
   E. Upright spin and inverted spin

19. The percentage of red cells recovered after thawing and deglycerolization of frozen blood is:
   A. 35%
   B. 50%
   C. 75%
   D. 85%
   E. 95%

20. Which of the following is *not* a clinical indication for frozen/deglycerolized red cells?
   A. An alloimmunized patient who has previously experienced nonhemolytic febrile transfusion reactions
   B. A patient with an IgA deficiency
   C. A patient who is allergic to plasma proteins
   D. Autologous transfusion
   E. None of the above

21. Which of the following is a cryoprotective additive?
   A. Glycerol
   B. Dimethyl sulfoxide
   C. Glucose
   D. Polyvinylpyrrolidone (PVP)
   E. All of the above

22 and 23

22. Under current regulations, frozen blood can be stored for up to **22.** ___ at **23.** ___

22.	23.
A. 21 days	A. 4° C
B. 35 days	B. 0° C
C. 90 days	C. −20° C
D. 1 year	D. −40° C
E. 3 years	E. −80° C

24. The *most common* application of deglycerolized red cells is:
   A. Autologous transfusion
   B. Prevention of febrile reactions caused by leukoagglutinins
   C. Prevention of febrile reactions caused by platelet antibodies
   D. Decreased sensitization to platelet antigens
   E. Prevention of dissemination of AIDS

25. The average total leukocyte count in a unit of deglycerolized red cells is:
   A. $0.1 \times 10^9/L$
   B. $0.3 \times 10^9/L$
   C. $0.5 \times 10^9/L$
   D. $5.0 \times 10^9/L$
   E. $8.8 \times 10^9/L$

26. Which of the following is *not* an advantage of deglycerolized red cells?
   A. Reduction of leukocytes
   B. Reduction of platelets
   C. Plasma protein removal
   D. Reduction of the incidence of cytomegalovirus
   E. Lower cost

27. The proper storage temperature for platelet concentrates for a 3-day period of time is ____ ° C.
   A. −1 to 0
   B. 1 to 6
   C. 10 to 15
   D. 20 to 24
   E. 37

28. The pH of stored platelet concentrates must *not* exceed:
   A. 4.5
   B. 5.5
   C. 6.0
   D. 7.0
   E. 7.5

29. According to AABB standards, ____ of random donor platelet concentrates must contain ____ platelets.
   A. $30\% - 1.5 \times 10^{10}$
   B. $30\% - 5.5 \times 10^{10}$
   C. $50\% - 1.5 \times 10^{10}$
   D. $50\% - 1.5 \times 10^{10}$
   E. $75\% - 5.5 \times 10^{10}$

30. The pH of platelet concentrates at maximum storage depends on:
   A. Type of plastic bag
   B. Concentration of platelets
   C. Method of preparation
   D. Type of anticoagulant that the initial blood was drawn in
   E. Volume of plasma

31. The best storage condition for platelet concentrates is:
   A. On a 6 rpm elliptical rotator
   B. On a 1 rpm elliptical rotator
   C. On a 2 rpm circular rotator
   D. On a 6 rpm circulator rotator
   E. All of the above, except A

32. Which of the following is *not* a possible consequence of the transfusion of platelet concentrates?
   A. Bacterial contamination
   B. Hemolytic transfusion reaction
   C. Pulmonary edema
   D. Febrile reactions to plasma proteins
   E. Graft-versus-host disease

33. Granulocyte transfusions are clinically appropriate for:
   A. Patients with severe neutropenia
   B. Patients who have infections
   C. Patients who have life-threatening systemic infections that are uncontrolled by antibiotics
   D. Patients needing granulocytes from a single unit of blood
   E. Patients about to undergo chemotherapy or radiation therapy

34. Graft-versus-host disease is caused by:
   A. Granulocytes
   B. Platelets
   C. Lymphocytes
   D. Erythrocytes
   E. Both A and C

35. Which of the following blood componenets has *not* been documented to cause GVHD?
   A. Single units of fresh plasma
   B. Fresh frozen plasma
   C. Stored whole blood
   D. Washed red cells
   E. Platelet concentrates

36. The types of patients at highest risk of developing GVHD are:
   A. Infants receiving intra-uterine transfusions
   B. Children with severe congenital AIDS
   C. Patients with acute leukemia receiving total body radiation
   D. Patients with solid tumors
   E. Patients with aplastic anemia receiving anti-thymocyte globulin therapy

37. The radiation source for irradiation of blood products is:
   A. I^{131}
   B. Ce^{137}
   C. C^{14}
   D. Te^{131}
   E. x-ray

38. The effect of radiation on lymphocytes is that it:
    A. Inhibits lymphocyte mitotic activity
    B. Inhibits lymphocyte blast transformation
    C. Affects locomotion
    D. Affects chemotaxis
    E. Both A and B

39. Single-donor plasma can appropriately be used for patients with:
    A. Dehydration
    B. Severe burns
    C. Hypovolemic shock
    D. Albumin deficiency
    E. Both B and C

40. An appropriate use of fresh-frozen plasma is:
    A. Volume replacement
    B. Protein replacement
    C. Coagulation replacement
    D. Carbohydrate and mineral supplementation
    E. Replacement of platelets

41. If a unit of fresh frozen plasma is stored at 1 to 6° C, it *must* be used within ____ hours after thawing.
    A. 2
    B. 4
    C. 8
    D. 12
    E. 24

42. Which of the following is a characteristic of cryoprecipitated antihemophiliac factor?
    A. Contains platelets
    B. Contains factor VIII
    C. Contains fibrinogen
    D. Contains fibronectin
    E. All of the above except A

43. How many bags of cryoprecipitate are required if the desired level of factor VIII is 60% and the patient's plasma volume is 2500 mL?
    A. 13
    B. 15
    C. 17
    D. 19
    E. 21

44. Once defrosted, cryoprecipitate must be administered within ____ hours of thawing.
    A. 2
    B. 4

C. 6
D. 12
E. 24

45. Transmission of viruses in cryoprecipitate may be eliminated by:
    A. Heating in the liquid form
    B. Heating in a lyopholized form
    C. Irradiating with ultraviolet light
    D. Solvent-detergent treatment
    E. All of the above

46. A major disadvantage of factor IX complex is the:
    A. High risk of hepatitis
    B. Lack of other coagulation factors
    C. Lack of platelets
    D. Need to adminster one hour after reconstitution
    E. Lack of albumin

47. Perfluorocarbons have been investigated as:
    A. Platelet substitutes
    B. Granulocyte substitutes
    C. Red blood cell substitutes
    D. Plasma substitutes
    E. Coagulation factors

48. One of the major disadvantages of stroma-free and polymerized hemoglobin is:
    A. Poor volume expansion
    B. Toxicity
    C. Decreased tissue oxygenation effects
    D. Difficulty of preparation
    E. High circulatory retention time

49. Neohemocytes are closer to being prototype artificial red cells because of the following characteristic(s):
    A. Lack of degradation of encapsulated hemoglobin
    B. Physiologically acceptable oxygen affinity
    C. Resistance to biodegradation
    D. Hemoglobin levels lower than 33%
    E. Both A and B

50. Recombinant DNA technology has been successful in the cloning and expression of all of the following except:
    A. Albumin
    B. Factor VIII
    C. Factor IX
    D. Factor X
    E. Antithrombin

ANSWERS

1. A	26. E
2. E	27. D
3. B	28. C
4. D	29. E
5. E	30. A
6. E	31. E
7. A	32. B
8. B	33. C
9. D	34. C
10. C	35. B
11. B	36. B
12. D	37. B
13. C	38. E
14. C	39. E
15. B	40. C
16. D	41. B
17. A	42. E
18. B	43. D
19. D	44. C
20. E	45. E
21. E	46. A
22. E	47. C
23. E	48. B
24. B	49. E
25. B	50. D

BIBLIOGRAPHY

Banzhaf, J.: Technical Quarterly (Am. Red Cross Blood Services, Rochester Region). Summer, 1988, pp 1-2.

Beissinger, R.L., Farmer, M.C., and Gossage, J.L.: Liposome-encapsulated hemoglobin as a red cell surrogate. Am. Soc. for Artificial Internal Organs, 32 (1):58-63, 1986.

Biotechnology. Parenterals 4 (5): 1-5, 1986.

Blomback, M.J., Chmielewska, et al.: Activation of blood coagulation, fibrinolytic and kallikrein systems during storage of plasma. Vox Sang. 47 (5):335-342, 1984.

Blumberg, N., et al.: A critical survey of fresh-frozen plasma use. Transfusion, 26 (6):551-513, 1986.

Boral, L.I.: Platelet transfusion therapy. Lab. Med., 16 (4):221-226, 1985.

Button, L., et al.: Rejuvenation of red cells drawn in Adsol to extend autologous red cell storage. Transfusion, 26(6):558, 1986.

Campbell, J. (Ed.): AABB News Briefs, 11 (6):3, 1988.

Castro, O.L.: Long-term cryopreservation of red cells from patients with sickle cell disease. Transfusion. 25(1):70-72, 1985.

Chang, T.M.: Artificial cells in medicine and biotechnology. Appl. Biochem. Biotechnol., 10:5-24, 1984.

Eisenstaedt, R.S.: Concurrent audit of fresh frozen plasma use. Abstract of a paper presented at the Annual American Association of Blood Banks Meeting. Transfusion 25(5):466, 1985.

Factor IX Complex Product Brochure. Berkeley, CA, Cutter Biological, May, 1986.

Fratantoni, J.C.: Comment on standardized procedures the regulatory process. Transfusion Vol. 26(1):36-37, 1986.

Gottschall, J.L., et al.: Studies of the minimum temperature at which human platelets can be stored with full maintenance of viability, Transfusion 26(5):460-462, 1986.

Gould, S. A., et al.: The development of polymerized pyridoxylated hemoglobin solution as a red cell substitute. Ann. Emerg. Med. 15(12):1416-1419.

Gould, S. A.: Fluosol-DA as a red-cell substitute in acute anemia. N. Engl. J. Med. 314(26):1653-1656, 1986.

Harley, K.M., et al.: Platelet temperature in transport under warm and cold conditions. Abstract of a paper to be presented at the Annual American Association of Blood Banks Meeting, Transfusion, 26, (6):558, 1986.

Hayward, J. A., et. al.: Polymerized liposmomes as stable oxygen-carriers. Fed. Eur. Biochem. Soc., 187(2):;261-266, 1985

Head, D.R.: Whole blood versus packed red cells. Transfusion, 25(6):591, 1985.

Hedlund, B.E., et al.: Polymerized Hemoglobins. In Transfusion Medicine: Recent Technological Advances, New York, Alan R. Liss, Inc., pp. 39-48, 1986.

Heldenbrant, C.M., et al.: Evaluation of two viral inactivation methods for the preparation of safer factor VIII and factor IX concentrates. Transfusion 25(6):510-515, 1985.

Henry, J.B. (Ed.): Clinical Diagnosis and Management by Laboratory Methods, 17th ed. Philadelphia, W.B. Saunders Co, 1982, pp. 1020-1022.

Hogan, V.A., et al.: A simple method for preparing neocyte-enriched Leukocyte-Poor Blood for Transfusion-Dependent Patients. Transfusion, 26(3):253-257, 1986.

Hogge, D.E., et al.: Platelet Storage for 7 Days in Second-Generation Blood Bags. Transfusion, 26(2):131-135, 1986.

Horowitz, B., et al.: Inactivation of viruses in labile blood derivatives. Transfusion 25, (6)523-527, 1985.

Huestis, D. W., Boue, J.R., and Case, J.: Practical Blood Transfusion, 4th ed. Boston, Little, Brown and Co., 1988, pp. 328-336.

Huggins, C.: Preparation and usefulness of frozen blood. Annual Review of Medicine. 36:499-503, 1985.

Hunt, C. A., et al.: Synthesis and evaluation of a prototypal artificial red cell. Science 230:1165B, 1985.

Hunt, C. A., and Burnette, R. R.: Lipid microencapsulation of hemoglobin. Appl. Biochem. Biotechnol. 10:147-149, 1984.

International Forum: What is the Prospective Impact of the Recombinant DNA Technique on the Production of Human Plasma Derivatives? Which are the Derivates Where Donor Plasma Could be Replaced? Vox Sang., 44:390-395, 1983.

Iwasaki, K. et al.: Efficacy and safety of hemoglobin-polyethylene glycol conjugate (pyridoxalated polyethylene glycol hemoglobin) as an oxygen-carrying resuscitation fluid. Artif. Organs. 10(6):470-474, 1986.

Janco, R.L., et al.: Perfluorochemical blood substitutes differentially alter human monocyte procoagulant generation and oxidative metabolism. Transfusion, 25(6):578-582, 1985.

Kahn, R. A., Allen, R. W., and Baldassare, J.: Alternate sources and substitutes for therapeutic blood components. Blood, 66(1):1-12, 1985.

Kevy, S.V., et al.: A seven year evaluation of extended storage of deglycerolized red cells. Abstract of Paper Presented at the Annual Meeting of the American Association of Blood Banks, Transfusion, 25(5):476, 1985.

Kim, H.C., et al.: The role of frozen-thawed-washed red blood cells (FTW-RBC) in preventing transfusion acquired CMV infection (TA-CMVI) in the neonate. Abstract of paper to be presented at the American Association of Blood Banks Annual Meeting, Transfusion, 25(5):472, 1985.

Lane, T.A., and Lamkin, G.E.: Glycogen metabolism in stored granulocytes. Transfusion, 25(3):246-250, 1985.

Lane, T.A., and Lamkin, G.E.: The effect of storage on degranulation by human neutrophils. Transfusion. 25(2):155-161, 1985.

Leitman, S.F., and Holland, P.V.: Irradiation of blood products: Indications and guidelines. Transfusion, 25(4):293-300, 1985.

Lowe, K. C.: Blood tranfusion or blood substitution? Vox Sang. 51(4):257-263, 1986.

Luff, R. D., et al.: Microwave technology for the rapid thawing of frozen blood components. Am. J. Clin. Pathol., Vol. No.:59-64, 1985.

McGill, M.: Blood product irradiation recommendations. Transfusion, 26(6): 542: 1986.

McLoud, B. C., Sassetto, R. J., Cole, E. R., and Pierce, M. I.: Factor VIII collection by pheresis, Lancet, Sept 27: 671-673, 1980.

McMican, A., Luban, N.L.C., and Sacher, R. A., Practical aspects of blood irradiation. Lab. Med., 18(5):299-303, 1987.

Menache, D.: Measures to Inactivate Viral Contaminants Of Pooled Plasma Products. Infection, Immunity and Blood Transfusion. New York, Alan R. Liss, Inc., 1985. pp. 407-423.

Menitove, et al.: Stability of protein C and protein S in blood components, Abstract of a paper presented at the Annual American Association of Blood Banks Meeting. Transfusion 25:466, 1985.

Meryman, H.T., and Hornblower, M.: The preparation of red cells depleted of leukocytes. Transfusion, 26(1):101-106, 1986.

Millward, B. L., and Hoeltge, G. A.: The historical development of automated hemapheresis. J. Clin. Apheresis, 1:25-32, 1982.

Mitra, G., et al.: Elimination of infectious retroviruses during preparation of immunoglobulins. Transfusion 26(4):94, 1986.

Moore, G.L., and Ledford, M.E.: Effects of 4000 Rad irradiation on the in vitro storage properties of packed red cells. Transfusion, 25(6):583-585, 1985.

Moss, G. S., et al.: Hemoglobin solution—from tetramer to polymer. Surgery 95(3):249-55, 1984.

Murphy, S.: Guidelines for platelet transfusion. JAMA 259(16):2453-2454, 1988.

National Institutes of Health. Fresh-Frozen Plasma: Indications and Risks. Connecticut Medicine, 49(5):295-297, 1985.

Oberman, H. A.: Transfusion Classics. Transfusion, 25:359, 1985.

Overby, L. R.: Challenges and Opportunities in Biotechnology. In Infection, Immunity, and Blood Transfusion. New York, Alan R. Liss, Inc., 1985, pp. 425-443.

Peetoom, F.: Closing: Transfusion Medicine, Recent Technological Advances. In Transfusion Medicine, Recent Technolgoical Advances. New York, Alan R. Liss, Inc., pp. 343-346.

Read, E.J., and Klein, H.G.: Fresh frozen plasma transfusion: A perspective survey. Abstract of AABB Meeting. Transfusion, 25(5):465, 1985.

Rock, G., et al.: Plasma Collection using an automated membrane device. Transfusion, 26(3):, 269-271, 1986.

Schwartz, G. J., and Diller, K. R.: Intracellular freezing of human granulocytes. Cryobiology, 21:654-660, 1984.

Sehgal, L.R., et al.: Polymerized pyridoxylated hemoglobin: Evolution of a new blood substitute. Am. Clin. Prod. Rev. 6(7):10-13, 1987.

Sehgal, L. R., et al.: Polymerized pyridoxylated hemoglobin: A red cell substitute with normal oxygen capacity. Surgery 95(4):433-438, 1984.

Sirchia, G., et al.: Leukocyte depletion of red cell units at the bedside by transfusion through a new filter. Transfusion, 27(3):402-405, 1987.

Snyder, E.L., et al.: The effect of mode of agitation and type of plastic bag on storage characteristics and in vivo kinetics of platelet concentrates. Transfusion, 26(2):125-130, 1986.

Snyder, A.J.: Why is fresh-frozen plasma transfused? Transfusion, 26:107-112, 1986.

Towell, B.L., et al.: A comparison of frozen and fresh platelet concentrates in the support of thrombocytopenic patients. Transfusion, 26(6):525-530, 1986.

Tremper, K. K., and Anderson, S. T.: Perfluorochemical emulsion oxygen transport fluids: A clinical review. Ann. Rev. Med. 36:309-313, 1985.

Tsuchida, E.: Liposome-embedded iron-porphyrins as an artificial oxygen carrier. Ann. N. Y. Acad. Sci. 446:429-442, 1985.

Turgeon, M. L.: Should a community hospital establish a frozen blood program? Med. Lab. September: 20-23, 1972.

Van Aken, W. G.: Future trends in blood component preparation. Vox Sang. 51(Suppl.1):67-71, 1986.

Widmann, F. K.: Technical Manual. (9th Ed.) Arlington, Va., American Association of Blood Banks, 1985. pp. 41-42, 44, 45, 46, 50, 52, 55, 269.

Yomtovian, R.: From ABO to HTLV: changing trends in blood transfusion safety. Minn. Med. 68:587-589, 1985.

PART FOUR

Clinical Conditions Associated with Immunohematology

10

Hemolytic Disease of the Newborn

At the conclusion of this chapter, the reader will be able to:

- Briefly define the cause (etiology) and consequences of hemolytic disease of the newborn (HDN).
- Describe the consequences of the coating of fetal erythrocytes with maternal antibody.
- Define the term "extramedullary hematopoiesis."
- Compare the consequences of hemolysis to the fetus versus those to the newborn baby.
- Describe the mechanism of the transfer of antibody from mother to fetus.
- Name the antibodies most frequently responsible for HDN in descending order of severity.
- Describe the mechanism of HDN.
- Explain how the fetus attempts to compensate for erythyrocyte hemolysis while in utero.
- Describe the in utero consequences of extensive hemolysis.
- Compare the physiologic activities of hemolysis in the fetus to the same process in the newborn infant.
- Name the major immunoglobulin class responsible for HDN.
- Briefly describe the mechanism of transplacental passage of an antibody.
- Name the specific IgG antibody types that cause HDN in descending order of severity.
- Rank the antibodies that cause HDN in order of severity.
- Explain the basic antigen-antibody reaction that produces HDN.
- List and briefly explain the factors that affect the production of antibodies in the maternal circulation.
- Name at least three causes of transplacental hemorrhage and the volume of fetal blood that is considered significant in fetal-maternal hemorrhage.
- Name six procedures generally used in prenatal testing.
- Describe the procedure of amniocentesis and the significance of the results.
- Name eight procedures used in postnatal assessment of potential HDN. Describe the significance of each procedure to the diagnosis.
- List the tests commonly performed in prenatal testing.
- Describe the general procedure and value of amniocentesis in the treatment of HDN.
- List the procedures that are useful in the postpartum diagnosis of HDN or the extent of fetal-maternal hemorrhage.
- Explain the relationship of the tests named in Chapter 13 to the assessment of HDN.
- Describe the etiology, genetic frequency, symptoms, physiology, laboratory diagnosis, and treatment of HDN caused by ABO incompatibility.

- Describe the cause of ABO-caused HDN.
- Calculate the genetic probability of ABO incompatibility between mother and fetus.
- Describe the symptoms and physiology of HDN caused by ABO incompatibility.
- List the laboratory procedures that are useful in the diagnosis of ABO incompatibility and describe the results in this type of HDN.
- Discuss the treatment procedures in HDN caused by ABO incompatibility.
- Describe the cause, genetic frequency, symptoms, physiology, laboratory diagnosis, and treatment of HDN caused by incompatibility.
- Explain the method of postpartum prevention of hemolytic disease due to the antigen.
- Describe the work of the major investigators in the study of HDN due to the Rh factor.
- Explain the types of responses to the $Rh_o (D)$ antigen.
- Apply the normal pattern of the immune response to the $Rh_o (D)$ antigen.
- Compare the relationship of HDN caused by ABO incompatibility to HDN caused by Rh incompatibility.
- Calculate the genetic probability of HDN caused by Rh_o in untreated women.
- Describe the role of antibody titer, antibody subclasses, and Gm allotypes to HDN caused by anti-D.
- Name and describe the prenatal tests that are significant in HDN caused by anti-D.
- Describe the prenatal treatments that could be used in severe cases of HDN.
- Explain the history of the development and the basis for modern prophylactic treatment against HDN due to anti-D.
- Calculate the appropriate number of vials of $Rh\ I_gG$ when given the Kleihauer-Betke value.
- List and describe the general and laboratory criteria for the administration of Rh IgG.
- Describe the etiology, genetic frequency, symptoms, physiology, laboratory diagnosis, and treatment of HDN caused by other blood group incompatibilities.
- Describe the role of other erythrocyte blood antigens in the causation of HDN.
- Explain the development of fetal antigens in major blood group systems associated with HDN.
- Describe the importance of laboratory assessment in HDN.
- Briefly compare the treatment of HDN caused by other blood group systems to HDN caused by either ABO or Rh_o incompatibility.

Hemolytic disease of the newborn (HDN) or erythroblastosis fetalis results from excessive destruction of fetal red cells by maternal antibodies. This condition in the fetus or newborn infant is clinically characterized by anemia and jaundice. If the hemoglobin breakdown product, bilirubin, which visibly produces jaundice, reaches excessive levels in the newborn infant's circulation, it accumulates in lipid-rich nervous tissue. This deposition of bilirubin (kernicterus) can cause mental retardation or death.

THE GENERAL CHARACTERISTICS OF HDN

Basic Physiology of HDN

In hemolytic disease of the newborn (Fig. 10-1), the erythrocytes of the fetus become coated with maternal antibodies that correspond to specific fetal antigens. This hemolytic process reduces the normal 45- to 70-day life span of fetal erythrocytes.

The fetal hematopoietic tissues (the liver, spleen and bone marrow) respond to hemolysis by increasing production of erythrocytes. Increased erythrocyte production outside the bone marrow, *extramedullary hematopoiesis*, can result in enlargement of the liver and spleen. There is also premature release from the bone marrow, pre-

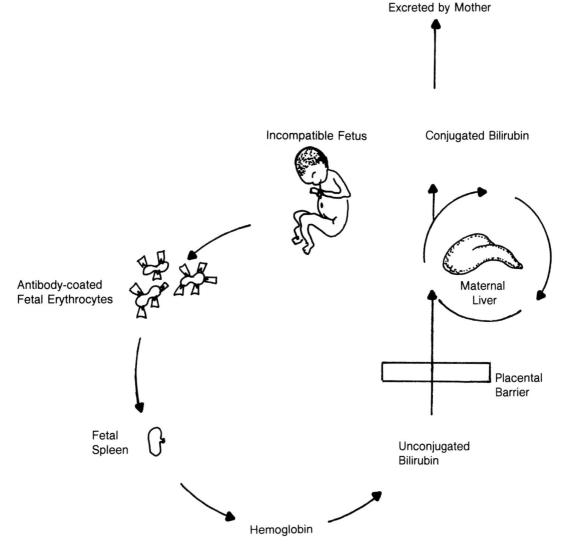

Excreted by Mother

Incompatible Fetus

Conjugated Bilirubin

Antibody-coated
Fetal Erythrocytes

Maternal
Liver

Placental
Barrier

Fetal
Spleen

Unconjugated
Bilirubin

Hemoglobin

Figure 10-1. Basic physiology of hemolytic disease of the newborn. If Rh_o (D) antigen-bearing erythrocytes enter the maternal circulation, these antigens are recognized as foreign by the Rh_o (D) negative mother. If antigenic stimulation or an anamnestic response caused by anti-D occurs in subsequent pregnancies, high titers of anti-D are produced in the maternal circulation. These anti-D antibodies can cross the placental barrier and attach to the D positive erythrocytes of the fetus in the current pregnancy. These antibody-coated erythrocytes have a shortened survival and the fetus suffers from anemia. The bilirubin resulting from erythrocyte (hemoglobin) breakdown is excreted through the maternal circulation and does not injure the fetus.

dominantly of many nucleated erythrocytes into the fetal circulation. If increased erythropoiesis cannot compensate for erythrocyte destruction, a progressively severe anemia develops. This severe anemia may cause the fetus to develop cardiac failure with generalized edema (hydrops fetalis), resulting in death in utero. In newborn in-fants, severe anemia can produce heart failure shortly after birth.

Less severely affected infants continue after birth to experience erythrocyte destruction, which generates large quantities of unconjugated bilirubin. Before birth, unconjugated bilirubin is normally bound to albumin and forms conjugated bilirubin in the mother's liver through the action of the enzyme glucuronidase. The newborn infant's immature liver does not efficiently synthesize glucuronidase during the first few days of life. This results in low amounts of the enzyme in the newborn infant's circulation. Additionally, the albumin, which is necessary to form conjugated bilirubin, is limited. This combination of factors in the newborn, who must excrete large quantities of bilirubin resulting from excessive hemolysis, can produce the threat of accumulation of free bilirubin in lipid-rich tissue of the central nervous system. Total plasma bilirubin levels approaching 20 mg/dL can cause mental retardation or death.

The Mechanism of Antibody Transfer from Mother to Fetus

The transfer of antibodies from the maternal circulation to the fetal circulation occurs through the placenta. The only immunoglobulin that is selectively transported to the fetus is IgG. Although the fetus produces some IgG, IgG in cord serum is derived almost entirely from the maternal circulation. Among the five classes of immunoglobulins in humans, only IgG is found in cord blood in a concentration equivalent to the concentration found in maternal blood. The other immunoglobulin classes, such as IgM, are either present in much lower concentrations in the newborn than in the mother or entirely absent.

In the first 12 weeks of gestation, only small amounts of IgG are synthesized. This concentration of IgG continues to rise until birth. Evidence suggests that the levels of the IgG subclass, IgG1, rise at an earlier stage of gestation than IgG3 subclass levels. At birth, IgG1 levels are higher than those of IgG3 compared to maternal concentrations. The fetal concentrations of IgG2 are distinctly lower than those of the other IgG subclasses.

The mechanism by which IgG passes through the placenta has not been definitely established; however, each immunoglobulin class is characterized by its heavy polypeptide chain. Therefore, the structure of IgG responsible for transplacental passage should reside in the (γ) chain. Most re-

search on the subject of transplacental passage supports the hypothesis that all IgG subclasses are capable of crossing the placental barrier between mother and fetus.

Blood Systems Involved in Causing HDN

The categories of HDN include virtually every blood group antibody that can occur as IgG (Table 10-1). In a survey of antibodies that have caused HDN, over 70 different antibodies were identified. Based on specific IgG antibody type, the causes of HDN in descending order of severity are:

1. Anti-D, either alone or in combination with anti-C or anti-E.
2. Other Rh antibodies, such as anti-c.
3. Other blood group system antibodies, such as anti-Kell, anti-Duffy, and anti-Kidd.
4. Antibody A and anti-B.

High titers of anti-A, B of the IgG type in group O mothers commonly cause a mild hemolytic disease of the newborn in approximately 1 in 150 births. Rarely is this form of HDN severe. This is chiefly because the A and B antigens are not fully expressed in the erythrocytes of the fetus and newborn.

Until the early 1970s, anti-D was the most frequent cause of moderate or severe forms of HDN. Before modern treatment for Rh_o(D)-induced HDN prevention, anti-D, either alone or in combination with anti-C, accounted for approximately 93% of the cases of non-ABO HDN. Other forms of HDN related to the Rh blood group system, such as anti-c and anti-E, or anti-C and anti-e, accounted for about 6% of the cases. Only a small fraction, approximately 1%, of the cases of HDN was caused by antibodies outside the Rh system, such as anti-Kell or anti-Duffy. Since the development of modern treatment, however, against immunization to the Rh_o(D) antigen, the frequency of HDN caused by anti-D has significantly decreased.

Table 10-1. Antibodies Causing HDN*

Blood Group System	Related Antigens	Severity of HDN
Rh	D	Mild to severe
	C	Mild to moderate
	c	Mild to severe
	E	Mild to severe
	e	Mild to moderate
Kell	K	Mild to severe
	k	Mild to severe
Duffy	Fy^a	Mild to severe
	Fy^b	Not implicated in HDN
Kidd	Jk^a	Mild to severe
	Jk^b	Mild to severe
Lutheran	Lu^a	Mild
	Lu^b	Mild
Lewis	Le^a	Rare
MNSs	M	Mild to severe
	N	Mild
	S	Mild to severe
	s	Mild to severe
P	PP_1P^k (Tj^a)	Mild to severe
I	Not a proven cause of HDN	
Xg	Xg^a	Mild
Colton	Co^a	Severe
	Co^{a-b}	Mild
Cartwright	Yt^a	Moderate to severe
	Yt^b	Mild
Diego	Di^a	Mild to severe
	Di^b	Mild to severe
Wright	Wr^a	Severe
Other antigens	At^a	Mild
	Batty	Mild
	Becker	Mild
	Berrens	Mild
	Biles	Moderate
	En^a	Moderate
	Evans	Mild
	Ge	Mild
	Gonzales	Mild
	Good	Severe
	Heibel	Moderate
	Hunt	Mild
	Jobbins	Mild
	Jr^a	Mild
	Lan	Mild
	Radin	Moderate
	Rm	Mild
	Ven	Mild
	Zd	Moderate

* Modified from Weinstein, L.: Irregular Antibodies Causing Hemolytic Disease of the Newborn Clin. Obstet, Gynecol. *25*(2):321–332, 1982.

Mechanism of HDN

HDN results from the production of antibodies in the mother that have been stimulated by foreign antigens. These immune antibodies subsequently react with fetal antigens if the latter are present. Erythrocytic antigens and leukocyte and platelet antigens can all induce maternal immunization by the formation of IgG antibodies.

The actual production of antibodies depends on a variety of factors: the genetic makeup of an individual, the antigenicity of a specific antigen, and the actual amount of antigen introduced into the maternal circulation.

GENETIC MAKEUP

For antibody formation to take place, the mother must genetically lack the trait and the fetus must genetically possess the trait, which has been inherited from the father. This genetic inheritance expresses itself in the mother as her being negative for an antigen, whereas the fetus possesses the antigen.

IMMUNOGENICITY

Antigens vary in terms of the number of receptor sites on the erythrocyte membrane and their immunogenic strength. Certain antigens, such D, c, and Kell, are known to be very potent in stimulating the immune system.

TRANSPLACENTAL HEMORRHAGE

Transplacental hemorrhage (TPH) can occur at any stage of pregnancy. Immunization resulting from TPH can result from negligible doses during the first 6 months in utero; however, significant immunizing hemorrhage usually occurs during the third trimester or at delivery. Fetal erythrocytes can also enter the maternal circulation as the result of physical trauma due to an injury, abortion, ectopic pregnancy, amniocentesis or normal delivery. Abruptio placentae, cesarean section, and manual removal of the placenta are often associated with a considerable increase in TPH. A significant fetal-maternal hemorrhage is considered to be 30 mL. or greater; evidence exists to support the theory that a minimal dose for inducing a primary immunization is probably less than 0.1 mL for some of the more immunogenic antigens.

ASSESSMENT OF HDN

Prenatal Testing

The following procedures are generally used in prenatal testing under various conditions:

1. ABO blood typing.
2. Rh testing for D and D^u.
3. Alloantibody screening; if negative, it should be repeated again at 34 weeks of gestation.
4. Alloantibody identification, if the antibody screening test is positive.
5. Antibody titer, if an alloantibody is present.
6. Amniocentesis.

AMNIOCENTESIS

Amniocentesis is an analysis of fluid from the amniotic cavity obtained by the transabdominal insertion of a needle. This analysis provides the physician with an assessment of fetal development and well-being. Using a prediction table, an estimate of cord hemoglobin concentration can be determined based on the optical density of the amniotic fluid during gestation. Other factors, such as genetic disorders and chromosomal abnormalities, can be determined through amniotic fluid.

Some of the clinical criteria used in deciding to perform an amniocentesis include the following:

1. If a previous infant had HDN, amniocentesis may be performed as early as 28 weeks of gestation, even if the antibody titer remains constant. If a previous child was severely afflicted, an amniocentesis may be performed as early as the 22nd week of gestation.
2. When the maternal antibody level accelerates before the 34th week of gestation.

The severity of hemolysis is related to the amount of bilirubin in the amniotic fluid as measured by spectrophotometry. The optical density (OD) of normal amniotic fluid forms a smooth curve at different wavelengths over the range of 400 to 600 nm. According to Liley, the OD of amniotic fluid at 450 to 460 nm in normal pregnancy is about 0.05 at 30 weeks and falls to about 0.02 at term. Fluid from an infant with severe HDN has a greatly increased optical density with a peak at 450 to 460, the so-called bilirubin bulge. There is a tendency for the bilirubin to decrease in mild cases of HDN as the pregnancy advances.

At 450 nm, the difference between the infant's OD and a baseline value is determined. This value is plotted on a Liley graph. On this graph, three zones are associated with the status of the severity of HDN. Zone 1 represents an unaffected state in which the fetus is considered not to be in danger. Zone 2 indicates that the fetus needs monitoring and the amniotic fluid should be retested. Zone 3 indicates that the fetus is in danger.

Amniotic fluid can also be analyzed to aid in making a decision regarding early delivery of the infant. Absorbance at 650 nm may be useful as a screen or as part of a battery of lung maturity estimates. If a fetus is under 34 weeks of gestation or immature for its gestational age, an intrauterine transfusion may be indicated rather than premature delivery.

Postpartum Testing

In addition to the clinical signs of anemia and jaundice in the newborn (Fig. 10-2), various laboratory procedures are helpful in addition to procedures 1 through 5 listed previously under Prenatal Testing. These postpartum procedures may be useful in determining the presence and assessing the severity of HDN, or quantitating the extent of fetal-maternal hemorrhage:

1. Hemoglobin and hematocrit determination of cord or infant blood.
2. Serum bilirubin of cord or infant blood.
3. ABO grouping and Rh typing of cord or infant blood.

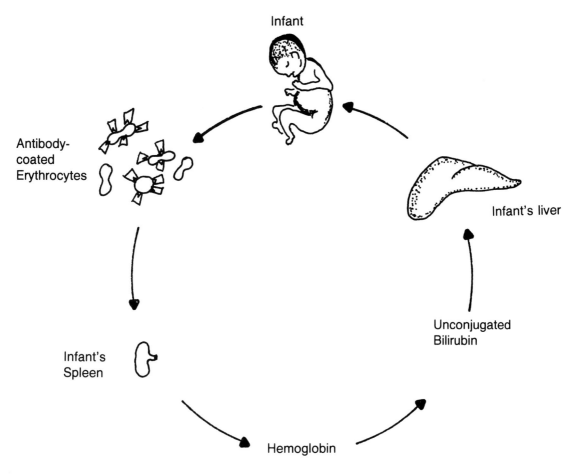

Figure 10-2. Postpartum effects of hemolytic disease of the newborn. After delivery, the accumulation of bilirubin can severely harm an infant. The liver of the newborn does not produce glucuronyl transferase, which is necessary for converting bilirubin to an excretable form. Consequently, bilirubin accumulates, and if not removed will be deposited in lipid-rich tissues such as the brain. Excessive bilirubin in the circulation also produces jaundice.

4. Direct antiglobulin test of cord or infant blood.
5. Antibody elution and identification, if the DAT is positive.
6. Peripherael blood smear.
7. The D^u rosette test.
8. The Kleihauer-Betke test.

Hemoglobin Determination

Most neonatologists refer to the cord hemoglobin as the reference criterion of the severity of the hemolytic process. The normal range for cord hemoglobin during the first day of life is 14.5 to 22.5 g/dL. Moderately afflicted infants suffering from HDN may have cord hemoglobins ranging from 10.5 g/dL to 14.5 g/dL. The cord hemoglobin levels in severely afflicted infants can range from 3.4 g/dL to 10.4 g/dL. Most infants with levels of cord hemoglobin concentration within the normal range do not require exchange transfusion.

Bilirubin Assay

An analysis of bilirubin is valuable in determining the severity of HDN because a relationship exists between cord bilirubin concentration and the severity of HDN. This relationship is less closely correlated than the relationship between cord hemoglobin levels and severity.

The normal infant's cord bilirubin level ranges from 0.7 to 3.5 mg/dL. A cord bilirubin of 4 mg/dL or more may be an indication for exchange transfusion. Severe cases of HDN frequently have cord bilirubin values in excess of 6.0 mg/dL.

DIRECT ANTIGLOBULIN TESTING (DAT)

About 40% of infants born with a positive DAT require no treatment; others need exchange transfusions to prevent kernicterus. The presence of a positive DAT is associated with hemolytic anemias, including HDN.

ABO AND RH TESTING

The relationship among specific ABO groups and Rh types and HDN is explained in the appropriate section of each discussion on HDN of various etiologies in this chapter. Problems in blood typing specific to the neonate or in the presence of a positive DAT are discussed in the procedures section for each test.

ANTIBODY ELUTION AND IDENTIFICATION

The coating of erythrocytes with antibodies can frequently be demonstrated through the use of an elution technique that removes the antibodies from the erythrocytic membrane. The quantity of antibody on fetal erythrocytes is not highly correlated with either the infant's cord hemoglobin concentration or the cord serum bilirubin concentration.

PERIPHERAL BLOOD SMEAR

Hypochromic erythrocytes and spherocytes are commonly seen in HDN. The number of immature nucleated erythrocytes is helpful in assessing the erythropoietic response to hemolysis.

D^u ROSETTE TEST

The D^u Rosette test (see Chapter 14) was developed and reported by Sebring and Polesky in 1982. This test will detect fetal-maternal hemorrhage of approximately 10 mL in the maternal circulation.

The principle of the test uses D$^+$ indicator erythrocytes to form identifiable rosettes around individuals D$^+$ fetal cells that may be in maternal circulation. The indicator erythrocytes bind to the free second antigenic determinant of the anti-D antibody, thus forming rosettes. Because this is a qualitative test, positive results must be followed by a quantitative procedure such as the Kleihauer-Betke test. This is particularly important in cases where D^u positive infant erythrocytes react as strongly as D$^+$ erythrocytes, or, if the mother is D^u positive, the rosette test is also positive.

The D^u rosette procedure has advantages over the conventional D^u test. The risk of false negatives is too great for the D^u test to be the only method used to detect significant fetal-maternal hemorrhage. The incidence of false negative results with an approximately 30 mL hemorrhage is 12%. Additionally, it is difficult to recognize Rh positive cells by the D^u procedure unless they constitute at least 2% of the total number of erythrocytes present.

KLEIHAUER-BETKE TEST

The Kleihauer-Betke test can detect a fetal-maternal hemorrhage as small as 7.5 mL of packed erythrocytes or 15 mL of whole blood. This procedure tests for fetal hemoglobin rather than the presence of erythrocytes. Fetal erythrocytes contain 53 to 95% hemoglobin F.

The principle of this procedure is that adult hemoglobin (hemoglobin A) is soluble in acid, while fetal hemoglobin (hemoglobin F) is insoluble at this low ph and not eluted. The disadvantages of this procedure include false positive results in cases of Rh negative mothers with high levels of fetal hemogloblin due to sickle trait or the hereditary persistence of fetal hemoglobin and the subjective nature of test interpretation.

HDN CAUSED BY ABO INCOMPATIBILITY

Etiology

In the White population, in 15% of all pregnancies, the mother has blood group O and the baby either blood group A or B. Although ABO incompatibilities between mother and baby occur frequently and represent a common form of HDN, the symptoms are usually mild and may not be clinically obvious. In cases where jaundice develops within 24 hours of birth, the incidence of HDN due to ABO incompatibility ranges from 1 in 70 to 1 in 180 with an estimated average of 1 in 150 births. The most frequent form of ABO incompatibility occurs when the mother is group O and the baby is group A or group B, usually group A. Although anti-A and anti-B are present in the absence of their corresponding antigens as environmentally stimulated (IgM) antibodies, infrequent IgG forms may be responsible for HDN caused by ABO incompatibility. Anti A,B can also be found in group O persons. This IgG antibody reacts with both A and B antigens. Consequently, it is primarily the antibody responsible for this type of HDN.

GENETIC FREQUENCY

The actual frequency of incompatible antigens can be determined by multiplying the maternal phenotype O with a frequency in the White population of 0.44 by the fetal gene frequency for A (0.27). This results in a chance combination of 0.12 or 12%. If the mother is group O, frequency 0.44 times the gene frequency for group B (0.07) produces a chance combination of 0.03 or 3%.

Signs, Symptoms, and Physiology

If a mother's first baby is mildly affected, subsequent ABO incompatible babies may be clinically unaffected; however, if the first child is severely affected, it is likely that subsequent ABO incompatible infants will also be severely affected. In the Black population, HDN caused by anti-B seems to be more severe than HDN caused by anti-A.

Anti-A and anti-B antibodies are usually 19S (IgM) in character and are unable to pass through the placental barrier. If antibodies of the IgG class are present, they are able to pass through the placental barrier.

The generally mild nature of this form of HDN may be due to several factors: fewer A and B antigen sites on the fetal/newborn erythrocytes, weaker antigen strength of fetal/newborn A and B antigens, and competition for anti-A and anti-B between tissues as well as erythrocytes. The number and strength of A and B antigen sites on fetal erythrocytes are less than on adult erythrocytic membranes. Newborn erythrocytes of blood group A_1 have an average of 300,000 A antigen sites compared to adult erythrocytes of blood group A_1, which have an average of 900,000 A antigen sites. Although A and B antigens are detectable before birth, the strength of the A and B antigens does not increase during fetal life; however, these antigens do gain in strength shortly after birth. Additionally, A and B substances are not confined to the red cells, so that only a small fraction of IgG anti-A and anti-B which crosses the placenta combines with the infant's erythrocytes.

Laboratory Diagnosis

Hemolytic disease caused by ABO incompatibility is clinically mild, with jaundice most frequently developing within 24 hours after birth. The laboratory profile of this form of HDN consists of:

1. ABO grouping of mother and baby
2. Direct antiglobulin test.
3. Antibody elution testing.
4. Hemoglobin assay.
5. Bilirubin assay.
6. Peripheral blood smear.

ABO GROUPING OF MOTHER AND BABY

ABO grouping most commonly reveals the mother to be group O and the baby to be group A or possibly group B.

DIRECT ANTIGLOBULIN TESTING

A DAT performed on cord or infant blood may be either negative or weakly positive. The lack of consistency in this test may be due to a weak antigen-antibody interaction which causes antibody to be removed during the washing phase of the DAT, an antibody titer that may be too low to be detectable, extensive intravascular hemolysis of coated erythrocytes, or variation in fetal erythrocyte antigen development.

ANTIBODY ELUTION

Antibody elution of cord blood may reveal the presence of immune anti-A or anti-B. An eluate is often more useful than the direct antiglobulin test in assessing HDN caused by ABO incompatibility. The demonstration of antibodies using an elution technique is positive in about one third of cases.

HEMOGLOBIN DETERMINATION

Hemoglobin may be slightly lower than in ABO compatible infants. Normal hemoglobin concentrations of cord and venous blood samples from newborn infants range from 15 to 20 g/dL.

BILIRUBIN ASSAY

The bilirubin assay may exceed the normal values of cord total serum bilirubin of 1 to 3 mg/mL. Hyperbilirubinemia may also be seen in conditions such as premature birth or maternal diabetes. HDN is judged to be clinically significant if the peak bilirubin level reaches 12 mg/dL or more.

PERIPHERAL BLOOD SMEAR MORPHOLOGY

This may reveal an anemia with erythrocyte abnormalities such as hypochromia, microspherocytosis, and reticulocytosis. Immature nucleated erythrocytes may be seen in small numbers.

Treatment

Except in the extremely rare cases of severe HDN produced by ABO incompatibility, phototherapy is the usual treatment. Phototherapy uses ultraviolet light that reacts with bilirubin near the surface of the skin. This process slowly decomposes/converts bilirubin into a nontoxic isomer, photobilirubin, which is transported in the plasma to the liver. There the molecules are rapidly excreted in the form of bile without being conjugated.

The need for exchange transfusion is rare in cases of ABO incompatibility because of the generally mild nature of this type of HDN. One of the risks of exchange transfusion in these cases is the triggering of yet more hemolysis. These hemolytic transfusion reactions may result from transfusing a baby with adult A or B cells that will interact with circulating maternal IgG anti-A,B in the baby's circulation.

HDN CAUSED BY Rh INCOMPATIBILITY

Etiology

In the early 1930s, Diamond, Blackfan and Baty made the classic observations that icterus gravis, hydrops fetalis, and anemia in the newborn represented different grades of clinical severity of the same unknown process. Unfortunately, they did not suspect that this syndrome was a manifestation of hemolytic anemia affecting the fetus. This process was originally referred to as erythroblastosis fetalis.

In 1938, Darrow suggested that this process was a hemolytic anemia caused by the transfer of immune bodies from the mother to the fetus. Because she had no data to support her hypothesis, she incorrectly selected fetal hemoglobin as the causative agent.

The developmental work on the Rh factor conducted by the major investigators, Landsteiner and Wiener, led Levine to establish that the Rh antigen was the immunizing agent in the blood and/or tissues of the fetus. He speculated that the Rh factor was not present in the mother but inherited by the fetus from the father. In 1941, Levine concluded, based on experimental and case study data, that the majority of cases of hemolysis in the fetus/newborn resulted from isoimmunization of an Rh negative mother by the Rh positive erythrocytes of the fetus.

Types of Responses to Rh Immunization

The immunization of Rh (D and D^u) mothers depends on both the dosage of Rh (D) positive erythrocytes and the mother's ability to respond to these foreign D antigens. About one third of all Rh (D) negative persons are classified as nonresponders. Nonresponders fail to form anti-D despite intentional repeated injections of Rh (D) positive erythrocytes.

In addition to the nonresponder status, two other categories of individuals exist: responders and hyperresponders. Responders and hyperresponders differ in terms of the type and quantity of anti-D antibody that they produce. Responders form anti-G, a component of anti-D. Hyperresponders produce extremely high titers of both IgM and IgG types of anti-D. Some hyperresponders may additionally produce antibodies to antigens to which they were never exposed. This hyperresponsive condition is referred to as augmentation. The Rh-augmented immune response is responsible for very rare cases of primary Rh immunization.

The normal pattern of immunization in an Rh_o (D) negative mother involves primary immunization due to a previously incompatible Rh (D) positive pregnancy or blood transfusion which stimulates the production of low titered anti-D, predominantly of the IgM class. Subsequent antigenic stimulation such as fetal-maternal hemorrhage in a woman pregnant with an Rh (D) positive fetus elicits a secondary (anamnestic) response, characterized by the predominance of increasing titers of anti-D of the IgG class.

Levine observed as early as 1943 that a condition of HDN due to ABO incompatibility between the mother and fetus reduced the chance of maternal immunization to the D antigen. Rh negative women with group O blood were more strongly protected than Rh women of other blood types to immu-

nization by the D antigen. In the most representative cases, a group O Rh negative mother pregnant with a group A Rh positive fetus is less likely to develop HDN due to anti-D. This situation exists presumably because the fetal erythrocytes that enter the maternal circulation contain both the A antigen and the D antigen. These cells react with the anti A,B in the maternal circulation and are destroyed before they can immunize the mother to the D antigen.

This observation led to the pioneering experiments which demonstrated that D negative individuals failed to produce anti-D antibodies after repeated injections of D positive cells that had been coated with anti-D antibodies in vitro. As a result of this work, the development and clinical use of Rh IgG in the prevention of HDN due to anti-D became a reality.

Genetic Frequency

Before the advent of modern prophylaxis to Rh_o (D), anti-D was the most frequent cause of severe HDN. Based on gene frequency, it is fairly easy to see why this situation existed.

When the homozygous Rh negative mother's genotype dd is crossed with a father's genotype of DD, the offspring will all have the genotype Dd, phenotype Rh positive. In cases where the father has a heterozygous genotype (Dd), a 50% probability exists for the offspring to be phenotypically Rh_o positive with half of the offspring having the genotype Dd and the other half having the genotype dd.

If the frequency of antigens in the general White population is taken into consideration, the theoretic probability that an Rh_o (D−) woman (0.16) with an Rh_o (D+) husband (0.84) will produce an Rh_o (D+) fetus is 0.134, or 13%. In reality, factors such as the ABO status of the mother and baby and the volume of transplacental hemorrhage will affect the rate of immunization in pregnant women without a history of prior pregnancies or blood transfusions. With the established rate of immunization, Rh_o (D) negative women who did not receive immunosuppressive therapy after their first Rh_o (D) positive infant and who are pregnant for the second time may demonstrate anti-D and have an affected infant.

Signs, Symptoms, and Physiology

Except in rare instances, the firstborn Rh positive infant of an Rh negative mother seldom shows clinical signs of HDN and may simply have a positive direct antiglobulin test. If severe HDN is observed in a firstborn RH_o (D) positive infant, it must always be suspected that the mother was previously immunized before the pregnancy by means of a previous blood transfusion, abortion, etc. Although the second Rh_o (D) can be severely affected, subsequent incompatible infants have no tendency for the disorder to become progressively more severe.

When the mother has been previously immunized and subsequently produces anti-D of the IgG type in response to a D positive fetus, the following activities occur: the passage of IgG Rh antibodies into the fetal circulation induces erythrocyte hemolysis and anemia of varying degrees of severity. This anemia may produce heart failure and hypoxia in the unborn child, causing stillbirth or rapid accumulation of bilirubin in the newborn.

THE EFFECT OF ANTIBODY TITER

Once an alloantibody such as anti-D has been identified in maternal serum, a rising antibody titer is evidence of a presently active immune response. The severity of HDN, however, does not correlate well with maternal anti-D antibody titer.

The discrepancy observed between the severity of HDN and the antibody titer may be due to differences in the nature of IgG antibodies. Fetal hemolysis is essentially due to antibodies of the IgG1 and IgG3 subclasses.

THE ROLE OF ANTIBODY SUBCLASSES

Antibodies of the IgG1, IgG2, IgG3, and IgG4 subclasses are all generally believed to be able to pass through the placental barrier. Because IgG subclasses have different properties such as their rate of trans-fer across the placenta and complement fixation, their hemolytic capacity varies.

Fetal hemolysis is primarily due to antibodies of the IgG1 and IgG3 subclasses. When IgG1 antibodies are absent, a lower frequency of severe forms of HDN is observed. The frequency of severe forms of HDN also decreases if IgG1 is found in association with IgG3. The molecular characteristics of IgG1 and IgG3 are undoubtedly responsible for their role in the hemolytic process.

The IgG1 antibodies transfer through the placenta earlier, have less difficulty in transfer, and have a longer half-life than IgG3 antibodies. Because IgG1 antibodies cross the placenta with greater ease and earlier (approximately 2 months before IgG3 antibodies), they are exposed to erythrocyte antigens for a longer period. This makes IgG1 antibodies more competitive in binding to erythrocytic antigens than IgG3 antibodies. Although both IgG1 and IgG3 antibodies bind to macrophages, IgG3 antibodies have a better binding and are more hemolytic when linked to erythrocytes.

Gm ALLOTYPES OF ANTI-D ANTIBODIES

A greater understanding of HDN due to anti-D has resulted from the accidental discovery of the Gm allotypic markers on the heavy chain of the IgG molecule. The structural differences among the immunoglobulin classes themselves and among the allotypes of IgG are situated at the level of the Fc fragment. Because of its placental transfer site and its macrophage binding site, the Fc fragment is responsible for the hemolytic properties of the anti-D antibodies.

In an analysis of the correlation between the severity of HDN and the type of anti-D antibodies, greater hemolytic action occurs when the IgG1 subclass is present. The greatest proportion of clinically severe cases had not only the IgG1 anti-D antibody, but within this class the antibody population marked by the G1m(4) allotype.

In cases of anemia (cord blood hemoglobin of less than 10 g/dL), the presence of G1m(1) and G1m(4) allotypes has been observed; however, when cord bilirubin and other criteria are used, severe forms of HDN are significantly higher when the G1m(4) allotype is present than when it is absent. The severity of hemolysis is not affected by the presence or absence of other allotypes. The prognostic value of anti-D antibody titers during pregnancy could be enhanced by a study of the IgG subclasses and their allotypes.

Laboratory Diagnosis

PRENATAL ASSESSMENT

Prenatal testing in the case of Rh_o (D) negative mothers has some special considerations in addition to the procedures already discussed in the section on assessment of HDN.

A detectable antibody titer (see Chapter 14, Special Procedures) is rarely detectable before 28 weeks of gestation in the first immunizing pregnancy. When anti-D develops during the first pregnancy, it is most commonly detected at about the 35th week of gestation or later. The titer is usually low. Rarely is there a significant rise in the anti-D titer if a subsequent Rh_o (D) fetus is present. If anti-D is detected and identified, attention should be paid to the presence of other alloantibodies of the Rh system or other alloantibodies such as anti-Duffy, anti-Kidd, and anti-S, which are common secondary antibodies in Rh immunization.

Amniocentesis may be performed in cases where the serum titer of anti-D is 1:16 or higher with a history of a previous stillbirth due to anti-D, a serum titer of 32 or higher in a pregnant women with a history of a previous child who needed an exchange transfusion, or a progressive rise of anti-D to 1:64 without a history of an affected fetus or child. In such cases, an initial amniocentesis would be done at 24 to 28 weeks of gestation or 6 to 8 weeks before the gestational age of previous fetal loss due to Rh_o (D). Two sequential amniotic specimens are required to assess change in the status of the fetus. The noninvasive monocyte monolayer assay is also believed to be efficient in predicting which infants are at risk of severe HDN, thus reducing the number of amnionteses required.

POSTPARTUM ASSESSMENT

The identification of HDN due to anti-D is characterized by the following test results:

1. *Rh blood typing* with Rh_o (D) or D^u positive results of the cord or infant's blood show the mother as Rh_o (D) and D^u negative.
2. *Direct antiglobulin test* is positive and the mother demonstrates a positive indirect antiglobulin test with anti-D the identified antibody.
3. *Antibody elution* of cord blood cells reveals the presence of anti-D.
4. *Hemoglobin* levels of cord blood may be moderately to severely decreased. Levels ranging from 10.5 to 14.5/dL are seen in moderately afflicted infants, while levels ranging from 3.4 to 10.4 g/dL are seen in severe cases.
5. *Bilirubin* levels on cord serum range from 3.5 mg/dL to more than 6.0 mg/dL in the most severely afflicted infants.
6. *Peripheral blood smears* demonstrate the presence of immature erythrocytes with a range of over 5 or 6 per 100 leukocytes.

Treatment

PRENATAL TREATMENT

Plasma Exchange. Plasma exchange is a therapeutic tool in the treatment of immune-mediated disease. An application of this can be in the treatment of pregnant women in whom a high antibody titer, coupled with a past history of delivering a stillborn infant due to HDN, indicates a significant possibility of another fetal loss due to HDN. Although results of this technique indicate that plasma exchange is a useful therapeutic tool in the treatment of high-risk HDN pregnancies, plasma exchange is not accepted by many clinicians for routine use. Some of the disadvantages include high cost, discomfort and inconvenience to the patient, and the non-selective removal of all plasma proteins.

Intraperitoneal and Intrauterine Transfusion. Severe intrauterine hemolysis in the fetus can be treated by intraperitoneal fetal transfusion (IPT) or intrauterine transfusion. In this procedure, blood is usually selected on the basis of compatibility with maternal serum and the matching of donor and maternal erythrocytes with respect to the antigen causing the hemolysis. Because of the high mortality in infants with severe HDN born before the thirtieth week of gestation, premature delivery may not be an option. Therefore, blood transfusion may be the only choice if the infant is to be saved.

One of the risks of transfusion is the introduction of other antigens into the circulation. Enhanced antibody production has been observed after intrauterine transfusion of common nonrhesus antigens which may also cause HDN, for example, Kidd (Jk) and Duffy (Fy). The risk may be greater for intravascular fetal transfusions in which a larger dose of antigen enters directly and more rapidly into the fetal vascular system, in contrast with the gradual absorption of antigen in IPT. Destruction of fetal erythrocytes could depend on whether the corresponding antigen had been inherited from the father. It has been suggested that the donor blood lack the Rh_o, Kell, Kidd, Duffy, and S antigens whenever any of these are absent from the maternal cells, even if the father also lacks them.

Antenatal Rh Immune Globulin. In 1900, Von Dungern initiated the first step in the prevention of HDN, when he discovered that active immunization is suppressed by a passive antibody. Forty years later, based on the pioneering work on the Rh_o factor by Landsteiner and Weiner, Levine demonstrated that a form of HDN was the direct result of an Rh_o incompatibility between an Rh_o negative mother and an Rh_o positive fetus. Later, three independent research teams demonstrated that a passive antibody, Rh IgG, could protect most Rh_o negative mothers from becoming immunized after the delivery of a Rh_o positive infant or similar obstetric conditions.

In 1968, Rh IgG was licensed for administration in the United States. Since that time, a dramatic decrease in the incidence of anti-D HDN has taken place. Although complete elimination may never occur because of the cases in which anti-D is formed prior to delivery, all pregnant Rh negative women should receive Rh IgG even if the Rh status of the fetus is unknown because fetal D antigen is present in fetal erythrocytes as early as 38 days from conception.

Administration of Rh immune globulin (Rh IgG) at 28 weeks gestation (antenatal) has decreased the incidence of primary immunization in Rh_o (D) negative women to 0.07%. In addition to this, the use of Rh IgG after conditions such as abortion, ectopic pregnancy, or antepartum hemorrhage has contributed to the decreased incidence of D antigen immunization. Antenatal treatment is most effective if initiated by the 28th week of gestation.

In the United States in 1980, more than 203,000 Rh negative primiparous women gave birth. In the absence of an antepartum program, among the future second births of these women, an estimated 300 infants will have Rh HDN attributable to antepartum sensitization. In about 2% of cases, an Rh negative mother is immunized by the time her first Rh positive infant is delivered.

Questions continue to remain concerning the cost-effectiveness of antepartum administration of Rh IgG. The major objection to this mode of treatment is the cost associated with the treatment of all pregnant Rh negative women who may be pregnant with an Rh positive fetus. Opponents to antenatal administration of Rh IgG cite that the value would be evident only if the mother conceived another Rh positive fetus or received an Rh positive transfusion. Other clinicians feel that the timing of administration and size of the dose need more research.

POSTPARTUM TREATMENT

Exchange Transfusion. Infants who are severely afflicted with HDN may require an exchange transfusion shortly after birth. An exchange transfusion removes bilirubin and circulating maternal antibodies from an infant's plasma and replaces antibody-coated erythrocytes with compatible donor cells.

Several criteria may be applied in determining whether or not an exchange transfusion is warranted. If the cord bilirubin is 5 mg/dL at birth, with the plasma bilirubin rising to above 11.5 mg/dL at 12 hours after birth and above 16 mg/dL after 24 hours, the need for an exchange transfusion is indicated. If the rate of increase in plasma bilirubin is more than 0.5 mg/dL/hour or anemia (hemoglobin below 14 g/dL) exists, exchange transfusion may be necessary. Prematurity is also a consideration. In premature infants, the threshold for bilirubin toxicity occurs at lower levels, along with decreased albumin binding capacity as well as a higher risk of acidosis, hypoglycemia, hypothermia, hypoxia, and sepsis.

The selection of blood, appropriate anticoagulants, and crossmatch procedures for exchange transfusions are discussed in the previous procedures section. The actual procedure of transfusion takes place by way of umbilical vessels.

The immediate effectiveness of a two-volume exchange transfusion is 45 to 50%; however, re-equilibration between bilirubin in plasma and extravascular bilirubin takes place. The plasma bilirubin tends to rise or rebound after an exchange transfusion, partly because of the entry of bilirubin from the extravascular spaces and partly because of continued production of bilirubin from residual maternal antibody coating newly released erythrocytes. If, following the first exchange transfusion, bilirubin threatens to exceed 20 mg/dL in a full-term infant, subsequent exchanges may be necessary. Additional exchanges are less effective in controlling the bilirubin level than are initial transfusions because they mainly remove bilirubin in the infant's plasma rather than removing the infant's Rh_o (D) positive erythrocytes. Phototherapy is used as an adjunct therapy in this situation.

Postpartum Prevention of HDN Caused by Anti-D. The frequency of HDN caused by anti-D has declined dramatically in the United States since the introduction of widespread postpartum administration of Rh immune globulin (Rh IgG) (Fig. 10-3). In 1968, Rh IgG began to become available to postpartum Rh negative women who had delivered an Rh positive infant. In a relatively short time, the incidence of immunization with the demonstration of anti-D dramatically dropped from 8% after the first pregnancy, with an additional 8% developing anti-D during their second pregnancy,

to 1 or 2%. Although postpartum administration of Rh IgG averts sensitization in most Rh_o (D) negative women with D positive incompatible pregnancies, it cannot help the 1 or 2% of mothers who are immunized due to significant prenatal fetal-maternal hemorrhage.

RELATED LABORATORY PROCEDURES. Up to 50% of Rh_o negative mothers with an incompatible fetus may demonstrate varying quantities of fetal erythrocytes after delivery (postpartum). One to 2% of women who received Rh IgG at the termination of their previous pregnancy have detectable Rh antibodies on delivery of a subsequent Rh positive infant. A major cause of these failures is the administration of inadequate amounts of Rh IgG. Various laboratory techniques can be used to detect the extent of fetal-maternal hemorrhage, such as the D^u rosette test, the Kleihauer-Betke acid elution test, an enzyme-linked antiglobulin test, or flow cytometry. A single vial of Rh IgG is sufficient to compensate for up to 30 mL of D antigen-bearing fetal erythrocytes.

With an assay such as the Kleihauer-Betke test, the number of vials of Rh IgG can be determined. In this procedure, the volume of fetal-maternal hemorrhage can be calculated by multiplying the percentage (%) of fetal cells by a factor of 50. The volume of fetal blood is divided by 30 to determine the number of vials of IgG needed.

Example:

1. Kleihauer-Betke reported as 3%
2. 3% × 50* = 150 mL of fetal blood
3. $\dfrac{150 \text{ mL}}{30}$ = 5.0 = 6** doses of Rh IgG

*Factor of 50 = 5000 mL (estimated maternal blood volume) × 1/100 (%)
**If the number to the right of the decimal point is less than 5, round down and add one vial. If the number to the right of the decimal point is 5 or greater, round up to the next number and then add one vial. Example: an answer of 2.4 will yield 3 doses and an answer of 2.9 will yield 4 doses.

CRITERIA FOR THE ADMINISTRATION OF Rh IgG. For prophylactic treatment using Rh IgG to be effective, appropriate amounts must be administered under the following general conditions to previously unsensi-

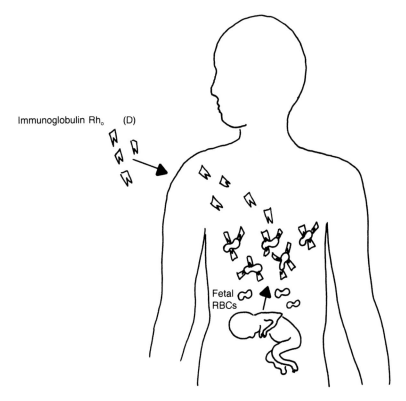

Figure 10-3. Prevention of a primary immune response to an Rh$_o$ (D) incompatible fetus. Prevention of sensitization of an Rh$_o$ (D) negative mother to an Rh$_o$ (D) positive can be accomplished by the antenatal or postnatal adminstration of immune globulin-D. The passively administered anti-D binds with the D antigen of the fetal erythrocytes. These cells are subsequently phagocytized and removed from the maternal circulation without foreign antigen recognition by the mother's immune system.

tized Rh (D) negative women within 72 hours of delivery or obstetric intervention:

1. After delivery of an Rh (D) positive infant.
2. After amniocentesis, abortion, miscarriage, or ectopic pregnancy.
3. Before delivery in selected cases (antenatal).

The laboratory criteria for Rh IgG administration are:

1. The mother is D and D^u negative.
2. The screening test for alloantibodies is negative for anti-D antibody.
3. The infant is D or D^u positive. In obstetric cases where the Rh cannot be determined, it must be assumed that this criteria has been met.

4. The direct antiglobulin test on cord cells or infant's cells, if available, is negative. If a positive DAT test result is obtained, an elution technique should be used to establish that anti-D is not the coating antibody.

OTHER BLOOD GROUP SYSTEMS

Etiology

Although the occurrence of HDN due to the D antigen has significantly decreased, the frequency of HDN due to other antigens has not and, in fact, is equally important to detect. Any fetal antigen that is recognized by the maternal immune system as foreign may prompt antigen-specific IgG production that can potentially result in fetal erythrocyte destruction. More than 40 antigens have been identified in cases of HDN. Sensitization to antigens of blood group systems other than ABO and Rh is reported to account for as high as 5% of all neonatal immune hemolytic disease. Although many of the cases of HDN caused by antibodies other than anti-D have been generally reported as clinically mild, some severe forms have been noted.

Signs, Symptoms, and Physiology

The frequency of various types of HDN due to alloantibodies reflects the antigen incidence in the general population. The developmental time of an antigen on fetal erythrocytes is another major determinant of its ability to stimulate immunization or react with corresponding maternal antibody.

RH ANTIGENS OTHER THAN D

Anti-c is less severe than anti-D. In severe cases, the cord hemoglobin average is 7.5 g/dL (rare). Most cases are in the range of 13 gm/dL. A history of previous blood transfusion is present in a substantial proportion of cases.

KELL ANTIGENS

Kell (K) antigen can be found to react as strongly on fetal erythrocytes of 10 weeks gestation and later as on adult erythrocytes. Cellano (k) is clearly detectable as early as 6 to 7 weeks of gestation. Kp^a can be detected as early as 16 weeks of gestation and as strongly as on adult erythrocytes.

Sensitization to subgroups (antithetical antigens of the Kell system (Kp^a, Kp^b, Js^a, and Js^b) has been reported to occur only occasionally and to result in mild HDN. Although anti Kp^b is generally reported to produce only mild hemolysis, cases of severe hemolysis have been reported.

DUFFY ANTIGENS

Both Fy^a and Fy^b have been found to be well developed during intrauterine life. At the earliest, Fy^a has been reported in a fetus

of 6 weeks of gestation and Fy^b in one of 6 ½ weeks. In these few cases, fetal erythrocytes have a weaker reaction than adult erythrocytes. At the twelfth week of gestation, Fy^a and Fy^b antigens were found on fetal erythrocytes in the same frequency and strength as on adult erythrocytes.

KIDD ANTIGENS

Kidd blood group antigens have been found to be well developed during intrauterine life. The Jk^b antigen has been found in fetuses as early as 6 to 7 weeks of gestation and Jk^a has been detected beginning at the tenth week of gestation. Both the Jk^a and Jk^b antigens occur in the same frequency and strength on fetal erythrocytes as on adult erythrocytes.

LEWIS ANTIGENS

Lewis antibodies are almost invariably IgM. It is rare to find an IgG Lewis antibody by indirect antiglobin test. Cases of HDN due to Lewis antigens are rare. One case of mild HDN and another case of a potent IgG anti-Le^a in cord serum have been reported. In the latter case, the cord bilirubin was 4.6 mg/dL and a positive direct antiglobulin test was obtained; however, the case was diagnosed as an ABO incompatibility. The anti-Le^a was not identified as contributing to the HDN caused by the ABO incompatibility.

LUTHERAN ANTIGENS

Antigens Lu^a and Lu^b have been reported as being more poorly developed on fetal erythrocytes than on adult erythrocytes, both in frequency and in strength. The Lu^a antigen was found at the earliest in a fetus of 14 weeks gestation and Lu^b was found in two cases at 10 weeks of gestation. The failure of these antigens to cause severe HDN is attributed to their weak expression during fetal development. Although the Lu^b antigen is of high frequency (99.8% in Whites), the antibody is IgM, IgA, or occasionally IgG.

In 1961, the first example of HDN due to Lu^a was identified. An example of mild HDN caused by anti-Lu^a in a primiparous woman has been reported. In this case, the bilirubin was 15.8 mg/dL when the infant was 4 days old and was treated with phototherapy.

OTHER ANTIGENS

Rare examples of other antigens, such as Lan, have been identified as the cause of mild HDN.

Antigen Lan belongs to the Langereis blood group system, a high incidence antigen. Anti-Lan is usually IgG and is stimulated by red cells. This antibody has been implicated in transfusion reactions and HDN.

Other examples of HDN have been attributed to the MNSs system. This system is normally a cold-reacting system; however, examples of anti-M and anti-U have been noted in rare cases of severe HDN which required exchange transfusion. Some of the cases, caused by anti-U, have been mild.

Laboratory Assessment

Laboratory assessment of HDN due to other blood group systems should follow the protocol outlined in the preceding sections on prenatal and postnatal testing. Evidence of an alloantibody in maternal serum, a positive direct anti-globulin test on cord cells, and the clinical symptoms of HDN are all important parameters in the assessment of this type of HDN.

Treatment

The prenatal treatment is in the manner described for $Rh_o(D)$, including serial amniocentesis when previous obstetric history and antibody titers are significant. Postnatal treatment of the infant may require exchange transfusion or phototherapy.

CHAPTER SUMMARY

Hemolytic disease of the newborn (HDN) or erythroblastosis fetalis is caused by excessive destruction of fetal erythrocytes by maternal antibodies. This process produces jaundice and can cause mental retardation or death in severe cases.

The General Characteristics of HDN

In HDN, the erythrocytes of the fetus or newborn are coated with maternal antibodies that correspond to specific fetal antigens. This action results in hemolysis with subsequent increased erythropoiesis both within the bone marrow and in the liver and spleen (extramedullary hematopoiesis). When the rate of erythrocytic hemolysis exceeds the ability to replace lost cells, anemia develops. The accumulated erythrocytic byproducts, specifically hemoglobin, are removed by way of the maternal circulation before birth; however, accumulation of these products can produce serious problems in the newborn infant.

The only immunoglobulin that is selectively transported through the placenta to the fetus is IgG. IgG in cord serum is derived almost exclusively from the maternal circulation.

The antibodies capable of causing HDN include blood group antibodies that can occur as IgG. Based on severity, the most common causes of HDN are anti-D alone or in combination with anti-C or anti-E; other Rh antibodies; other blood group system antibodies, such as anti-Kell, anti-Duffy, and anti-Kidd; and anti-A and anti-B. Most cases of HDN due to anti-A or anti-B are clinically mild.

For HDN to occur, the mother must lack the antigen that is expressed on the fetal erythrocyte. This antigen must be introduced into the maternal circulation as either the primary immunizing event or the result of transplacental hemorrhage (TPH).

Assessment of HDN

Prenatal assessment of potential cases of HDN include the following tests: ABO grouping D and D^u testing, a screening test for alloantibodies with the identification and titering of any antibodies, and amniocentesis. Amniocentesis is performed only when certain clinical criteria exist. Two sequential amniotic samples must be obtained for the data to be useful in the assessment of fetal well-being.

Postpartum testing should include the tests suggested for prenatal testing, if not previously performed, as well as several other tests. A hemoglobin, hematocrit, serum bilirubin, and direct antiglobulin test (DAT) should be performed on cord blood if indicated on the basis of the prenatal testing results and clinical status of the infant. If the DAT is positive, an antibody elution and identification should be performed. A peripheral blood smear from the infant is an additional assessment tool. The mother's blood can also be tested by the D^u rosette test or Kleihauer-Betke test.

HDN Caused by ABO Incompatibility

ABO blood group incompatibility between mother and fetus occurs frequently and represents a common form of HDN; however, the symptoms are usually mild. The occurrence of this cause of HDN is most frequent if the mother is group O and the baby group A. Any pregnancy can be affected. Treatment using phototherapy is usually sufficient in this form of HDN.

HDN Caused by Rh Incompatibility

The history of HDN due to anti-D demonstrates that HDN was recognized as a clinical entity as early as the 1930s. This manifestation of hemolytic anemia was originally referred to as erythroblastosis fetalis. The major investigators of this process were Landsteiner, Wiener, and Levine.

Immunization to Rh (D and D^u) mothers depends on both the dosage of Rh (D) positive erythrocytes and the mother's ability to respond to these foreign D antigens. The normal pattern of immunization involves primary immunization due to a previously incompatible Rh (D) positive pregnancy or blood transfusion which stimulates the production of low titered anti-D, predominantly of the IgM class. Subsequent antigenic stimulation, such as fetal-maternal hemorrhage during pregnancy with an Rh (D) positive fetus, elicits a secondary (anamnestic) response. This response is characterized by the predominance of increasing titers of anti-D of the IgG class.

The incidence of HDN due to anti-D was the second most common cause of HDN before modern prophylaxis. Usually, the first-born infant is unaffected. Although the second D positive infant can be severely afflicted, subsequent incompatible infants have no tendency for the disorder to become progressively more severe.

A rising alloantibody titer, such as anti-D, is evidence of a presently active immune response. The severity of HDN does not directly correlate with the antibody titer. Fetal hemolysis is primarily due to antibodies of the IgG1 and IgG3 subclasses. The greatest proportion of clinically severe cases have an anti-D antibody of the IgG1 subclass with the G1m(4) allotype.

Laboratory assessment of anti-D HDN follows the protocol discussed in the assessment of HDN. Because of the progressive nature of this type of HDN in second and additional pregnancies, amniocentesis is frequently performed.

HDN due to anti-D may be treated prenatally by prenatal plasma exchange, prenatal intraperitoneal and intrauterine transfusion, or antenatal prophylaxis. Postpartum treatment includes exchange transfusion of the infant in severe cases. Prevention of HDN due to anti-D has significantly decreased the incidence of this form of HDN. In previously nonimmunized women, the administration of immune globulin D is advised. It is important that the woman meet the criteria for this prophylaxis. The dosage of immune globulin must be sufficient to protect adequately against immunization. The Kleihauer-Betke test is frequently used to assess the extent of fetal-maternal hemorrhage. The dosage can be determined on the basis of this assessment.

Other Blood Group Systems

The frequency of HDN due to other blood group antigens continues to exist. More than 40 antigens have been identified as causing HDN. Depending on the antigen strength and other variables, the severity of the disorder can range from mild to severe. Kell, Duffy, Kidd, Lewis, and Lutheran are major categories of antigens in this category.

Laboratory assessment of this form of HDN is consistent with the general protocol for assessment. Treatment is similar to Rh_o treatment; however, prophylactic measures are not currently available.

REVIEW QUESTIONS

1. In hemolytic disease of the newborn, the mother's ___ is directed against fetal ___.
   A. Antigen——antibody
   B. Antibody——antigen
   C. Antigen——antigen
   D. Antibody——antibody
   E. Bilirubin——lipid-rich nervous tissue

2. The normal life span of fetal erythrocytes is ___ days.
   A. 30–45
   B. 45–70
   C. 70–95
   D. 95–120
   E. over 120

3. Extramedullary hematopoiesis results in increased:
   A. Leukocyte production
   B. Bilirubin production
   C. Normal erythrocyte production
   D. Liver and spleen size
   E. None of the above

4. Which of the following is *not* true of unconjugated bilirubin?
   A. Results from erythrocyte destruction
   B. Is bound to albumin by the action of glucuronidase
   C. Becomes conjugated with albumin
   D. Is attracted to tissue proteins
   E. Is a problem to the fetus

5. The antibody class implicated in hemolytic disease of the newborn is:
   A. IgM
   B. IgG
   C. IgD
   D. IgE
   E. IgA

6. The most severe form of hemolytic disease of the newborn is associated with:
   A. Anti-A
   B. Anti-B
   C. Anti-D
   D. Anti-K
   E. Anti-c

7. Production of maternal antibodies depends on all of the following factors *except*:
   A. Lack of a specific antigen in the mother
   B. Presence of a specific antigen in the fetus
   C. Presence of a specific antibody in the fetus
   D. Immunogenic strength of an antigen
   E. The quantity of transplacental hemorrhage

8. Prenatal testing routinely includes all of the following, *except*:
   A. ABO grouping
   B. Rh_o (D) typing
   C. D^u testing if D is negative
   D. Screening for irregular antibodies
   E. Amniocentesis

9. The normal cord hemoglobin (at birth) is:
   A. 0.7–3.4 mg/dL
   B. 3.4–10.4 g/dL
   C. 10.5–14.5 g/dL
   D. 14.5–22.5 g/dL
   E. over 22.5 g/dL

10. A cord bilirubin of ___ may be an indication for exchange transfusion.
    A. 0.1–0.5 mg/dL
    B. 0.5–1.0 mg/dL
    C. 1.0–2.5 mg/dL
    D. 2.5–4.0 mg/dL
    E. over 4.0 mg/dL

11. Both the D^u rosette test and the Kleihauer-Betke test are performed on a:
    A. Baby's cord blood specimen
    B. Baby's circulating blood specimen
    C. Mother's circulating blood specimen
    D. Both A and B
    E. Both A and C

12. The purpose of both the D^u rosette test and the Kleihauer-Betke test is to detect:
    A. Maternal D antigen
    B. Maternal D antibody
    C. Fetal D antigen
    D. Fetal D antibody
    E. Fetal-maternal hemorrhage

13. The most frequent cause of ABO hemolytic disease of the newborn is:
    A. Mother group O, baby group A
    B. Mother group O, baby group B
    C. Mother group A, baby group O
    D. Mother group A, baby group B
    E. Mother group B, baby group A

14. Hemolytic disease of the newborn due to ABO incompatibility is usually milder than other types due to all of the following factors *except*:
    A. There are fewer A and B antigen sites on fetal erythrocytes
    B. Fetal A and B antigens have weaker antigenic strength
    C. The presence of the D antigen has a protective effect
    D. Competition for anti-A and anti-B exists between the tissues and erythrocytes
    E. Only a small fraction of IgG anti-A and anti-B combines with fetal erythrocytes

15. Rh sensitization is *least* likely to occur in an Rh negative woman if her ABO type is ___:
    A. A
    B. B
    C. O
    D. AB

16. The typical laboratory profile of hemolytic disease of the newborn caused by ABO incompatibility is:
    A. Mother group O, baby group A, DAT negative, cord bilirubin 3.0 mg/dL
    B. Mother group A, baby group O, antibody elution from cord blood-positive, cord bilirubin 1.0 mg/dL
    C. Mother group O, baby group A, DAT strongly positive, cord bilirubin 10.0 g/dL.
    D. Mother group O, baby group B, DAT strongly positive, cord hemoglobin 10.0 g/dL
    E. Mother group A, baby group O, antibody elution negative cord hemoglobin 10.0 g/dL

17. All of the following characteristics are typical of hemolytic disease of the newborn caused by the D antigen *except*:
    A. Depends on the dosage of D antigen on fetal erythrocytes
    B. Depends on the mother's ability to respond to foreign D antigens

C. Usually does not occur in the first pregnancy
D. May require an exchange transfusion
E. Has a laboratory profile of a positive DAT, decreased cord hemoglobin, and increased total cord bilirubin

18. Antenatal Rh immune globulin should be administered at:
    A. 12 weeks gestation
    B. 24 weeks gestation
    C. 28 weeks gestation
    D. 32 weeks gestation
    E. After delivery

19. Rh immune globulin provides ___ protection against fetal D antigen.
    A. Active
    B. Passive
    C. Antigen-stimulated
    D. Antibody-stimulated
    E. No

20. An exchange transfusion is warranted if the:
    A. Cord bilirubin is 2.5 mg/dL, plasma bilirubin 10.0 mg/dL at 12 hours, and 10.0 mg/dL at 24 hours
    B. Cord bilirubin is 5.0 mg/dL, plasma bilirubin 11.5 mg/dL at 12 hours, and 16.0 mg/dL at 24 hours
    C. Increase in plasma bilirubin is more than 0.2 mg/dL/hour
    D. Infant is full-term
    E. Both B and D

21. If an Rh_o (D) negative woman recently delivered an Rh_o (D) positive baby and the Kleihauer-Betke test result is 5%, how many vials of immunoglobulin D should be administered?
    A. 6
    B. 7
    C. 8
    D. 9
    E. 10

22. Which of the following does *not* partially meet the criteria for postpartum administration of immune globulin D?
    A. Mother D negative, infant D positive, cord cell elution revealed anti-Kell
    B. Mother D negative, alloantibody screen-anti-c, infant D positive, DAT-negative

C. Mother D negative, alloantibody screen-negative, infant D negative, DAT-negative.
D. Mother D negative, infant's type unknown, alloantibody screen-positive (anti-K)
E. None of the above

23. In addition to the A, B, and D antigens, hemolytic disease of the newborn can be caused by:
   A. No other antigens
   B. Only c antigen
   C. c and Kell antigens
   D. More than 20 different antigens
   E. More than 40 different antigens

24-25. Match the following (an answer may be used more than once):
24. Anti-Lu[a]
25. Anti-M
   A. Has been reported to produce severe forms of HDN
   B. Has been reported to produce mild forms of HDN
   C. Has not been identified as a cause of HDN

ANSWERS

1. B	14. C
2. B	15. C
3. D	16. A
4. D	17. A
5. B	18. C
6. C	19. B
7. C	20. B
8. E	21. D
9. D	22. C
10. E	23. E
11. C	24. B
12. E	25. A
13. A	

Bibliography

Adams, M. M., et al.: Cost implications of routine antenatal administration of Rh immune globulin. Am. J. Obstet. Gynecol., 149(6):633-38, 1984.

Barrie, J. U., and Quinn, M. A.: Selection of donor red cells for fetal intravenous transfusion in severe haemolytic disease of the newborn. The Lancet, i (8441):1327-1328, 1985.

Bergstrom, H., et al.: Demonstration of Rh antigens in a 38-day-old fetus. Am. J. Obstet. Gynecol., 99:130-133, 1967.

Bowman, J. M.: Prevention of rhesus isoimmunization. Am. J. Obstet. Gynecol., 148(8):1151-1153, 1984.

Bowman, M. (Ed): Rh₀ (D) Immune Globulin. Berkeley, CA, Cutter Biological, 1984.

Bradshaw, D. A.: Red blood cell antibody testing of obstetric patients. Lab. Med., 18(2):77-81, 1987.

Branch, D. R.: Fetal death due to extreme maternal Rh immune augmentation. Transfusion, 21(3):281-284, 1981.

Buck, S. A.: Hemolytic Disease of the Newborn. In Modern Blood Banking and Transfusion Practices, D. H. Pittiglio (Ed.). Philadelphia, F. A. Davis, pp. 399-421.

Caswell, A. K., and Caswell, M.: Antenatal treatment to prevent Rh immunization. Lab. Med., 14(10):655-658, 1983.

Characteristics of Blood Group Antibodies (Product Brochure). Miami, FL, Baxter Healthcare Corp., 1987.

Cheng, M. S., and Lukomskyj, L.: Postpartum Dᵘ-positive women and Rh immune globulin. Lab. Med., 17(12):748-749, 1986.

Chibber, G., et al.: Rh Isoimmunization following abdominal trauma: A case report. Am. J. Obstet. Gynecol., 149(6):692, 1984.

Culver, P. L., Brubaker, D. B., Sheldon, R. E., Martin, M., and Richter, C. A.: Anti-At[a] causing mild hemolytic disease of the newborn. Transfusion, 27(5):468-470, 1987.

Dacus, J. V., and Spinnato, J. A.: Severe erythroblastosis fetalis secondary to Anti-Kp[b] sensitization. Am. J. Obstet. Gynecol., 150(7):888-889, 1984.

Davey, M. G.: Nonresponders and hyperresponders to Rh antigens. Proceedings of a symposium on Rh antibody mediated immunosuppression. Ortho Diagnostics, 1976.

Dopp, S. L., and Isham, B. E.: Anti-U and hemolytic disease of the newborn. Transfusion, 23(3):273, 1983.

Drozda, E. A., and Ciotola, R.: Unexpected hemolytic disease of the newborn. Lab. Med., 15(7):486-487, 1984.

Dube, V. E., and Zoes, C. S.: Subclinical hemolytic disease of the newborn associated with IgG anti-Lu[b]. Transfusion, 22(3):251-253, 1982.

Fudenberg, H. H., et al.: Basic and Clinical Immunology. 2nd Ed. Los Altos, CA; Lange Medical Publications, 1978. p.63.

Greenwalt, T. J.: Rh Isoimmunization. JAMA, 251(10):1318-1320, 1984.

Henry, John B. (Ed.): Clinical Diagnosis and Management by Laboratory Methods, 17th Ed. Philadelphia, W. B. Saunders Co., 1982, pp. 503-506, 694, 1055-1059.

Inderbitzen, P. E., and Windle, B.: An example of HDN probably due to anti-Lu[a]. Transfusion, 22(6):542, 1982.

Kolins, J.: Dᵘ and rosetting tests for FMH. Diagn. Med., 23, May, 1984.

Krauss, J. S., et al.: Detection of fetomaternal hemorrhage in a mother with sickle trait and hereditary persistence of fetal hemoglobin. Transfusion, 23(6):530-531, 1983.

LaFerla, J. J., and Butch, S.: Fetal Rh blood group determination in pregnancy termination by dilatation and evacuation. Transfusion, 23(1):67-68, 1983.

Mellbye, N.: Presence and origin of human IgG subclass proteins in newborns. Vox Sang., 24:206-215, 1973.

Mollison, P. L.: Blood Transfusion in Clinical Medicine. 5th Ed. Oxford, Blackwell Scientific Publications, 1983.

Nance, S., Nelson J., Horenstein, J., O'Neill, P., and Garratty, G.: Predictive value of amniocentesis versus monocyte monolayer assays in pregnant women with Rh antibodies (Abstract of paper presented at the 39th Annual Meeting of the American Association of Blood Banks). Transfusion, 26(6):570, 1986.

Nance, S. J., Nelson, J., O'Neill, P., Lam, H., and Garratty, G.: Quantitation of fetal-maternal hemorrhage by flow cytometry. Transfusion, 26(6):571, 1986.

Nance, S. J., Nelson J., O'Neill, P., and Garratty, G.: Correlation of monocyte monolayer assays, maternal antibody titers, and clinical course in hemolytic disease of the newborn (Abstract of paper presented at the 37th Annual Meeting of the American Association of Blood Banks). Transfusion, 24:415, 1984.

Page, P. L.: Hemolytic disease of the newborn due to anti-Lan. Transfusion, 23(3):256-257, 1983.

Parinaud, J., et al.: IgG subclasses and Gm allotypes of anti-D antibodies during pregnancy: Correlation with the gravity of the fetal disease. Am. J. Obstet. Gynecol., 151(8):1111-1115, 1985.

Pittiglio, D. H. (Ed.): Modern Blood Banking and Transfusion Practices. Philadelphia, F. A. Davis, 1983. pp. 399-421.

Riley, J. Z., et al.: Detection and quantitation of fetal maternal hemorrhage utilizing an enzyme-linked antiglobulin test. Transfusion, 22(6):472-474, 1982.

Roitt, I.: Essential Immunology. 4th Ed., Oxford, Blackwell Scientific Publications, 1983. pp. 41.

Sbarra, A. J.: Amniotic fluid optical density, lecithin-sphingomyelin ratio, and phosphatidylglycerol comparisons. Am. J. Obstet. Gynecol., 148(8):1151-1153, 1984.

Sebring, E. S., and Polesky, H. F.: Detection of fetal maternal hemorrhage in Rh immune globulin candidates. Transfusion, 22(6):468-471, 1982.

Shah, V. P., and Gilja, B. K.: Hemolytic disease of newborn due to anti-Duffy (Fy[a]). N.Y. State J. Med., 244-245, Feb. 1983.

Shirey, R. S., et al.: The association of anti-P and early abortion, Transfusion, 27(2):189-191, 1987.

Toivanen, P., and Hirvonen, T.: Antigens: Duffy, Kell, Kidd, Lutheran and Xg[a] on fetal red cells. Vox Sang., 24:372-376, 1973.

Tovey, L. A., and Taverner, J. M.: A case for the antenatal administration of anti-D immunoglobulin to primigravidae. Lancet, i:878-881, 1981.

White, P., Hendrick, E., and Mark D. Kolins, M.D.: Fetomaternal hemorrhage revisited. Lab. Med., 16(7):428-430, 1985.

Widmann, F. K. (Ed.): Technical Manual (Ninth Ed.) Washington, D.C., American Association of Blood Banks, 297-324, 1985.

Yesus, Y. W.: Hemolytic disease of the newborn due to anti-C and anti-G masquerading as anti-D. Am. J. Clin. Pathol., 84(6):769-772, 1985.

11

Transfusion Reactions

At the conclusion of this chapter, the reader will be able to:

- Define the term "transfusion reaction."
- State the most frequent cause of fatal transfusion reactions.
- Cite at least one example for each of the following types of transfusion reactions: immediate hemolytic, immediate non-hemolytic, delayed hemolytic, and delayed nonhemolytic.
- State the most severe form of a transfusion reaction.
- Name the factors that determine whether a transfusion reaction will be acute or delayed and intravascular or extravascular.
- State the most frequent cause of an acute hemolytic transfusion.
- Name the nonantibody cause or causes of acute hemolytic reactions.
- Explain the clinical manifestations of an acute hemolytic transfusion reaction.
- Describe the most common initial symptoms of an acute hemolytic reaction in an unanesthetized patient.
- Explain the in vivo consequences of the interaction between antigens and their corresponding antibodies.
- Cite the most serious physiologic result of an acute hemolytic transfusion reaction.
- Discuss the rationale of a delayed hemolytic transfusion reaction.
- List the characteristics of a delayed hemolytic transfusion reaction, including the usual consequence of such a reaction.
- Describe the reasons for immediate post-transfusion jaundice.
- Cite one of the ways in which this type of reaction can be prevented.
- Name the most frequent cause of febrile transfusion reaction.
- Describe the clinical manifestations of febrile (non-hemolytic) transfusion reactions.
- State the immediate reactions to plasma constituents.
- Cite the most common cause of transfusion-related sepsis.
- Describe the consequences of contaminated blood in transfusion.
- Discuss the features of graft-versus-host disease including etiology and prevention.
- Explain cardiopulmonary and embolic reactions to blood transfusion.
- List and briefly describe some of the other adverse reactions to the infusion of blood or blood components.
- Describe the protocol for the investigation of a transfusion reaction.
- Arrange the steps in a post-transfusion workup in the appropriate sequence.
- List the supplementary tests that can be performed in a transfusion reaction workup.
- Resolve transfusion-associated problems with the appropriate action or explanation.

DEFINITION AND CAUSES

The term *transfusion reaction* generally refers to the adverse signs and symptoms produced by incompatibility between a patient and a unit of donor blood or a blood component. Typically, visible signs occur during or shortly after a transfusion; however, conditions such as shortened post-transfusion survival of erythrocytes, allergic response, and disease transmission also constitute transfusion reactions.

When a physician makes the clinical judgment to transfuse a patient, the expected benefits of the product must be weighed against the known risks. The risk of a transfusion reaction is minimal but not unimportant. Although one estimate of the fatality rate due to blood transfusion is approximately 1 per million units transfused, the rate of all types of adverse reactions to transfused blood or blood components is assessed at about 1 in every 200 transfusions.

The vast majority of fatal transfusion reactions result from misidentification or clerical errors rather than technical limitations. Causes of fatal reactions in order of frequency are:

1. Misidentification of patients
2. Mislabelling of blood samples
3. Errors in laboratory records
4. Mistakes in blood typing
5. Inaccurate antibody screening or crossmatching

Transfusion reactions can be divided into hemolytic and non-hemolytic types. Hemolytic reactions are associated with the infusion of incompatible erythrocytes. Transfusion reactions can be further classified into acute (immediate) or delayed in their manifestations (Table 11-1).

Acute hemolytic reactions occur during or immediately after blood has been transfused; delayed reactions may not express themselves until 7 to 10 days post-transfusion. Many reactions demonstrate both extravascular and intravascular hemolysis.

Table 11-1. Types of Transfusion Reactions

Type of Reaction	Manifestations
Immediate hemolytic	Intravascular hemolysis of erythrocytes
Delayed hemolytic	Extravascular hemolysis of erythrocytes
Immediate Nonhemolytic	Febrile reactions Anaphylaxis Urticaria Noncardiac pulmonary edema Fever and shock Congestive heart failure Myocardial failure
Delayed Nonhemolytic	Graft-versus-host disease Post-transfusion purpura Iron overload Alloimmunization to erythrocytes, leukocytes, and/or platelet antigens or plasma proteins Infectious diseases

Acute hemolytic reactions are the most serious and potentially lethal. The major crossmatch should demonstrate incompatibility because this type of response represents the combination of patient antibodies with antigens possessed by the infused erythrocytes. If an antibody is capable of activating complement and is sufficiently active in vivo, intravascular hemolysis occurs, producing a rapid increase of free hemoglobin in the circulation. The cause of the immediate clinical symptoms is uncertain, but they may be due to products released by the action of complement on the erythrocytes, which triggers multiple shock mechanisms.

Delayed reactions occur in the extravascular spaces and are associated with decreased red cell survival because of the coating of the red cells (a positive DAT, which promotes phagocytosis and premature removal of the red cells by the mononuclear phagocytic system). If an antibody does not activate complement or does so very slowly, extravascular hemolysis occurs. Most IgG antibody-coated erythrocytes are destroyed extravascularly, mainly in the spleen. Antibodies commonly associated with extravascular hemolysis include anti-E, anti-c, anti-K, and anti-Jk[a].

Factors that influence whether a transfusion reaction will be acute or delayed include:

1. Number of incompatible erythrocytes infused
2. Antibody class or subclass
3. Achievement of the optimal temperature for antibody binding

ACUTE HEMOLYTIC REACTIONS

Etiology

The most common cause of an acute hemolytic transfusion reaction is transfusion of ABO-incompatible blood. In patients with pre-existing antibodies caused by prior transfusion or pregnancy, other blood groups may be responsible. Infusion of incompatible erythrocytes in the presence of pre-existing antibodies initiates an antigen-antibody reaction with the activation of the complement, plasminogen, kinin, and coagulation systems. Other initiators of acute hemolytic reactions include bacterial contamination of blood or the infusion of hemolyzed erythrocytes.

Signs and Symptoms

Reactions can occur with the infusion of as little as 5 mL or less of incompatible blood. The most common initial symptoms are fever with or without chills that mimics a febrile, nonhemolytic reaction due to leukocyte incompatibility. Lower back pain, flushing of the face, shortness of breath, pain at the infusion site and hypotension are also symptoms. Oliguria and anuria may be present but not necessarily caused by a transfusion reaction. Complications of trauma or hemorrhage, such as inadequate blood volume restoration, can also cause oliguria and anuria. In addition to the signs of shock, the release of thromboplastic substances into the circulation can induce disseminated intravascular coagulation (DIC) and acute renal failure.

The only signs of a hemolytic reaction in patients under general anesthesia may be hypotension or excessive bleeding from the operative site. Most fatalities due to acute hemolytic transfusion reactions occur in anesthetized or unconscious patients; the immediate cause of death is uncontrollable hypotension.

An acute hemolytic transfusion reaction is a medical emergency. If a reaction is suspected, the transfusion should be stopped immediately. It is important that the attending physician maintain the patient's blood volume with intravenous electrolytes supplemented with mannitol or furosemide and maintain urinary flow at 1 to 3 mL per minute.

The laboratory investigation of a suspected acute hemolytic transfusion reaction is described later in this chapter.

Physiology

The in vivo results of the interaction of antigens and antibodies are that the neuro-endocrine system is stimulated, complement is activated, and hemostasis mechanisms may be altered. Complement activation may produce accelerated intravascular destruction of erythrocytes and altered hemostasis can result in disseminated intravascular coagulation.

THE NEURO-ENDOCRINE RESPONSE

The neuro-endocrine response associated with an acute hemolytic transfusion reaction results from the antigen-antibody complex activation of blood coagulation factor XIIa (Hageman factor), which in turn acts on the kinin system to produce bradykinin. Bradykinin has the physiologic effect of increasing capillary permeability and dilating the arterioles. Hypotension results, with subsequent stimulation of the sympathetic nervous system. Norepinephrine and other catecholamines secreted by the sympathetic nervous system produce vasoconstriction in various organs, including the kidneys, lungs, and skin. Serotonin and histamines released by mast cells (tissue basophils) and platelets mediate many of the clinical symptoms of an acute hemolytic reaction.

COMPLEMENT ACTIVATION AND INTRAVASCULAR HEMOLYSIS

An antigen-antibody complex has the ability to activate complement. If this activation proceeds to completion, intravascular hemolysis occurs. If activation does not proceed to completion, the erythrocytes become coated with complement. These coated red blood cells are usually phagocytized by the cells of the mononuclear phagocytic system and catabolized through the process of extravascular destruction (see Delayed Hemolytic Reactions, this chapter) but, in some cases, complement-coated erythrocytes survive normally. Renal damage resulting from nonfatal hemolysis is believed to be caused by the presence of antibody-coated cell membrane (stroma).

Intravascular destruction of erythrocytes (Fig. 11-1) accounts for less than 10% of normal erythrocytic destruction. If antigen-antibody complexes activate complement and produce rapid lysis of erythrocytes,

hemoglobin is released directly into the blood stream and undergoes dissociation into alpha-beta dimers, which are quickly bound to the plasma globulin, haptoglobin. The formation of the large molecular haptoglobin-hemoglobin complex prevents urinary excretion of plasma hemoglobin. This stable complex is removed from the circulation by the hepatocytes, in which it is processed by the cells in a manner similar to normal intact (extravascular) erythrocytic breakdown. Because haptoglobin is removed from the circulation as part of the haptoglobin-hemoglobin complex, the level of plasma haptoglobin decreases with hemolysis. Once plasma haptoglobin is depleted in the blood circulation, unbound hemoglobin alpha and beta dimers are rapidly filtered by the kidney's glomeruli, reabsorbed by the renal tubular cells, and converted to hemosiderin. Renal tubular uptake can process up to 5 g of filtered hemoglobin per day. Once the capacity for renal tubular uptake has been exceeded, however, free hemoglobin and methemoglobin begin to appear in the urine. Hemoglobin appears in the urine when plasma-free hemoglobin (unbound to haptoglobin) reaches 25 mg/dL or more. The renal processing of filtered hemoglobin can produce excretion of the following:

1. Hemoglobin alone, if hemolysis is severe,
2. Hemosiderin by itself.
3. Both hemosiderin and hemoglobin. If desquamated tubular cells contain hemosiderin granules, this is evidence of a previous condition of hemoglobinemia.

Hemoglobin which is neither bound by haptoglobin nor directly excreted in the urine is oxidized to methemoglobin. The heme groups in methemoglobin are released and taken up by another transport protein, hemopexin. This complex is removed from the circulation by hepatocytes and catabolized. Heme groups in excess of the hemopexin-binding capacity combine with albumin to form methemalbumin until more hemopexin is available. Once this needed hemopexin becomes available, the complex is subsequently phagocytized by hepatocytes.

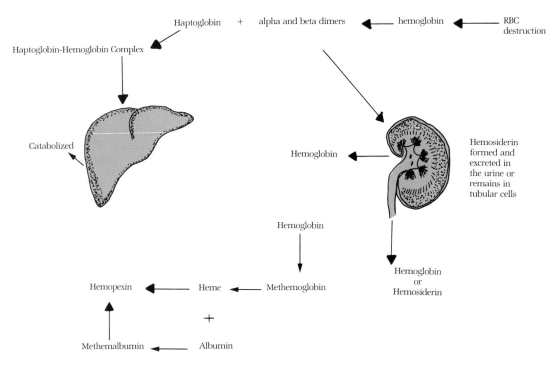

Figure 11-1. Intravascular metabolism of erythrocytes.

The combined depletion of haptoglobin and hemopexin and the presence of methemalbuminemia and hemosiderinuria can be seen in conditions such as intravascular hemolysis. The presence of methemalbumin accompanied by hemopexin depletion *without* hemosiderinuria is associated with bleeding into the tissues, such as intraabdominal bleeding in ectopic pregnancy.

HEMOSTASIS AND DISSEMINATED
INTRAVASCULAR COAGULATION

Antigen-antibody complexes can activate the intrinsic coagulation mechanism by way of factor XIIa or directly by the presence of erythrocyte stroma. Plasma activators of plasminogen include plasma kallikrein, activated plasma thromboplastin antecedents (factor XI), and activated Hageman factor (factor XIIa).

Through its lysis of fibrin, plasmin is responsible for forming degradation or fibrin split products consisting of intermediate fragments that exert an antithrombin effect, inhibit the hemostasis system through interference with fibrin monomer polymerization, and interfere with platelet function.

Pathologic Activation of Coagulation Factors. Primary and secondary fibrinolysis are recognized as extreme complications of various intravascular and extravascular disorders and may lead to life-threatening consequences. Primary fibrinolysis is associated with conditions in which gross activation of the fibrinolytic mechanism with subsequent fibrinogen and coagulation factor consumption occurs. The important characteristic of primary fibrinolysis is that no evidence of fibrin deposition appears. Primary fibrinolysis occurs when large amounts of plasminogen activator enter the circulatory system.

Although the same clinical conditions may also induce secondary fibrinolysis or disseminated intravascular coagulation (DIC), the distinction between the two is essentially in the demonstration of fibrin formation. In secondary fibrinolysis, excessive clotting and fibrinolytic activity occur. Increased amounts of fibrin-split (degradation) products (FSPs) and fibrin monomers are detectable because of the action of thrombin on the fibrinogen molecule. This fibrinolytic process is due only to excessive clotting; therefore, it is a secondary condition.

DISSEMINATED INTRAVASCULAR COAGULATION (DIC). Initiation of DIC can be caused by several factors, most commonly tissue thromboplastin introduced into the circulation. This introduction of tissue thromboplastin activates the extrinsic coagulation pathway and platelets, which may result in intravascular consumption of factors V, VIII, fibrinogen, and platelets in the formation of intravascular thrombi. Antithrombin III also appears to be consumed during this process and a deficiency of antithrombin III may contribute to further thrombosis.

DIC may initially occur with varying degrees of thrombosis and hemorrhage, but bleeding is usually the major symptom, particularly in acute cases. The process involves coagulation factors, platelets, vascular endothelial cells, fibrinolysis, and plasma inhibitors. This major breakdown of the hemostatic mechanism occurs when the procoagulant factors outweigh the anticoagulant mechanisms. The generation of microthrombi can cause small blood vessel obstruction and tissue necrosis. Abnormal secondary bleeding is produced by the FSPs, which are produced in time by the increased destruction of fibrinogen. The FSPs disrupt fibrin monomer polymerization by exerting an antithrombin effect and preventing normal platelet function.

The stimuli that can induce DIC may ultimately result in abnormal levels of protein C. Monitoring of patients reveals that protein C antigen and activity decrease progressively during the initial stages of DIC and remain at a low level for 24 to 48 hours before gradually returning toward normal in nonfatal cases.

THROMBIN. Mechanisms involved in DIC result in the formation of thrombin in the circulating blood. Among its many feedback reactions, thrombin indirectly participates in the activation of the fibrinolytic system secondary to DIC and activates protein C. The latter reaction is accelerated by the presence of the endothelial cell cofactor, protein S. Once the generation of excess thrombin is decreased by the action of activated protein C and other regulatory mechanisms, the coagulation process can return to normal. This negative feedback mechanism has the potential to slow down the formation of excess thrombin and stop DIC.

Prevention

Acute hemolytic transfusion reactions can be prevented by the proper identification of patients and patient samples, and error-free laboratory record-keeping, blood grouping, and crossmatching. The autologous-donor patient must also be carefully identified. Multiple crosschecks should be a routine procedure to prevent inadvertent misidentification of the patient and/or donor unit.

DELAYED HEMOLYTIC REACTIONS

Etiology

Delayed hemolytic transfusion reactions can occur from two days to several months post-transfusion. This type of hemolytic reaction is underdiagnosed, under-reported, and under-rated in terms of complications, and is far more frequent than the acute hemolytic reaction.

Delayed hemolytic transfusion reactions may be of two types. They may represent an anamnestic antibody response in a previously immunized recipient on secondary exposure to transfused erythrocyte antigens or result from primary alloimmunization. In an anamnestic response, the antibodies are to antigens to which recipients have been previously immunized by transfusion or pregnancy.

The incidence of primary alloimmunization, excluding D antigen, is 1 to 6% for each unit of blood transfused. Antibodies implicated in delayed hemolytic reactions are anti-E, anti-C, anti-M, anti-Lu^a, anti-K, anti-Ce, anti-Jk^a, anti-Jk^b, anti-k, anti-Fy^a, anti-U, and anti-Co^b.

Signs and Symptoms

The most common clinical sign is fever. The triad of anemia, fever, and recent transfusion suggests a delayed hemolytic reaction. Symptoms can range from an asymptomatic state to oliguria or renal shutdown in less than 10% of cases to DIC in very rare cases. Commonly, the accidental discovery of a positive DAT in a subsequent crossmatch reveals that a patient has antibody-coated erythrocytes in the circulation.

In a patient demonstrating an anamnestic response, fever, post-transfusion jaundice, and a sudden drop in the hemoglobin and packed cell volume (hematocrit) with no evidence of hemorrhage or hemodilution may occur within as few as 2 days post-transfusion. A patient exhibiting primary alloimmunization may suffer from a sudden drop in hemoglobin and packed cell volume (hematocrit) several weeks post-transfusion.

Physiology

An anamnestic antibody response usually begins to occur from 2 or 3 to 7 days post-transfusion. Despite a visibly compatible crossmatch, transfused erythrocytes are removed from the circulating blood and the products of the *extravascular hemolysis* of erythrocytes, such as bilirubin, increase.

In primary alloimmunization, antibody production begins no earlier than 7 to 10 days posttransfusion, but it is several weeks or months before antibodies can be detected clinically. *In vivo* erythrocyte survival, however, is shortened, with the degree of the decrease depending on the quantity of antibody produced and the quantity of transfused erythrocytes remaining.

Because the antibody produced in a delayed transfusion reaction is largely of the IgG class, it rarely causes *intravascular* hemolysis as seen in an acute hemolytic reaction. The pathologic destruction of erythrocytes is by *extravascular* hemolysis.

When an erythrocyte is phagocytized and digested by the macrophages of the reticuloendothelial system, the hemoglobin molecule is disassembled (Fig. 11-2). The resulting components are iron, protoporphyrin, and globin. Iron is transported in the plasma by transferrin to be recycled by the red bone marrow in the manufacture of new hemoglobin. Globin is catabolized in the liver into its constituent amino acids and enters the circulating amino acid pool. The porphyrin ring is broken at the alpha methene bridge by the heme oxidase enzyme. The alpha carbon leaves as carbon monoxide. The tetrapyrrole (bilirubin) resulting from the opened porphyrin ring is carried by plasma albumin to the liver, where it is conjugated to form glucuronide and excreted in the bile. Both unconjugated (prehepatic) and conjugated (posthepatic) bilirubin are present in the plasma. Bilirubin glucuronide is excreted into the gut, converted by bacterial action, and excreted in the feces as stercobilinogen. A small amount of urobilinogen is reabsorbed into the blood circulation and excreted in the urine.

In the case of a suspected delayed hemolytic transfusion reaction, demonstrating the existence of hemolysis by measuring haptoglobin, hemoglobin or bilirubin in serum, and hemoglobin, hemosiderin or urobilinogen in urine may be confirmatory. Often these tests are ordered later than the time at which maximally abnormal findings exist. Increased extravascular catabolism can produce a decreased haptoglobin level, increased indirect bilirubin, and the presence of hemosiderin in urinary epithelial cells.

Prevention

The blood specimens used for compatibility testing should be *no more* than 3 days old at the time of transfusion if a patient has been previously transfused or pregnant within the preceding 3 months. Although a patient's serum may not demonstrate alloantibodies when antibody attachment and hemolysis first occur, circulating antibody concentrations usually reach detectable levels within several days; however, this may not be the case if the alloantibody produced has been completely absorbed onto the erythrocytes. A low-titered primary immune response may fail to demonstrate detectable levels of the antibody in the patient's serum compared to the level of antibody produced from an anamnestic response.

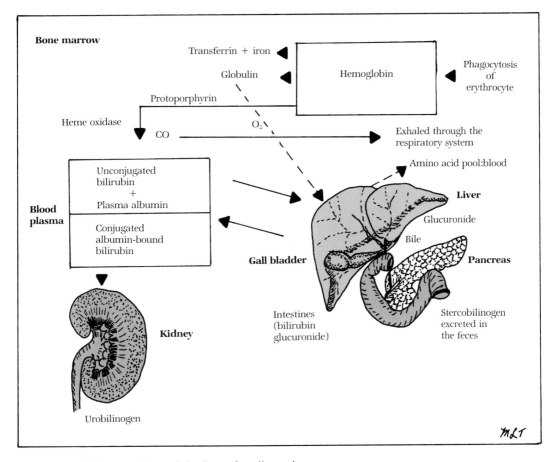

Figure 11-2. Extravascular catabolism of erythrocytes.

Elution and identification of antibody are necessary if a positive DAT has been newly discovered. If the patient's serum is negative for alloantibodies or questionable, and the DAT is positive, crossmatching should be done using an eluate. When a positive DAT is present, performing an elution is necessary to identify the specificity of the immunoglobin absorbed on the cells. A stronger reaction may be achieved by using enhancement media such as LISS. Stronger serum reactions may also be observed by using selected cells that are homozygous for antigens in systems such as Rh, Duffy, and Kidd. Antibodies in these systems sometimes react more strongly with red cells that are homozygous for the corresponding antigen.

After the accelerated destruction and removal of incompatible donor erythrocytes, a delayed hemolytic transfusion reaction is no longer characterized by either a positive

DAT or positive eluates. The persistence of a positive DAT with autologous antibodies characterizes a warm acquired hemolytic anemia (discussed in Chapter 6).

IMMEDIATE NONHEMOLYTIC REACTIONS

In this section, reactions that are not usually associated with erythrocyte hemolysis are discussed. Nonhemolytic reactions, like hemolytic reactions, may be of an immediate or delayed nature.

Febrile Reactions

ETIOLOGY

The most common type of febrile transfusion reaction is that due to cytotoxic antibodies or leukoagglutinins (leukocyte antibodies). If these antibodies are present in the recipient's plasma, a reaction occurs between the antibodies and the antigens present on the cell membrane of transfused leukocytes or platelets. In one study, granulocytes were found to be responsible for 91% of leukocyte reactions. Patients who have received multiple platelet transfusions have a high incidence of febrile reactions. Nonspecific leukoagglutinins, as well as those of HLA origin, have been implicated in febrile reactions. Although cytotoxic antibodies and leukoagglutinins can often be demonstrated in patients with febrile reactions, the cause of many of these reactions is obscure and cannot be readily documented by laboratory testing. Frequently the diagnosis is by exclusion of other causes. Leukoagglutinins have also been implicated in a specific type of delayed reaction referred to as the *noncardiac pulmonary edema syndrome*.

SIGNS AND SYMPTOMS

The most common symptom is fever, often accompanied by chills, which begins during or soon after transfusion. Although a nonhemolytic febrile reaction is rarely harmful, fever may be one of the clinical symptoms of a hemolytic transfusion reaction. Evidence of chills and fever should be investigated as a *potential* hemolytic transfusion reaction.

The fever associated with a febrile non-hemolytic reaction is defined as a rise in body temperature of 1° C or more, occurring in association with the transfusion of blood or components and with no other explanation. Febrile reactions may be mild to severe and may begin early in the transfusion to an hour or two after the transfusion has been completed. Fever is more common in patients receiving granulocytes than in those receiving other blood products and tends to occur more often in repeatedly transfused patients and in women who have had multiple pregnancies.

PREVENTION

Documenting the existence of leukoagglutinins may be helpful in patients who are expected to need additional transfusions. Tests such as leukoagglutinin and micro-lymphocytotoxicity assays can be performed. With or without documentation of the existence of specific antibodies, the use of leukocyte-poor preparations (see Chapter 9) is recommended *only* after a patient has had two or more febrile nonhemolytic reactions.

Platelet Reactions

Two types of immediate reactions to transfused platelets have been documented. These are febrile reactions and hemolytic reactions.

FEBRILE ETIOLOGY

Febrile reactions to platelet transfusions are probably related to the presence of large numbers of leukocytes in the platelet concentrate component.

FEBRILE SIGNS, SYMPTOMS, AND PREVENTION

Refer to previous discussion of febrile reactions.

HEMOLYTIC ETIOLOGY

The hemolytic reaction to platelet components is related to the common practice of transfusing ABO-incompatible platelets when group-specific platelets are not available.

Transfusions which are not group-specific are generally considered safe and are accepted as clinically effective. Transfusions of incompatible platelets are not, however, without risks related to passively transfused antibodies. In a typical platelet concentrate, a relatively small volume of plasma (commonly 50 to 70 mL) and few erythrocytes (less than 0.1 mL) may be present. Two hemolytic reactions, one fatal, have been reported. Both were related to isoagglutinins present in group O platelet concentrates. One pediatric patient was a group A who received 200 mL of plasma in two aliquots containing a hemolytic anti-A (1:16) and an IgG anti-A (1:32,000). The second patient, who was group B, received between 50 and 70 mL of O plasma with a titer (1:16,000) of anti-B.

HEMOLYTIC SIGNS

In the group A patient, in addition to the patient's pre-existing sepsis, a classic case of DIC resulted and the patient expired. In the group B patient, the platelet concentrate produced hemolysis of 40% of the patient's erythrocytes.

HEMOLYTIC PREVENTION

The use of group-specific or group-compatible platelets is preferred. In cases of ABO-incompatible platelet preparations, however, it is recommended that as much plasma as possible be removed. Observation of patients during transfusion of any blood product is important in the identification of *immediate* transfusion reactions.

Reactions to Plasma Constituents

Immediate reactions to plasma constituents may be classified as *allergic, anaphylactoid,* or *anaphylactic* in nature.

ALLERGIC AND ANAPHYLACTOID REACTIONS

Etiology. Although the mechanism of this type of reaction is unclear, most authorities agree that it is a reaction to soluble constituents in donor plasma. There is more discomfort than danger. Allergic reactions are the second most common type of transfusion reaction. When the reaction is extensive or produces edema, it is referred to as anaphylactoid. Anaphylactoid reactions are not uncommon following intramuscular injection of serum immune globulins that have detectable amounts of IgA.

Signs and Symptoms. This type of reaction develops during or shortly after transfusion. Allergic reactions are manifested by urticaria (hives), itching, and local erythema, but usually no fever. If the cutaneous reaction is extensive or produces oral, pharyngeal, or laryngeal edema, it is known as an anaphylactoid reaction.

Prevention. Laboratory investigation usually yields little information; however,

reactions can be well controlled with antihistamines. In repeated or severe reactions, washed or deglycerolized frozen erythrocytes are recommended.

ANAPHYLACTIC REACTIONS

Etiology. Anaphylactic reactions occur in IgA-deficient patients who have developed anti-IgA antibodies. Patients lacking IgA have an increased risk of forming anti-IgA antibodies. Anti-IgA antibody formation can result from immunization due to previous transfusions or pregnancy; however, patients often have anti-IgA without a known source of stimulation.

IgA deficiency is the most frequent of all of the selective deficiencies of serum immunoglobins, occurring in about 1 in 700 persons. In these patients, 10% develop antibodies to IgA protein and can suffer acute anaphylactic reactions when infused with blood products containing the protein. Anti-IgA antibodies exist in 86% of patients with anaphylactic or anaphylactoid reactions.

Fortunately, anaphylactic reactions due to anti-IgA are very rare. Other potential causes of anaphylactic reaction are the presence of antibodies to soluble plasma antigens or to drugs contained in transfused blood, such as penicillin.

Signs and Symptoms. Anaphylactic reactions are dramatic and rapid in their onset. Clinical signs are seen suddenly after exposure to the IgA protein, often before 10 mL of plasma have been infused. Symptoms include nausea, abdominal cramps, emesis, and diarrhea. Transient hypertension is followed by hypotension. Shock and loss of consciousness follow. Medical assistance must be sought immediately if anaphylaxis is suspected.

It is important to distinguish an anaphylactic reaction from other immediate reactions. In an anaphylactic reaction, symptoms become obvious after the infusion of only a few milliliters of blood or plasma, and fever is absent.

Prevention. Demonstration of antibody to IgA remains a research procedure, but evidence can be obtained by documenting the absence of serum IgA in the patient through immunodiffusion or immunoelectrophoresis techniques.

Avoiding exposure to IgA is mandatory in previously immunized IgA-deficient patients. These patients *must* be transfused with blood components that lack IgA. In some cases, it may be possible to collect and store frozen autologous components for known IgA-deficient patients. When that is not possible, files of such donors are maintained by the AABB Rare Donor File, the Irwin Memorial Blood Bank (San Francisco), the American National Red Cross (Washington), and the Canadian Red Cross (Toronto, Ontario, Canada).

Bacterial Endotoxemia and Sepsis

ETIOLOGY

Although transfusion reactions are rarely due to bacterial contamination of whole blood and other selected components, an increased number of deaths caused by bacterial contamination of platelet concentrates have been reported to the FDA since 1980. In contrast to a report in 1980, when two fatalities were attributed to contaminated blood or blood components in the previous 2½ years, six deaths due to bacterial contamination of platelet concentrates were reported between January 1980 and December 1983. A report in 1986 stated that, in a three-month period, four episodes of bacterial sepsis related to contaminated random donor platelet concentrates were observed at one medical center. Platelet concentrates that, by contemporary standard practice, are stored at room temperature are now the most common cause of transfusion-related sepsis.

Bacterial endotoxemia in whole blood or blood components stored under refrigeration is usually due to the endotoxins produced by psychrophilic (cold-growing) gram-negative bacteria, such as the *Pseudomonas* species. In products such as platelet concentrates stored at room temperature, bacterial isolates have included *Salmonella heidelberg*, the *Corynebacterium JK* group, *Staphylococcus epidermidis* and *Staphylococcus aureus.*

SIGNS AND SYMPTOMS

The appearance of signs and symptoms caused by bacterial endotoxemia begins within 30 minutes and may follow the infusion of as little as 50 mL of blood. Initial symptoms may include characteristic shaking chills, severe hypotension, pain in the abdomen, generalized muscle pain, vomiting, and bloody diarrhea. The manifestation of shock syndrome is unusual because it appears as dry flushed skin and fever. Renal failure and possibly DIC may follow. If this type of transfusion reaction is not immediately recognized and treated, it can be fatal. Treatment usually consists of the administration of broad-spectrum antibiotics, fluid replacement, respiratory support, corticosteroids, and vasopressors to maintain blood pressure and urinary output.

Reactions caused by recent bacterial contamination are usually manifested within minutes of completing a transfusion. Fever, chills, and hypotension are common symptoms. Antibiotic treatment of the patient must be initiated immediately. Other forms of treatment should be consistent with the patient's clinical condition.

PREVENTION

Maintenance of sterility is essential to the prevention of bacterial contamination. Caution must be exercised before and during blood collection and component preparation. Unit dose dispensing of small quantities of blood to neonatal patients has not led to bacterial contamination. Storage temperature and length of storage are critical considerations. The length of storage time currently approved for platelet concentrates is being questioned.

It is important to inspect blood and blood components visually before issue. If a unit has a brownish or purple discoloration, bacterial contamination should be strongly suspected. Units should also *not* be issued if clots are apparent or if the interface between plasma and erythrocytes has a fuzzy or blurred appearance. Plasma should be inspected for an opaque or muddy look as evidence of bacterial contamination.

Current regulations impose only limited sterility constraints on perishable products such as packed erythrocytes and fresh-frozen plasma. It is essential to monitor the sterility of blood products resulting from aseptic donations. The effectiveness of available methods has been questioned because the integrity of a closed system may be destroyed. Accidental contamination during sterility testing can never be totally excluded; however, a safer technique using a simple, permanently closed system has been recently described.

Circulatory Overload

ETIOLOGY

Circulatory overload can result from rapid transfusion of large volumes of blood without equivalent blood loss. It can also occur after transfusion of small amounts of blood to patients with abnormal cardiac function and reserve.

SIGNS AND SYMPTOMS

Typical symptoms include severe head-ache, dyspnea, cyanosis, and congestive heart failure. Pulmonary edema can subsequently develop as a result of congestive heart failure. In infants with high cardiac reserve function, the prodromal symptoms may be hidden, with complication emerging rapidly and proving fatal.

PREVENTION

The use of packed erythrocytes rather than whole blood substantially reduces the risk of circulatory overload. In patients who are not actively bleeding or who are susceptible to circulatory overload, such as those with chronic heart disease, blood should be administered slowly. The usual rate of blood administration, 200 mL/hour, should be reduced to 100 mL/hour, although prolonging the time does increase the risk of bacterial growth. In addition, it is preferable to have the patient in a sitting rather than a reclining position. Some clinicians prefer to divide full units of packed red cells in half. One divided unit can be transfused while the other remains refrigerated. The attending physician may also order the administration of a diuretic medication to reduce fluid retention. In patients with low hematocrits (15 to 20%), phlebotomy of whole blood followed by the transfusion of packed red cells may be useful in increasing oxygen-carrying capacity without expanding blood volume. The protocol for this technique must be approved by the blood bank director and medical staff.

Other Immediate Adverse Effects

Rapid transfusion of 10 or more units of citrated blood can elevate plasma citrate levels. Clinical and experimental studies have demonstrated that rapid transfusion with citrated bank blood components can cause hypocalcemic myocardial depression.

Hypocalcemia is usually self-compensated, with no need for calcium therapy. Acute cardiac failure and cardiac arrest are rare and have been observed primarily in association with exchange transfusion in infants.

Two additional complications that can precipitate arrhythmias are hyperkalemia (an increase in plasma potassium) and transfusion of a large volume of cold blood, which lowers body temperature.

DELAYED NONHEMOLYTIC REACTIONS

Graft-Versus-Host Disease

ETIOLOGY

When immunocompetent lymphocytes are transfused from a donor to a recipient who is not capable of rejecting them, the transfused or *grafted* lymphocytes recognize the antigens of the host as foreign and react immunologically against them. Instead of the usual transplantation reaction of host against graft, the reverse graft-versus-host reaction occurs and produces an inflammatory response.

In a normal lymphocyte transfer reaction, the results of a graft-versus-host reaction are usually not serious because the recipient is capable of destroying the foreign lymphocytes. If the recipient, however, cannot reject the transfused lymphocytes, they may cause uncontrolled destruction of the host's tissues and eventually death. Engraftment/multiplication of donor lymphocytes in an immunosuppressed recipient is a real possibility because lymphocytes capable of mitosis can be found in stored blood products.

Graft-versus-host reactions occur in immunodeficient or immunosuppressed patients. Cases of transfusion-related graft-versus-host disease have increased significantly in the past two decades. This reaction has been reported after blood transfusion in bone marrow transplant recipients following total body irradiation, adults receiving intensive chemotherapy for hematologic malignancies, and infants with severe congenital immunodeficiency. Graft-versus-host disease has occurred in infants who have received intrauterine transfusions followed by exchange transfusion. Patients at risk are those with severe lymphocytopenia (less than 500 lymphocytes/μl) and bone marrow suppression.

SIGNS AND SYMPTOMS

Post-transfusion symptoms begin within 3 to 30 days of transfusion. Because of lymphocytic infiltration of the intestine, skin, and liver, mucosal destruction including ulcerative skin and mouth lesions, diarrhea, and liver necrosis occur. Other clinical signs include jaundice, fever, anemia, weight loss, skin rash, and splenomegaly.

The stronger the antigen difference, the more severe the reaction. Nearly 90% of patients with post-transfusion graft-versus-host disease die of acute complications of the disease. The usual immediate mechanism of death is generalized infection.

PREVENTION

Irradiated blood and blood components may be used to avoid graft-versus-host disease.

Noncardiac Pulmonary Edema Syndrome

ETIOLOGY

This disorder is characteristically a complication of granulocyte transfusion. It has occurred, however, after the transfusion of whole blood or plasma, and there are isolated reports of its occurring after cryoprecipitate infusion. The precise cause is not known, but leukoagglutinins have been implicated. The incidence of noncardiac pulmonary edema increases with parity in women.

Two mechanisms have been postulated. In one mechanism, the reaction between donor leukoagglutinins and recipient leukocytes produces leukocyte aggregates that are trapped in the pulmonary microcirculation and produce changes in vascular permeability. If granulocyte concentrates are administered, the reaction involves recipient leukoagglutinins that aggregate the transfused granulocytes. An alternate proposed mechanism is the activation of complement to generate the anaphylatoxins C3a and C5a. These complement components stimulate the release of histamine and serotonin from tissue basophils and platelets in addition to directly aggregating granulocytes. Directly aggregated granulocytes produce leukocytic emboli that lodge in the microvascular circulation of the lungs.

SIGNS AND SYMPTOMS

The reaction may be mild and respond to supportive therapy but it is characteristically severe and delayed, occurring 1 to 6 hours after transfusion. Respiratory distress can begin after the infusion of amounts of blood too small to produce hypervolemia. Clinical signs include chills, fever, dyspnea, nonproductive cough, hypotension, and cyanosis. Blood eosinophilia is common.

PREVENTION

Washed or frozen-deglycerolized units of blood may be used to avoid some of these reactions because leukocytes are almost completely eliminated.

Post-Transfusion Purpura

ETIOLOGY

Post-transfusion purpura is a rare event that may develop after the administration of blood or platelet-containing components.

Most patients have been women, most of whom appear to have been immunized by previous pregnancies or, less frequently, by previous transfusions. The severe thrombocytopenia that develops in the disorder is associated with platelet alloantibodies. Almost all affected patients have been shown to be P1^{A1} negative with anti-P1^{A1} antibodies in their plasma at the time of thrombocytopenia. This antibody was directed against platelet membrane glycoprotein III. P1^{A1} antigen is present in 98.3% of the U.S. population. The P1^{A1} antibody destroys not only the transfused platelets but the patient's own P1^{A1} negative platelets. The mechanism of destruction of the patient's own platelets or of P1^{A1} negative platelets from normal donors during the acute phase of post-transfusion purpura is unknown. In three cases, the patients were P1^{A1} positive with an antibody specificity that may have been anti-P1^{A2}.

Signs and Symptoms

Clinical signs generally manifest themselves about a week after transfusion due to a sudden decrease in the patient's platelet count. This severe thrombocytopenia produces generalized purpura. In addition to purpura and petechiae, occult or obvious hemorrhage may be present.

Prevention

In patients with severe thrombocytopenia who need treatment, exchange plasmapheresis is a possible mode of therapy. The thrombocytopenia in this disorder is usually self-limiting. Platelet transfusions are usually not beneficial.

Iron Overload

Etiology

A delayed effect of multiple transfusions of erythrocytes in nonbleeding, chronically anemic patients is iron overload from transfusion hypersiderosis or hemosiderosis. Patients at risk of iron overload include those with hemoglobinopathies, such as the thalassemias, and aplastic or sideroblastic anemias. Every unit of erythrocytes contains approximately 250 mg of iron. When patients have received more than 100 transfusions, significant iron deposition may occur.

Signs and Symptoms

Deposits of iron in parenchymal cells cause damage to many organs, most significantly the liver, heart, and endocrine glands. Dysfunctions of specific body systems, such as jaundice or cardiac dysfunction, represent manifestations of this condition.

Prevention

Iron-chelating agents may be useful in reducing body storage iron; however, it has not been proven that such treatment can reverse the tissue damage that has already occurred, nor has it been demonstrated that consistent long-term iron balance can be achieved with this therapy. A recent approach to reducing the risk of transfusion-induced iron overload is transfusion with erythrocytes that have been enriched with younger erythrocytes, *neocytes.* Neocytes survive longer in the circulation and result in a greater interval between transfusions, with subsequent reduction in the total iron infused over an extended period of time.

Other Delayed Adverse Effects

Two significant consequences of blood transfusion are immunization to foreign antigens and the transmission of disease. Immunization to antigens is described in detail in Chapter 3. Because the transmission of disease through transfusion is critical, it is discussed separately in Chapter 12.

LABORATORY INVESTIGATION OF TRANSFUSION REACTIONS

Investigation of possible transfusion reactions is important to the immediate and long-term safety of patients. Although the protocol may vary depending on the patient's signs and symptoms, the generally accepted procedure for investigation of a transfusion reaction includes the steps outlined in the following sections.

Immediate Steps

1. Check the identification of the patient and the transfused unit of blood or component. Notify the appropriate persons if any clerical or identification error exists. If a discrepancy is noted, check to see if any other patients are at risk.
2. Obtain a post-transfusion blood specimen from the patient. Label it as the post-transfusion specimen. Obtain the discontinued bag of blood, administration set, and any attached IV solutions.
3. Visually examine the patient's post-transfusion serum or plasma for hemolysis. In a properly drawn specimen, a pink color indicates that intravascular hemolysis may have taken place. If massive hemolysis has occurred, free hemoglobin will be apparent at once. It may be detectable with the onset of clinical signs and symptoms. Free hemoglobin is cleared from the plasma in 5 to 12 hours.
4. Perform a direct antiglobulin test on an anticoagulated post-transfusion blood specimen from the patient. If the transfused red cells are not immediately destroyed, the direct AHG test will be positive with a mixed-field appearance. If the post-transfusion specimen is positive, the pretransfusion DAT should also be checked. If only the DAT on the post-transfusion test is positive, the patient's erythrocytes have been coated with antibody or complement. Procedures for investigation of a positive DAT should be followed to determine the cause.
5. Perform an ABO grouping and Rh typing of the patient's pretransfusion and post-transfusion blood specimens, and of a specimen from the bag or a segment attached to the transfused unit. If a discrepancy exists between the ABO group or Rh type of the patient's pretransfusion and post-transfusion specimens or the donor unit, an error in patient identification, specimen la-

beling, or donor unit identification, or other clerical error, is responsible. The results must be crosschecked against all past records as well as the labelling of the blood product itself. Any other patient specimens drawn at approximately the same time should be rechecked if the possibility of having another patient at risk exists.

Follow-Up Steps

Depending on the patient's signs and symptoms (see examples), additional testing may be indicated. Procedures include the following:

1. Repeat the crossmatch with the pretransfusion and post-transfusion specimens. An incompatible crossmatch with the pretransfusion specimen indicates that an error existed in the patient or donor specimen during pretransfusion testing. If the crossmatch is incompatible *only* with the post-transfusion specimen, a patient identification problem or an anamnestic reaction may be responsible, depending on the time interval between the transfusion and the reactions.
2. Repeat the alloantibody screening tests on the pretransfusion and donor units as well as on the post-transfusion specimen. If either the pretransfusion or donor unit specimen has a previously unreported alloantibody, check for clerical errors in the pretransfusion testing. If the post-transfusion specimen has an antibody not present in the pretransfusion specimen, an anamnestic reaction or passive administration of antibody in a recently infused blood component should be suspected.
3. If any of the alloantibody screening tests are positive, identify the antibody. The presence of an alloantibody does not necessarily indicate that it is the cause of the reaction; the corresponding antigen must also be present. Test the patient or donor erythrocytes for the corresponding antigen.
4. Request the collection of a urine sample from the patient as soon as pos-

sible. Intact red cells indicate hemorrhage into the urinary tract—not hemolysis. Test the urine specimen for the presence of free hemoglobin. If the urine specimen is not collected for several days, it may be tested for hemosiderin.

Additional Tests

If routine testing fails to provide information and immune hemolysis is suspected, the following tests may be helpful:

1. Antibody screening and compatibility tests with enhancement media or by increasing the ratio of serum to cells.
2. DAT and alloantibody screening tests on several post-transfusion specimens collected from the patient at daily or frequent intervals.
3. Monitoring of hemoglobin / hematocrit levels. In a nonbleeding patient, a unit of packed erthrocytes should produce an increase of 1 g / dL or packed cell volume (hematocrit) of 3%.
4. Genotyping of the erythrocytes of the patient's pre-transfusion specimen and the donor cells. The patient's postreaction specimen must be examined for the presence of cells bearing foreign antigens. If an antigen can be found that is present on the donor cells and absent on the patient's cells, its presence or absence in the post-transfusion sample indicates the degree to which the transfused cells have survived and remain in the circulation.

5. Testing of post-transfusion serum samples for the presence of unconjugated bilirubin. A rising bilirubin may be detectable as early as 1 hour post-transfusion. Peak levels occur at 3 to 6 hours. The degree of hyperbilirubinemia depends on the extent and rapidity of hemolysis and the rate of bilirubin excretion.
6. Measure of serum haptoglobin in pre- and post-transfusion patient specimens. When haptoglobin is fully saturated, free hemoglobin appears in the plasma. A decline in haptoglobin is useful in detecting chronic hemolysis. If studies are performed several days after a hemolytic episode, normal levels may be restored because haptoglobin is an acute-phase reactant that may regenerate rapidly after depletion.

Tests for Fibrinolysis (DIC)

Because the manifestations of fibrinolysis and DIC are extremely variable, diagnosis depends on laboratory testing. The key feature is an elevation of circulating fibrinogen-fibrin split products (FSPs).

Typical results in DIC include prolonged activated partial thromboplastin time (APPT), prothrombin time (PT), and thrombin time. Fibrinogen levels and the total platelet count may vary, although thrombocytopenia and a decrease in fibrinogen are common. Excessive fibrinolysis with the release of FSPs occurs secondary to intravascular fibrin formation. While the presence of FSPs is characteristic, the finding of FSPs is not specific for DIC and cannot be used as the sole criterion for diagnosis.

CASE STUDIES OF TRANSFUSION REACTIONS

Case 1

An 18-year-old man was admitted with multiple injuries after he and a passenger, another 18-year-old man, were in a motor vehicle accident. After receiving 50 mL of the first unit of blood, the patient developed shaking chills and became hypotensive. The unit of blood was immediately discontinued and the blood bank was asked to recheck the crossmatch (STAT).

LABORATORY TESTING

Clerical Check. No evidence of blood bank clerical errors.

Hemoglobinemia. Slight hemolysis observed.
Direct Antiglobulin Test. Patient pretransfusion specimen: Negative
Patient post-transfusion specimen: Weakly positive (mixed field)

Recheck of Blood Grouping

	Anti–A	Anti–B	Anti–A,B	Anti–D	A_1 Cells	B Cells	Int.
Patient:							
Pretransfusion	4+	Neg	4+	3+	Neg	4+	A+
Post–transfusion	Neg	Neg	Neg	3+	4+	4+	O+
Donor segment	4+	Neg	4+	2+	Neg	3+	A+

Recheck of Crossmatching

Patient pretransfusion specimen and donor segment: Compatible (immediate spin)

Patient post-transfusion specimen and donor segment: Incompatible (immediate spin)

INTERPRETATION

This is a life-threatening emergency because the patient has the signs of an acute hemolytic transfusion reaction. The emergency room physician and the medical director of the blood bank were immediately notified and treatment was initiated. A rapid check of the passenger's blood status revealed that he was group A and was incorrectly receiving group O blood. The patient was group O and had received group A blood. Further investigation revealed that the original patient blood specimen labels had been reversed when the emergency room personnel handed the already drawn tubes of blood to the phlebotomist.

CONCLUSION

Acute hemolytic transfusion reaction.

Case 2

A 38-year-old woman was admitted for thoracic surgery. She had received 2 units of packed red blood cells following the birth of her third child 10 years ago. During her present hospitalization, she developed a fever 72 hours after receiving 3 units of blood during surgery. On her fifth postoperative day, she began to appear mildly jaundiced and experienced a sudden drop in her hemoglobin and hematocrit, with no evidence of hemorrhage. A transfusion reaction workup was ordered.

LABORATORY TESTING

Clerical Check. No evidence of blood bank clerical errors.

Hemoglobinemia. Absent from fifth-day post-transfusion specimen.

Direct Antiglobulin Test
Patient post-transfusion specimen: Positive (polyspecific and IgG antisera)
Patient pretransfusion specimen: Negative

Recheck of Blood Grouping

	Anti–A	Anti–B	Anti–A,B	Anti–D	A_1 Cells	B Cells	Int.
Patient:							
Pretransfusion	Neg	Neg	Neg	3+	4+	4+	O+
Post–transfusion	Neg	Neg	Neg	3+	4+	4+	O+
Donor segment 1	Neg	Neg	Neg	2+			O+
Donor segment 2	Neg	Neg	Neg	4+			O+
Donor segment 3	Neg	Neg	Neg	3+			O+

Recheck of Crossmatching

Patient pretransfusion specimen and donor segment: Compatible

Patient post-transfusion specimen and donor segment 1: Compatible

Patient post-transfusion specimen and

donor segment 2: Incompatible (microscopically in AHG)

Patient post-transfusion specimen and donor segment 3: Incompatible (microscopically in AHG)

Alloantibody Screening

Patient pretransfusion specimen: Negative

Genotyping

Patient	E negative e positive	Genotype: ee
Donor #1	E negative e positive	Genotype: ee
Donor #2	E negative e positive	Genotype: Ee
Donor #3	E negative e positive	Genotype: EE

Patient post-transfusion specimen: Weakly positive (AHG)

Alloantibody Identification

Patient post-transfusion specimen: Anti-E (enzyme technique only)

Eluate of patient red blood cells: Anti-E (enzyme technique only)

INTERPRETATION

This patient exhibits the signs and symptoms of a delayed hemolytic transfusion reaction caused by anti-E. The rapid development of the antibody suggests an anamnestic response. Previous exposure to the E antigen, which the patient lacks, may have occurred during pregnancy or prior transfusion. The patient was transfused with two units of donor blood possessing the E antigen 5 days before development of signs and symptoms of a reaction. If future transfusions are required, the patient should receive blood that lacks the E antigen.

CONCLUSION

Delayed hemolytic transfusion reaction.

Case 3

A 69-year-old women was being transfused because of a low postoperative hematocrit. She had a history of anemia and had received multiple previous transfusions. She had experienced a febrile transfusion reaction 4 years ago while receiving washed red cells, but had received two units of blood two years ago while in surgery without demonstrating a reaction. During the present episode, she displayed signs and symptoms of a reaction 20 minutes after the initiation of the infusion of a unit of centrifuged red cells. Her temperature rose from 97.5° F to 102.9° F and her blood pressure rose from 130/70 to 150/80. She also experienced chills. The unit of blood was discontinued and 3/4 of it was returned to the blood bank.

LABORATORY TESTING

Clerical Check. No evidence of blood bank clerical errors.

Hemoglobinemia. Absent from post-transfusion specimen.

Direct Antiglobulin Test

Patient post-transfusion specimen: Negative

Recheck of Blood Grouping

	Anti–A	Anti–B	Anti–A,B	Anti–D	A₁ Cells	B Cells	Int.
Patient:							
Pretransfusion	Neg	Neg	Neg	2+	4+	4+	O+
Post–transfusion	Neg	Neg	Neg	2+	4+	4+	O+
Donor segment	Neg	Neg	Neg	2+			O+

INTERPRETATION

There is no evidence of a hemolytic transfusion reaction. This patient exhibits the signs and symptoms of a febrile transfusion reaction. It is recommended that she receive leukocyte-depleted red blood cells if future transfusions are indicated.

CONCLUSION

Febrile transfusion reaction, probably due to leukoagglutinins.

Case 4

A 58-year-old woman was admitted with the diagnosis of a fractured hip and anemia. She had no prior history of transfusion, but was the mother of three children. Two hours and 45 minutes after initiation of the infusion of a unit of packed red cells, the patient's blood pressure rose from 128/70 to 180/90 and her temperature rose from 98.7° F to 100.6° F. She did not exhibit chills. The transfusion was discontinued and 1/3 of the unit was returned to the blood bank.

LABORATORY TESTING

Clerical Check. No evidence of blood bank clerical error.

Direct Antiglobulin Test.
Patient post-transfusion specimen: Negative

Hemoglobinemia. Absent from post-transfusion specimen.

Recheck of Blood Grouping

	Anti–A	Anti–B	Anti–A,B	Anti–D	A₁ Cells	B Cells	Int.
Patient:							
Pretransfusion	Neg	Neg	Neg	3+	2+	1+	O+
Post–transfusion	Neg	Neg	Neg	3+	2+	1+	O+
Donor segment	Neg	Neg	Neg	2+			O+

INTERPRETATION

There is no evidence of a hemolytic transfusion reaction. This patient exhibits the signs and symptoms of a mild febrile transfusion reaction. If a subsequent transfusion produces a similar reaction, it is recommended that she receive leukocyte-depleted red blood cells.

CONCLUSION

Febrile transfusion reaction, probable leukoagglutinins.

Case 5

An 81-year-old man was admitted with a diagnosis of chronic anemia. He had no history of previous transfusion. One hour after the initiation of the infusion of a unit of packed red blood cells, he developed hives and his blood pressure increased from 140/70 to 168/76. His temperature remained normal. Approximately 35 mL of blood remained in the donor unit that was returned to the blood bank.

LABORATORY TESTING

Clerical Check. No evidence of blood bank clerical error.

Direct Antiglobulin Test
Patient post-transfusion specimen: Negative

Hemoglobinemia. Absent from post-transfusion specimen.

Recheck of Blood Grouping

	Anti–A	Anti–B	Anti–A,B	Anti–D	A₁ Cells	B Cells	Int.
Patient:							
Pretransfusion	Neg	3+	3+	Pos	3+	Neg	B+
Post–transfusion	Neg	3+	3+	Pos	3+	Neg	B+
Donor segment	Neg	3+	3+	Pos			B+

INTERPRETATION

There is no evidence of a hemolytic transfusion reaction. This patient demonstrates the signs and symptoms of an allergic reaction to the foreign proteins in the donor plasma. If additional transfusions are required; the patient should receive a plasma protein-deficient red blood cell product or be premedicated with an antihistamine.

CONCLUSION

Allergic reaction to plasma protein.

Case 6

A 25-year-old man, a burn patient, had previously received multiple transfusions and had a clinical diagnosis of burn / wound sepsis. Ten minutes after the initiation of an infusion of whole blood, he demonstrated an increased pulse rate (from 112 to 118) and an increased body temperature (from 100° F to 102.4° C). The unit of blood was discontinued and 3/4 of it was returned to the blood bank.

LABORATORY TESTING

Clerical Check. No evidence of clerical error.
Direct Antiglobulin Test
Patient post-transfusion specimen: Negative
Hemoglobinemia. Absent from post-transfusion specimen.

Recheck of Blood Grouping

	Anti–A	Anti–B	Anti–A,B	Anti–D	A_1 Cells	B Cells	Int.
Patient:							
Pretransfusion	Neg	4+	4+	Neg	4+	Neg	B–
Post–transfusion	Neg	4+	4+	Neg	4+	Neg	B–
Donor segment	Neg	4+	4+	Neg			B–

INTERPRETATION

There is no evidence of a hemolytic transfusion reaction. Although the possibility of a febrile reaction to donor leukocytes cannot be totally excluded, the patient's signs and symptoms are probably due to an endogenous fever.

CONCLUSION

Endogenous fever.

CHAPTER SUMMARY

Definition and Causes

The term transfusion reaction generally refers to the adverse signs and symptoms produced by incompatibility between a patient and a unit of donor red blood cells or blood component. When a physician makes the clinical judgment to transfuse a patient, the expected benefits of the product must be weighed against the known risks. The risk of a transfusion reaction is minimal but not unimportant. The vast majority of fatal transfusion reactions result from misidentification or clerical errors rather than technical limitations. Transfusion reactions can be divided into hemolytic and nonhemolytic types and can be acute or delayed in their manifestation. Acute hemolytic reactions occur during or immediately after blood has been infused; delayed reactions may not express themselves until 7 to 10 days post-transfusion. Acute hemolytic reactions are the most serious and potentially lethal.

Factors that influence whether a transfusion reaction will be acute or delayed include the number of incompatible erythrocytes infused, the antibody class or subclass, and the achievement of the optimal temperature for antibody binding.

Acute Hemolytic Reactions

The most common cause of an acute hemolytic transfusion reaction is transfusion of ABO-incompatible blood. The signs and symptoms of a reaction can occur with the infusion of as little as 10 to 15 mL of incompatible blood. The most common initial symptoms are fever and chills, which mimic a febrile, nonhemolytic reaction due to leukocyte incompatibility. Back pain, shortness of breath, pain at the infusion site, and hypotension are also symptoms. The release of thromboplastic substances into the circulation can induce shock or disseminated intravascular coagulation (DIC) and acute renal failure. Prevention of acute hemolytic reactions rests in the proper identification of patients and patient samples, along with error-free laboratory record-keeping, blood grouping, and crossmatching.

Delayed Hemolytic Reactions

Delayed hemolytic transfusion reactions can occur from two days to several months post-transfusion. This type of hemolytic reaction is underdiagnosed, under-reported, and under-rated in terms of complications and is far more frequent than acute hemolytic reactions. A delayed hemolytic transfusion reaction may represent an anamnestic antibody response in a previously immunized recipient on secondary exposure to transfused erythrocyte antigens or it may result from primary alloimmunization. The most common clinical sign is fever. The triad of anemia, fever, and blood transfusion within the last 3 months suggests a delayed hemolytic reaction. However, symptoms can range from an asymptomatic state to oliguria or renal shutdown in less than 10% of cases to DIC in very rare cases. Accidental discovery of a positive DAT in a subsequent crossmatch commonly reveals that a patient has antibody-coated erythrocytes in the circulation. To prevent a delayed transfusion reaction, patient specimens used for compatibility testing should be no more than 3 days old at the time of transfusion if a patient has been previously transfused, pregnant within the past 3 months, or of unknown transfusion status.

Immediate Nonhemolytic Reactions

Febrile reactions are the most prevalent type of immediate nonhemolytic reaction. Febrile reactions are most commonly due to cytotoxic antibodies or leukoagglutinins. The most frequent symptom is fever, often accompanied by chills, which begins during or soon after transfusion. Although a nonhemolytic febrile reaction is rarely harmful, fever may be one of the clinical symptoms of a hemolytic transfusion reaction. Evidence of chills and fever should be investigated as a potential hemolytic transfusion reaction. To prevent a reaction, documenting the existence of antibodies may be helpful in patients who are expected to need additional transfusions. Tests such as leukoagglutinin and microlymphocytotoxicity assays can be performed. With or without documentation of the existence of specific antibodies, however, leukocyte-poor preparations should be administered only after a patient has had two or more febrile nonhemolytic reactions.

Two types of immediate reactions to transfused platelets have been documented: febrile reactions and hemolytic reactions. Febrile reactions to platelet transfusions are probably related to the presence of large numbers of leukocytes in the platelet concentrate component. A hemolytic reaction to platelet components is related to the common practice of transfusing ABO-incompatible platelets when group-specific platelets are not available. Transfusions which are not group-specific are generally considered safe and are accepted as clinically effective. Transfusions of incompatible platelets are not, however, without risks related to passively transfused antibodies. The use of group-specific platelets is preferred but in cases of ABO-incompatible platelet preparations, removal of as much plasma as possible provides an acceptable product.

Immediate reactions to plasma constituents may be classified as allergic, anaphylactoid, or anaphylactic in nature. Although the mechanism of allergic and anaphylactoid reactions is unclear, most authorities agree that it is a reaction to soluble constituents in donor plasma. Allergic reactions are manifested by urticaria, itching, and local erythema. If the cutaneous reaction is extensive or produces oral, pharyngeal, laryngeal edema, it is known as an anaphylactoid reaction. Reactions can be well controlled with antihistamines. In repeated or severe reactions, washed or deglycerolized frozen erythrocytes are recommended. Anaphylactic reactions occur in IgA-deficient patients who have developed anti-IgA-antibodies. Patients lacking IgA have an increased risk of forming anti-IgA antibodies. Anti-IgA antibody formation can result from immunization due to previous transfusions or pregnancy; however, patients often have anti-IgA without a known source of stimulation. Fortunately, anaphylactic reactions due to anti-IgA are very rare. Other potential causes of an anaphylactic reaction are the presence of antibodies to soluble plasma antigens or to drugs contained in transfused blood such as penicillin. Anaphylactic reactions are dramatic. Symptoms include flushing of the skin, dyspnea, coughing, laryngeal edema, bronchospasm, and severe hypotension. Shock and loss of consciousness follow. These symptoms are seen soon after exposure to the IgA protein. Avoiding exposure to IgA is mandatory in previously immunized IgA-deficient patients. These patients must be transfused with blood components that lack IgA.

Bacterial sepsis is rarely due to bacterial contamination of whole blood and other selected components, but an increased number of deaths caused by bacterial contamination of platelet concentrates have been reported since 1980. Platelet concentrates stored at room temperature are now the commonest cause of transfusion-related sepsis. Bacterial endotoxemia in whole blood or blood components stored under refrigeration is usually due to the endotoxins produced by psychrophilic gram-negative bacteria. Appearance of symptoms due to bacterial endotoxemia begins shortly after the introduction of the endotoxin into the patient's circulation. Initial symptoms may include flushing and dryness of the skin, abdominal cramps, generalized muscle pain, vomiting, and diarrhea. Progressively more severe symptoms include high fever, hemoglobinuria, shock, renal failure, and possibly DIC. In septic reactions, symptoms are usually apparent within minutes of completing a transfusion. Fever, chills, and hypotension are common symptoms. Maintenance of sterility is essential to the prevention of bacterial contamination. Storage temperature and length of storage are also critical considerations. It is equally important to visually inspect blood and blood components before issue.

Circulatory overload can result from rapid transfusion of large volumes of blood without equivalent blood loss. It can also occur after transfusion of small amounts of blood to patients with abnormal cardiac function and reserve. Typical symptoms include severe headache, dyspnea, cyanosis, and pulmonary edema. Congestive heart failure can consequently develop. In infants with high cardiac reserve function, the prodromal symptoms may be hidden, with complications emerging rapidly and proving fatal. Circulatory overload can be prevented through the use of packed erythrocytes rather than whole blood.

The rapid transfusion of 10 or more units of citrated blood can elevate plasma citrate levels. Clinical and experimental studies have demonstrated that rapid transfusion with citrated bank blood components can cause hypocalcemic myocardial depression. Hyperkalemia is another theoretic complication. Additionally, transfusing a large volume of cold blood can lower body temperature.

Delayed Nonhemolytic Reactions

Graft-versus-host disease can develop when immunocompetent lymphocytes are transfused from a donor to a recipient who is not capable of rejecting the transfused or grafted lymphocytes. In a normal lymphocyte-transfer reaction, the results of a graft-versus-host reaction are usually not serious because the recipient is capable of destroying the foreign lymphocytes, but if the recipient cannot reject the transfused lymphocytes, the grafted lymphocytes may cause uncontrolled destruction of the host's tissues and eventually death. Post-transfusion symptoms begin within 3 to 30 days after transfusion. Because of lymphocytic infiltration of the intestines, skin, and liver, mucosal destruction including ulcerative skin and mouth lesions, diarrhea, and liver destruction result. Other clinical symptoms include jaundice, fever, anemia, weight loss, skin rash, and splenomegaly. Irradiated whole blood, packed erythrocytes, and blood components should be used in susceptible patients.

Noncardiac pulmonary edema syndrome is chiefly a complication of transfused granulocytes. The reaction may be mild and respond to supportive therapy, but the reaction is characteristically severe and delayed, occurring 1 to 6 hours after transfusion. Respiratory distress can begin after the infusion of amounts of blood too small to produce hypervolemia. Clinical symptoms include chills, fever, dyspnea, nonproductive cough, hypotension, and cyanosis. Washed or frozen deglycerolized red cells eliminate this complication.

Post-transfusion purpura is a rare event that may develop following the administration of blood or platelet containing blood components. The severe thrombocytopenia that develops in the disorder is associated with platelet alloantibodies. Clinical symptoms generally manifest themselves about a week after transfusion due to a sudden decrease in the patient's platelet count which produces generalized purpura. In addition to purpura and petechiae, occult or obvious hemorrhage may be present. In patients with severe thrombocytopenia who need treatment, exchange plasmapheresis is a possible mode of therapy.

Iron overload is a delayed manifestation in patients who have received multiple transfusions over an extended period of time. Deposits of iron in parenchymal cells cause damage to many organs, most significantly the liver, heart, or endocrine glands. Symptoms typical of dysfunction of the specific body systems, such as jaundice or cardiac dysfunction, are manifestations of this condition. Iron-chelating agents may be useful in reducing body iron storage and transfusion with neocytes may be useful.

Two additional significant consequences of blood transfusion can be immunization to foreign antigens and transmission of disease.

Laboratory Investigation of Transfusion Reactions

The investigation of possible transfusion reactions is important to the immediate and long-term safety of patients. Although specific details of the protocol may vary from one blood bank to another, the general approach to the investigation of a transfusion reaction includes immediate steps such as checking the identification of the patient and of the transfused unit of blood or component. Additional testing is needed if routine testing fails to provide information and immune hemolysis is suspected.

REVIEW QUESTIONS

1. A transfusion reaction includes:
   A. Incompatibility between red cell antigens and antibodies.
   B. Shortened posttransfusion survival of erythrocytes
   C. An allergic response
   D. Infection with a blood borne disease
   E. All of the above
2. The *most* frequent cause of fatal transfusion reactions is:
   A. Mislabelling of blood samples
   B. Errors in laboratory records
   C. Misidentification of patients
   D. Crossmatching that failed to detect antibodies

E. Reactions to leukocytes

3–6. Match the type of transfusion reaction with the appropriate condition:

A. Immediate hemolytic
B. Immediate nonhemolytic
C. Delayed hemolytic
D. Delayed nonhemolytic

3. Urticaria

4. Hemolysis of erythrocytes during or immediately after blood infusion

5. Graft-versus-host disease

6. Hemolysis of erythrocytes 7 to 10 days post-transfusion

7. Infectious diseases

8. The most severe form of a transfusion reaction is:

A. Intravascular hemolysis
B. Extravascular hemolysis
C. Iron overload
D. Urticaria
E. Febrile reactions

9. The factor/factors that determine(s) whether a transfusion reaction will be acute or delayed and intravascular or extravascular is/are:

A. The volume of incompatible erythrocytes infused
B. Antibody class and subclass
C. Achievement of an optimal temperature for antibody binding
D. Distribution of antibodies on erythrocytes
E. All of the above

10. The *most frequent* cause of an acute hemolytic transfusion reaction is:

A. Anti-I
B. Anti-A, anti-B
C. Anti-Le^a
D. Anti-K
E. Anti-D

11. Nonantibody causes of *acute* hemolytic reactions include:

A. Leukocytes
B. Platelets
C. Bacterial contamination
D. Infusion of hemolyzed erythrocytes
E. Both C and D

12. The *most* common initial symptoms of an *acute* hemolytic reaction in unanesthetized patients are:

A. Fever and chills
B. Shock and urticaria
C. Pain in the lower back and hypotension

D. Pain in the lower back and urticaria
E. Hypotension and fever

13. In vivo interaction between antigens and antibodies results in:

A. Activation of factor XIIa
B. Production of bradykinin
C. Complement activation
D. Accelerated intravascular hemolysis
E. All of the above.

14. Of the reactions listed, the most serious consequence of an *acute* hemolytic transfusion reaction is:

A. Graft-versus-host disease
B. Urticaria
C. Alloimmunization to erythrocytic antigens
D. Disseminated intravascular coagulation
E. Iron overload

15. Delayed hemolytic transfusion reactions may represent:

A. An anamnestic antibody response to leukocyte antigens
B. An anamnestic antibody response to erythrocyte antigens
C. Primary alloimmunization to erythrocyte antigens
D. Primary alloimmunization to leukocyte antigens
E. Both B and C

16. Characteristics of a delayed hemolytic transfusion reaction include:

A. Anemia, fever, and transfusion history
B. Jaundice
C. Renal shutdown
D. Positive direct antiglobulin test (DAT)
E. None of the above

17. Antibody production in primary alloimmunization to erythrocyte antigens begins ___ following transfusion.

A. Within 1 day
B. Within 2 days
C. Within 3 days
D. About 5 days
E. About 7-10 days

18. The usual consequence(s) of a delayed hemolytic transfusion reaction is/are:

A. Shortened erythrocyte survival in vivo
B. Intravascular destruction of erythrocytes

C. Extravascular destruction of erythrocytes
D. A positive DAT
E. All of the above, except B

19. To prevent delayed transfusion reactions, blood specimens used for compatibility testing should be *no more* than ____ old, if a patient has been recently transfused.
    A. 1 day
    B. 2 days
    C. 3 days
    D. 5 days
    E. 7 days

20. The *most frequent* cause of febrile transfusion reaction is the presence of ____ in the recipient.
    A. Erythrocyte antigens
    B. Erythrocyte antibodies
    C. Leukocyte antigens
    D. Leukocyte antibodies
    E. Bacterial contamination

21. The type of cell *most frequently* responsible for febrile transfusion reactions is the:
    A. Erythrocyte
    B. Lymphocyte
    C. Granulocyte
    D. Platelet
    E. Thrombocyte

22. A febrile transfusion reaction is defined as a rise in body temperature of ____ occurring in association with the transfusion of blood or components and *without* any other explanation.
    A. 1° C or more
    B. 1° F or more
    C. 5° C or more
    D. 5° F or more
    E. 10° F or more

23. With or without documentation of the existence of specific antibodies, the AABB recommends leukocyte-poor preparations only after a patient has had at least ____ febrile nonhemolytic transfusion reactions.
    A. One
    B. Two
    C. Three
    D. Four
    E. Five

24. Transfusion reactions to platelet concentrates can be:
    A. Febrile reactions

B. Hemolytic reactions
C. Immediate
D. Delayed
E. All of the above

25. Immediate reactions to plasma constituents may be ____ in nature:
    A. Allergic
    B. Anaphylactoid
    C. Anaphylactic
    D. Both A and B
    E. All of the above

26. The *most common* cause of transfusion-related sepsis is:
    A. Whole blood
    B. Platelet concentrates
    C. Packed red cells
    D. Leukocyte concentrates
    E. Fresh-frozen plasma

27. Graft-versus-host disease can be a consequence of transfusion if ____ are transfused into a recipient who is not capable of rejecting them.
    A. Granulocytes
    B. Platelets
    C. Lymphocytes
    D. Erythrocytes
    E. Both A and C

28. The patients susceptible to graft-versus-host disease are:
    A. Immunodeficient
    B. Immunosuppressed
    C. Adolescents
    D. Elderly
    E. Both A and B

29. Symptoms of graft-versus-host disease begin with ____ after transfusion.
    A. 1-2 days
    B. 2-3 days
    C. 3-30 days
    D. 2-3 months
    E. 1 year

30. Graft-versus-host disease can be prevented by:
    A. Fresh whole blood
    B. Blood stored for more than 10 days
    C. Irradiated blood products
    D. Fresh-frozen plasma
    E. None of the above

31. Noncardiac pulmonary edema is characteristically a complication of transfused:
    A. Erythrocytes
    B. Platelets
    C. Lymphocytes

D. Granulocytes

E. Plasma

32. Post-transfusion purpura typically occurs in patients who are:

A. Pl^{A1} positive without Pl^{A1} antibodies in their plasma

B. Pl^{A1} negative without Pl^{A1} antibodies in their plasma

C. Pl^{A1} positive with Pl^{A1} antibodies in their plasma

D. Pl^{A1} negative with Pl^{A1} antibodies in their plasma

E. None of the above

33. In the investigation of a transfusion reaction, the first step should be:

A. Obtain a post-transfusion specimen

B. Repeat the initial crossmatch

C. Check the identification of the patient and transfused unit

D. Visually examine a fresh blood specimen from the patient

E. Perform an ABO blood typing on the initial blood specimen

34–38. Arrange the following steps in a post-transfusion workup in the appropriate sequence.

A. Check the identification of the patient and transfused unit

B. Repeat the pretransfusion crossmatch

C. Perform a DAT

D. Perform an ABO and Rh grouping

E. Obtain a post-transfusion specimen from the patient and visually examine it for hemolysis

34. __

35. __

36. __

37. __

38. __

39. Supplementary tests for a transfusion reaction workup can include:

A. Alloantibody screening

B. Genotyping of patient and donor erythrocytes

C. Serum bilirubin assay on post-transfusion specimen

D. Urine examination for the presence of free hemoglobin

E. Serial post-transfusion DATs

40–43. Match the following conditions with the appropriate action or explanation. (Use an answer only once).

40. An ABO discrepancy is detected.

41. Crossmatch is incompatible only with post-transfusion specimen

42. Antibody detected in post-transfusion specimen only

43. Antibody detected in pretransfusion specimen only

A. Crosscheck past records and the labeling of blood products

B. Error in patient or donor during pretransfusion testing

C. A possible anamnestic response

D. Prior alloimmunization

ANSWERS

1.	E	23.	B
2.	C	24.	E
3.	B	25.	E
4.	A	26.	B
5.	D	27.	C
6.	C	28.	E
7.	D	29.	C
8.	A	30.	C
9.	E	31.	D
10.	B	32.	D
11.	D	33.	C
12.	A	34.	A
13.	E	35.	E
14.	D	36.	C
15.	E	37.	D
16.	D	38.	B
17.	E	39.	E
18.	E	40.	A
19.	B	41.	B
20.	D	42.	C
21.	C	43.	D
22.	A		

BIBLIOGRAPHY

Barton, J.C.: Nonhemolytic, noninfectious transfusion reactions. *Sem. Hematol. 18*:95-121, 1981.

Bashour, T.T., et al.: Hypocalcemic acute myocardial failure secondary to rapid transfusion of citrated blood. *Am. Heart J., 108*(4–Part 1):1040-1042, 1984.

Bauer, J. D.: Transfusion Reactions: *Clinical Laboratory Methods.* 9th Ed. St. Louis, C.V. Mosby, 1982, pp. 432-430.

Braine, H.G., et al.: Bacterial sepsis secondary to platelet transfusion: An adverse effect of extended storage at room temperature. *Transfusion, 26*(4):391, 1986.

Burdick, J.F. et al.: Severe Graft-versus-host disease in a liver-transplant recipient. *Med. Intelligence, 318*(11):689-691, 1988.

Campbell, J. (Ed.): Changes to 12th Edition Standards G 2.000. AABB News Briefs, *11*(6):1988.

Deeg, H. J., and Storb, R.: Graft-versus-host-disease. Ann. Rev. Med., *35*:11-24, 1984.

Dunstan, R.A., and Rosse, W.F., Posttransfusion purpura. Transfusion, *25*(3):219-222, 1985.

Gerhan, S.L.: Investigation of an apparent delayed transfusion reaction. *Lab. Med., 17*(10):607-609, 1986.

Gueguen, M., et al.: A new method for monitoring the sterility of blood donation. *Transfusion, 26*(3):293-295, 1986.

Heal, J.M., et al.: Bacterial proliferation in platelet concentrates. Transfusion, *26*:(4) 388, 1986.

Hoogan, V.A., et al.: A simple method for preparing neocyte-enriched leukocyte-poor blood for transfusion-dependent patients. Transfusion, *26*(3):253-257, 1986.

Huestis, D.W., Boue, J.R., and Case, J.: Practical Blood Transfusion, 4th Ed. Boston, Little, Brown and Co., pp. 249-268, 1988.

Lee, C.L., and Henry, J.B., Blood banking and hemotherapy. In *Clinical Diagnosis and Management by Laboratory Methods.* 17th Ed. Edited by J. B. Henry. Philadelphia, W.B. Saunders, 1984, pp. 1046-48.

Leitman, S.F., and Holland, P.V.: Irradiation of blood products. *Transfusion, 25*(4):293-300, 1985.

Leparc, G. F. and Schmidt, P. J. Stop transfusion reaction. Diagnos. Med., 1984:49-53.

Mollison, P.L.: Blood transfusion in clinical medicine. 6th Ed. Oxford, Blackwell Scientific Publications, 1979. p. 617.

Moore, G.L., and Ledford, M.E.: Effects of 4000 rad irradiation on the in vitro storage properties of packed red cells. *Transfusion, 25*(6):583-585, 1985.

Moore, S.B., et al.: Delayed hemolytic transfusion reactions, *Am. J. Clin. Pathol., 74*:94-97, no. 1, 1980.

Novak, R.W.: Immediate transfusion reactions in the pediatric population. *Lab. Med., 18*(6):388-390, 1987.

Myhre, B., et al.: Wrong blood, A needless cause of surgical deaths. *Anesth. Analg., 60*:77-78, 1981.

Petz, L.D., and Swisher, S.N.: Clinical Practice of Blood Transfusion. New York; Churchill Livingstone, 1981, pp. 783-801.

Pierce, R.N., et al.: Hemolysis following platelet transfusions from ABO-incompatible donors. Transfusion, *25*(1):60-62, 1985.

Roitt, I. M.: Essential Immunology. 5th Ed., Oxford, Blackwell Scientific Publications, 1984. p. 277.

Rosenfield, R. E.: Two types of delayed hemolytic transfusion reactions. Transfusion, *25*(2):182, 1985.

Squires, J.E., et al.: A delayed hemolytic transfusion reaction due to anti-Co[b]. Transfusion, *25*(2):137-139, 1985.

Strauss, R.G.: Sterility and quality of blood dispensed in syringes for infants. Transfusion, *26*(2):163-166, 1986.

Szymanski, I.O.: Sterility of single-donor apheresis platelets. Transfusion, *25*(3):290, 1985.

Tizard, I.R.: Immunology: An Introduction. Philadelphia, W.B. Saunders, 1984. p. 335.

Turgeon, M.L.: Clinical Hematology. Boston, Little, Brown and Co., 1988. pp. 107-110.

Widmann, F. K.: *Technical Manual,* 9th Ed. Arlington, Va., 1985. p. 325-337.

Widmann, F. K.: The hazards of transfusion. In Modern Blood Banking and Transfusion Practices. Edited by D.H. Pittiglio. Philadelphia, F.A. Davis, 1983, pp.362, 376-378.

12

Transfusion-Acquired Infectious Diseases

At the conclusion of this chapter, the reader will be able to:

- List at least three factors that have contributed to a reduction in accidental transmission of infectious agents in blood or blood products.
- List the factors that influence the acquisition of an infectious disease through blood or blood components.
- Name the diseases that can be transmitted through blood or blood components.
- List the patient-related factors that influence the actual development of a blood-borne disease if a potentially infectious virus is present in transfused blood or a blood component.
- State the most cost-effective method of preventing the transmission of viral agents via transfusion.
- Cite the incidence of transfusion-acquired hepatitis B and non-A, non-B hepatitis.
- Describe the characteristics of each of the forms of hepatitis, including features such as the average incubation time and symptoms.
- List the direct and surrogate tests that are useful in the detection of hepatitis.

- Discuss the characteristics, including etiology and symptoms, of cytomegalovirus.
- Explain the characteristics of Epstein-Barr virus infection.
- Name the human T-cell leukemia-lymphoma viruses that are transmitted through blood transfusion.
- Analyze the difference between the immunodeficiency virus (HIV) and other blood-borne viruses.
- Briefly describe the signs and symptoms of HIV infection.
- Describe the methods that are effective in reducing the incidence of blood-borne HIV infection.
- State the blood product that can be responsible for the transmission of parvovirus.
- Name the parasitic diseases that can be transmitted via blood or blood components.
- Rank the blood-borne parasitic disease in order of frequency in the United States.
- Name the bacterial disorders that can be acquired through blood transfusion.
- State the most significant reason for the decrease of transfusion-acquired syphilis.

Chapter Outline

BACKGROUND

Many potentially infectious agents can be acquired through blood transfusion. Careful interviewing of blood donors, serologic screening of donated blood, the use of plastic collection bags, and refrigerated storage methods have all helped to reduce accidental transmission of infectious agents. However, the possibility of initially acquiring or reactivating an infectious agent is a constant danger. Factors that can influence the acquisition of a disease from blood include:

1. Overall incidence of an agent or organism in the donor population
2. Pathogenicity of the agent
3. Actual presence of a large enough dose of the agent or organism in the transfusion to produce an infection
4. Immune status of the recipient
5. Physical condition of the recipient
6. Age of stored blood
7. Type of blood component received
8. Availability of a sensitive screening assay for the presence of the agent/organism
9. Donor screening (appropriate interview) or serologic screening such as HIV, if available

Viral agents, parasitic organisms, and bacteria can be transmitted through blood or blood components (Table 12-1). Viral diseases, such as non-A, non-B hepatitis and acquired immunodeficiency syndrome (AIDS), are presently a serious health hazard and may be acquired through transfusion. Although parasitic and bacterial diseases are less common on the North American continent than elsewhere, their significance should not be underrated. Two major parasitic infections, malaria and American trypanosomiasis, are the predominating transfusion-acquired parasitic diseases among patients in the Americas. However, cases of transfusion-acquired babesiosis have recently been documented in southern New England, and toxoplasmosis is increasingly being recognized as a hazard. In areas of the world where parasitic diseases are endemic, various parasites may be transmitted through blood transfusion. Transfusion-acquired bacterial in-

Table 12-1. Examples of Agents and Diseases Acquired Through Transfusion

Category	Agent	Disease
Viruses	Hepatitis A	Hepatitis A
	Hepatitis B and delta agent	Hepatitis B
	Non-A, non-B hepatitis	Non-A, non-B hepatitis
	Parvovirus	
	Cytomegalovirus	
	Epstein-Barr virus	Infectious mononucleosis
	HTLV (Human T-cell leukemia virus)	
	Type I	Potential T-cell leukemia
	Type III	AIDS
Parasites	Malaria species	Malaria
	Trypanosoma cruzi	American trypanosomiasis
	Babesia microti	Babesiosis
	Toxoplasma gondii	Toxoplasmosis
Bacteria	Treponema pallidum	Syphilis

fections, primarily syphilis, have become less of a risk than in the past but continue to be a problem in underdeveloped countries.

TRANSFUSION-ASSOCIATED VIRUSES

General Characteristics

Since the discovery of the Australian antigen (hepatitis B surface antigen, HB_sAg) in 1966 and the establishment of its relationship to post-transfusion hepatitis, numerous transfusion-associated viruses have been identified. The transmission and potential disorders caused by some of these viruses have become apparent only recently.

Transmission of viruses through blood transfusion is a challenging problem to control. Apparently healthy donors may be suffering from subclinical infections, may be in a carrier state as seen in hepatitis B, or may harbor a latent infection such as cytomegalovirus. If viral antigens or antibodies are not detected by screening methods in donor blood and the virus is stable in stored blood or blood products, transmission of the virus is likely. Untreated blood products, such as factor VIII concentrate prepared from pools of plasma derived from many donors, have an extremely high incidence of transmitting infectious viruses. Depending on the virus and the particular type of blood product, transmission through transfusion can be associated with the cel-

lular components of blood, usually leukocytes, or the plasma alone.

Not all transfusion-acquired viruses manifest themselves as clinical disorders. For a virus present in blood to infect a patient, the recipient must be susceptible to that virus. The immune status of the patient is influenced by age, nutritional status, and previous viral exposure. Whether or not the patient has been previously exposed or is harboring the virus in a dormant condition are also determining factors in the actual development of disease.

General Prevention of Virus Transmission

Prevention of viral transmission and diseases associated with blood transfusion requires knowledge of the infectious agent in terms of isolation of the virus, identification of associated antigens and/or antibodies, and the mechanism of transmission. In addition to this knowledge, methods for reducing transmission must be recognized and applied. Present methods to reduce the transmission of transfusion-associated viruses include:

1. Self-exclusion of high-risk blood donors through interviewing
2. Serologic screening of donor blood
3. Chemical or physical treatment of blood and blood components

Careful selection of donors and screening of blood for either viral antigens such as hepatitis B surface antigen, or the presence of antibodies, such as cytomegalovirus antibodies, represent the major means of providing transfusion products that are free of viruses. In the case of newly recognized transfusion-acquired viral diseases, such as AIDS, the importance of excluding high-risk populations and the efforts to develop a serologic antibody screening test as quickly as possible illustrate how important donor selection and screening are to maintaining a safe blood supply.

By understanding the mode of transmission of an infectious virus, physical or chemical treatments of blood or components may be effective in eliminating or reducing the level of the virus present. Methods of preparation, such as freezing and deglycerolizing red cells, are known to reduce viral contamination. Heat inactivation may be appropriate for plasma components if the virus can be destroyed without compromising the biologic activity of the component.

Several developing methods to reduce the transmission of viral disease include:

1. Vaccination, if suitable vaccines are available. This method has proven effective in the prevention of transmission of hepatitis B in high-risk populations, such as health care professionals. Vaccination, however, is rarely possible because of the lack of identification of the virus or because efficacy of vaccination has not been proven.
2. The addition of an antibody, possibly even a monoclonal antibody, to blood in an attempt to reduce the infectivity of blood or blood components.
3. Gene cloning and commercialization of recombinant DNA blood products. Three human gene products of importance to transfusion therapy have been cloned and expressed in microorganisms: albumin (1981), hepatitis B vaccine (1981), and factor VIII (1984). Hepatitis B vaccine is now available, and the commercialization of the other products is expected in the near future.

A major issue in prevention of viral disease is cost. The cost of screening blood and of alternative preparations or safe substitutes must be determined for each viral agent. Significant factors in determining when screening should be used or what alternatives are appropriate are definition of the population "at risk" and assessment of the impact of the resulting clinical disease.

General Characteristics of Hepatitis

ETIOLOGY

Transfusion-associated hepatitis continues to be one of the major complications of blood transfusion. Post-transfusion hepatitis may be caused by hepatitis A virus (rare), hepatitis B virus with or without the delta agent, the non-A, non-B hepatitis virus(es), or cytomegalovirus (CMV). The viruses for type A and type B viruses, the delta agent, and CMV have been isolated and identified. The agents that cause non-A, non-B hepatitis have not yet been identified, and it is not clear whether non-A, non-B hepatitis represents one, two, or many diseases.

INCIDENCE

Estimates of the frequency of post-transfusion hepatitis vary from 0.16 cases per 1000 units transfused to as high as one in four recipients. In institutions using blood from volunteer donors who have been screened for hepatitis B surface antigen by third-generation tests, hepatitis B infections probably account for less than 10% of transfusion-acquired hepatitis cases. Another 10 to 14% of cases may be caused by cytomegalovirus. The remaining 80% are attributable to the one or more agents currently referred to as the non-A, non-B viruses.

SIGNS AND SYMPTOMS

As a clinical disease, hepatitis can occur in two forms, acute and chronic. Symptoms of hepatitis are extremely variable. The disease can be mild, transient, and completely asymptomatic or severe, prolonged, and ultimately fatal. Viral hepatitis can be in any of the following forms:

1. Typical acute hepatitis with icterus (jaundice). In this form the disease has four phases: incubation, preicteric phase, icteric phase, and convalescence. The incubation period, from the time of exposure and the first day of symptoms, ranges from a few days to many months. The average time is 25 days (range of 15 to 45 days) in hepatitis A (infectious hepatitis), 75 days (range of 40 to 180 days) in hepatitis B, and 50 days (range of 15 to 150 days) in the non-A, non-B form of hepatitis.
2. Fulminant acute hepatitis. This rare form of hepatitis is associated with hepatic failure.
3. Subclinical hepatitis without icterus. This form of hepatitis includes cases in persons with demonstrable antibodies in their serum but no reported history of hepatitis.
4. Chronic hepatitis. This form of hepatitis is accompanied by hepatic inflammation and necrosis which lasts for at least 6 months. It occurs in about 10% of hepatitis B and 10 to 60% of non-A, non-B types of hepatitis; however, it does not occur with hepatitis A.

Hepatitis B

Hepatitis B virus is the classic example of a virus acquired through blood transfusion. In part, this observation led to the name "serum hepatitis" by which hepatitis B was previously known. Hepatitis B serves as a model when considering transfusion-transmitted viral infections.

ETIOLOGY

In 1966 the Australia antigen now called the hepatitis B surface antigen, was discovered. This permitted the biochemical and epidemiologic characterization of the virus. Soon after discovery of the virus, the relationship between the presence of the antigen in donor blood and post-transfusion hepatitis was documented.

VIRAL CHARACTERISTICS

The hepatitis B virus is a complex DNA virus that belongs to a new class called the hepadna viruses. Much is known about the structure of the hepatitis B surface antigen (HB$_s$Ag). The intact virus is a double-shelled particle referred to as the *Dane particle.* It has an outer-surface component of HB$_s$Ag and an inner-core component, the hepatitis B core antigen (HB$_c$Ag). Inside of this core is the genome of the hepatitis B virus, a single molecule of partially double-stranded deoxyribonucleic acid (DNA) (Fig. 12-1).

The unique structure of the DNA of hepatitis B virus is one of the major distinguishing characteristics of the hepadna class of viruses. The DNA is circular and double-stranded, but one of the strands is incomplete, leaving a single-stranded or gap region that comprises 10 to 50% of the total length of the molecule. The other DNA strand is nicked (the 3 and 5 ends are not joined). The entire DNA molecule is small, and all of the genetic information for producing both the surface and core antigens is on the complete strand. In addition to the DNA configuration, the core of virus also contains an enzyme which is a DNA-dependent DNA polymerase. This polymer-

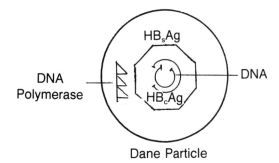

Dane Particle

Figure 12-1. Hepatitis B virus. The intact hepatitis B virus (HBV) consists of a double-shelled particle referred to as the Dane particle. It has an outer surface component of hepatitis B surface antigen (HB$_s$Ag) and an inner core component of hepatitis B core antigen (HB$_c$Ag). Inside the core is the genome, a single molecule of partially double-stranded DNA, which contains the genetic information. One of the DNA strands is incomplete, leaving a single-strand or gap region which comprises 10 to 50% of the total length of the molecule.

ase acts to complete the single-stranded region of the DNA.

EPIDEMIOLOGY

In the past, hepatitis B was one of the most frequent clinical infections transmitted by blood transfusion. Hepatitis B is largely a disease spread by the parenteral route through blood transfusion, needle-stick accidents, and contaminated needles, although the virus can be transmitted in the absence of obvious parenteral exposure. About half of the patients with acute type B hepatitis have a history of parenteral exposure. Inapparent parenteral exposure involves close intimate or sexual contact with an infectious individual. Hepatitis B virus has been found in saliva, semen, and other biologic fluids of hepatitis B virus carriers. Urine and stool are not believed to be infectious. Because hepatitis B virus does not seem capable of penetrating the skin or mucous membranes, some break in these barriers is required for disease transmission.

INCIDENCE

The incidence of transfusion-acquired hepatitis B has been severely reduced since high-risk donor groups, such as paid donors, prison inmates, and military recruits have been eliminated as a major source of donated blood. This shift to an all-voluntary donor supply probably accounts for a 50 to 60% reduction in transfusion-related hepatitis. The overall incidence of hepatitis B, however, is high among patients who have received multiple transfusions, those who have received blood components prepared from multiple-donor plasma pools, dialysis patients, drug addicts, and medical personnel.

SIGNS AND SYMPTOMS

The clinical response following exposure to hepatitis B virus is influenced by numerous factors including the dose of the agent and individual immunologic host response ability. The most frequent clinical response to hepatitis B virus is an asymptomatic or subclinical infection.

In patients developing clinical symptoms of transfusion-associated hepatitis B, jaundice, and abnormal transaminase (ALT/SGPT) levels last from a few weeks to 6 months after a single transfusion episode if other causes of hepatotoxicity are ruled out. There is rarely any doubt about the diagnosis in patients with a classical serologic response associated with hepatitis B virus infection, even in the absence of significant symptoms. Less clear is the asymptomatic patient with negative HBV serology, who a few weeks after a transfusion has a mild elevation of transaminase levels that persists for a week or two.

Hepatitis B leads to chronic infection, and some chronically infected persons have been shown to have the viral DNA actually incorporated into their liver cells' DNA. This integration may be an important factor in the eventual development of liver cell cancer (hepatocellular carcinoma), a well-known long-term outcome of chronic HBV infection.

CARRIER STATE

Carriers can be divided into two categories based on differing infectivity, depending on the presence in their serum of another antigen, hepatitis B e antigen (HB_eAg) or its antibody, anti-HB_e.

1. About one in four carriers has HB_eAg in his/her serum. It is likely that he/she has recently become a carrier and that his/her blood is highly infectious.
2. The more commonly identified carriers have anti-HB_e in their serum and are at a later stage of infection. The patients are less infectious but may transmit infection through blood transfusion. HB_sAg-positive carriers become anti-HB_e positive carriers at a rate of about 5 to 10% per year. All HB_sAg-positive individuals must be excluded from giving blood for transfusion.

LABORATORY TESTING—SEROLOGIC MARKERS

Several serologic markers for hepatitis B virus infection have been defined. These markers include:

1. Hepatitis B surface antigen (HB$_s$Ag).
2. Hepatitis B e antigen (HB$_e$Ag).
3. Antibody to the hepatitis B core antigen (anti-HB$_c$).
4. Antibody to hepatitis B e antigen (anti-HB$_e$).
5. Antibody to hepatitis B surface antigen (anti-HB$_s$).

Hepatitis B Surface Antigen (HBsAg). The first laboratory screening of donor blood for hepatitis was the detection of what is now known as hepatitis B surface antigen (HB$_s$Ag). This screening procedure for the presence of the major coat-protein of the virus (HB$_s$Ag) in donor serum is considered the most reliable method of choice for preventing the transmission of hepatitis B virus through blood transfusion, and has in fact produced a dramatic decrease in post-transfusion hepatitis B. The national average for HB$_s$Ag in random donors as reported by the Centers for Disease Control is 0.3% (6% for male homosexuals).

The initial detectable marker that can be found in serum during the incubation period of hepatitis B is HB$_s$Ag. The titer of HB$_s$Ag rises and generally peaks at or shortly after the onset of elevated transaminase (ALT/ SGPT) levels. Clinical improvement of the patient's condition with a decrease in serum transaminase is parallelled by a fall in the titer of HB$_s$Ag, which subsequently disappears. However, there is variability in the duration of HB$_s$Ag positivity and in the relationship between clinical recovery and the disappearance of HB$_s$Ag (Fig. 12-2).

Among persons infected with hepatitis B virus and detectable HB$_s$Ag in their serum, not all of the HB$_s$Ag represents complete Dane particles. HB$_s$Ag positive serum also contains two other virus-like structures. These are incomplete spherical and tubular forms, consisting entirely of HB$_s$Ag and devoid of any HB$_c$Ag, DNA, or DNA polymerase. The incomplete HB$_s$Ag particles can be present in serum in extremely high concentrations and form the bulk of the circulating HB$_s$Ag.

Test protocols for HB$_s$Ag range from immunodiffusion and its electrophoretic modifications to solid-phase assays including reverse passive hemagglutination (RPHA), radioimmunoassay (RIA), more correctly called immunoradiometric assay (IRMA), enzyme-linked immunosorbent assays (ELISA), and fluorescent immunoassays (FIA). One of the most popular methods is the enzyme immunoassay procedure.

Hepatitis B e Antigen (HB$_e$Ag). A hepatitis B-related antigen, the hepatitis B e antigen (HB$_e$Ag), is found in the serum of some patients who are HB$_s$Ag positive. It is rarely found in the absence of HB$_s$Ag. HB$_e$Ag appears to be associated with the hepatitis B virus core; however, the relationship between HB$_e$Ag and the structure of hepatitis B virus is unclear. HB$_e$Ag appears to be a reliable marker for the presence of high levels of virus and a high degree of infectivity. A specific immunoassay for HB$_e$Ag is available.

Hepatitis B Core Antibody (Anti-HB$_c$). Testing for antibody to the core of the virus (anti-HB$_c$) may provide some additional advantage because it may lead to the identification of a donor recently recovered from a hepatitis B virus infection, who may still be infectious.

During the course of most hepatitis B virus infections, the Hb$_s$Ag forms immune complexes with the antibodies produced as part of the recovery process. Because HB$_s$Ag contained in these complexes is usually undetectable, HB$_s$Ag disappears from the serum of up to 50% of symptomatic patients. During this phase, an indicator of a recent hepatitis B infection is anti-HB$_c$, the antibody to the core antigen. The period between the disappearance of detectable HB$_s$Ag and the appearance of detectable antibody to HB$_s$Ag (anti-HB$_s$) is called the *anti-core window* or hidden antigen phase of hepatitis B virus infection. This window phase may last for a few weeks, several months, or a year, during which time anti-HB$_c$ may be the only serologic marker. Usually, anti-HB$_c$ alone probably means immunity from remote infection.

The most recent assay to be developed is the test for IgM antibody to hepatitis B core antigen (anti-HB$_c$ IgM). This test is considered a reliable marker during the so-called "core window period" when most other markers may be absent. The IgM anti-HB$_c$ titer rises rapidly in the acute phase and becomes negative in most patients in 3 to 9 months, although it may persist for

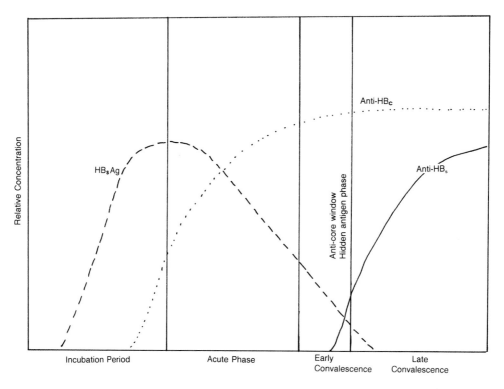

Figure 12-2. Representative profile of hepatitis B serum markers. HB$_s$Ag = hepatitis B surface antigen, anti-HB$_c$ = hepatitis B core antibody; anti-HB$_s$ = anti-core window or hidden antigen phase.

many years. The presence of anti-HB$_c$ IgM in the absence of HB$_s$Ag in the serum indicates a recent episode of type B hepatitis.

In a comparison of testing for antibody to the core antigen and the presence of surface antigen, one study demonstrated:

Results	No. of Patients	Anti-HB$_c$	HB$_s$Ag
Random donors	209	7 (3%)	0
Homosexuals			
High–risk	39	14 (36%)	0
Low–risk	13	2 (15%)	0

Anti-HB$_c$ occurs in 3 to 5% of persons. Of 100 anti-HB$_c$-positive persons, 97 will have anti-HB$_s$, two will have HB$_s$Ag, and one may have only anti-HB$_c$.

ANTIBODIES TO HB$_e$Ag AND HB$_s$Ag

Antibodies to HB$_e$Ag (anti-HB$_e$) and Hb$_s$Ag (anti-HB$_s$) develop during convalescence and recovery from HBV infection. Theoretically, development of anti-HB$_e$ in a case of acute hepatitis is the first serologic evidence of the convalescent phase, but most patients probably never demonstrate anti-HB$_e$. Antibody to HB$_s$AG (anti-HB$_s$),

unlike anti-HB$_c$ and anti-HB$_e$, does not arise during the acute disease but rather during convalescence. Anti-HB$_s$ is a serologic marker (Table 12-2) of recovery and immunity. Anti-HB$_s$ is probably the major protective antibody in this disease. Thus, hepatitis B immune globulin is so named because it contains high levels of anti-HB$_s$.

PREVENTION

The most important factors in preventing transfusion-acquired hepatitis B are donor interviewing (refer to Chapter 8), screening

Table 12-2. Serologic Markers for Hepatitis B Viral Infection*

	HB_sAg	anti–HB_s	anti–HB_c	anti–HB_c IgM
Early (asymptomatic)	+	−	−	−
Acute or chronic	+	−	+	+‡
Acute or chronic	+	+	+	+‡
Carrier	+	−	±	−
Characteristic of window phase†	−	−	+	−
Immediate recovery	−	−	+	+
Long after infection	−	−	+	−
Long after infection (i.e., immunity)	−	+	−	−
Immunization with HB_sAg	−	+	−	−

* The incidence of markers for hepatitis B viral exposure is 3.5 to 10% in the general population and 60 to 68% for homosexual men.
† This pattern most often means immunity or window phase.
‡ Presence of the IgM fraction classically connotes a recent infection.
Modified from Hoofnagle, J. H.: Type A and Type B Hepatitis. Lab. Med. *14(11)*: 713, 1983.

of donor blood, use of hepatitis-free products when possible, and appropriate use of blood and blood components (refer to Chapter 9). Elimination of high-risk donors has accounted for at least a 50% reduction in the incidence of hepatitis. Routine testing of donated blood for HB_sAg has further reduced the incidence by 20 to 30%. Testing for anti-HB_c detects almost 100% of Hb_sAg-positive persons, the rare asymptomatic donor who is in the core window phase, and the large number of donors who have had subclinical hepatitis B infections and are now immune.

The use of a vaccine against hepatitis B, licensed since 1982, is warranted for high-risk persons, among whom are technologists who handle patient blood specimens. Vaccination offers a new approach to preventing transfusion-acquired hepatitis in patients who are likely to need ongoing transfusion therapy, such as nonimmune patients with hemophilia, sickle cell anemia, or aplastic anemia. Additionally, avoidance of high-risk blood components, such as untreated factor VIII prepared from multiple donor pools, reduces the incidence of hepatitis B. Hepatitis B vaccine is also a vaccine against cancer (hepatic carcinoma). It is probably the first such vaccine and is very important to third-world countries.

In cases of accidental needlestick exposure or exposure of mucous membranes or open cuts to HB_sAg positive blood, hepatitis B immune globulin (HBIG) should be administered within 24 hours of exposure and again 25 to 30 days later. The protocols for ACIP (CDC) also require hepatitis B vaccine in this setting, unless the patient has been previously vaccinated, with positive serologic antibody markers. Infants born to mothers with acute hepatitis B in the third trimester or with HB_sAg at the time of delivery should be given HBIG as soon as possible and no later than 24 hours after birth. Persons who are either HB_sAg positive or who have anti-HB_s need not be given HBIG.

Delta Hepatitis

ETIOLOGY

Another transfusion-acquired hepatitis virus is the *delta agent,* but one cannot contract delta hepatitis without hepatitis B infection. This agent was first described in 1977 as the cause of either acute or chronic hepatitis. Delta infection may increase the severity of both acute and chronic hepatitis B infections and probably partially suppresses HBV replication. The possibility of an acute delta hepatitis should be considered in cases of acute hepatitis in B carriers.

VIRAL CHARACTERISTICS

The delta agent is an RNA virus. This agent is unique because it can replicate only in hepatitis B virus-infected hosts. The delta agent consists of viral RNA coated in HB_sAg produced by hepatitis B virus, its "helper" virus. Therefore, the delta virus infects only patients who are HB_sAg-positive.

EPIDEMIOLOGY AND INCIDENCE

In Italy and the Middle East, delta infection is common and found in HB_sAg carriers. In the United States, northern Europe, and Asia, infection is uncommon and occurs only in persons with multiple parenteral exposures, such as hemophiliacs and intravenous drug addicts.

SIGNS AND SYMPTOMS

Infection with delta hepatitis can occur in several conditions, and the symptoms are typical of either acute or chronic hepatitis. These situations are:

1. Acute delta hepatitis with a concurrent acute type B hepatitis.
2. Acute delta hepatitis in a chronic HB_sAg carrier.
3. Chronic delta hepatitis in a chronic HB_sAg carrier.

LABORATORY TESTING

The delta agent appears in the circulating blood as a particle with a core of delta antigen and a surface component of HB_sAg. A person with delta hepatitis has detectable delta antigen in the liver and antibody to the delta agent in the serum; however, serologic assays are not generally available.

Hepatitis A Virus

ETIOLOGY

Hepatitis A virus is very rarely the cause of post-transfusion hepatitis.

VIRAL CHARACTERISTICS

The hepatitis A virus is a small RNA virus that belongs to the picornavirus class. The structure is that of a simple nonenveloped virus with a nucleocapsid designated the hepatitis A antigen (HA Ag). Inside the capsid is a single molecule of single-stranded RNA (Fig. 12-3). It is believed that the RNA has a positive polarity and that proteins are translated directly from the RNA, as is the case with messenger RNA.

EPIDEMIOLOGY

The hepatitis A virus is transmitted by the fecal-oral route. Infection is noted for occurring in isolated outbreaks or as an epidemic, but may also occur sporadically.

INCIDENCE

Because of short viremia, the lack of a carrier state, and the high prevalence of immunity in recipients, hepatitis A is very rarely a transfusion-acquired hepatitis. The incidence of infection is not increased among health-care workers or dialysis patients. Hepatitis A virus is the cause of about 20% of viral hepatitis cases in adults in the United States and other industrialized countries.

SIGNS AND SYMPTOMS

Most nonimmune adult patients infected with hepatitis A virus exhibit jaundice and other clinical symptoms within 4 to 6 weeks after exposure. This leads to donor self-exclusion and limits the entrance of infected blood into the blood supply.

LABORATORY TESTING

Hepatitis A antigen is usually not detectable in serum. However, antibody to hepatitis A virus is almost always detectable with the onset of symptoms. The antibody titer rises quickly and persists for long periods, probably for life. The initial antibody response consists almost entirely of IgM type antibody, followed by IgG type antibody. Within 3 to 6 months after exposure, the IgM antibody to the hepatitis A

Hepatitis A Virus

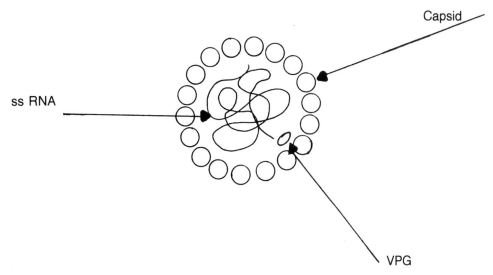

Figure 12-3. Hepatitis A virus. The protein capsid is composed of four viral polypeptides. Inside the capsid is a single-strand molecule of RNA, which has a genomic viral protein (VPG) on the 5′ end.

virus reaches undetectable levels. Immunoassays for hepatitis A IgM antibody are available.

PREVENTION

After close personal contact with a person with hepatitis A or if travelling to an endemic area, individuals should receive immune globulin intramuscularly. If a person remains in an endemic area for more than 3 months, he/she should receive immune globulin injections every 5 months.

Non-A, Non-B Hepatitis

ETIOLOGY

Non-A, non-B hepatitis was first recognized in 1974. If viral hepatitis is suspected in a patient, hepatitis B and hepatitis A, cytomegalovirus, and Epstein-Barr virus must be eliminated as causes before non-A, non-B hepatitis is considered. Cytomegalovirus and Epstein-Barr virus are discussed in later sections of this chapter.

VIRAL CHARACTERISTICS

The virus or viruses responsible for non-A, non-B hepatitis have not been identified. Epidemiologic studies, however, suggest that at least two forms of non-A, non-B hepatitis exist, which may indicate that more than one viral agent is responsible for non-A, non-B hepatitis. The existence of at least two transfusion-associated non-A, non-B viruses is also indicated by multiple episodes of acute hepatitis in treated hemophiliacs and by chimpanzee studies.

EPIDEMIOLOGY

Transmission of the virus or viruses is by both parenteral and nonparenteral routes. Epidemic water-borne acute non-A, non-B hepatitis has an epidemiology similar to that of hepatitis A virus. Blood or blood component transfusion and accidental needlesticks also comprise a clearly documented route of transmission. Blood donors and patients incubating acute non-A, non-B hepatitis are primary sources in the transmission of this form of post-transfusion hepatitis. The carrier state further increases the transmission of the virus.

INCIDENCE

Non-A, non-B hepatitis is the principal cause of post-transfusion hepatitis and is also the major source of hepatitis among dialysis patients. In prospective studies prior to surrogate testing in the United States, approximately 1 in 10 transfusions appears to cause transfusion-acquired hepatitis. These cases of hepatitis are of the non-A, non-B variety in 80 to 90% of the cases. Between 25 and 50% of sporadic hepatitis cases in the United States that are unrelated to parenteral exposure are of the non-A, non-B variety. These cases are serologically and epidemiologically unrelated to hepatitis A or hepatitis B.

SIGNS AND SYMPTOMS

Several different patterns of non-A, non-B hepatitis exist. Transfusion-associated non-A, non-B hepatitis can be divided into short- and long-incubation types, with incubation periods of short duration ranging from 1 to 5 weeks and those of longer duration ranging from 7 weeks to 6 months. Many infections are inapparent and are detected by mild elevation of transaminase (ALT/SGPT) levels. Less than 25% of infected patients develop jaundice.

In prospective studies, non-A, non-B hepatitis associated with transfusion has usually been defined by transaminase (alanine aminotransferase ALT/SGPT) levels 2.5 times the upper limit of normal on two or more separate occasions. Elevation of ALT can be due to a variety of causes, including medications, alcohol intake, and obesity.

The diagnosis of the non-A, non-B form of hepatitis has a guarded prognosis. Between 20 and 40% of patients with this disease develop chronic persistent or chronic active hepatitis, followed by a slowly pro-

gressive, frequently asymptomatic disease eventually leading to cirrhosis.

LABORATORY TESTING

No reliable diagnostic markers (Table 12-3) for detecting the presence of non-A, non-B hepatitis presently exist. Serologic antigen-antibody systems have not proved repeatable or specific. Elevated ALT levels and the absence of hepatitis A and hepatitis B markers are of little value in diagnosing or monitoring individual patients.

Surrogate Testing ALT and Hepatitis B Core Antibody Testing. Because of the lack of specific antigen or antibody tests for non-A, non-B type viruses, two procedures have been implemented as surrogate tests: the ALT and hepatitis B core antibody testing.

Routine testing of donor blood for ALT has been advocated as a means of reducing transfusion-acquired non-A, non-B hepatitis. In one blood center, the chance of non-A, non-B hepatitis occurring in a recipient was eight times greater if the donor's serum ALT was greater than 45 IU/L above normal. However, 62% of transfusion-acquired non-A, non-B hepatitis cases occurred in recipients of blood below the cutoff value. The effectiveness of ALT screening is difficult to assess because of the high proportion of false-positive and false-negative results involved when ALT is used as an index of non-A, non-B hepatitis infectivity. The test is not specific and is influenced by a large number of physiologic variables. ALT testing is probably not a cost-effective way to prevent transfusion-acquired hepatitis.

The relationship between the presence of antibody to hepatitis B core antigen (anti-HB_c) in donor blood and the development of hepatitis in recipients of that blood was studied. Of 193 recipients of at least 1 unit of blood positive for anti-HB_c, 11.9% developed non-A, non-B hepatitis, compared with 4.2% of recipients of only anti-HB_c negative blood. Donor anti-HB_c status was not significantly associated with the development of hepatitis B in the recipient and was negatively associated with the development of cytomegalovirus hepatitis. Where enzyme immunoassay (EIA) testing for antibody to hepatitis B core antigen (anti-HB_c)

Table 12-3. Characteristics of Acute Viral Hepatitis

	Type A Travelers	Type B Hospital Personnel	Delta	Non–A, Non–B Post–transfusion
Agent	Hepatitis A	Hepatitis B	Delta agent	Unknown
	RNA	DNA	RNA	Unknown
Antigens	HA Ag	HB$_s$Ag, HB$_c$Ag, HB$_c$Ag, HB$_e$Ag	Delta	Unknown
Antibodies	Anti–HAV	Anti–HB$_s$, anti–HB$_c$, anti–HB$_e$	Anti–delta	Unknown
Epidemiology	Fecal–oral	Parenteral	Parenteral	Parenteral Nonparenteral
Incubation period (in days)	15–45	40–180	30–50	15–150

Adapted from Hoofnagle, Jay H.: Type A and Type B Hepatitis, *Lab. Med., 14* (11): 715, 1983.

was used as a surrogate test for non-A, non-B hepatitis, the EIA testing identified a subset of donors whose results were not consistent over multiple donations. This inconsistency must be considered when donors are notified of results because the significance of these findings as they relate to the utility of the anti-HB$_c$ assay as a surrogate marker for non-A, non-B hepatitis remains unclear. Recent investigations, however, have shown that removing blood from donors with anti-HB$_c$Ag from the blood supply may reduce post-transfusion non-A, non-B hepatitis.

PREVENTION

Data from two major investigations has indicated that eliminating the use of blood containing anti-HB$_c$Ag could lower the incidence of post-transfusion non-A, non-B hepatitis.

Until the agent of non-A, non-B hepatitis is characterized, it is unlikely that a specific assay will be developed. As an alternative, there is some evidence that it may be possible to identify donors belonging to "high-risk" populations. It is questionable that using anti-HB$_c$ as a marker for high risk donors is generally applicable.

Cytomegalovirus

In 1966, it was first reported that cytomegalovirus infection was associated with

what is now referred to as post-transfusion mononucleosis. Infants infected with cytomegalovirus can become severely ill, with symptoms including pneumonia and hepatitis. Cytomegalovirus may be associated with transfusion-associated hepatitis and is one of the most important causes of the congenital viral infections in the United States that may cause death in premature infants.

ETIOLOGY

The first descriptive report of histologic changes characteristic of the changes now associated with cytomegalovirus infection was published in 1904, when protozoan-like cells in the lungs, kidneys and liver of a syphilitic fetus were seen. In the 1920s, it was suggested that the large protozoan-like cells with intranuclear inclusions seen in some histologic preparations were not protozoal in origin, but it was not until 1956 that the cytomegalovirus was isolated in the laboratory. In 1966, the actual isolation of the virus after transfusion and the observation of elevated antibody titers were noted.

VIRAL CHARACTERISTICS

Human cytomegalovirus is classified as a member of the herpes family of viruses. There are presently five recognized human herpesviruses: herpes simplex I, herpes simplex II, varicella-zoster virus, Epstein-Barr virus, and cytomegalovirus. All of the herpesviruses are relatively large, enveloped DNA viruses which undergo a replicative cycle involving DNA expression and nucleocapsid assembly within the nucleus. The viral structure gains an envelope, when the virus buds through the nuclear membrane, that is altered to contain specific viral proteins.

These viruses are susceptible to lipid solvents, freezing, and heat, and viral isolates are not well preserved at 4° C, 20° C, or higher temperatures. Variables such as the location of the virus (intracellular versus extracellular), the presence of host cells, and soluble substances such as antibodies or complement have made studying the stability of the virus in biologic situations difficult. If the virus is present in blood, urine, and breast milk, it may be more stable than laboratory isolates of the virus.

Although the herpes family produces diverse clinical diseases, the viruses share the basic characteristics of being cell-associated. The requirements for cell association vary, but all five viruses may spread from cell to cell, presumably by way of intercellular bridges, and in the presence of antibody in the extracellular phase. This common characteristic may play a role in the ability of the virus to produce subclinical infections which can be reactivated under appropriate stimuli.

EPIDEMIOLOGY

Cytomegalovirus infection is endemic worldwide. Many cases are congenital infections in newborn infants; however, dissemination of the virus may be by oral, respiratory, and venereal routes or parenterally by organ transplantation or by the transfusion of fresh blood. A complete characterization of the transmission of cytomegalovirus from person to person has not been established, but transmission appears to require close, intimate contact with secretions or excretions (primarily urine, respiratory secretions, tears, feces, and genital secretions of infected persons). The most likely mode of acquisition is venereal, through contact with infectious virus in body secretions.

It has been recognized for more than 15 years that transfusion of blood from healthy asymptomatic blood donors is occasionally followed by active cytomegalovirus infection in the recipient. There is strong evidence to incriminate peripheral blood leukocytes and transplanted tissues as sources of cytomegalovirus.

INCIDENCE

The incidence of primary infection during childhood is low, but the rate of exposure to the virus may be accelerated during the first years of life in toddlers and children in day care centers. During adolescence the infection rate rises significantly. By adulthood, most persons have experienced asymptomatic contact with cytomegalovirus, as demonstrated by the fact that 35 to 100% of adults have detectable antibodies to cytomegalovirus by age 35. Serologic evidence further demonstrates that adult women have higher rates of antibody responses than men of the same age. The incidence of viral exposure and subsequent antibody formation (seropositivity) varies greatly depending on the socioeconomic status and living conditions of the population surveyed.

Less than 1% of normal healthy adults excrete the virus in their urine, but persons experiencing acquired infection, reinfection with the same or different strains of cytomegalovirus, or reactivation of a latent infection can excrete the virus in titers as high as 10^6 infective units/mL in the urine and/or saliva for weeks or months. There is an average infection rate of 13% after transfusion to immunocompetent recipients, with most infections being asymptomatic.

LATENT INFECTION

Persistent infections characterized by periods of reactivation are frequently termed *latent* infections, although this condition has not been clearly defined for cytomegalovirus. True viral latency is defined by the presence of the genetic information in an unexpressed state in the host cell. An operational definition of latency can include the conditions of a dynamic relationship between the virus and the host, along with evidence of latency and reactivation of a latent infection.

Evidence that cytomegalovirus produces latent infections in humans is circumstantial and indirect. The mechanism of latency and the identity of the host cells which harbor the latent virus remain undocumented. Leukocytes from the peripheral blood of patients with active cytomegalovirus infections have been cultured, with subsequent recovery of cytomegalovirus; however, attempts to recover the virus from the leukocytes of healthy donors have been unsuccessful except in one report. In animal models, the virus is present and recoverable from neutrophilic leukocytes in active infections, but it is also believed that splenic B lymphocytes and possibly monocytes may harbor latent infections. Additionally, salivary gland, heart, and prostate tissue may be sites of latent infection. The types of cells and the mechanism of latency remain to be demonstrated in humans. The estimated cytomegalovirus carrier rate among blood donors, which is defined as the number of seroconversions (patients changing from being negative for antibodies to the virus to demonstrating antibodies) per 100 units of blood transfused ranges from 1 to 12%.

PATIENTS AT RISK

Cytomegalovirus is known to cause transfusion-related infections, especially in premature infants, and can be a frequent cause of morbidity and mortality in recipients of organ transplants and patients receiving immunosuppressive chemotherapy. Because cytomegalovirus can persist latently, active infections may develop under a variety of conditions such as pregnancy and immunosuppression, or after organ transplantation. In practice, the greater the degree of immunosuppression, the more likely the patient is to suffer from a cytomegalovirus infection, primary or reactivated. Children with leukemia and premature infants of less than 1200 g birthweight fare badly, with fatal infections reported.

Patients with the highest risk of mortality from cytomegalovirus infections are transplant-seronegative patients who receive tissue from a seropositive donor. Cytomegalovirus is the most commonly recognized pathogen in the first 6 months after renal transplantation. Infections in cardiac transplant recipients have been reported to occur in association with increased pulmonary superinfections in addition to the clinical signs and symptoms of primary infection. Active cytomegalovirus infection is a major cause of morbidity and often mortality in AIDS patients.

The risk of developing cytomegalovirus infection is greatest for patients who are exposed to cellular blood components from a large number of donors. In heavily transfused patients, blood transfusion becomes a significant risk factor. The transfusion of granulocytes carries a high risk of viral infection in immunocompromised bone marrow recipients, with interstitial pneumonia occurring in 38 to 44% of cases. The relative importance of blood transfusion as a risk factor in organ transplantation patients varies according to the organ or tissue transplanted. The greatest majority of infections in patients are transmitted by the donor kidney or arise from the reactivation of the recipient's latent virus.

Infections in immunosuppressed patients may result in disseminated multisystem involvement including pneumonitis, hepatitis, gastrointestinal ulceration, arthralgias, meningoencephalitis, and retinitis. Interstitial pneumonitis, frequently associated with cytomegalovirus infection, is a major cause of death following allogeneic bone marrow transplantation. In premature infants, acquired cytomegalovirus infection can result in atypical lymphocytosis, hepatosplenomegaly, pneumonia, or death.

SIGNS AND SYMPTOMS

The classic congenital cytomegalovirus syndrome is manifested by a high incidence of neurologic symptoms. Psychomotor retardation is seen in 51 to 75% of survivors. Hearing loss is observed in 21 to 50% of cases and visual impairment in 20% of cases. Infants without symptoms at birth may develop hearing impairment and neurologic impairment at a later date.

In most patients, cytomegalovirus infection is asymptomatic, with jaundice being rare. Infections occurring in healthy immunocompetent adults usually result in seroconversion. Occasionally a self-limited, heterophile-negative mononucleosis-like syndrome occurs. The symptoms include sore throat and fever, chills, profound malaise, and myalgia. Lymphadenopathy and splenomegaly may be observed.

Infrequent complications of cytomegalovirus infection in previously healthy adults include interstitial pneumonitis, hepatitis, Guillain-Barré syndrome, meningoencephalitis, myocarditis, thrombocytopenia, and hemolytic anemia. However, transfusion-acquired cytomegalovirus infections may cause not only a mononucleosis-like syndrome but hepatitis and an increase in rejection of transplanted organs.

Three types of cytomegalovirus infections are possible in blood transfusion recipients:

1. Primary infection occurs when a previously unexposed (seronegative) recipient is transfused with blood from an actively or latently infected donor. This type of infection is accompanied by the presence of cytomegalovirus in the blood and urine, a transient virus-specific IgM antibody response, and eventual seroconversion to produce IgG antibodies to the virus. Primary infections may be symptomatic, but the great majority are not.
2. Reactivated infections are produced when a seropositive recipient is transfused with blood from either a cytomegalovirus antibody positive or negative donor. Donor leukocytes are thought to trigger an allograft reaction, which in turn reactivates the recipient's latent infection. Such infections may be accompanied by significant increases in IgG antibodies to the virus but no detectable IgM response. Some reactivated infections exhibit viral shedding as their only manifestation. Reactivated infections are largely asymptomatic.
3. Reinfection may be caused by a strain of cytomegalovirus in the donor's blood that is different than the one originally infecting the recipient. A significant antibody response is observed in this situation and viral shedding occurs. Whether or not an IgM response occurs is unknown. Although it is difficult to differentiate a reactivated infection if both patient and donor are cytomegalovirus antibody positive before transfusion, reinfections can be documented if isolates can be obtained from both donor and recipient.

ALTERATIONS IN THE IMMUNE SYSTEM

Cytomegalovirus is known to alter the immune system as well as producing overt manifestations of infection. A cytomegalovirus infection interferes with the host's immune responsiveness in both normal and immunocompromised individuals. This diminished responsiveness results in a decreased proliferative response to the cytomegalovirus antigen which persists for several months. In patients with cytomegalovirus mononucleosis, alterations of T lymphocyte subsets produce an increase in the absolute number of suppressor (T8) lymphocytes and a decrease in helper (T4) lymphocytes. These subset abnormalities persist for months.

Questions have been raised regarding cytomegalovirus as a potentially oncogenic virus because viral antigens and/or nucleic acid have been found in human malignancies, including adenocarcinoma of the colon, carcinoma of the cervix, cancer of the prostate, and Kaposi sarcoma. Cytomegalovirus does have transforming properties in vitro. However, even though considerable circumstantial evidence exists linking cytomegalovirus to human malignancies (especially Kaposi's sarcoma), a direct cause-and-effect relationship has not been established.

LABORATORY TESTING

In cytomegalovirus infection, hematologic examination of the blood usually reveals a characteristic leukocytosis. A slight lymphocytosis with over 20% variant lymphocytes is common. Clinical chemistry assays may demonstrate abnormal liver function tests. Tests for heterophil, Epstein-Barr virus, and toxoplasma antibodies are negative. Elevated concentrations (titers) of several antibodies may occur. These include antinuclear antibody (ANA), rheumatoid factor (RA) antibodies, and nonspecific cold agglutinins. Another assessment of infection is the demonstration of inclusion bodies in leukocytes in urinary sediment.

A definitive diagnosis can be made only by isolating the cytomegalovirus from urine or blood samples or demonstrating of a rise in antibody titer. Human cytomegalovirus is indistinguishable by negative staining electron microscopy from its close relatives, herpes simplex and varicella, the cause of chickenpox. Viral culture is the method of choice for confirming cytomegalovirus infection.

Serologic Markers

In cells infected by cytomegalovirus, several antigens appear at varying time intervals postinfection. Before replication of viral DNA takes place, immediate-early antigens and early antigens are present in the nuclei of infected cells. Immediate-early antigens appear within one hour of cellular infection, and early antigens are present within 24 hours. At about 72 hours postinfection or at the end of the viral replication cycle, late antigens are demonstrable in the nucleus and cytoplasm of infected cells.

The immune antibody response to these various antigens differs in incidence and significance. The presence of antibodies against immediate-early and early antigens is associated with active infection of either a primary or reactivated nature.

Antibody to early antigen undergoes a relatively rapid decline after recovery but can persist for up to 250 days and may identify patients with recent infections as well as active infections. The presence of antibody to early antigen is strongly associated with viral shedding. Antibodies to late antigens persist in high titer long after the recovery from an active infection.

Screening of Blood Donors

The morbidity and mortality due to transfusion-acquired cytomegalovirus infection in high-risk patients have prompted serious efforts to provide convenient screening methods. The prevalence of cytomegalovirus antibody varies with age and geographic location but ranges from 40 to 100%.

The incidence of antibodies against cytomegalovirus-induced immediate-early antigens, early antigens, and late antigens was studied in a population of healthy blood donors. Antibodies to immediate-early antigens were found in 9.6%, antibodies to early antigens in 10.2%, and antibodies to late antigens in 76% of the donors. The incidence of antibodies to cytomegalovirus-induced immediate-early and early antigens increased with age and was higher in women than men.

In another study, 51% of donors were seronegative for cytomegalovirus antibodies. The highest percentage of seronegative findings (60%) was among donors 18 to 35 years old. This age group represented 57% of the donors. If viruric donors are a source of transfusion-acquired cytomegalovirus in high-risk patients, screening blood for early antigen antibodies is warranted. In another study of random donors, 28% had antibodies to cytomegalovirus; however, among the 52 homosexual donors who were eligible on the basis of their medical histories, the following results were obtained:

High risk: Of 39 patients, 35 (90%) were seropositive

Low risk: Of 13 patients, 10 (77%) were seropositive

A study at a San Francisco clinic showed 94% of homosexual men and 43% of random donors to have cytomegalovirus antibodies.

Laboratory Procedures

Procedures for the identification of cytomegalovirus infections include:

1. Viral cultures of urine and/or blood.
2. ELISA technique for IgG type antibodies
3. Passive latex agglutination (PLA)
4. Indirect immunofluorescence (IFA)
5. Enzyme-linked antigen assay (ELA)
6. A microtiter complement fixation (CF) test
7. Enzyme immunoassay tests (EIA)
8. Indirect hemagglutination (IHA)

In one investigation comparing IHA, IFA, EIA, and PLA techniques of blood testing within 1 week of collection, the passive latex agglutination technique (PLA) was rated best overall because it was technically the easiest and required the least hands-on and turnaround times. The short turnaround time (10 minutes) rendered the latex techniques a more flexible test for blood bank use because both scheduled and emergency screening of donors could be accommodated. The comparatively high reagent cost of the kit could be offset by time savings. IHA, EIA, ELISA, and PLA were found suitable for donor screening.

Results of EIA Testing of Random Donors. IgG antibody tests have the disadvantage of cross-reacting with Epstein-Barr, varicella, and herpes simplex viruses. IgM screening by IFA and ELA does not always identify the viruric donor.

PREVENTION

Most transfusion-acquired infections need not be prevented. Those occurring in immunocompetent patients rarely give rise to serious disease. Of patients who are immunosuppressed, only seronegative patients appear to be at significant risk of developing cytomegalovirus infections. The use of cytomegalovirus-seronegative blood has been recommended for transfusion of selected premature babies and for recipients of bone marrow transplants. Transmission of this virus by transfusion of blood or components containing white cells is assuming increasing importance in patients with severely impaired immunity who require supportive therapy.

Transfusion-acquired cytomegalovirus infections can be prevented by using blood from donors unlikely to carry the virus, such as those negative for antibodies. Effective antibody screening, leukocyte-depleted blood products, and immune globulin containing passively acquired cytomegalovirus antibodies are all methods of prevention. Immune globulin was found to prevent infections in seronegative patients who did not receive granulocytes. This treatment is promising for preventing cytomegalovirus infections in high-risk patients. Resolution of the mechanism of latency or inapparent infections is critical to the further prevention of transfusion- and transplantation-associated cytomegalovirus infection.

Health care professionals are among the groups that are becoming increasingly concerned about the risks associated with exposure to cytomegalovirus. Nosocomial transmission from patients to health care workers has not been documented, but observance of good personal hygiene and hand-washing offers the best measure for preventing transmission.

Epstein-Barr Virus

The Epstein-Barr virus (EBV) can be transfusion-acquired. This virus can produce infectious mononucleosis, with hepatitis as the most frequent complication. EBV infection is an infrequent consequence of blood transfusion and does not cause as much of a problem in blood recipients as does cytomegalovirus.

ETIOLOGY

The Epstein-Barr virus was first discovered in 1964 as the cause of infectious mononucleosis. This same virus is associated with Burkitt's lymphoma, a malignant tumor of the lymphoid tissue occurring mainly in African children.

VIRAL CHARACTERISTICS

EBV is a human herpes DNA virus which has been isolated with increasing regularity. This virus is found in association with blood leukocytes. In infectious mononucleosis, the virus infects B lymphocytes; however, the variant lymphocytes produced in response to infection and seen in an examination of the peripheral blood have T cell characteristics. Among the habitats of the persisting virus in the carrier state is the B-lymphocyte in lymph nodes and peripheral blood.

EPIDEMIOLOGY

Although the Epstein-Barr virus appears to be transmitted primarily by close contact with infective oral-pharyngeal secretions, the virus has been reported to be transmitted by blood transfusion and transplacental routes.

Patients at risk include those who lack antibodies to the Epstein-Barr virus. The frequency of seronegative recipients is nearly 100% in early infancy and declines with increasing age, more or less rapidly depending on socioeconomic conditions, to less than 10% in young adults. Probably because approximately 90% of adult patients already have protective neutralizing antibodies in their serum, most blood transfusion recipients are immune to the virus. If multiple transfusions are received, antibody to the Epstein-Barr virus will be present in one or more of the donations and may have a protective effect. Thus, there is little chance to transmit the virus under ordinary conditions.

Despite the various factors that reduce the transmission of Epstein-Barr virus, cases of transfusion-associated infectious mononucleosis or infectious mononucleosis-like illnesses have been recorded. The Epstein-Barr virus is only a minor problem for immunocompetent individuals but can become a major problem for immunologically compromised patients. Infectious mononucleosis or infectious mononucleosis-like illness following blood transfusion may often be due to concomitant cytomegalovirus infections rather than the Epstein-Barr virus. Therefore, transmission of Epstein-Barr virus may occur only under rather limited conditions:

1. If a single unit of blood is transfused from a donor who is in the viral incubation period. Although transfusion of additional units of blood should theoretically protect the recipient unless the blood came from seronegative donors, on rare occasions single units of blood or platelet-rich plasma from donors who were incubating the virus produced viremia and infectious mononucleosis-like symptoms in recipients from 2 to 17 days later.
2. When the donor is seropositive, based on a test for antibodies to Epstein-Barr viral capsid antigen, but lacks Epstein-Barr neutralizing antibodies or possesses them at a level too low to protect the recipient. Multiple transfusions of blood would probably reduce or eliminate this possibility.
3. When the recipient has a T lymphocyte deficiency which might permit the donor's B lymphocytes, including EBV genome-carrying B cells, to outlast the period of a blood donor's passive antibody protection (approximately 4 weeks). The lymphomas observed in severely immunosuppressed patients could then arise from the recipient's or donor's B lymphocytes.

INCIDENCE

Immunosuppressed patients have a higher prevalence of Epstein-Barr infection. The incidence ranges from 35 to 47%. As occurs with other herpesviruses, there is a carrier state after primary infection. More than 90% of blood donors have antibodies to Epstein-Barr virus and thus are carriers of the virus.

SIGNS AND SYMPTOMS

Infectious mononucleosis is a self-limiting lymphoproliferative disorder. It is a fairly common acute disorder and is usually benign. Although anyone can suffer from this condition, it typically affects young adults. However, an increasing number of older adult cases is being recognized.

The incubation period of infectious mononucleosis is from 10 to 50 days and, once fully developed, it lasts for 1 to 4 weeks. Clinical manifestations include extreme fatigue, sore throat, fever, and cervical lymphadenopathy. Splenomegaly occurs in about 50% of cases. Jaundice is infrequent, although the most common complication is hepatitis.

LABORATORY TESTING

In addition to clinical symptoms, hematologic and serologic laboratory testing is necessary to establish a diagnosis. Leukocyte counts range from 10 to 20 $\times$ 10^9/L in about two thirds of patients. About 10% of the patients with this disorder demonstrate leukopenia. Differential leukocyte examination may reveal neutrophilia, although mononuclear cells usually predominate as the disorder develops. Typical relative lymphocyte counts range from 60 to 90%. Variant lymphocytes with a variety of morphologic features are characteristic and persist for 1 to 2 months or as long as 4 to 6 months.

A definite diagnosis of infectious mononucleosis is established by serologic antibody testing. The antibodies present are heterophil and Epstein-Barr virus antibodies. Other tests may detect viral capsid and nuclear antigens.

Heterophil antibodies may be present in a normal person in low concentrations (titers); however, a titer of 1:56 or greater is clinically significant in suspected cases of infectious mononucleosis. Heterophil antibodies are defined as antibodies that are stimulated by one antigen and react with entirely unrelated antigens. Infectious mononucleosis antibodies are one type of heterophil antibody that has a variety of characteristics, which include:

1. Reaction with horse, ox, and sheep erythrocytes
2. Absorption of beef erythrocytes
3. No absorption by guinea pig kidney cells

Rapid slide tests are now available using the principle of agglutination of horse erythrocytes. The use of horse erythrocytes appears to increase the sensitivity of the test.

An assay for IgM and IgG antibodies to the antigens of the Epstein-Barr virus is available. Antibodies to viral antigen develop within the first 2 weeks of disease onset. Other antibodies appear later. Allo-Anti-i is the most clinically significant antibody because it can cause hemolytic anemia.

PREVENTION

Transfusion of blood products which contain few viable lymphocytes should reduce the chance of transfusing Epstein-Barr virus to patients at risk. These blood components may be leukocyte-depleted or irradiated products.

Investigating Post-Transfusion Hepatitis

The viral agents discussed in the preceding sections can be the direct cause of hepatitis or lead to hepatitis as a complication, but documenting transfusion-acquired hepatitis in transfusion recipients is difficult. Two approaches to documentation are available: prospective follow-ups and retrospective assessments.

In prospective follow-ups, serologic and biochemical evaluation of a transfusion recipient could be conducted at periodic intervals following transfusion. In actual practice, prospective follow-ups are not realistic because of cost. In retrospective studies, the identification of clinical cases of hepatitis could be correlated with the patient's transfusion history of the previous 6 months; however, numerous donors may be implicated.

In attempting to identify the cause of the hepatitis, hepatitis B is typically suspect. The incidence of HB_sAg in follow-up donor samples is rare. Because all donors have been tested previously, seroconversion indicates that, at the time of the implicated donation, the level of circulating HB_sAg was below the detectability of the test used (most third-generation tests detect about $1 \times 10^{-9}g$ HB_sAg/mL) or that the original test was done incorrectly. In implicated donors, the presence of anti-HB_c alone or in combination with an elevated transaminase (ALT/SGPT) level is used by some centers as a reason to permanently defer a donor. If a donor is the only source of blood or a component given to a patient, that donor must be permanently deferred (refer to Chapter 2).

Unless a specific viral agent, such as cytomegalovirus, can be demonstrated in both patient and donor serum, the cause is only speculative. In the case of an unidentified viral agent, such as non-A, non-B hepatitis, diagnosis is by exclusion rather than identification.

Human T-Cell Leukemia-Lymphoma Virus (HTLV)

The HTLV group of viruses is composed of types I, II, and III. The group of retroviruses classified as human immunodeficiency viruses HIV-1 (also called HTLV-III, LAV-1 or ARV) and HIV-2 (also called LAV-2 or HTLV-IV) are the known etiologic agents for acquired immunodeficiency syndrome (AIDS). It should be noted that HTLV-IV has not yet been demonstrated to cause AIDS.

HTLV-I

HTLV-I was first isolated in 1978 in a Black man residing in the southeastern United States. HTLV-I is associated with acute adult T-cell leukemia. Although HTLV-I is known to produce malignant transformation, the exact mechanism by which the transformation occurs is not known. Two cases of malignant transformation have been described in patients previously well but known to have HTLV-I antibodies for 5 to 10 years. It has been demonstrated that the T helper lymphocytes of seropositive but clinically normal, unaffected individuals can release HTLV-I viral particles in vitro when co-cultured with normal lymphocytes.

HTLV-I is usually cell-associated, and transmission through blood transfusion has been documented only for whole blood and cellular components. The association of human retroviruses, the HTLV group, with overt malignant lymphoma/leukemia raises the concern of possible transmission of neoplasia by blood transfusion. When blood from 41 seropositive but healthy individuals was transfused into seronegative recipients, it induced seroconversion in 63% of the recipients. However, seroconversion did not occur in any of 14 recipients of fresh-frozen plasma derived from seropositive donors, and thus far none of these patients has developed clinical disease.

Serologic studies of family members of affected patients have revealed a high intrafamilial incidence of HTLV-I antibodies, often in the total absence of clinical disease. The incidence of HTLV-I infection is variable, but in certain areas of the world as many as one in four adults shows serologic evidence of infection. However, few adults subsequently develop malignancies.

The spectrum of disease associated with HTLV-I infection ranges from the chronic, asymptomatic carrier form to the chronic form, to the typical acute forms. It is hypothesized that immunologic status, age, and genetic and environmental conditions are all important factors. HTLV-I infection is common in Japan and the Caribbean.

Consideration may need to be given to identifying and excluding infected donors, particularly in areas where the incidence of infection is high. Because blood transmission of HTLV-I has been recognized in Japan, even though actual clinical disease resulting from transfusion has not been established at the present time, the Japanese Blood Centers screen donated blood for HTLV-I antibodies. HTLV-I screening was also recently instituted by the American Red Cross Blood Centers.

HUMAN IMMUNODEFICIENCY VIRUS (HIV)

Etiology. Over the last several years, one of the most publicized transfusion-acquired viruses has been HIV. HIV-1 and HIV-2 are responsible for the clinical disease acquired immunodeficiency syndrome (AIDS).

Viral Characteristics. HIV is a type D retrovirus that belongs to the lentivirus subfamily. Since the discovery of HIV, much has been learned about the impact of viruses on human cells. The virus is composed of structural proteins and glycoproteins that occupy the core and envelope regions of the particle. HIV appears to have genes that could encode for at least six proteins.

Retroviruses carry a single, positive-stranded RNA and use a special enzyme, called *reverse transcriptase,* to convert viral RNA into DNA. This reverses the normal process of transcription where DNA is converted to RNA, hence the term *retrovirus.*

The life cycle of the HIV consists of five phases:

1. The virus attaches and penetrates target cells that express the CD4 receptor. After penetration, the virus loses its protein coat, exposing the RNA core.
2. Reverse transcriptase converts viral RNA into proviral DNA.

3. The proviral DNA is integrated into the genome (genetic complement) of the host cell.
4. New virus particles are produced as the result of the normal cellular activities of transcription and translation.
5. These new particles bud from the cell membrane. Once the viral genome is integrated into host cell DNA, the potential for viral production always exists and the viral infection of new cells can continue.

HIV has a marked preference for the helper-inducer (T4) subset of lymphocytes. It displays an affinity for these cells because the CD4 surface marker protein on these cells serves as a receptor site for the virus. In addition to lymphocytes, cells such as those found in the central nervous system have a similar receptor. Recent studies have demonstrated that immunologic activation of T helper cells latently infected with HIV induces the production of multiple viral particles leading to cell death. The extensive destruction of T cells and possibly other factors lead to the gradual depletion of the helper-inducer type of lymphocytes. Defects in immunity are believed to be partially related to this T-cell depletion. Progressive defects in the immune system include a severe B cell failure, defects in monocyte function, and defects in granulocyte function.

Epidemiology. Transmission of HIV is believed to be restricted to contact with body fluids such as blood or seminal fluid. (See Chapter 1). Although the virus is considered to be predominantly sexually transmitted, it can be transmitted through the parenteral route by transfusion with infected blood (if the blood has not been screened for HIV) or in drug addicts through needles contaminated with the virus. Posttransfusion AIDS is now well documented from both cellular blood components and untreated cell-free preparations, such as factor VIII concentrate and plasma.

Incidence. Pediatric AIDS occurs in children under age 13, primarily infants and toddlers. Of these cases of AIDS, 91% have been in children under 3 years. The majority are born to parents in a high-risk group or have a parent with AIDS. The next most

common cause in these cases is transfusion-associated AIDS.

Transfusion-acquired AIDS in patients with no other risk factors accounted for only 1 to 2% of the cases reported to the Centers for Disease Control. Transfusion-associated AIDS is defined as AIDS in persons with no other known risk factor for AIDS who were transfused with blood or blood components within 5 years of the onset of illness. In a study of 90,000 donors who made 240,000 blood donations, each multiply tested donor averaged 2.6 seronegative donations. During the period of the study, 4 seroconverters were detected with an interval of 2 to 4 months between seronegative and seropositive donations. Donor interviews revealed that two donors were male homosexuals; the other two had no risk factors.

Signs and Symptoms. The mean period between viral transmission and diagnosis has been reported to be 27 months. The range is believed to be from 15 to 57 months (possibly longer). HIV produces an infection that ranges from asymptomatic to the terminal end-stage complications of AIDS.

Typically, patients in the early stages of HIV infection are either completely asymptomatic, or may show mild, chronic lymphadenopathy. The early phase may last from many months to many years after viral exposure. Clinical signs and symptoms of the later phase include extreme weight loss, fever, and multiple secondary infections. End-stage AIDS is characterized by the occurrence of neoplasms and/or opportunistic infections. Opportunistic infections noted with the greatest frequency are caused by *Pneumocystis carinii, cytomegalovirus, M. avium—intracellulae, Cryptosporidium, Entamoeba, toxoplasmosis, M. tuberculosis,* herpes simplex virus, and *Legionella. Histoplasma capsulatum* is being recognized with increasing frequency. The most frequent malignancy observed is an aggressive, invasive variant of Kaposi's sarcoma, discovered in many cases on autopsy. Malignant B cell lymphomas are being recognized with increasing frequency in patients with AIDS or at high risk for AIDS. AIDS is presently considered fatal, although several experimental treatments are being tested.

Laboratory Testing. A common denominator of HIV infection is a deficiency of a specific subset of thymus-derived (T) lymphocytes, designated by the phenotypic marker T 4. T lymphocyte subset distribution is altered, with a decrease in the helper-inducer T cells and an increase in suppressor-cytotoxic T cells. In this disorder, both leukopenia and lymphocytopenia exist. A decreased lymphocyte proliferative response to soluble antigens and mitogens also exists. Defective natural killer (NK) cell activity can also be observed. Various other ancillary findings including polyclonal hypergammaglobulinemia, elevated levels of alpha interferon, alpha $(\alpha)_1$ thymosin, beta microglobulin, and reduced levels of T cell growth factor or interleukin-2 have been noted.

SEROLOGIC TESTING. Development of first-generation serologic tests was rapid and has had a significant effect on reducing the transmission of HIV by blood. Serologic tests, whether current or under development, detect antibodies to HIV and are capable only of determining whether an individual has had prior HIV exposure. Newer research techniques are directed at HIV antigen detection. HIV located inside of T4 lymphocytes does not produce a protein in excess like HB_sAg. The quantity of viral protein in the blood of persons infected with HIV is very low. Antibodies to HIV are present in much greater quantity, and with present techniques, it is much easier to detect.

INTERPRETATION OF RESULTS. A positive test result means only that the antibody to HIV virus is present. In AIDS patients, 85 to 90% do have a positive HIV antibody test as well as increased antibody titers to viruses such as cytomegalovirus, Epstein-Barr virus, hepatitis A and B, and *Toxoplasma gondii;* and circulating immune (antigen-antibody) complexes can be found.

Several problems are associated with the use of crude viral preparations as antigen targets. Because the AIDS virus represents an enveloped particle, its membrane shares many antigenic similarities with the cell line used as virus producer. These include T-cell antigens, HLA antigens, and other potential targets of the humoral response that can produce false positive results. The sensitivity of ELISA tests with respect to disease detection is also subject to inherent difficulties. Examples of false-negative results can include:

1. AIDS patients with diminished antibody titer associated with late-stage disease or loss of the virus envelope accompanying purification procedures.
2. Patients who lack detectable antibody for approximately 6 weeks after infection. Virus-positive, antibody-negative individuals would go undetected in an initial screening assay.

At present, blood samples from donors that are initially reactive to HIV antibody testing are rechecked in duplicate to rule out technical errors. If, on repeat testing, one or more of the duplicates is positive, the sample is considered "repeatably reactive," and the unit of blood is not used for transfusion. To rule out false-positive results, it is necessary to confirm repeatably reactive test results by an alternative protocol. The most commonly used confirmatory procedure is the Western Blot technique.

WESTERN BLOT PROCEDURE. Before a blood donor is notified of "anti-HIV reactivity" tests demonstrating positive results, the results should be both reproducible and confirmable by at least one additional test. The most frequently used confirmatory test is the Western blot test, an alternative procedure to establish the presence of antibody to HIV in serum or plasma. When the test is positive in conjunction with a positive ELISA test, it can be regarded as confirmatory. The test appears to work best with samples that contain high levels of antibody.

In the Western blot procedure, purified HIV viral antigens are electrophoresed on SDS gels and the separated polypeptides are then transferred onto sheets of nitrocellulose paper. The nitrocellulose paper is incubated with the serum specimen. Any antibody that binds to the separated peptides present on the nitrocellulose paper is detected by a secondary anti-human antibody and is conjugated to a suitable enzyme marker and incubated with the appropriate enzyme substrate. Antibody specificities against known viral components (generally the core component and envelope component) are considered true positive results, while antibody specificities against nonviral cellular contaminants are nonspecific, false-positive results. The Western blot is a time-consuming and expensive methodology open to considerable interpretation.

To confirm antibody reactivities in a more objective manner than the Western blot methodology, the development of an immunofluorescent test has been sought which can accurately and rapidly confirm an initially reactive serum specimen. The simplicity of the test reflects its format: an HIV-induced cell line and an uninfected control cell line are separately deposited onto a microscope slide. The serum specimen to be tested is incubated on each cell spot, followed by incubation with a goat anti-human antibody conjugated to fluorescein isothiocyanate (FITC), and the microscope slides are examined with an ultraviolet microscope. It is possible to distinguish true from false-positive test results. A dipstix version has also been developed for clinical laboratories, physicians' offices, and field testing conditions.

SECOND AND THIRD-GENERATION TESTING METHODS. Second-generation methods are currently under development. These tests are similar to the first-generation tests in format and principle, with the exception that the antigen sources are recombinant DNA-derived products rather than crude or purified viral antigens. Sensitivities of gene-derived assays may not be significantly improved, but the specificity of second-generation tests may be superior because the problems associated with antibody reactivities against cell-substrate components will be nonexistent. Third-generation tests are needed for the detection of actual infectious viral particles. Cell culture methods provide information regarding the presence of the virus; however, to be specific for HIV, a virus capture assay is needed to detect viral antigens in cell culture specimens.

Prevention. The first step in prevention of transfusion-acquired HIV is careful screening of blood donors. Blood donor medical history standards have recently undergone extensive revision (refer to Chapter 2).

In addition to interviewing, screening of blood donors for HIV and hepatitis B core antibody is essential. Serum transaminase values demonstrate no significant changes; therefore, the risk factors for NANB hepatitis and HIV infection in blood donors are likely to be independent. The U.S. Public Health Service has recommended that all donated blood and plasma be tested for HIV, and additionally recommends that blood or serum from donors of organs, tissues, or semen intended for human use be similarly tested. The test results should be used to evaluate the appropriateness of such materials from these donors. Organs, tissues, and semen obtained from HIV persons must be considered potentially infectious.

The National Hemophilia Foundation currently recommends that pediatric hemophiliacs receive cryoprecipitate. Patients who have never previously received factor VIII should receive heat-treated products if no other alternative exists. (Refer to Chapter 9 for a discussion of the future applications of biotechnology in the production of factor VIII.) Treatment of blood components can be an additional preventive method if biologic activity of the needed component is not compromised. HIV has been demonstrated to be efficiently inactivated by formalin, beta-propiolactone, ethyl ether, detergent, and ultraviolet light plus psoralen. The results are reassuring as to the potential safety of various biologic products.

Guidelines from the Centers for Disease Control for clinical and laboratory personnel who work with AIDS patients and blood specimens suggest that the same precautions be used as when the risk of hepatitis B infection is present. Specifically, patient-care and laboratory personnel should avoid direct contact of the skin and mucous membranes with potentially infectious materials (see Chapter 1).

Parvovirus

The parvovirus-like virus of humans has been shown to be transmitted in factor VIII concentrates. Transmission of the virus has been demonstrated in concentrates prepared from donor pools but not from single-donor cryoprecipitate or whole blood. The significance of transmission is uncertain; however, the fact that this virus is transmitted by blood should be kept in mind when considering the transmission of other agents. It is presently believed that the resulting viremia is transient.

TRANSFUSION-ACQUIRED PARASITES

Transmission of parasitic infections through blood transfusion is infrequent in developed countries. Although deaths caused by transfusion-acquired malaria are rare, fatal cases have occurred in the United States and elsewhere. In many underdeveloped nations where diseases such as African trypanosomiasis (sleeping sickness) are endemic, transfusion-acquired parasitism is a significant problem in nonimmune recipients.

On the North American continent, four parasitic diseases can be seen with greater frequency than others. These are malaria (*Plasmodium* species), Chagas' disease (*Trypanosoma cruzi*), babesiosis (*Babesia microti*), and toxoplasmosis (*Toxoplasma gondii*). In underdeveloped, primarily tropical countries a variety of transfused-acquired parasitic diseases has been observed. In addition to African sleeping sickness (*Trypanosoma brucei rhodesiense* or *Trypanosoma brucei gambiense*), transfusion-acquired parasites include *Wuchereria bancrofti*, *Loa loa*, and *Mansonella ozzardi*.

Malaria Species

ETIOLOGY

In 1884, two human subjects demonstrated that malaria could be transmitted through blood. The first case of accidental transmission through blood transfusion was described in 1911. The modern tendency is to refer to the various types of malaria by the names of their causative agents: *Plasmodium vivax* (*P. vivax*), *Plasmodium fal-*

ciparum (*P. falciparum*), *Plasmodium malariae* (*P. malariae*) and *Plasmodium ovale* (*P. ovale*). The life cycle of *Plasmodium* is in both humans and mosquitoes.

INCIDENCE

Although a program coordinated by the World Health Organization from 1960 to 1970 was partially successful in eradicating malaria, the incidence of this disease has progressively increased. The number of cases of malaria reported worldwide increased 2.5 times between 1972 and 1977. In part, the spread of malaria is associated with increased population shifts and travel between temperate and tropical parts of the world.

The resurgence of malaria over most of the tropics continues to endanger the health of developing countries and represents a serious problem for other countries, such as the United States. The total number of people living in endemic areas of malaria in 1982 was 1600 million. The population distribution in these endemic areas is as follows:

1. Southeast Asia   920 million
2. Africa   282 million
3. Eastern Mediterranean   170 million
4. The Americas   130 million
5. Western Pacific   74 million
6. Between Europe and Asia   40 million

Species distribution of *Plasmodium* indicates that *P. vivax* is the predominant species worldwide, *P. falciparum* is almost entirely confined to the tropics and subtropics, and *P. malariae* occurs primarily in subtropical and temperate areas where other species of malaria are found. *P. ovale* is rather widely distributed in tropical Africa and replaces *P. vivax* in frequency on the West African coast. *P. ovale* has also been reported in South America and Asia.

It has been estimated that during the period from 1950 to 1982, the total number of recorded cases of transfusion-acquired malaria exceeded 3500. Transfusion-acquired malaria is particularly high in Bangladesh, Brazil, India, Iran, and Mexico. In the United States, 26 cases of transfusion-acquired malaria were reported from 1972 to

1981. A worldwide survey (1973 to 1980) of transfusion-acquired malaria demonstrated that *P. vivax* (together with a few cases of *P. ovale*) was the most common (42%), followed by *P. malariae* (38%) and *P. falciparum* (20%).

TRANSMISSION

Induced malaria is a term that can be applied to accidental or deliberate inoculation of malarial parasites by either a mosquito bite or injection into a human host. Three types of transmission are possible:

1. Transfusion malaria, which is accidentally related to whole blood, blood components, or organ transplants.
2. Accidental "needle" malaria due to the unintentional introduction of parasites by a contaminated needle.
3. Congenital malaria in the newborn who became infected by the transplacental route from the mother.

The Disease Phase in the Mosquito. The disease cycle of malaria is initiated when a female mosquito of various species of anopheline mosquitoes bites an infected human. The infected blood of the person, which may contain male and female gametocytes, is drawn into the stomach of the mosquito. In the mosquito, the male or microgametocyte undergoes maturation and results in the production of microgametes.

Concurrently, the female or macrogametocyte matures into a macrogamete, which may be fertilized by the microgamete to become a zygote. The active zygote is referred to as an ookinete, and after constricting as an oocyst. The growth and development of the oocyte results in the production of a large number of thread-like sporozoites, which circulate throughout the body of the mosquito. The sporozoites that enter the salivary glands of the mosquito are ready to be inoculated into the next person bitten by the mosquito.

The length of this cycle depends upon factors such as the species of *Plasmodium* and the ambient temperature. It may range from as short as 8 days in *Plasmodium vivax* (*P. vivax*) to as long as 35 days in *P. malariae*.

The Disease Phase in Humans. Sporozoites injected into the bloodstream of a human by an infected mosquito leave the circulatory system within a period of 40 minutes and invade the liver cells of the human host. In the cells of the liver, all four species undergo an asexual multiplication phase. This asexual multiplication produces thousands of tiny merozoites in each infected cell. Subsequent rupture of the infected liver cells releases the merozoites into the circulation.

In the circulation, an asexual cycle takes place within the erythrocytes. This process, referred to as schizogony, results in the formation of from 4 to 36 new parasites in each infected erythrocyte within 48 to 72 hours. At the end of this schizogonic cycle, the infected erythrocytes rupture, liberating merozoites, which in turn infect new erythrocytes.

Usually, after a patient has become clinically ill, gametocytes appear in circulating erythrocytes. Gametocytes, derived from merozoites, grow but do not divide and finally form the male and female gametocytes. Gametocytes circulate in the blood for some time and, if ingested by an appropriate species of mosquito, undergo the sexual cycle, gametogony, which develops into sporogony in the mosquito.

SIGNS AND SYMPTOMS

There are usually no symptoms of malaria until several continuous life cycles have been completed. The simultaneous rupturing of erythrocytes liberates toxic products that characteristically produce chills followed by a fever in a few hours. A patient's temperature may rise to 104° or 105° F. The symptoms last from 4 to 6 hours and recur at regular intervals, depending on the type of malaria.

LABORATORY TESTING

Examination of blood smears is inappropriate for the screening of asymptomatic blood donors. Serologic techniques for diagnosis of malaria include indirect hemagglutination (IHA) test, ELISA, and indirect fluorescent antibody (IFA) tests.

French investigators assessed their 5-year rule, which refers to the amount of time that should elapse after leaving a malarious area before a person can safely be accepted as a blood donor. In this study, potential blood donors who had visited areas where malaria was present had the following rates of positive reactions using the IFA antibody method.

1. Within the past 5 years   14.0%
2. More than 5 years   4.5%

Screening for the presence of malarial parasites can be performed using automated flow cytometry. With this technique, erythrocytes are stained with acridine orange. Mature erythrocytes contain no DNA and do not fluoresce with this stain. Malaria-infected erythrocytes contain DNA and fluoresce.

PREVENTION

Current donor standards of the AABB require that travelers be excluded for 6 months after returning from endemic areas and that persons who have had malaria be deferred for 3 years after therapy (refer to Chapter 2 for complete details). A general consensus supports the view that a single infection with *P. falciparum* does not survive in a human host for more than 2 years; *P. vivax* and *P. ovale* usually die out within 3 years. The survival times of *P. falciparum* and *P. vivax* may be longer in persons who live in endemic areas most of their lives, and infections may be delayed in their reappearance in immune carriers. *P. malariae* may exist with or without symptoms for up to 40 or 50 years. The Centers for Disease Control have proposed that the country of birth of the donor be included as part of the oral and written information required from blood donors to facilitate the detection of those who lived for long periods in malarious areas of the world. The 3-year time limit is a compromise. To retain as many donors as possible, the risk of some cases of transfusion malaria has to be accepted in the hope that the 3-year limit will minimize the occurrence of *P. falciparum* and *P. vivax* infection.

Because the incidence of malaria worldwide and that of transfusion-acquired malaria have increased to the highest level in the past 25 years, careful interviewing of donors supplemented by serologic screening may become necessary in the future. The importance of donor screening for malarial antibodies was recognized in the 1984 recommendation of the Committee of Ministers of the Council of Europe and also in the regulations of the UK National Blood Transfusion Service. An advantage of the wider use of serologic screening lies in the fact that blood donors who might have been rejected because of the mere suspicion of a previous infection may not be accepted. Screening suspected asymptomatic carriers, however, increases the cost of processing donor blood and the volume of laboratory work in donor processing.

SPECIAL NOTES

The ideal policy of detecting and excluding parasitized donors is often impossible in areas where malaria is endemic. In one report, the population of one town in Nigeria is nearly 100% parasitized with *Plasmodium*, mostly *Falciparum*. In this circumstance, it is impossible to exclude a donor because of malaria except for those with an active infection. To prevent transfusion-induced malaria, chloroquine prophylaxis is given routinely to all blood recipients. This prophylaxis is also given to all postoperative patients since surgery often activates latent malaria because little, if any, chloroquine resistance has been observed in this particular area. However, in areas with drug resistance, routine prophylaxis is withheld and treatment is administered only to patients in whom symptoms appear after transfusion.

The geographic extension of *P. falciparum* strains resistant to chloroquine has been quite rapid since 1960. Resistant strains of *P. falciparum* species have appeared in large areas of Southeast Asia and also in several countries of Central and South America. Protection of recipients of whole blood in these situations depends on the use of sulphadoxine-pyrimethamine or mefloquine.

Chagas' Disease

ETIOLOGY

Trypanosoma cruzi (*T. cruzi*) is a parasitic blood and tissue protozoan. This organism has an intracellular state in cardiac muscle and other tissues as well as a trypanosome form in the circulating blood. *T. cruzi* is the causative agent of *Chagas' disease* or *American trypanosomiasis.*

INCIDENCE

More than 12 million people live in areas in which *T. cruzi* is endemic. Chagas' disease is a serious medical and health problem within the endemic belt of the disease, between northern Argentina and southern Mexico. Of the 65 million people who live within this endemic area, at least 20 million are infected with *T. cruzi.* The risk of transmitting the disease in endemic areas of Chile is between 1 and 7%. Although rare, cases of Chagas' disease have been reported in the United States.

The disease is most commonly seen and most severe in children under 5 years. Older children and adults have milder, subacute, or chronic forms, which generally follow an acute attack.

TRANSMISSION

From the southern parts of the United States through Mexico and Central America and as far south as Argentina, various wild rodents, opossums, and armadillos may be infected and capable of producing disease in humans. Infected potential vectors have been shown to exist farther north.

T. cruzi develops in a large number of insects, but reduviid bugs are considered the only important vectors. Only those species that invade houses and habitually defecate during the process of feeding or immediately thereafter are major vectors of the human disease. Most cases of Chagas' disease occur in rural and periurban areas where poor housing conditions, combined with the vector's adaptation to human dwellings, influence the persistence of the domestic cycle, which includes the vector living in intimate contact with man and domestic animal reservoirs.

The trypanosomes develop in the hindgut of the insect and are carried in the feces. The parasite is spread into the skin by scratching near the bite where deposits of infective feces are. The disease may also be transmitted congenitally. Blood transfusion is apparently the second most important mechanism of *T. cruzi* transmission. If no prophylactic measures are taken, the risk of receiving contaminated blood depends on the prevalence of the infection among blood donors and the number of transfusions received.

SIGNS AND SYMPTOMS

Studies of Chagas' disease indicate that this infection induces a strong immune response, which reduces the infection to subclinical levels. But the infection is lifelong, with progression to clinical symptoms, especially in the myocardium.

At the site of infection, the organisms proliferate, producing an erythematous area known as a chagoma. This lesion occurs most frequently on one side of the face but may appear elsewhere on the body. Incubation varies from 4 to 116 days after exposure. Organisms appear in the blood (in small numbers in persons over 1 year) at about 10 days or persist during the acute stage. Clinical symptoms of the acute stage include generalized malaise, chills, high fever, muscular aches and pains, and increasing exhaustion. An acute attack may terminate in a few weeks or the patient may enter the chronic stage of the infection. Variable periods of remission may occur. Exacerbations marked by fever and the appearance of trypanosomes in the circulating blood may serve to separate the two stages of the disease, or the chronic phase may be initially asymptomatic. Lymphadenopathy and splenomegaly are common findings.

Drugs are effective in the early stages of infection and cure from 50 to 90% of cases. If treatment is not administered, 5 to 40% of infected persons (depending on geographic area) enter a silent, latent period of 10 or more years. These patients may subsequently develop the clinical manifestations of cardiopathy, megaesophagus, and/or megacolon which characterize the chronic stage of the disease.

LABORATORY TESTING

Confirmation of a suspected case of Chagas' disease can be made through direct blood smear examination, blood culture, animal inoculation, or serologic testing for specific IgM antibodies. Trypanosomes are seldom seen in the circulating blood.

Chronic infections can be detected by the presence of antibodies against *T. cruzi*. Procedures include complement fixation, direct agglutination, indirect hemagglutination (IHA), indirect immunofluorescence (IFA), or ELISA tests. A radioimmunoassay (RIA) has been developed for immunologic diagnosis of Chagas' disease in humans.

The Machado test for diagnosis of Chagas' disease is a complement fixation reaction, using as antigen an extract of the spleen of puppies severely infected with *T. cruzi*. This test is used extensively in the endemic areas of South America and gives a high percentage of positive reactions in patients in the chronic stage of the disease. Direct agglutination is a very sensitive method for the diagnosis of acute cases. High sensitivity and reproducibility of the indirect hemagglutination procedure have been demonstrated.

PREVENTION

To prevent transmission of *T. cruzi* in countries where the organism is prevalent, serologic tests should be mandatory for blood donors. In nonendemic areas, screening of donors from endemic areas should be conducted.

Immunologic studies have shown that a chronic, asymptomatic *T. cruzi* infection is characterized by common antigens shared by the parasite and the human host. Unfortunately, this has an adverse effect on the development of a protective vaccine.

Other Parasitic Diseases

In addition to malaria and *T. cruzi,* a variety of parasitic diseases can be ac-

quired through blood transfusion. Two of these diseases, toxoplasmosis (*T. gondii*) and babesiosis (*Babesia* species), are of importance to blood bank technologists.

TOXOPLASMOSIS (TOXOPLASMA GONDII)

The hazard of transfusion-transmitted toxoplasmosis has been recently recognized in connection with the use of leukocyte concentrates given to patients. Patients at risk are those who are receiving immunosuppressive agents or corticosteroids.

Etiology. *Toxoplasma* has been recognized as a tissue coccidium. *Toxoplasma gondii* was first discovered in a North African rodent and has been observed in numerous birds and mammals around the world, including humans. It is a parasite of cosmopolitan distribution that is able to develop in a wide variety of vertebrate hosts. The definitive hosts are the domestic cat and certain other feline animals.

Incidence. Human infections are common in many parts of the world. The incidence rates vary from place to place for unknown reasons. The highest recorded rate (93%) occurs in Parisian women who prefer undercooked or raw meat, and a 50% rate of occurrence exists in their children.

Transmission. Domestic cats are the source of the disease, producing oocysts which are present in their feces. Accidental ingestion of oocysts by humans and animals, including the cat, produce a proliferative infection in the body tissues. Fecal contamination of food, and water soiled hands, inadequately cooked infected meat, and raw milk can be important sources of human infection.

All mammals, including humans, can transmit the infection transplacentally. Transplacental transmission usually takes place in the course of an acute but inapparent or undiagnosed maternal infection. In addition to transplacental transmission, transmission by means of tachyzoites in blood transfusion has been observed, and transmission by means of other body fluids is a theoretic possibility.

THE DISEASE CYCLE IN CATS. Reproduction of *T. gondii* takes place in the intestinal epithelium of cats by both schizogony and gametogony, with the resulting oocysts passed in the feces. This is referred to as the enteric cycle. The cat, as well as humans and other animals, may also have the extraintestinal or proliferative forms in the body tissues (tachyzoites and bradyzoites).

THE DISEASE CYCLE IN HUMANS. The proliferative stage in humans and animals produces the parasites as tachyzoites, which are rapidly multiplying forms characteristic of an acute infection. In the slowly multiplying encysted forms characteristic of chronic infections, the parasitic forms are referred to as bradyzoites. Tachyzoites and bradyzoites comprise the extraintestinal or tissue phase of the cycle, which is the only phase known to exist in humans.

In adults and children other than newborn babies, the disease is usually asymptomatic. A generalized infection probably occurs. When symptoms are seen, they are frequently mild. The disease picture may simulate infectious mononucleosis, with chills, fever, headache, lymphadenopathy, and extreme fatigue. A chronic form of toxoplasmic lymphadenopathy has been described.

T. gondii presents a special problem in immunosuppressed or otherwise compromised hosts. Some of these patients have developed reactivation of a latent toxoplasmosis. This has been observed in Hodgkin's and non-Hodgkin's types of lymphoma as well as recipients of organ transplants. Reactivation of cerebral toxoplasmosis is not uncommon in patients with AIDS. Primary infection may be promoted by immunosuppression. This was the case in two cardiac transplant patients who were seronegative before surgery but received organs from donors who had serologic evidence of acute toxoplasma infection.

Symptoms of the disease vary with most patients demonstrating subclinical or nonspecific illness. Although spontaneous recovery follows acute febrile disease, the organism can localize and multiply in any organ of the body or the circulatory system.

Laboratory Testing. Serologic screening for *T. gondii* can be by indirect fluorescent antibody (IFA), hemagglutination (IHA), and enzyme-linked immunosorbent assay (ELISA). Antibodies are demonstrable within the first 2 weeks after infection, rise to high levels early in the infection, and fall

slightly but persist at an elevated level for many months before declining to low levels after many years. Absolute diagnosis must be established by biopsy, necropsy, or intraperitoneal inoculation into mice.

Prevention. Screening of blood donors or potential organ donors for *T. gondii* would prevent the transmission of this parasite to immunocompromised patients.

BABESIOSIS

Human babesiosis was first recognized and reported in Europe in 1957. Since that time, human infections by *Babesia* have been reported from North America and Europe. Accidental transmission of *Babesia* is now known as a possible consequence of blood transfusion.

Etiology. European cases of human babesiosis have been demonstrated to be caused by *B. divergens* (*bovis*), a parasite of cattle. The patients diagnosed in Europe had been associated with land grazed on by cattle with babesiosis. Human babesiosis in North America is usually caused by *B. microti,* a parasite of rodents.

Incidence. In all the European cases, babesiosis occurred in persons who had been splenectomized prior to infection. It is likely that the splenectomy affected patient susceptibility to infection and the severity of illness. North American infections have most often occurred in persons with intact spleens. The majority of North American infections have been associated with people living in or visiting the Cape Cod islands of Nantucket, Martha's Vineyard, Shelter Island, or Long Island. Three asymptomatic cases have been reported in Mexico and another from the state of Georgia. One case of babesiosis has been reported in a splenectomized patient in California.

Transmission. *Babesia* are transmitted by various species of ixodid ticks, in which a sexual multiplicative cycle occurs. Feral mice are reservoir hosts of *B. microti.* Most cases of *Babesia* infection occur in late summer and early fall. It is believed that ticks must feed for at least 12 hours before they transmit the infective organisms.

A carrier state is difficult to confirm in immunologically competent adults. It is known, however, that *Babesia* remain infective in blood drawn from donors with subclinical disease after 14 days of storage.

Of the two confirmed cases of transfusion-associated babesiosis in the United States, one patient received 2 units of packed red cells from a donor who had camped on Cape Cod a week before donation. In the second case, a patient with idiopathic thrombocytopenia who had been treated with corticosteroids had a splenectomy. This patient received 20 units of platelet concentrates from 17 donors, one of whom was a summer resident of Nantucket.

Signs and Symptoms. Five of seven European patients infected with *B. divergens* (*bovis*) died after a rapidly progressive illness characterized by fever, anemia, jaundice, and renal failure. Most cases of babesiosis in North America have occurred in non-splenectomized patients, and the infection has been self-limited, with an incubation period of 1 to 4 weeks. In these cases, the disease was characterized by gradual onset of malaise followed by fever, headache, chills, sweating, arthralgias, myalgias, fatigue, and weakness. The incubation period of *B. microti* varies from 1 to 4 weeks. However, severe and fatal cases have occurred in persons who underwent splenectomy or were treated by corticosteroids and immunosuppressive drugs.

Chloroquine, which has anti-inflammatory properties, provides symptomatic relief in most cases but seems to have no effect on the degree of parasitemia or its duration.

Laboratory Testing. Human infection is diagnosed by identifying the intraerythrocytic parasites in Giemsa-stained blood films. However, blood film examination is not sensitive enough, and the duration of the asymptomatic carrier state is uncertain.

Serologic testing with the indirect immunofluorescent antibody test (IIF) is useful in diagnosis. Specific serologic tests require the *B. microti* antigen, which is not always easily available.

Prevention. The only recognized control measure is to avoid tick-infested areas. Exclusion of febrile donors who have visited endemic areas or those who have an anti-*Babesia* IFA titer of 1:16 or higher may reduce the risk of accidentally transmitted babesiosis.

TRANSFUSION-ASSOCIATED BACTERIA

Transfusion reactions due to contamination of donated blood by bacteria such as *Staphylococcus* and *Pseudomonas* were not uncommon in the past. Proper collection, refrigerated storage, disposable containers, and a 24-hour expiration time for components collected or processed in an open system has almost eliminated bacterial contamination and growth in blood and blood components. The exception to this situation is the increased incidence of bacterial contamination in platelet concentrates stored for up to 7 days at room temperature (discussed in Chapter 9).

Transfusion-acquired blood-borne diseases, such as syphilis, are also less of a hazard due to testing of donor blood and refrigeration. However, syphilis may be acquired under certain circumstances.

Syphilis

ETIOLOGY

The etiologic agent of syphilis, *Treponema pallidum* (*T. pallidum*) is a thin, spiral-shaped bacterium. Following World War II, the reported incidence of early syphilis in the U.S. declined each year until 1958, when the rate once again began to rise progressively.

TRANSMISSION

Treponema pallidum is usually acquired by the venereal route. However, during the first half of this century, syphilis was a major blood-borne infectious disease which was easily transmitted through the prevailing method of direct donor-to-patient blood transfusion. The hazard of transmission of syphilis or of yaws (*Treponema pertenue*) has not disappeared in some tropical countries, where the organization of blood banks is deficient and direct blood transfusion prevails in emergency situations.

INCIDENCE

Very few cases of transfusion-acquired syphilis have been reported in recent years.

Refrigerated blood storage decreases accidental transmission of the microorganism because *Treponema pallidum* has a short survival in stored blood. Spirochetes do not appear to survive in citrated blood at 4° C for more than 72 hours.

SIGNS AND SYMPTOMS

After a variable incubation period of 10 days to several months, the primary lesion or chancre appears. This begins as a small nodule that enlarges, forming a relatively painless ulcer. Pus is usually absent and the primary lesion heals spontaneously.

The systemic nature of the disease becomes apparent 6 to 8 weeks after the appearance of the initial chancre, when a generalized rash involving both skin and mucous membranes occurs. During this secondary phase, there may be involvement of the central nervous system, eyes, bones, and liver. *T. pallidum* is more likely to be present in the blood during the secondary stage of syphilis, with symptoms of fever, skin rash, and lymphadenopathy. After a period of weeks to months, the lesions of secondary syphilis resolve spontaneously and the individual enters a latent syphilitic phase. In latent syphilis, serologic tests are reactive but clinical signs or symptoms are absent. One third of untreated latent syphilis cases subsequently develop tertiary syphilis, including neurosyphilis.

LABORATORY TESTING

The serologic diagnosis of syphilis can be demonstrated with reagin tests or specific treponemal antigen tests. The reagin tests use a nonspecific antigen which is lipid in character. These tests detect IgG or IgM antibodies produced by the infected host as a result of the interaction of lipids from either the host or spirochetes, or both, with the immune system of the host. Reagin tests use as antigens defined mixtures of cardiolipin, cholesterol, and lecithin. Two commercially available reagin tests are the VDRL (developed by the Venereal Disease Research Laboratories) and RPR (rapid plasma reagin). Positive reagin tests for syphilis occur in a number of other diseases including leprosy, systemic lupus erythematosus, and malaria.

Reactive (positive) reagin tests can be confirmed with two specific treponemal antigen tests: the fluorescent treponemal antibody absorption test and microhemagglutination techniques. The fluorescent treponemal antibody absorption test (FTA-ABS) uses as the antigen a killed suspension of *T. pallidum* spirochetes. The microhemagglutination assay for *T. pallidum* test is based on agglutination by specific antibodies in the patient's serum with sheep erythrocytes sensitized to *T. pallidum* antigen.

CHAPTER SUMMARY

Background

A variety of blood-borne diseases can be acquired through transfusion. Methods such as careful interviewing of blood donors, serologic screening of blood, use of plastic collection bags, and refrigeration have all contributed to a reduction in accidental transmission of infectious agents, but the possibility of initially acquiring or reactivating an infectious agent is a constant danger. Acquisition of a blood-borne disease is influenced by the overall incidence of an organism in the donor population, the pathogenicity and amount of the agent in the blood, the immune status of the recipient, the physical condition of the recipient, and the age and type of the blood.

Viral agents, parasitic organisms, and bacteria can be transmitted through blood or blood components. Various viral diseases can be transmitted by transfusion. Blood-borne viral diseases include hepatitis B, non-A, non-B hepatitis; *Cytomegalovirus* infection, infectious mononucleosis, and human immunodeficiency syndrome (HIV). Two major parasitic infections, malaria and American trypanosomiasis, are the predominating transfusion-acquired parasitic diseases among patients in the Americas. Transfusion-acquired babesiosis has recently been documented in southern New England, and toxoplasmosis is increasingly being recognized as a hazard. Transfusion-acquired bacterial infections, primarily syphilis, have become less of a risk than in the past, but continue to be a problem in underdeveloped countries.

Transfusion-Associated Viruses

In the past, hepatitis B was one of the most frequent clinical infections transmitted by blood transfusion. Hepatitis B is largely a disease spread by the parenteral route through blood transfusion, needle-stick accidents, and contaminated needles, although the virus can be transmitted in the absence of obvious parenteral exposure. The incidence of transfusion-acquired hepatitis B has been severely reduced since high-risk donor groups such as paid donors, prison inmates, and military recruits have been eliminated as a major source of donated blood. Carriers can be divided into two categories based on differing infectivity, depending on the presence in their serum of another antigen, hepatitis B_e antigen ($HB_e Ag$) or its antibody (anti-HB_e). Several serologic markers for hepatitis B virus infection have been defined. These markers are hepatitis B surface antigen ($HB_s Ag$), Hepatitis B_e antigen ($HB_e Ag$), antibody to the hepatitis B core antigen (anti-HB_c), antibody to hepatitis B_e antigen (anti-HB_e), and antibody to hepatitis B surface antigen (anti-HB_s).

The existence of at least two transfusion-associated non-A, non-B viruses is suspected. Transmission of the virus or viruses is by both parenteral and nonparenteral routes. Blood donors as well as patients incubating acute non-A, non-B hepatitis are primary sources in the transmission of this form of post-transfusion hepatitis. Non-A, non-B hepatitis is the principal cause of post-transfusion hepatitis and is also the major source of hepatitis among dialysis patients. No reliable diagnostic markers for detecting the presence of non-A, non-B hepatitis presently exist. Because of the lack of specific antigen or antibody tests for non-A, non-B type viruses, two procedures have been implemented as surrogate tests: ALT and hepatitis B core antibody testing.

Cytomegalovirus infection was previously associated with what is now referred to as post-transfusion mononucleosis. Cytomegalovirus is known to cause trans-fusion-related infections, especially in premature infants, and can be a frequent cause of morbidity and mortality in recipients of organ transplants and patients receiving immunosuppressive chemotherapy. In practice, the greater the degree of immunosuppression, the more likely the patient is to suffer from a cytomegalovirus infection, primary or reactivated. The risk of developing cytomegalovirus infection is greatest for patients who are exposed to cellular blood components from a large number of donors. In heavily transfused patients, blood transfusion becomes a significant risk factor.

The Epstein-Barr virus (EBV) can be transfusion-acquired. Although the virus can produce infectious mononucleosis with hepatitis as the most frequent complication, it is an infrequent consequence of blood transfusion and does not cause as much of a problem in blood recipients as does cytomegalovirus. Immunosuppressed patients have a higher prevalence of EBV infection.

Over the last several years, one of the most publicized transfusion-acquired viruses has been the human T cell leukemia-lymphoma virus, also referred to as the HTLV-III, LAV virus, or human immunodeficiency virus (HIV). HIV-1 and HIV-2 are responsible for acquired immunodeficiency syndrome (AIDS). Transmission of HIV is believed to be restricted to contact with body fluids such as blood or seminal fluid. This virus can be transmitted through a parenteral route by transfusion with infected blood. Post-transfusion AIDS is now well documented, from both cellular blood components and untreated cell-free preparations such as factor VIII concentrate and plasma. Transfusion-associated AIDS is defined as occurring in persons with no other known risk factor for AIDS who were transfused with blood or blood components within a minimum of 5 years before the onset of illness. Treatment of blood components can be an additional preventive method, if biologic activity of the needed component is not compromised. HIV has been demonstrated to be efficiently inactivated by formalin, beta-propiolactone, ethyl ether, detergent, and ultraviolet light.

The parvovirus-like virus of humans has been shown to be transmitted in factor VIII concentrates. Transmission of the virus has been demonstrated in concentrates prepared from donor pools but not from single-donor cryoprecipitate or whole blood. The significance of transmission is uncertain.

Transfusion-Acquired Parasites

Transmission of parasitic infections through blood transfusion is infrequent in developed countries. On the North American continent, four diseases can be seen with greater frequency than other parasitic diseases: malaria (*Plasmodium* species), Chagas' disease (*Trypanosoma cruzi*), babesiosis (*Babesia microti*), and toxoplasmosis (*Toxoplasma gondii*). In underdeveloped, primarily tropical countries, a variety of transfusion-acquired parasitic diseases such as African sleeping sickness (*Trypanosoma brucei rhodesiense* or *Trypanosoma brucei gambiense*), *Wuchereria bancrofti, Loa loa,* and *Mansonella ozzardi* have been observed.

Transfusion-Associated Bacteria

Transfusion reactions due to contamination of donated blood by bacteria such as *Staphylococcus* and *Pseudomonas* were not uncommon in the past. Proper collection, refrigerated storage, and a 24-hour expiration time for components collected or processed in an open system has almost eliminated bacterial contamination and growth in blood and blood components. The exception to this situation is the increased incidence of bacterial contamination in platelet concentrates stored for up to seven days at room temperature.

Transfusion-acquired blood-borne diseases such as syphilis are also less of a hazard due to testing of donor blood and refrigeration. Very few cases of transfusion-acquired syphilis have been reported in recent years. Refrigerated blood storage decreases accidental transmission of the microorganism because *Treponema pallidum* has a short survival in stored blood.

REVIEW QUESTIONS

1. Which of the following is *not* a factor in the acquisition of an infectious disease through blood or blood component transfusion?
   A. Incidence of the organism or agent in the donor population
   B. ABO and Rh type of the donor
   C. Pathogenicity of the agent/organism
   D. Physical and immune status of the patient
   E. Type of blood component received
2. Which of the following infections can be potentially transmitted through blood or blood component transfusion?
   A. Non-A, non-B hepatitis
   B. AIDS
   C. Malaria
   D. Syphilis
   E. All of the above
3. If a potentially infectious virus is present in a transfusion, actual development of a clinical disorder depends on all of the following patient-related factors *except:*
   A. Overall susceptibility
   B. Previous exposure to bacterial organisms
   C. Nutritional status
   D. Previous exposure to that particular virus
   E. Age
4. The most cost-effective method of preventing transmission of viral agents by transfusion is:
   A. Serologic screening of donor blood
   B. Chemical treatment of blood and blood components
   C. Physical treatment (e.g., filters) of blood and blood components
   D. Self-exclusion of high-risk donors through interviewing
   E. Use of aseptic donor blood collection techniques
5. Hepatitis B accounts for approximately ____% of cases of transfusion-acquired hepatitis.
   A. 5
   B. 10
   C. 25
   D. 75
   D. 95

6. Non-A, non-B hepatitis accounts for approximately ____% of cases of transfusion-acquired hepatitis.
   A. 10
   B. 20
   C. 40
   D. 60
   E. 80

Questions 7–9. Match the following average incubation times (in days) with the appropriate form of hepatitis.

7. Hepatitis A
8. Hepatitis B
9. Non-A, non-B hepatitis
   A. 5
   B. 25
   C. 50
   D. 75
   E. 150

10. Which type of hepatitis does *not* have a chronic form?
    A. Hepatitis A
    B. Hepatitis B
    C. Non-A, non-B hepatitis

11. Another name for hepatitis B infection is:
    A. Infectious hepatitis
    B. Serum hepatitis
    C. Australia antigen
    D. Dane particle
    E. Cytomegalovirus

12. The most frequent clinical response to hepatitis B virus is:
    A. Jaundice within 25 days
    B. Jaundice within 75 days
    C. Asymptomatic infection
    D. Subclinical infection
    E. Both C and D

13. The first laboratory screening test of donor blood is for the detection of:
    A. HBc
    B. HBs Ag
    C. HBe
    D. Anti-HB$_e$
    E. Anti-CMV

14. Which surface marker is a reliable marker for the presence of high levels of hepatitis virus and a high degree of infectivity?
    A. HB$_e$Ag
    B. Hb$_s$Ag
    C. HB$_c$Ag
    D. Anti-HB$_s$Ag
    E. Anti-HB$_e$

15. The serologic marker during the "window period" of type B hepatitis is:
    A. Anti-HB$_s$
    B. Anti-HB$_c$
    C. Anti-HB$_e$
    D. HBsAg
    E. CMVAg

16. Which of the following is a characteristic of the delta agent?
    A. A DNA virus
    B. Replicates only in hepatitis B-virus infected hosts
    C. Infects patients who are HB$_c$Ag positive
    D. Frequently found in the United States
    E. Both A and B

17. Which of the following viruses is rarely implicated in transfusion-associated hepatitis?
    A. Hepatitis A
    B. Hepatitis B
    C. Non-A, non-B
    D. Cytomegalovirus
    E. Epstein-Barr

18. Post-transfusion hepatitis is most frequently due to:
    A. Delta agent
    B. Non-A, non-B hepatitis
    C. Hepatitis A
    D. Hepatitis B
    E. Cytomegalovirus

19. The specific diagnostic test for non-A, non-B hepatitis is:
    A. Absence of anti-HAV and anti-HB$_s$Ag
    B. An increase in serum ALT
    C. Detection of non-A, non-B antibodies
    D. Anti-HB$_c$
    E. None available

20. Surrogate testing for non-A, non-B hepatitis consists of:
    A. HB$_s$Ag and ALT
    B. Anti-HB$_c$ and ALT
    C. HB$_s$Ag and anti-HB$_c$
    D. Anti-HB$_s$ and anti-HB$_c$
    E. HB$_s$Ag and anti-HB$_s$

21. Fill in the blank. Human cytomegalovirus is classified as a ____ virus.
    A. Herpes
    B. Hepadna
    C. Retrovirus
    D. RNA

E. HTLV

22. Transfusion-related cytomegalovirus infections can occur in:
    A. Premature infants
    B. Seronegative patients who have received seropositive organ transplants
    C. Seronegative patients receiving immunosuppressive chemotherapy
    D. Healthy adults
    E. All except D

23. Cytomegalovirus can be assessed in the laboratory by:
    A. Demonstrating inclusion bodies in leukocytes in urinary sediment
    B. A positive heterophil antibody test
    C. The presence of Epstein-Barr antibodies
    D. A positive test for *Toxoplasma* antibodies
    E. Surrogate testing

24. Fill in the blank. The presence of antibodies against immediate-early and early CMV antigens is associated with ____ infection.
    A. Chronic
    B. Active
    C. Latent
    D. Carrier state
    E. Both A and C

25. Characteristics of Epstein-Barr virus include:
    A. Transfusion-associated malignancy
    B. Transfusion-associated infectious mononucleosis
    C. Transplacental transmission
    D. An RNA virus
    E. Both B and C

26. Transfusion-associated Epstein-Barr virus infections have a higher prevalence in:
    A. Infants
    B. Adolescents
    C. Healthy adults
    D. Immunosuppressed patients
    E. All of the above

27. Which of the following human T-Cell leukemia-lymphoma viruses is/are known to be transmitted through blood transfusion?
    A. Type I
    B. Type II
    C. Type III
    D. Both A and C

E. Both B and C

28. The immunodeficiency virus (HIV) differs from viruses such as hepatitis because:
    A. T4 lymphocytes are depleted
    B. Reverse transcriptase is present
    C. Helper-inducer lymphocytes are depleted
    D. It carries a single, positive-stranded RNA genome
    E. All of the above

29. The mean period (in months) between viral transmission and the development of AIDS symptoms is:
    A. 3
    B. 6
    C. 12
    D. 15
    E. 27

30. First-generation tests for HIV screening detect the presence of ____ in a donor.
    A. Antigen
    B. Antibody
    C. Viral capsid
    D. Genome
    E. Lymphocyte alterations

31. Parvovirus has been shown to be transmitted in:
    A. Whole blood
    B. Packed red blood cells
    C. Leukocyte concentrates
    D. Factor VIII concentrates
    E. Single-donor cryoprecipitate

32. One of the four disease-causing parasites seen with the greatest frequency in North America is:
    A. *Trypanosoma brucei rhodesiense*
    B. *Trypanosoma cruzi*
    C. *Trypanosoma brucei gambiense*
    D. *Mansonella ozzardi*
    E. *Wuchereria bancrofti*

33. The occurrence of transfusion-acquired malaria is ____ in the United States.
    A. Non-existent
    B. Decreasing
    C. Remaining the same
    D. Increasing
    E. Epidemic

34 and 35. The multiplication of the ____ phase of the malarial parasite takes place in the human ____.

34.
    A. Sexual
    B. Asexual

35.
   A. Blood stream
   B. Intestine
   C. Liver
   D. Salivary glands
   E. Erythrocytes
36. Using the IFA method, ____% of potential donors have a positive reaction within 5 years of leaving an endemic malarial area.
   A. 50
   B. 28
   C. 14
   D. 7
   E. 4.5
37. *Trypanosoma cruzi* produces:
   A. Malaria
   B. Chagas' disease
   C. American trypanosomiasis
   D. African sleeping sickness
   E. Both B and C
38. Toxoplasmosis infection has been recognized in conjunction with ____ transfusions.
   A. Whole blood
   B. Packed erythrocytes
   C. Leukocytes
   D. Factor VIII
   E. AHF factor
39. Transfusion-acquired babesiosis has been recognized primarily in:
   A. South America
   B. Central America
   C. North America
   D. Cape Cod
   E. Cats
40. One of the most significant reasons for the decrease of transfusion-acquired syphilis is:
   A. Decreased incidence in donors
   B. More sensitive testing methods
   C. Refrigerated blood storage
   D. Better donor interviewing methods
   E. None of the above

9. C	25. E
10. A	26. D
11. B	27. D
12. E	28. E
13. B	29. E
14. A	30. B
15. B	31. D
16. B	32. B
17. A	33. D
18. B	34. B
19. E	35. C
20. B	36. C
21. A	37. E
22. E	38. C
23. A	39. D
24. B	40. C

BIBLIOGRAPHY

Alpaugh, K., Beckwith, D., et al.: A donor population classified for viral exposure and infection: Cytomegalovirus and hepatitis B, with an addendum on HTLV-III test results. Lab. Med., *16*(8): 485-488, 1985.

Barbara, J.A.J., and Tedder, R.S.: Viral infections transmitted by blood and its products. Clin. Haematol., *13*(3): 693-707, 1984.

Beck, J.W., and Davies, J.E.: The Flagellates (Mastigophora). In Medical Parasitology, 2nd ed. St. Louis, C.V. Mosby, 1976, pp. 45-53.

Borek, D. A., et al.: The use of hepatitis B marker prevalence in regional blood center employees as a guide to vaccination policy. Transfusion *24*(5): 408, 1984.

Brady, M.T.: Cytomegalovirus infections: Occupational risk for health professionals. *Am. J. Infect. Contr. 14*(5): 197-203, 1986.

Bruce-Chwatt, L.J.: Transfusion associated parasitic infections. Infection, Immunity, and Blood Transfusion. New York, Alan R. Liss, 1985. pp.101-125.

Bruce-Chwatt, L.J.: Transfusion malaria. *Lancet, ii*: August 3, 1985. p.271.

Camazine, B.: Transfusion-associated malaria. *Lancet, ii*: July 6, 37, 1985.

Centocor Product Bulletin, Uncovering the Hidden Antigen Phase of Hepatitis B Infection, 1986.

Decker, R. H. (Ed.): *Hepatitis Forum.* North Chicago, Abbott Laboratories, winter, 1985-86.

Dialogues in Medicine, AIDS and the HTLV-III test: Current considerations, *Lab. Med. 16*(8): 489-492, 1985.

Feng, C.S., et al.: A comparison of four commercial test kits for detection of cytomegalovirus antibodies in blood donors. Transfusion. *26*(2): 203-204, 1986.

Fiesthumel, S., et al.: Cytomegalovirus (CMV) infection in blood donors: Correlation of serologic markers with viral shedding. American Red Cross Blood Services, Syracuse, New York. (Abstract of

ANSWERS

1. B	5. B
2. E	6. E
3. B	7. B
4. D	8. D

Paper presented at the 39th Annual American Association of Blood Banks Meeting, October, 1986.) Transfusion, 26(6): 554, 1986.

Fody, E. P., and Johnson, D. F.: The serologic diagnosis of viral hepatitis. J. Med Tech, 4(2): 54-58, April, 1987.

Gitnick, G.: Non-A, non-B hepatitis: Etiology and clinical course. Lab. Med., 14(11): 721-726, 1983.

Gudino, M., et al.: Exclusion of HTLV-III antibody positive donors does not decrease the number of donors with elevated ALT Levels. Abstract of a paper to be presented at the 39th Annual AABB Meeting. Transfusion, 26(6): 551, 1986m.

Hanson, M., and Polesky, J.F.: Comparison of Anti-HTLV-III LAV tests. Abstract of paper to be presented at the 39th Annual AABB Annual Meeting. Transfusion, 26: 553, 1986.

Henle, W. and Henle, G.: Epstein-Barr virus and blood transfusions. Infection, Immunity, and Blood Transfusion. New York, Alan R. Liss, 1985. pp.201-209.

Henry, J.B. (Ed.): Clinical Diagnosis and Management by Laboratory Methods, 17th ed. Philadelphia, WB Saunders, 1982, p.1049.

Hollard, P. V. et al.: Anti-HTLV-III testing of blood donors: Reproducibility and confirmability of commercial test kits. Transfusion, 25: 395, 1985.

Hoofnagle, J. H.: Type A and Type B Hepatitis. Lab. Med., 14(11): 705-716, 1983.

Ito, S., et al.: Clinical value of the Guanas screening test in donor blood for prevention of posttransfusion Non-A, Non-B Hepatitis. Hepatology, 8(2): 383-384, 1988.

Johnson, B., et al.: Transfusion malaria: Serologic identification of infected donors. MMWR, 32: 222-229, 1983.

Kelly, R. T.: Spirochetes and Spiral Bacteria. In Henry, J.B. (Ed.): Clinical Diagnosis and Management by Laboratory Methods, 17th ed. Philadelphia, W.B. Saunders, 1982, p. 1139.

Kleinman, S., and Arens, L.: One year analysis of anti-HTLV-III prevalence and incidence of seroconversion. (Abstract of paper to be presented at the 39th Annual AABB Annual Meeting) Transfusion, 26: 553, 1986.

Kline, W.E., Schuller, R., and Bowman, R.J.: Comparison of assays for detecting Anti-HBcAg. (Abstract of paper to be presented at the 39th Annual AABB Meeting) Transfusion, 26(6) 552, 1986.

Kline, W.E., et al.: Anti-HBcAg screening in blood donors: Test performance and potential impact on the blood supply. (Abstract of paper to be presented at the 39th Annual AABB Meeting). Transfusion, 26(6): 552, 1986.

Koff, W. C., and Hoth, D. F.: Development and testing of AIDS vaccines. Science, 241: 426-432, 1988.

Koziol, D.E., et al.: Antibody to Hepatitis B core antigen as a paradoxical marker for non-A, non-B Hepatitis agents in donated blood. Ann. Intern. Med., 104: 488-495, 1986.

Lamberson, H.V.: Cytomegalovirus (CMV): The agent, its pathogenesis, and its epidemiology. Infection, Immunity, and Blood Transfusion. New York, Alan R. Liss, 1985. pp.149-173.

Lombardo, J. M.: HIV-1 testing: An overview, Am. Clin. Prod. Rev. 10, 12-18, Nov., 1987.

Markell, E.K, et al.: Medical Parasitology. 6th Ed. Philadelphia, W.B. Saunders, 1986. pp.112-117, 131-138.

MMWR: Testing donors of organs, tissues, and semen for antibody to human T-lymphotropic virus type III / lymphadenopathy-associated virus. MMWR, 34(20): 294, 1985.

Musianim, M., et al.: Serological screening for the prevention of transfusion-acquired cytomegalovirus infections. J. Infection, 9: 148-152, 1984.

Nath, N., Wilkinson, S., and Dodd, R. Y.: Use of a control serum containing a low level of HB$_s$Ag for monitoring proficiency in screening for HB$_s$Ag. Transfusion, 26(6): 519-524, 1986.

Noall, R., Williams, A., et al.: Inconsistent Anti-HBc assay results in blood donors. (Abstract of paper to be presented at the 39th Annual AABB Meeting). Transfusion, 26(6): 552, 1986.

Nevalainen, D. E.: Viral hepatitis: Yesterday, today, and tomorrow. Lab. Med., 14(11): 698, 1983.

Overby, L. R.: Challenges and opportunities in biotechnology. Infection, Immunity, and Blood Transfusion, New York, Alan R. Liss, 1985. pp.425-443.

Papsidero, L., et al.: Acquired immune deficiency syndrome: Detection of viral exposure and infection. Am. Clin. Prod. Rev., 4: 17-23, 1986.

Peetoom, F., and the Cooperative Study Group: Use of an enzyme immunoassay for detection of antibody to human immunodeficiency virus in low risk populations. Transfusion, 26(6): 591, 1986.

Polesky, H. F., and Hanson, M.: Transfusion-associated hepatitis: A dilemma. Lab. Med., 14(11): 717-720, 1983.

Polesky, Herbert F.: Hepatitis. In Pittiglio, D.H.: Modern Blood Banking and Transfusion Practice. Philadelphia, FA Davis, 1983, pp. 385-397.

Quinnan, G.V., et al.: Inactivation of human T-Cell lymphotropic virus, Type III by heat, chemical, and irradiation. Transfusion, 26(5): p.481, 1985.

Schiff, E. (Ed): Hepatitis Forum. North Chicago, Abbott Laboratories, Sept., 1987.

Schmidt, Paul J. Member Advisory on HTLV-1 and HIV-2, Arlington, Va: American Association of Blood Banks, Feb. 23, 1988. pp 1-3.

Schmunis, G.A.: Chagas' Disease and Blood Transfusion. Infection, immunity, and blood transfusion. New York, Alan R. Liss, 1985. pp.127-145.

Swenson, S., and Gilcher, R. O.: Hepatitis profile testing on donors with history of hepatitis. (Abstract of the 39th Annual Meeting of the American Association of Blood Banks). Transfusion, 26(6): 588, 1986.

Tarleton, R.L., et al.: Diagnosis of Chagas' disease in humans using a biotin-^{3}H-avidin radioimmunoassay. Am. J. Trop. Med. Hyg. 33: 34-40, 112-117, 360-361, 1984.

Taswell, H.F., et al.: Comparison of three methods for detecting antibody to cytomegalovirus. Transfusion, 26(3): 285-289, 1986.

Tegtmeier, G.E.: Cytomegalovirus and blood transfusion. Infection, Immunity, and Blood Transfusion. New York, Alan R. Liss, 1985. pp.175-199.

Testing Donors of Organs, Tissues, and Semen for An-

tibody to Human T-Lymphotropic Virus Type III /
Lymphadenopathy-Associated Virus. MMWR
34(20): 294, May 24, 1985.

Turgeon, M. L.: *Clinical Hematology*. Boston, Little,
Brown and Co., 1988. pp. 212-219.

Wyler, D.J.: Malaria-Resurgence, resistance and research. N. Engl. J. Med. *308*: 875-878, 1983.

Yomtovian, R.: From ABO to HTLV changing trends
in blood transfusion safety. *Minn. Med. 68*: 587-
589, 1986.

Part Five

Procedures in Blood Banking

13

Routine Blood Banking Procedures

At the conclusion of this chapter, the reader will be able to:
- Cite the most frequent source of pretesting error.
- Describe how systematic errors can be eliminated in blood banking.
- Name at least five possible causes of technical errors that can produce false positive results.
- Name at least five possible causes of technical errors that can produce false negative results.
- Name at least five possible causes of technical errors that can produce false positive *or* false negative results.
- Describe the safety techniques that should be adhered to in laboratory practice.
- Discuss the general principles of basic procedures in blood banking.
- Describe the proper type of specimen needed for each procedure.
- Prepare the necessary reagents for each procedure.
- Describe the quality control steps needed for each procedure.
- Perform the stated procedure.
- Calculate any results needed for reporting a procedure.
- State the reference values for each procedure.
- Describe the sources of error and clinical applications for each procedure.

Chapter Outline

GENERAL CONSIDERATIONS IN BLOOD BANK TESTING

The procedures in Chapters 13 and 14 are presented in a format that is consistent with the guidelines set forth by the National Committee for Clinical Laboratory Standards (NCCLS). This format includes:

1. Procedure title and specific method
2. Test principle, including type of reaction and the clinical reasons for the test
3. Specimen collection and preparation
4. Reagents, supplies, and equipment
5. Quality control
6. Procedure
7. Calculations
8. Reporting results
9. Procedure notes, including sources of error, clinical applications, and limitations
10. References

Accuracy in Pretesting

To eliminate the *most* frequent source of pretesting error, a patient must be positively

413

identified when a blood specimen is obtained. This specimen must be properly collected and labelled (see Chapter 2 for a complete discussion of patient specimen collection and identification). Hemolyzed specimens should not be used for testing.

Blood and blood components must also be correctly collected, labelled and stored (see Chapters 2 and 9 for a complete discussion of collection and storage of blood and blood products).

Accuracy in Blood Bank Testing

Inaccuracies in testing can be systematic or sporadic. Systematic errors can be eliminated by a continuing quality assurance program that monitors equipment, reagents, and other factors.

The manufacturer's directions for the use of reagent antisera and cells must be followed precisely. For each new lot, package inserts should be saved and the directions reviewed because changes are occasionally introduced. Reagents should be checked for turbidity or an abnormal appearance at each time of use. Contaminated reagents can produce erroneous results.

Test protocols must be *strictly* followed. Techniques such as the sequence of addition of test cells or serum and the time and temperature of incubation must be exact. Sporadic or isolated errors in technique can produce false-positive and/or false-negative results. Other possible causes of technical errors are listed as follows:

Possible causes of false-positive errors:

1. Addition of the wrong antiserum to a test tube
2. Overcentrifugation of a serum-cell mixture
3. Dirty glassware
4. Hemolyzed patient serum or reagent RBCs
5. Inadequate dispersal of centrifuged serum-cell mixture

Possible causes of false-negative errors:

1. Omitting patient or donor serum from the test mixture

2. Omitting antiserum from the test mixture
3. Failure to identify hemolysis of red blood cells by the patient's serum as a positive reaction
4. Inappropriately warming a cell-serum mixture
5. Undercentrifugation of a serum-cell mixture
6. Vigorous shaking of a centrifuged serum-cell mixture

Possible causes of false-positive *or* false-negative errors:

1. Incorrect labelling of test tubes
2. Addition of the wrong antiserum
3. Erroneous reading or interpretation of results
4. Inaccurate recording of results
5. Contamination of antiserum or reagent red cells
6. An inaccurate serum-cell ratio in a test mixture

Safety in Blood Bank Testing

All specimens should be treated with caution. During the testing of specimens and the handling of blood specimens or blood products, disposable gloves should be worn. Other precautions such as disinfection of work areas and equipment, consistent with the Universal Blood and Body Fluid Precautions (see Chapter 1) must be followed.

TITLE: ANTIBODY SCREENING (INDIRECT ANTIGLOBULIN OR INDIRECT COOMBS' TEST) WITH AUTO-CONTROL

Principle

The antibody screening test is a qualitative test for detection of unexpected alloantibodies in recipient or donor serum. Serum from patients, for example a surgical or obstetric patient, or from blood donors, is tested against two or three group O reagent screening cells that represent a variety of blood group antigens.

Detection of an antibody depends on the method, medium, and temperature of reactivity as well as the titer of the antibody. Hemolysis or agglutination of reagent red blood cells in the presence of serum at any stage of the test demonstrates the presence of an antibody (a positive test) with specificity to a corresponding antigen on the reagent red blood cells. The absence of hemolysis and/or agglutination indicates that the serum being tested does not contain detectable antibodies directed at antigens present on the reagent red cells being used. Preliminary specificity of an antibody can be established using two or three screening cells; however, the exact specificity of an antibody or antibodies can be established only by further testing with an additional panel of reagent red cells and comparing the reaction patterns with the known antigens of the panel.

A positive reaction indicates that an antibody is present in the serum being tested. If the antibody is not an autoantibody, a specific blood group antibody directed against an antigenic determinant that is absent from the patient's own erythrocytes, may have been produced as a result of previous transfusions or pregnancies. Infrequently, an antibody may be present that reacts with all red cells tested, including the patient's own cells. This pattern of reactivity is typical of acquired hemolytic anemia.

Specimen

No special preparation of the patient is required before specimen collection. The patient must be positively identified when the specimen is collected. The specimen shall be labelled at the bedside and the label must include the patient's full name, the date when the specimen is collected, and the patient's hospital identification number. The time of collection and the phlebotomist's initials should be written on the required form.

Blood should be drawn by an aseptic technique and the specimen should be tested as soon as possible. The required specimens are 5 to 7 mL of clotted blood (red top evacuated tube) and 7 mL of EDTA blood (lavender top evacuated tube). The presence of hemolysis in the specimen makes it unsuitable for testing.

Antibodies that depend on the binding of complement for their detection may not be detected if aged serum or plasma from an anticoagulated sample are used for antibody detection testing. Samples for antibody screening may be used up to 48 hours after collection. The specimen must be stored at 1 to 6° C for 7 days.

Reagents, Supplies, and Equipment

10 × 75 mm disposable test tubes
Disposable pipettes, $4\frac{5}{8}''$ plastic or Pasteur
Normal saline (0.9%)
Bovine albumin* (optional)
Antiglobulin reagent antiserum*
Coombs' control or check cells (IgG-sensitized cells)*
Reagent red blood cells I*
Reagent red blood cells II*
Patient requisition and patient cumulative cards
Centrifuge
37° C waterbath or heat block
Test tube rack
High intensity lamp/optical magnifying lens
Microscope (optional)
* Should be refrigerated when not in use

Quality Control

The test reagents should be monitored daily or at the time of use as described in Chapter 1 and according to the Daily Reagent Quality Assurance procedure outlined in this chapter.

An autocontrol, a mixture of patient's erythrocytes and serum, must be tested simultaneously with each antibody screening test.

All negative antiglobulin reactions must be tested with Coombs' control/check cells. A positive test result at this point will confirm that active antiglobulin was added to the test system and was present when the original antiglobulin test was interpreted as negative. If a positive result is *not* obtained with the control cells, the test is invalid and must be repeated.

Procedure

PRELIMINARY

1. Compare information on specimen with request form; full name, full hospital number, and date. If this information is *not identical*, obtain a new specimen.
2. Prepare a 2 to 4% suspension of patient's red cells (see Preparation of Red Cell Suspensions, later in this chapter).
3. Centrifuge the clotted specimen for 5 minutes at 2500 rpm.
4. Determine if the patient has been previously tested by checking past records in a cumulative patient file.

ANTIBODY SCREENING

1. Label three 10 × 75 mm test tubes:
   1. I
   2. II
   3. AUTO
2. Using a disposable pipette, add 2 drops of the patient's serum to each tube.
3. Add 2 drops of bovine albumin to each tube (optional).
4. Add 1 drop of reagent red blood cells I to the tube labelled I and 1 drop of reagent red blood cells II to the tube labeled II.
5. Add 1 drop of the patient's red cell suspension to the tube labelled AUTO.
6. Mix all tubes and centrifuge for 15 seconds at 3400 rpm.
7. Gently resuspend the cells in all 3 tubes and examine macroscopically for agglutination or hemolysis. Record the results as immediate spin (IS) reactions. Positive reactions should be graded from 1 to 4+ at each stage of observation (see Grading Agglutination Reactions, this chapter).

Complete hemolysis precludes further testing and must be interpreted as a positive result. If partial hemolysis is observed, record and proceed. All positive and negative tests should be continued through all phases of testing.

8. Incubate all 3 tubes for 30 minutes at 37° C.
9. Centrifuge all 3 tubes for 15 seconds at 3400 rpm.
10. Gently resuspend the cells in all 3 tubes and examine macroscopically for agglutination or hemolysis. Record results as 37° C reactions.
11. Wash each tube 3 times. Decant completely after the last wash.
12. Add 2 drops of antiglobulin (AHG) reagent to each tube.
13. Mix each tube and centrifuge for 15 seconds at 3400 rpm.
14. Gently resuspend the cells and examine macroscopically with the aid of magnification (microscopic examination is optional). Record results as antiglobulin (AHG) reactions.
15. To each tube that exhibits no agglutination add 1 drop of Coombs' check cells. Mix well and centrifuge for 15 seconds at 3400 rpm. Resuspend the cells and examine macroscopically for agglutination. Record these results as control cells (CC).

Reporting Results

Agglutination or hemolysis of any screening cell suspension in the immediate-spin, 37° C, or antiglobulin (AHG) phase indicates a positive reaction. The absence of hemolysis or agglutination constitutes a negative test and indicates the absence of detectable antibodies to specific antigens present on the reagent erythrocytes.

If a pattern of positive and negative reactions is observed with one of the two reagent erythrocytes, antibody identification can be simplified by eliminating antibodies specific for antigens present on the nonreactive cell (see Chapter 6 for the technique of preliminary antibody identification). If one or both reagent screening cells is / are positive, a panel of reagent red cells should be tested to identify the alloantibody (see Alloantibodies: Antibody Panel Testing in Chapter 14).

If the autocontrol demonstrates a positive reaction, the serum contains an autoantibody. The presence of an autoantibody can conceal an underlying alloantibody in the serum. Autoabsorption (see sections on absorption of cold and warm agglutinins in Chapter 14) may be required to test the serum for the presence of alloantibodies.

If the patient has been recently transfused, a mixed-field reaction in the autocontrol suggests that an alloantibody directed at an antigen present on surviving donor cells is present.

Procedure Notes

Because some antibodies exhibit dosage, practitioners may prefer to use three reagent screening cells instead of two. The use of three cells allows for a greater variety of antigens, particularly cells having homozygous expression of certain antigens. In other cases, one pooled reagent erythrocyte screening cell is used in place of the two or three individual donor reagent erythrocytes. Pooled screening cells do not provide optimum sensitivity for antibody detection and cannot be used when screening potential blood recipients. However, pooled reagent erythrocytes are acceptable for antibody screening tests on blood donors.

The basic screening cell procedure can be modified with enhancement media, such as albumin, enzymes, polybrene (hexadimethrine bromide), or LISS. If albumin is used as an enhancer, the reactivity of low-titered antibodies may be increased by washing the reagent erythrocytes once with normal saline, decanting the saline completely, and using the "dry button" of cells for the test. If using a low ionic strength test procedure, the cell suspensions should be prepared according to the manufacturer's directions.

In the absence of hemolysis in the pretest specimen or due to bacterial or chemical contamination, hemolysis may demonstrate that an antigen-antibody reaction has occurred. With the exception of the ABO antibodies that are not detected using group O screening erythrocytes, antibodies capable of producing hemolysis have specificities for the P, Lewis, Kidd, or Vel blood group systems.

Limitations

The detection of antibodies in serum can be compromised if the ratio of serum to cells in the test or the length of incubation is incorrect. Failure to detect alloantibodies in a serum can result from:

1. Low-titered antibodies that are too weak to be detected by the test methods and/or media being used.
2. The lack of an antigen on the screening cells to an antibody in the serum.
3. The lack of complement in the test system, e.g., use of plasma or aged serum, which prevents the detection of complement-dependent antibodies.

In rare cases, the presence an antibody directed at one of the antibiotics in the reagent red cell suspending medium may cause false-positive reactions. Antibodies to both neomycin and chloramphenicol have been reported. False-negative reactions can result from as little as 1/10,000 of a drop of the original serum remaining after cell washing. This produces some neutralization of antiglobulin reagent.

REFERENCES

Beattie, K.M., Ferguson, S.J., Burnie, K.L., et al.: Chloramphenicol antibody causing interference in antibody detection and identification tests, *Transfusion,* 16: 174-177, 1976.

Gamma Biologicals, Inc., Houston, Texas: *Reagent Red Blood Cells,* package insert, January, 1986.

Huestis, D., et al., *Practical Blood Transfusion,* 3rd Ed. Boston, Little, Brown and Co., 1982, pp. 106-107.

Issitt, P.: *Applied Blood Group Serology,* 2nd Ed. Oxnard, CA, Spectra Biologics, 1975, pp. 273-274.

Mollison, P.L.: *Blood Transfusion in Clinical Medicine,* 6th Ed. Oxford, Blackwell Scientific Publications, 1979, p. 556.

Turgeon, M.L., and Bender, J.: Routine Analysis, Corning, NY, Corning College Press, 1982.

TITLE: ABO BLOOD GROUPING (FORWARD TYPING)

Principle

The ABO blood groups (A, B, AB, and O) represent the antigens expressed on the erythrocytes of each group. When an antibody and its corresponding antigen are combined in vitro, clumping of the erythrocytes expressing the antigen results. An antibody and its corresponding antigen are not normally present in the same blood specimen.

Human erythrocytes expressing either A or B antigens agglutinate in the presence of reagent antisera containing IgM anti-A or anti-B. Thus, anti-A will agglutinate all erythrocytes expressing the A antigen; anti-B will agglutinate all erythrocytes containing the B antigen. Determination of ABO grouping is important in pretransfusion studies of patients and donors as well as in specialized cases such as obstetric patients.

Specimen

No special preparation of the patient is required before specimen collection. The patient must be positively identified when the specimen is collected. The specimen must be labelled at the bedside and the label must include the patient's full name, the date when the specimen is collected, and the patient's hospital identification number. The time of collection and the phlebotomist's initials should be written on the required form.

Blood should be drawn by an aseptic technique and the specimen should be tested as soon as possible. Approximately 5 to 7 mL of blood should be collected in a plain (red top) evacuated tube or the specimen may be collected in an EDTA (lavender top) evacuated tube. Newborn or infant samples may be collected in pediatric blood specimen containers or as red cells in normal saline. Cord blood specimens are also appropriate. In forensic laboratories, other types of specimens may be used.

The blood sample should be tested as soon as possible. If a delay in testing is necessary, the blood should be refrigerated.

Reagents, Supplies and Equipment

Commercial blood grouping antisera: Anti-A and Anti-B
10 × 75 mm disposable test tubes
Normal saline (0.9% NaCl)
Disposable pipettes, 4 ⅝" plastic or Pasteur
High intensity lamp/optical magnifying lens
Centrifuge

Quality Control

Reagent antisera should be tested daily with erythrocytes of known antigenicity (see Daily Reagent Quality Assurance, this chapter).

Procedure

1. Check the patient's name and identification numbers on the blood specimen and requisition.
2. Prepare a 2 to 4% suspension of the patient's red cells in normal saline (see Preparation of Red Cell Suspensions, this chapter).
3. Label two 10 × 75 mm test tubes—one with the letter A, the other with the letter B.
4. To the tube labeled A, add 1 drop of anti-A antiserum.
5. To the tube labeled B, add 1 drop of anti-B antiserum.
6. Using a disposable pipette, add 1 drop of the cell suspension to each of the 2 test tubes.
7. Mix well and centrifuge both test tubes for 15 seconds at 3400 rpm.
8. Resuspend the cells with gentle agitation and examine macroscopically for agglutination (see Grading Agglutination Reactions, this chapter).

Reporting Results

Agglutination of erythrocytes with a specific antiserum is interpreted as a positive (+) test result and indicates the presence of the corresponding antigen. No agglutination of the erythrocytes produces a negative (0) test indicating that the corresponding antigen is not present.

The various agglutination patterns and their respective interpretations are presented in Table 13-1.

Procedure Notes

Each manufacturer provides, with each package of antiserum, detailed instructions for the use of anti-A and anti-B. These directions vary in details; therefore, it is important to follow the directions for the specific antiserum in use.

Procedures that apply to all tests for ABO grouping include the following:

1. Do not rely on the color of dyes to identify reagent antisera. All tubes must be properly labelled.
2. Do not perform tests at temperatures higher than room temperature (20 to 24° C).
3. Perform observations of agglutination with a well-lighted background, not a warm viewbox.
4. Record results immediately after observation.
5. Remember that contaminated blood specimens, reagents, or supplies may interfere with the test results.

If a patient has been recently transfused with nongroup-specific blood, mixed-field agglutination may be observed. If large quantities of nongroup-specific blood have been transfused, determination of the correct ABO grouping may be impossible. Discrepancies in forward typing can result from conditions such as weak antigens, altered expression of antigens due to disease, chimerism, or excessive blood group substances. Excess amounts of blood group specific soluble substances present in the plasma in certain disorders, for example carcinoma of the stomach and pancreas, neutralize the reagent anti-A or anti-B, leaving no unbound antibody to react with the patient's erythrocytes. This excess of blood group specific substance produces a false-negative or weak reaction in the forward grouping. If the patient's erythrocytes are washed with saline, the substance should be removed and a correct grouping can be observed.

Incorrect typing can also result from additional antigens due to:

1. Polyagglutinable red cells
2. Acquired B-like antigen; acquired A-like antigen
3. Complexes attached to red cells
4. Agents causing nonspecific erythrocyte agglutination
5. Antibody-sensitized red cells—effect of colloids and anti-antibodies, e.g., hemolytic disease of the newborn, incompatible transfusions, or autoimmune processes.

Limitations

Antisera prepared from human sources are capable of detecting A_1 and A_2 groups; however, weak subgroups of A may only be detected with anti-A,B reagent antiserum or monoclonal products. Except in the case of newborn and very young infants, a reverse cell typing should also be performed to verify the results of forward typing.

Table 13-1. Reactions of Patient Erythrocytes and Known Antisera

Antisera		Interpretation
Anti-A	Anti-B	Blood Group
0	0	O
+	0	A
0	+	B
+	+	AB

REFERENCES

Beattie, K.M.: Discrepancies in ABO Blood Groupings: A Seminar on Problems Encountered in Pre-Transfusion Tests. Washington, D.C., AABB, 1972.

Blood Group Antigens and Antibodies as Applied to the ABO and Rh Systems, Ortho Diagnostics, Raritan, NJ, 1969, pp. 15-32.

Huestis, D. et al.: *Practical Blood Transfusion*, 3rd Ed. Boston, Little, Brown and Co., 1982, pp. 163-164.

Issitt, P.: *Applied Blood Group Serology*, 2nd Ed. Oxnard, CA, Spectra Biologics, 1975, pp. 75-86.

Turgeon, M. L., and Bender, J.: Routine Analysis. Corning, NY, Corning College Press, 1982.

Widmann, F. K. (Ed.): *AABB Technical Manual*, 9th Ed. Arlington, VA, American Association of Blood Banks, 1985, pp. 113-121.

TITLE: ABO BLOOD GROUPING (REVERSE TYPING)

Principle

The reverse (serum) grouping procedure to confirm ABO blood grouping is based on the presence or absence of the antibodies, anti-A and anti-B, in serum. If these antibodies are present in serum, agglutination should be demonstrated when the serum is combined with reagent erythrocytes expressing either A or B antigens.

Reverse typing is a crosscheck for forward typing. Because of the lack of synthesized immunoglobulins in newborn and very young infants, this procedure is not performed on specimens from these patients.

Specimen

No special preparation of the patient is required before specimen collection. The patient must be positively identified when the specimen is collected. The specimen must be labelled at the bedside and the label must include the patient's full name, the date when the specimen is collected, and the patient's hospital identification number. The time of collection and the phlebotomist's initials should be written on the required form.

Blood should be drawn by an aseptic technique and the specimen should be tested as soon as possible. Approximately 5 to 7 mL of blood should be collected in a red top (no anticoagulant) or lavender top (EDTA) evacuated tube.

The blood sample should be tested as soon as possible. Hemolysis is undesirable. If a delay in testing is necessary, the blood should be refrigerated.

Reagents, Supplies, and Equipment

Reagent erythrocytes: A_1 and B (A_2 optional)
10 × 75 mm disposable test tubes
Disposable pipettes, 4 ⅝" plastic or Pasteur
High intensity lamp/optical magnifying lens
Centrifuge

Quality Control

Reagent erythrocytes should be tested daily with known antisera (see Daily Reagent Quality Assurance, this chapter).

Procedure

1. Label two 10 × 75 mm test tubes—one with the letter *A*, the other with the letter *B*. Label each with the last three digits of the laboratory number. Note: the letters A and B should be underlined to denote reverse grouping.
2. To each of the two test tubes add 2 drops of the serum or plasma to be tested, using a disposable pipette.
3. To the tube labeled *A*, add 1 drop of the thoroughly mixed A_1 reagent erythrocytes.
4. To the tube labeled *B*, add 1 drop of the thoroughly mixed B reagent erythrocytes.
5. Mix well and centrifuge both test tubes for 15 seconds at 3400 rpm.
6. Resuspend the cells by gentle agitation and examine macroscopically for agglutination; record results.

Reporting Results

Agglutination indicates that an antibody specific for either the A or B antigen is present in the serum or plasma being tested.

The blood group of the individual, based on the presence or absence of agglutination, is presented in Table 13-2.

Procedure Notes

A hemolyzed specimen is unsuitable for this test. As in the forward typing, testing must be conducted at room temperature or colder. If the expected results of both forward and reverse typing are not demonstrated, either a variation in the patient or a technical error may exist.

Discrepancies in serum (reverse) grouping (see Chapter 4 for a full discussion) can be due to unexpected or missing antibodies. A brief summary of these situations follows.

Causes of unexpected antibodies:

1. Passively acquired isoagglutinins
2. Alloantibodies
3. Rouleaux formation
4. Auto anti-I; iso anti-I
5. Anti-A$_1$ in A$_x$, A$_2$, and A$_2$B bloods
6. Anti-H in A$_1$B, A$_1$, B and Bombay bloods
7. Anti-IA and/or iA

Causes of weak or missing antibodies:

1. Deteriorated reagent erythrocytes
2. Hypogammaglobulinemic or elderly patients
3. Newborn infants
4. Chimerism
5. Rare variants of A or B

RESOLUTION OF TECHNICAL ERROR

When results of cell and serum tests for ABO do not agree, the discrepancy must be investigated. If the blood is from a donor unit, the unit must not be released for transfusion until the discrepancy is resolved. When the blood is from a potential recipient, it may be necessary to administer group O erythrocytes of the appropriate Rh group before the investigation is complete. Note: It is important to obtain enough of the patient's blood before transfusion that testing can be continued on a sample free of transfused cells.

If the forward and reverse groups do not agree, several immediate steps can be taken. These include the following:

1. Check the quality control results of the antisera and reagent erythrocytes.
2. Recheck the specimen and requisition for accuracy.
3. Recheck the labelling of the erythrocyte preparation.
4. Repeat both the forward (including anti-A,B antiserum) and reverse grouping tests, if the results are the same as the original:
   A. Incubate all test tubes at room temperature for 15 to 30 minutes. This may enhance weak reactions.
   B. Reverse-group the serum, including an autocontrol. Incubate these tubes at 4° C for 15 minutes.

This testing may reveal the reason for the original discrepancy. A summary of possible reactions and their causes is presented in Table 13-3.

If this additional testing fails to reveal the source of the discrepancy, the following steps should be taken:

1. Obtain a new blood specimen. This should identify discrepancies due to contaminated or misidentified samples.
2. Wash the patient's erythrocytes 3 or 4 times.

Additional Erythrocyte Testing

1. Repeat the forward grouping on a 2 to 5% saline suspension of washed cells. Testing of the red blood cells should include anti-A,B, anti-A$_1$, or anti-H, as appropriate to the problem.

Table 13-2. Reactions of Patient Serum and Reagent Erythrocytes

A$_1$ Cells	B Cells	Antibody	Blood Group
+	+	Anti-A and Anti-B	O
0	+	Anti-B	A
+	0	Anti-A	B
0	0	Neither	AB

Table 13-3. Results in ABO Typing

| | Antisera | | | Reagent RBCs | |
Phenotype	Anti-A*	Anti-B	Anti-A,B	A$_1$	B
A$_{sub}$B with anti-A$_1$	Neg	Pos	Pos	2+	Neg
A$_{sub}$B with no anti-A$_1$	Neg	Pos	Pos	Neg	Neg
A with acquired B	Pos	Pos	Pos	Neg	Pos
A$_{sub}$ no anti-A$_1$	Neg	Neg	Pos	Neg	Pos
A$_x$ with anti-A$_1$	Neg	Neg	Pos	Pos	Pos
A$_3$	Pos (m.f.)	Neg	Pos	Neg	Pos
O with autoagglutinins	Pos	Pos	Pos	Pos	Pos
O with In-polyagglutinable	Pos	Neg	Pos	Pos	Pos
Cord blood AB with weak A antigen	Neg	Pos	Pos	—	—
Cord blood A with weak A antigen	Neg	Neg	Pos	—	—

* Human anti-A detects Group A$_1$ and A$_2$; BioClone anti-A detects subgroups of A.

2. Perform a DAT on the washed erythrocytes.

Additional Serum Testing. Test the serum with three examples of A$_1$, A$_2$, and O screening cells. A group B cell and auto control should also be used. It may be helpful to test group O (or ABO compatible) cord cells if anti-I is suspected. If necessary, incubate cell and serum tests at least 30 minutes at room temperature and at 4° C before concluding that the results are negative. Group O and autologous control cells are especially important for tests incubated at 4° C, to prevent misinterpretation of positive reactions due to autoantibodies or alloantibodies reactive at these temperatures.

ANTI-A$_1$

Anti-A$_1$ in the serum of A or A$_2$B individuals usually agglutinates the A$_1$ cells used for serum grouping tests. An antibody can be considered to be anti-A$_1$ if it agglutinates all the A$_1$ cells and none of the A$_2$ or O cells (Table 13-4). Anti-A$_1$ sometimes causes incompatibility on crossmatches. If, on carefully temperature-controlled tests, the antibody is reactive at 35° C, it should be considered clinically significant, and only A$_2$ or O erythrocytes should be used for transfusion.

UNEXPECTED ALLOANTIBODIES

Reverse grouping may demonstrate the presence of an unexpected non-ABO anti-body. In these cases, either the A or B reagent cell may express the corresponding antigen. If the group O screening cells as well as additional examples of A$_1$ and B cells are negative, the antigen is uncommon. If the group O cells are positive, the procedure for alloantibody screening and identification should be performed.

WEAK OR MISSING ANTIBODIES

In patients with agammaglobulinemia or hypogammaglobulinemia, expected isoantibodies may be weak or absent. In addition, ABO antibodies decrease in strength as individuals grow older; thus, in elderly patients, the agglutinins may be difficult to detect. Testing at 4° C may be necessary to demonstrate their presence. If this is done, a control of the patient's own cells and serum is essential to prove that ABO antibodies and not cold-reacting autoagglutinins are being detected.

Table 13-4. Reactions of Anti-A$_1$

Reagent Cells	Reactions
1. A$_1$ cell	3+
2. A$_1$ cell	3+
3. A$_1$ cell	3+
4. A$_2$ cell	Neg
5. A$_2$ cell	Neg
6. A$_2$ cell	Neg
7. O cell	Neg
8. O cell	Neg
9. O cell	Neg

Limitations

Reverse grouping must be conducted with forward grouping. By itself, the test is not definitive for ABO grouping.

Reverse grouping performed on cord blood or the serum of a very young infant may give misleading results until the child is approximately 6 months old. Antibodies found in the infant's circulation before this time are usually of maternal origin.

REFERENCES

Beattie, K.M.: Discrepancies in ABO Blood Groupings: A Seminar on Problems Encountered in Pre-Transfusion Tests. Washington, D.C., AABB, 1972.
Blood Group Antigens and Antibodies as Applied to the ABO and Rh Systems, Ortho Diagnostics, Raritan, NJ, 1969, pp. 15-32.
Gamma package inserts for anti-A, anti-B. Gamma Biologicals, Inc., Houston, Texas, January, 1986.
Huestis, D. et al.: *Practical Blood Transfusion,* 3rd Ed. Boston, Little, Brown and Co., 1982, pp. 163-164.
Issitt, P.: *Applied Blood Group Serology,* 2nd Ed. Oxnard, CA, Spectra Biologics, 1975, pp. 75-86.
Turgeon, M. L., and Bender, J.: Routine Analysis. Corning, NY, Corning College Press, 1982.
Widmann, .F. K. (Ed.).: *AABB Technical Manual,* 9th Ed. Arlington, VA, American Association of Blood Banks 1985, pp. 113-121, 123.

TITLE: D (Rh$_o$) TYPING

Principle

Human erythrocytes are classified as Rh positive or Rh negative depending solely on the presence or absence of the D antigen. Agglutination will be observed if reagent antiserum containing anti-D is mixed with erythrocytes expressing the D antigen. Determination of the D antigen status of patients is important in pretransfusion and prenatal testing because of the immunogenicity of the D antigen. If a D (Rh) negative person is exposed to the D antigen through transfusion or pregnancy, sensitization is likely to occur. This could subsequently result in incompatible crossmatches or hemolytic disease of the newborn.

Specimen

Approximately 5 to 7 mL of blood should be collected in a red top (no anticoagulant) evacuated tube or a specimen may be collected in a lavender top (EDTA) evacuated tube. Newborn or infant samples may be collected as red cells in normal saline or from a clotted cord sample.

The blood sample should be tested as soon as possible. If a delay in testing is necessary, the specimen should be refrigerated.

Reagents, Supplies, and Equipment

Commercial blood typing antisera: Anti-D (Rh$_o$) for slide and / or rapid tube tests
Commercial blood typing antisera: Rh control serum
10 × 75 mm disposable test tubes
Normal saline (0.9% NaCl)
Disposable pipettes, 4 ⅝″ plastic or Pasteur
High intensity lamp / optical magnifying lens
Centrifuge

Quality Control

Reagent antisera should be tested daily with erythrocytes of known antigenicity (see Daily Reagent Quality Assurance, this chapter).

Every specimen tested for the D antigen should have a control run concurrently. Each manufacturer provides, with each package of antiserum, detailed instructions for use. These directions vary in details; therefore, it is important to follow the directions for the specific antisera in use.

Procedure

1. Label two tubes:
   1. D
   2. D control
2. Prepare a 4% suspension of the erythrocytes (see Preparation of Red Cell Suspensions, this chapter).

3. Place 1 drop of anti-D (anti-Rh₀) slide and/or rapid tube antiserum into the test tube labeled D. To the test tube labeled D control, add 1 drop of Rh control.
4. Add 1 drop of the red cell suspension to be tested to each tube.
5. Mix well and allow both tubes to incubate at room temperature for 2 to 5 minutes.
6. Centrifuge for 15 seconds at 3400 rpm.
7. Resuspend the cells by gentle agitation and examine macroscopically for agglutination (see Grading Agglutination Reactions, this chapter).
8. Record results.

Reporting Results

Agglutination of the erythrocytes indicates the presence of the D antigen (i.e., Rh-positive). No agglutination indicates that the D antigen is not expressed (i.e., Rh negative). Erythrocytes that appear to be Rh negative must be tested for the D^u antigen if the specimen is from a blood donor. D^u testing is no longer performed on specimens from potential recipients.

If the D control shows agglutination, the test results are invalid. Rh negative blood must be used for transfusion in such cases.

Procedure Notes

Testing for D antigen may be performed using the slide instead of the tube technique. The test erythrocyte suspension, however, must be 40 to 50% and several sources of false-positive reactions, such as rouleaux, are associated with the slide method.

False-negative results can be encountered with the tube technique if the red blood cell suspension is too strong. Conversely, a false-negative result with the slide technique can be encountered if the suspension is too weak.

If a positive autocontrol is demonstrated, saline or chemically modified anti-D antisera should be used. These reagents should also be used if the erythrocytes have im-

munoglobulins attached (a positive direct antiglobulin test).

Problems that can be encountered in Rh typing and their respective probable explanations are presented in Table 13-5.

Limitations

Contaminated blood specimens or the presence of materials such as undissolved salt particles or silica may interfere with the test results. Cases of false positive results with chemically modified anti-D have also been reported.

REFERENCES

Gamma Package Insert for Anti-D. Gamma Biologicals, Inc., Houston, Texas, January, 1986.

Issitt, P.: *Applied Blood Group Serology*, 2nd Ed. Oxnard, CA, Spectra Biologics, 1975, pp. 115-152.

Jones, E.C., Sinclair, M., Unrau, L. and Grawe, G.: False-positive results with chemically modified anti-D. Transfusion, *27*: 142-144, 1987.

Turgeon, M. L., and Bender, J.: Routine Analysis, Corning, NY, Corning College Press, 1982.

Widmann, F. K. (Ed.): *AABB Technical Manual,* 9th Ed. Arlington, VA, American Association of Blood Banks, 1985, p.144.

TITLE: D^u TYPING

Principle

The D^u antigen is a variant of the D antigen. The presence of D^u can be demonstrated by an indirect antiglobulin (Coombs) technique, i.e., incubating a red blood cell suspension at 37° C with anti-D antisera. The erythrocytes of donors or selected patients, for example maternity patients, that appear to be Rh₀ negative by direct methods must be further tested for the presence of the D^u antigen.

Specimen

Approximately 5 to 7 mL of blood should be collected in a red top (no anticoagulant) evacuated tube or a specimen may be col-

Table 13-5. Problems in Rh Typing

Procedure	Reactions Observed With: Anti-D (Rh$_o$)	Rh Control	Cell Suspension	Probable Explanations
Slide	Positive	Positive	Serum or plasma	Abnormal serum protein*, positive DAT*
	Weakly positive	Negative	Serum or plasma	D^u†
				Mixture or Rh positive and Rh negative cells (post-transfusion)
Modified tube	Positive	Positive	Saline	Positive DAT**
	Positive	Positive	Serum or plasma	Abnormal serum protein*, positive DAT**
	Weakly positive	Negative	Saline, plasma or serum	D^u†
				Weakly expressed D (Rh$_o$) antigen, mixture of Rh positive and Rh negative cells (post-transfusion)
D^u (AHG phase)	Positive	Positive	Saline, plasma, or serum	Positive DAT**
	Weakly positive	Negative	Saline, plasma, or serum	Low-grade D^u
				Weakly expressed D (Rh$_o$) antigen, postpartum specimen from a large fetal-maternal hemorrhage, mixture of Rh positive and Rh negative cells (post-transfusion)

* If washed cells are used, valid results can be obtained.
** Use anti-Rh$_o$ (D) for saline tube test to obtain valid results.
† D^u produced by genetic suppression of D antigen (high-grade D^u).
Modified from Ortho Brochure, Ortho Diagnostics, Inc., Raritan, New Jersey. 1976.

lected in a lavender top (EDTA) evacuated tube. Newborn or infant samples may be collected as red cells in normal saline or from a clotted cord sample.

The blood sample should be tested as soon as possible. If a delay in testing is necessary, the sample should be refrigerated.

Reagents, Supplies, and Equipment

Commercial blood typing antisera: Anti-D (Rh$_o$) for slide and/or rapid tube tests
Commercial blood typing antisera: Rh control serum
10 × 75 mm disposable test tubes
Test tube racks
Normal saline (0.9% NaCl)
Disposable pipettes, 4 ⅝″ plastic or Pasteur
37° C waterbath or heat block
Centrifuge
Cell washer (optional)
High intensity lamp/optical magnifying lens

Quality Control

A negative control AUTO control is tested concurrently with every specimen tested for the D antigen.

Procedure

1. Label two tubes:
   1. D
   2. D control
2. Prepare a 2 to 4% suspension of the erythrocytes to be tested (see Preparation of Red Cell Suspension, later in this chapter).
3. Place 1 drop of anti-D (anti-Rh$_o$) slide and/or rapid tube antiserum into the test tube labeled D. To the test tube labeled D control, add 1 drop of Rh control.
4. Add 1 drop of the red cell suspension to be tested to each tube.
5. Mix well and allow both tubes to incubate at 37° C for 15 minutes.

6. Wash the cells three times with normal saline. Decant the final wash.
7. Add 2 drops of antiglobulin broad-spectrum antisera to each tube.
8. Centrifuge for 15 seconds at 3400 rpm.
9. Resuspend the cells by gentle agitation and examine macroscopically for agglutination (see Grading Agglutination Reactions, later in this chapter). Record results.
10. Add 1 drop of Coombs control cells to all negative tubes.
11. Centrifuge and examine for agglutination. If the Coombs control cells do not agglutinate, repeat the D^u testing. This step verifies the activity of AHG antisera. Coombs control cells must agglutinate in all tubes that were initially negative.

Reporting Results

If the D^u test and control are negative, the blood is Rh negative, D^u negative. If the D^u test is positive and the control is negative, the individual has the D^u variant (see Chapter 5) and is Rh negative, D^u positive. For purposes of blood donation, such persons are considered Rh positive. However, as a blood recipient, an individual is regarded as Rh negative, D^u negative, and only Rh negative blood is used for transfusion.

If the control is positive, the test is invalid. In such cases, the patient may have a positive direct antiglobulin test, and the D^u type cannot be determined.

Procedure Notes

Mixed-field agglutination in a D^u test from a postpartum woman may indicate a mixture of maternal Rh negative and fetal Rh positive cells.

Some D^u variant individuals may have anti-D. Their cells may also stimulate the production of anti-D in an Rh negative person.

Limitations

If the erythrocytes are coated with immunoglobulins, that is, demonstrate a positive direct antiglobulin test (DAT), the D^u test cannot be performed.

REFERENCES

Epley, K.M., and Klina, L.M.: One step D^u test. Transfusion, 26(6): 570, 1986.

Huestis, D.W., Bove, J.R., and Case, J.: Practical Blood Transfusion. Boston, Little, Brown and Co., 1988, pp. 169-209.

Issitt, P.: Applied Blood Group Serology, 2nd ed. Oxnard, CA, Spectra Biologics, 1975, pp. 273-274.

Schmidt, P.J., Klein, R.E., and Sherwood, N.C.: D^u confirmation, Transfusion, 26(4): 1986, pp. 364-365.

Turgeon, M. L., and Bender, J.: Routine Analysis. Corning, NY, Corning College Press, 1982.

Widmann, F. K. (Ed.): AABB Technical Manual, 9th Ed. Arlington, VA, American Association of Blood Banks, 1985, p. 206.

TITLE: COMPATIBILITY TESTING (CROSSMATCHING)

Principle

Pretransfusion compatibility testing combines a potential recipient's blood specimen with a blood specimen from an intended donor. The major crossmatch consists of combining a sample of the recipient's serum with a sample of erythrocytes from the intended donor. This mixture is tested at various temperatures and with enhancement media. If an antibody is present in the potential recipient that has specificity for an antigen on the donor red cells, agglutination or hemolysis should be exhibited.

Specimen

No special preparation of the patient is required before specimen collection. The patient must be positively identified when the specimen is collected. The specimen must be labelled at the bedside and the label must include the patient's full name, the date when the specimen is collected, and the patient's hospital identification number. The time of collection and the phlebotomist's initials should be written on the required form.

Blood should be drawn by an aseptic technique and the specimen should be tested as soon an possible. Approximately 5 to 7 mL of blood should be collected in a plain red top or lavender top (EDTA) evacuated tube. Hemolysis renders the specimen unsuitable for testing. If a delay in testing is necessary, the blood should be refrigerated.

If a patient's specimen is older than approximately 48 hours, complement-dependent antibodies may not be detected. If a patient has never been transfused or pregnant, most blood banks prefer to use a specimen no more than 48 hours old. If a patient has been previously transfused or pregnant, most blood banks require that the specimen be less than 24 hours old. In massively transfused (10 units or more) patients, the general rule of thumb is that a new specimen should be drawn after each 10 units of transfused blood. In cases of transfusion with other than group specific blood, a new specimen must be drawn before switching back to the patient's own blood type.

All specimens must be retained under refrigeration for 7 days after transfusion of a unit of blood.

Reagents, Supplies, and Equipment

Commercial antiglobulin (AHG) reagent (broad-spectrum or IgG)
Commercial 22% albumin (optional)
10 × 75 mm disposable test tubes
Disposable pipettes, 4 ⅝″ plastic or Pasteur
Scissors
Test tube rack
Normal (0.9%) saline
37° C waterbath or heat block
High intensity lamp/optical magnifying lens
Centrifuge

Quality Control

Reagent erythrocytes should be tested daily with known antisera (see Daily Reagent Quality Assurance, this chapter). All negative AHG reactions must be tested with IgG sensitized erythrocytes and pro-duce a positive reaction. If the AHG control cells do not agglutinate, the compatibility test is invalid.

Procedure

PRELIMINARY

1. Compare the information on the patient's specimen with the information on the test requisition: name, identification number, date. If this information is not identical, obtain a new specimen.
2. Centrifuge the clotted specimen for 5 minutes at 2000 rpm.
3. Check past blood bank records to determine if the patient has ever been screened for antibodies or previously transfused.
4. Perform an ABO grouping (forward and reverse), Rh typing, and alloantibody screen on the recipient's specimen. Record all test results in the blood bank log as well as on the crossmatch requisition.
5. Check data on previous records. If the ABO and Rh are not identical, obtain a new specimen for repeat testing.
6. Procure the whole blood or packed cells to be crossmatched from the blood bank refrigerator. Check all identification on the units, for example, group and Rh, expiration date; and the physical characteristics of the units, for example, absence of hemolysis or abnormal color.
7. Detach a segment from the unit of blood. Cut the ends of the segment and drain the contents into a 10 × 75 mm test tube. Label the tube with the donor unit identification number. Recheck the number.
8. Wash the donor specimen 3 times with normal saline. Decant the last wash completely and prepare a 3% suspension of the erythrocytes.
9. Enter the donor number and expiration date on the test requisition. If the donor unit has not been retyped on entering the blood bank inventory, an

ABO grouping and Rh typing should be performed.

COMPATIBILITY PROCEDURE

The compatibility test can be divided into three phases: room temperature (immediate spin), 37° C, and AHG. In some blood banks, only the immediate spin phase is performed if a patient demonstrates a negative antibody screen in the AHG phase using two or three group O screening cells. The following is an example of a typical crossmatch configuration including all phases.

Room Temperature (Immediate Spin) Phase

1. Label two 10 × 75 mm test tubes. One tube should have the patient's last name and donor number; the other should be labeled AUTO (control).
2. To tube 1 add:
    2 drops of patient serum
    1 drop of donor's washed cells
    2 drops of 22% bovine albumin (optional)
    To the AUTO tube add:
    2 drops of patient serum
    1 drop of patient's washed cells
    2 drops of 22% bovine albumin (optional)
3. Mix and centrifuge for 15 seconds at 3400 rpm.
4. Gently resuspend the cell button and read macroscopically (see Grading Agglutination Reactions, this chapter). If agglutination is observed, do not proceed with the next phases. Agglutination at this phase is considered to indicate an *incompatible* crossmatch. Additional testing may not strengthen the degree of agglutination.
5. Record results. If compatible, proceed with the next phase.

37° C Phase

1. Incubate the 2 tubes from the IS phase for 30 minutes at 37° C.
2. Centrifuge for 15 seconds at 3400 rpm.
3. Gently resuspend the cell button and read macroscopically (see Grading Agglutination Reactions, this chapter).

4. Record results.

Antiglobulin Phase (AHG)

1. Wash the 2 test tubes from the 37° C phase three times with normal saline.
2. After the last wash, decant all saline and add 2 drops of AHG reagent.
3. Mix and centrifuge for 15 seconds at 3400 rpm.
4. Gently resuspend the cell button and examine macroscopically and microscopically.
5. Record results.
6. If either or both of the tubes demonstrate no agglutination, add one drop of IgG sensitized (Coombs control or check cells) to the tube.
7. Centrifuge the tubes for 15 seconds at 3400 rpm and observe and grade for agglutination. *Agglutination must occur.* The test is invalid if the control cells do not agglutinate, and the test must be repeated.
8. Record results.

Reporting Results

A compatible crossmatch is indicated by the absence of agglutination and/or hemolysis at any stage of the crossmatch. The absence of agglutination indicates that the patient has no demonstrable antibodies with a specificity for any of antigens on the donor erythrocytes.

Procedure Notes

If incompatibility is demonstrated by agglutination or hemolysis at any stage of the crossmatch, the donor unit should not be used for transfusion. Exceptions might include "least compatible" units in patients with autoantibodies.

If the patient has a positive antibody screen or demonstrates an incompatibility with a donor unit, the antibody specificity should be determined as soon as possible. After antibody identification, corresponding units that are negative for the antigen to the patient's antibody can be crossmatched.

The crossmatch will detect the following:

1. ABO incompatibility
2. Most alloantibodies directed against common antigens

If a patient exhibits strong rouleau formation, a saline replacement technique may be used.

SALINE REPLACEMENT TECHNIQUE

1. Recentrifuge the serum-cell mixture when rouleau formation is suspected.
2. Remove the serum.
3. Replace the serum with an equal volume of saline (2 drops) and mix.
4. Centrifuge the saline-cell mixture.
5. Resuspend the saline-cell mixture and examine for agglutination. *Rouleaux* will disperse. *True agglutination* will remain.

Limitations

Low-titered antibodies in the patient's serum may not be detectable in the pretransfusion compatibility test. These antibodies may be demonstrable with enhancement methods such as enzyme treatment. In some cases, a delayed hemolytic transfusion reaction may become apparent in 7 to 10 days, if the transfused unit has the antigen corresponding to the patient's antibody.

A crossmatch will not:

1. Prevent immunization of the patient.
2. Guarantee normal survival of transfused erythrocytes.
3. Detect all unexpected alloantibodies in a patient's serum.

REFERENCES

Baumgarten, R.K.: Elimination of the crossmatch, *Transfusion, 27*(5): 445, 1987.
Shulman, Ira A.: The abbreviated crossmatch, College of American Pathologists check sample, *Immunohematology, 30*(2): 2-4, 1987.
Turgeon, M. L., and Bender, J.: Routine Analysis. Corning, NY, Corning College Press, 1982.

TITLE: CORD BLOOD WORKUP

Principle

Blood drained from the umbilical cord is tested for ABO group, Rh type, and the presence of IgG antibodies on the erythrocytes (DAT). This protocol is followed if the infant's mother is group O or D (Rh$_o$) negative and in other cases where the possibility of hemolytic disease of the newborn (HDN) exists.

Specimen

Approximately 5 to 7 mL of blood should be collected in a red top (no anticoagulant) and 3 to 5 mL in a lavender top (EDTA) evacuated tube.

Routinely collected cord blood specimens may be marked HOLD. In cases of potential HDN, the specimen is usually marked STAT. If the specimen is marked HOLD, it should be stored at 1° to 6° C for a minimum of 4 days in a special container for cord blood specimens.

Reagents, Supplies, and Equipment

See ABO, Rh, and DAT procedures, described in this chapter.

Quality Control

See ABO, Rh, and DAT procedures, described in this chapter.

Procedure

1. When a specimen of cord blood arrives, the requisition and blood samples must be checked to ensure that the information on the specimen matches the information on the requisition.
2. If the specimen is STAT, it should be tested for ABO and Rh antigens and a

direct antiglobulin test (DAT) should be performed.

3. If the DAT is positive, bilirubin and CBC tests should be performed immediately. An elution (see Elution Techniques in Chapter 14) should be performed on the DAT-positive cells.

Reporting Results

See ABO, Rh, and DAT procedures, described in this chapter.

Procedure Notes

It is important to wash cord blood cells appropriately. Cord blood specimens should be washed at least four times before forward blood typing to remove residual proteins. Reverse typing should be omitted because any detectable antibodies are usually of maternal origin.

Washing the erythrocytes with saline or adding a drop or two of saline to the test tube will free the aggregated erythrocytes in case of rouleau formation.

Limitations

Failure to remove Wharton's jelly or residual protein from a cord blood specimen may produce a false negative DAT.

REFERENCE

Turgeon, M. L. and Bender, J.: Routine Analysis. Corning, NY, Corning College Press, 1982.

TITLE: DAILY REAGENT QUALITY ASSURANCE

Principle

A comprehensive quality assurance system requires that blood bank reagents be tested on the day of use to ensure that the antisera and reagent erythrocytes are ap-

propriately reactive. Such a system incorporates both positive and negative controls into the procedures recommended by the manufacturer. Any deviation from the expected results warrants investigation before use of the reagent.

Reagents, Supplies, and Equipment

Commercial antisera: Anti-A, anti-B, anti-AB, anti-D (modified slide / tube test), Rh control, 22% albumin, and antiglobulin (AHG)

Reagent red blood cells: A_1, A_2, B, group O antibody screening cells, and IgG-sensitized erythrocytes, e.g., Coombs control / check cells.

10×75 mm test tubes

Test tube racks

Normal saline (0.9% NaCl)

Disposable pipettes: 4 $\frac{5}{8}$" plastic or Pasteur, 1 mL graduated serologic, 5 mL graduate serologic

Safety bulb pipettor

37° C waterbath or heat block

Centrifuge

Cell washer (optional)

High intensity lamp / optical magnifying lens

PROCEDURE

PRELIMINARY

1. Prepare a 1:10 dilution of IgG sensitized red blood cells (Coombs' control / check cells) by adding 0.1 mL of red blood cells to 0.9 mL of saline.
2. Prepare a 1:50 dilution of anti-D by adding 0.1 mL of anti-D to 4.9 mL of saline.

ANTISERA AND REAGENT RED BLOOD CELL CONTROLS

1. Label a set of 10×75 mm test tubes with the numbers 1 through 15.
2. Add undiluted reagent antisera to the labelled tubes as follows:
   A. To tubes 1, 2, and 3, add 1 drop of anti-A.

B. To tubes 4, 5, and 6, add 1 drop of anti-B.

C. To tubes 7, 8, and 9, add 1 drop of anti-AB.

D. To tubes 10 and 11, add 1 drop of anti-D.

E. To tube 12, add 1 drop of Rh control.

F. To tubes 13 and 14, add 1 drop of AHG.

G. To tube 15, add 1 drop of saline.

3. Add undiluted reagent red blood cells to the labelled tubes as follows:

A. To tubes 1, 4, 7, 10, 12, and 13, add 1 drop of A₁ cells.

B. To tubes 2, 5, and 8, add 1 drop of A₂ cells.

C. To tubes 3, 6, and 9, add 1 drop of B cells.

D. To tube 13, add 1 drop of A₁ cells.

4. Add 1 drop of diluted IgG sensitized red blood cells to tubes 11, 14, and 15.

5. Centrifuge all of the tubes at 3400 rpm for 15 seconds or 1000 rpm for 1 minute.

6. Gently resuspend the cell button and examine macroscopically for agglutination and grade the strength of agglutination.

7. Record the results (see Fig. 1–1).

SCREENING CELLS AND AHG REAGENT CONTROL

1. Label four test tubes with the numbers 16 through 19.

2. Add the following reagents as follows:

A. To tubes 16 through 19, add 2 drops of albumin.

B. To tubes 16 and 17, add 1 drop of screening cells I.

C. To tubes 18 and 19, add 1 drop of screening cells II.

D. To tubes 16 and 18, add 1 drop of dilute anti-D.

E. To tubes 17 and 19, add 2 drops of saline.

3. Centrifuge tubes 16 through 19 at 3400 rpm for 15 seconds.

4. Gently resuspend the cell button and examine macroscopically. Record the results as the (IS) room temperature phase.

5. Incubate all of the tubes (16 through 19) for 30 minutes at 37° C.

6. Centrifuge these tubes. Gently resuspend the cell button and examine macroscopically. Record these results as the 37° C phase.

7. Wash the contents of each tube 3 times.

8. To each tube, add 2 drops of AHG.

9. Centrifuge at 3400 rpm for 15 seconds. Gently resuspend the cell button and examine macroscopically. Record the results as the AHG phase.

10. To all negative reactions, add 1 drop of IgG sensitized red blood cells. Centrifuge at 3400 rpm for 15 seconds. Gently resuspend the cell button and examine macroscopically. These reactions must demonstrate agglutination or the test is invalid.

REFERENCES

Quality Control in Blood Banking, Ortho Diagnostics, 1973.

Widmann, F. K. (Ed.): *AABB Technical Manual,* 9th Ed. Arlington, VA, American Association of Blood Banks, 1985, pp. 374-377.

TITLE: DIRECT ANTIGLOBULIN (COOMBS') TEST

Principle

The direct antiglobulin test is based on the principle that antiglobulin antibodies induce in vitro agglutination of erythrocytes with immunologically bound antibodies. After erythrocytes are washed to remove free plasma protein from the test mixture, they are tested directly with reagents containing anti-IgG and anti-C3d (broad spectrum/polyspecific). Monospecific antisera, for example anti-IgG, anti-C3d, and anti-C4, that are specific for immunoglobulins or complement components, may also be used. The DAT procedure is clinically important in the diagnosis of conditions such as hemolytic anemia or delayed hemolytic transfusion reactions.

Specimen

No special preparation of the patient is required before specimen collection. The patient must be positively identified when the specimen is collected. The specimen must be labelled at the bedside, and the label must include the patient's full name, the date when the specimen is collected, and the patient's hospital identification number. The time of collection and the phlebotomist's initials should be written on the required form.

Blood should be drawn by an aseptic technique and tested as soon as possible. The specimen should consist of 5 to 7 mL of clotted blood (red top evacuated tube) and 7 mL of EDTA blood (lavender top evacuated tube). Newborn or infant samples may be collected as red cells in normal saline or from a cord blood sample.

If a delay in testing occurs, the specimen must be refrigerated. Antibodies dependent for their detection upon the binding of complement may not be detected if aged serum or plasma from an anticoagulated sample is used. Hemolysis of the specimen is undesirable.

Reagents, Supplies, and Equipment

Antiglobulin serum (polyspecific or monospecific)
IgG sensitized erythrocytes (Coombs control cells)
10 × 75 mm disposable test tubes
Disposable pipettes, 4⅝″ plastic or Pasteur
Normal saline (0.9%)
Test tube rack
Centrifuge
Cell washer (optional)
High intensity lamp/optical magnifying lens

Quality Control

In addition to the daily reagent quality assurance check, each test must have a saline control run concurrently to rule out autoagglutination. Coombs control/check cells must be added to each test that does not exhibit agglutination. Agglutination of the Coombs control cells verifies the reactivity of the antiglobulin antiserum.

Procedure

1. Prepare a 2% saline suspension of the patient's erythrocytes (see Preparation of Red Cell Suspension, later in this chapter).
2. Label one 10 × 75 test tube with the letters DAT. Label a second 10 × 75 test tube as DAT Control.
3. Using a disposable pipette, add 1 drop of the red cell suspension to each tube.
4. Wash the contents of both tubes three times. If they are washed by hand, fill both tubes with saline and resuspend the red cells, centrifuge at 3400 rpm for 30 seconds and decant. Repeat three times. Be sure saline is completely decanted after the final wash. Note: Washing should be rapid to prevent elution of the antibody into the saline.
5. Add 2 drops of antiglobulin serum to the tube labelled DAT.
6. Add 2 drops of saline to the tube labelled DAT Control.
7. Resuspend the red cells completely in both tubes and mix well.
8. Centrifuge at 3400 rpm for 15 seconds.
9. Gently resuspend the red cells and examine macroscopically and microscopically for agglutination. Grade the reaction and record results. Note: Following AHS addition, the test should be spun and read immediately.
10. Verify the AHG activity if the DAT tube demonstrated no agglutination:
    A. Add 1 drop of Coombs control cells to the DAT tube.
    B. Centrifuge at 3400 rpm for 15 seconds.
    C. Gently resuspend the red cells and examine macroscopically and microscopically for agglutination.
    D. Agglutination *must* be present. If agglutination is not present, the test is invalid and must be repeated.

Reporting Results

A negative test is demonstrated by the absence of agglutination in the DAT test tube. A positive test is manifested by the presence of agglutination. If a cord blood specimen is positive, the attending physician and the nursery should be notified immediately.

Procedure Notes

A positive DAT, typically a mixed-field pattern, may be seen following an incompatible transfusion, for example delayed hemolytic transfusion reaction. Additionally, a positive DAT may be exhibited in various disorders including autoimmune hemolytic anemia, lymphoma, chronic lymphocytic leukemia, collagen disorders such as SLE; other diseases such as carcinoma, hepatic disease, or infectious mononucleosis; and illness caused by drugs, such as penicillin and cephalothin.

Several assumptions are made when interpreting a positive DAT, including the following:

1. The test results are obtained from a properly collected, uncontaminated blood specimen.
2. The red cells are properly washed.
3. The antiglobulin reagent is potent and uncontaminated.

A positive DAT does not imply overt hemolysis; it may occur in healthy persons. The DAT may be negative in individuals with immune hemolytic anemia. In these cases, additional testing should be performed to determine the possible causes of hemolysis. In some circumstances, an alloantibody in the serum may be unrelated to a positive DAT. Patterns of reactivity with AHG antisera vary, depending on the cause. Table 13-6 summarizes some of the typical patterns of AHG reactivity.

To interpret the cause of a positive DAT, the results of the DAT, alloantibody screening test, elution studies, and evidence of hemolysis, such as a decreasing hematocrit, can be combined. Examples of such interpretation are given as follows:

Table 13-6. Examples of Cases of Positive DATs

Disorder	AHG Pattern
Hemolytic disease of the newborn (HDN)	Anti-IgG
Delayed hemolytic transfusion reaction	Anti-IgG
Warm autoimmune hemolytic anemia	Anti-IgG or IgG with anti-C3
Cold autoimmune hemolytic anemia	Anti-C3
Acquired hemolytic anemia	Anti-IgG, Anti-IgG + Anti-C3, Anti-C3 only
Collagen vascular disease	Anti-C3, weak reactions
Chronic lymphocytic leukemia	Anti-IgG
Penicillin antibodies	Anti-IgG

SITUATION 1

Anti-IgG (negative) and anti-C3d (positive)
Antibody screen (negative)
Eluate (negative)
No evidence of hemolysis
Interpretation: Normal individual, immune disorders, drug-Induced.

SITUATION 2

Anti-IgG (negative) and anti-C3d (positive)
Antibody screen (negative)
Eluate (negative)
Hemolysis
Interpretation: Drug-induced warm autoimmune hemolytic anemia (rare)

SITUATION 3

Anti-IgG (negative) and anti-C3d (positive)
Antibody screen (positive)
Eluate (negative)
Interpretation: Cold agglutinin syndrome, paroxysmal cold hemoglobinuria

SITUATION 4

Anti-IgG (positive) and anti-C3d (positive or negative)
Antibody screen (negative)
Eluate (negative)

No evidence of hemolysis
Interpretation: Drug-induced

SITUATION 5

Anti-IgG (positive) and anti-C3d (positive
or negative)
Antibody screen (negative)
Eluate (negative)
No evidence of hemolysis
Interpretation: Drug-induced

SITUATION 6

Anti-IgG (positive) and anti-C3d (positive
or negative)
Antibody screen (negative)
Eluate (Positive)
    or
Anti-IgG (positive) and anti-C3d (positive
or negative)
Antibody screen (positive)
Eluate (positive)
Interpretation: Warm autoimmune hemo-
         lytic anemia, Drug Induced
         (methyldopa or deriva-
         tives), transfusion reaction,
         hemolytic disease of the
         newborn, antenatal IgG (D)

SITUATION 7

Anti-IgG (positive) and anti-C3d (negative)
Antibody screen (negative)
Eluate (negative)
    or
Anti-IgG (positive) and anti-C3d (negative)
Eluate (negative)
Screening with A$_1$ and/or B red blood cells
(positive or negative)
Eluate with A$_1$ and/or B red blood cells
(positive or negative)
Interpretation: Hemolytic disease of the
         newborn, passively ac-
         quired antibody, placental
         transfer of drug antibody

SITUATION 8

Anti-IgG (positive) and anti-C3d (negative)
Antibody screen (positive)
Eluate (positive)
Interpretation: Passively acquired anti-
         body

Limitations

False-positive results may be observed in
the DAT due to:

1. Contamination of the AHG antisera or
   supplies
2. Overcentrifugation
3. Bacterial contamination of specimen
   or reagents
4. Fibrin clot in cell suspension
5. Overzealous reading of serum-cell
   mixture
6. Anti-formaldehyde antibodies
7. Variables in sample procurement such
   as drawing the specimen from a line
   containing 5% or 10% dextrose, using
   a clotted specimen rather than an anticoagulated sample or drawing too
   small a sample in the anticoagulated
   tube

False-negative results usually result from
technical error. They are infrequently
caused by a true failure of the antibody-
coated red cells to react with the antiglobulin serum. Common causes of false-negative reactions include:

1. Failure to add antiglobulin reagent
2. Inadequate washing of red blood cells
3. Inactivation of AHG sera by exogenous gamma globulin
4. Weak or inactive AHG
5. Lack of broad-spectrum specificity of
   the AHG
6. Mixing tubes by inverting uncovered
   tubes with the finger
7. Decreased reactivity of antiserum
   due to storage
8. Elution of antibody into the supernatant on standing, with subsequent
   neutralization of AHG
9. Low pH of saline solution (pH less
   than 6.0)
10. Saline, autoclaved and stored in plas-
    tic containers

REFERENCES

Bruce, M., Watt, A.H., Hare, W., Blue, A., and Mitchell,
    R.: A serious source of error in antiglobulin testing.
    Transfusion, *26*(2):177-181, 1986.

Dzik, W.H., and Darling, C.A.: Positive direct antiglobulin test (DAT) due to anti-formaldehyde antibodies. Transfusion, *26*(6):578, 1986.

Grindon, A.J., and Wilson, M.J. False-positive DAT caused by variables in sample procurement. Transfusion, *21*(3):313-314, 1981.

Huestis, D., et al.: Practical Blood Transfusion, 3rd ed. Boston, Little, Brown & Co., 1982, pp 101-116.

Issitt, P.: Applied Blood Group Serology 2nd ed. Oxnard, CA, Spectra Biologies, 1975, pp 273-274.

Widmann, F.K. (Ed): AABB Technical Manual, 9th Ed. Arlington, VA, American Association of Blood Banks, 1985, p 206.

TITLE: GRADING AGGLUTINATION REACTIONS

Principle

Uniformity in reading reactions is an important aspect of quality assurance. Table 13-7 represents a consistent method of grading agglutination.

REFERENCE

Widmann, F.K. (Ed.): AABB Technical Manual, 9th Ed. Arlington, VA, American Association of Blood Banks, 1985.

Table 13-7. Grading Agglutination Reactions

Grade	Description
Negative	No aggregates
Mixed-field (MF)	Few isolated aggregates, mostly free-floating cells, supernatant appears red
Weak	Tiny aggregates that are barely visible macroscopically, many free erythrocytes, turbid and reddish supernatant
1+	A few small aggregates just visible macroscopically, many free erythrocytes, turbid and reddish supernatant
2+	Medium-sized aggregates, some free erythrocytes, clear supernatant
3+	Several large aggregates, some free erythrocytes, clear supernatant
4+	All of the erythrocytes are combined into one solid aggregate, clear supernatant

TITLE: INSPECTION OF DONOR BLOOD

Principle

Each unit of donor blood must be examined when crossmatched and *immediately* before issue to a patient. This inspection must be recorded.

Quality Control

Blood should be rejected for transfusion if:

1. The color is abnormal. Abnormal conditions include purple discoloration of the red cells, or brown or red plasma.
2. Alterations in the physical appearance are present. Clots or hemolysis render a unit unsuitable for transfusion.
3. Contamination is suspected. Cloudy plasma may indicate bacterial contamination.
4. Blood or plasma is present at the sealing ports or tubing. Improper sealing can produce bacterial contamination of a unit.

Questionable units of blood must be quarantined until disposition. Evaluation of a questionable unit should include inverting it gently a few times to mix the cells and plasma. Undetected hemolysis, clotting, or other alterations may exist in the undisturbed red blood cell mass. Abnormal blood that cannot be released for transfusion should be returned to the collection center (if imported) or properly disposed of (if drawn in-house).

REFERENCE

Widmann, F.K.: AABB Technical Manual, 9th Ed. Arlington, VA, American Association of Blood Banks, 1985.

TITLE: PREPARATION OF RED CELL SUSPENSIONS

Principle

The concentration of erythrocytes in a saline suspension is important to the accuracy of testing in the blood bank. With experience, most technologists are able to visually prepare a suspension of the proper concentration; however, students and technologists who work infrequently in the blood bank should follow the methods for preparing an accurate suspension.

Specimen

No special preparation of the patient is required before specimen collection. The patient must be positively identified when the specimen is collected. The specimen must be labelled at the bedside and the label must include the patient's full name, the date when the specimen is collected, and the patient's hospital identification number. The time of collection and the phlebotomist's initials should be written on the required form.

Blood should be drawn by an aseptic technique and tested as soon as possible. The specimen should consist of 7 mL of EDTA blood (lavender top evacuated tube). Newborn or infant samples may be collected as red cells in normal saline or from a cord blood sample.

Reagents, Supplies, and Equipment

Large disposable test tubes or 10 × 75 mm test tubes
Disposable pipettes: 1 mL, 5 mL, 10 mL, or $4\frac{5}{8}''$ plastic or Pasteur
Normal saline (0.9%)
Rubber stoppers or plastic covering
Test tube rack
Centrifuge

Procedure

Preparation of an accurate 2% red blood cell suspension is as follows:

1. Place 1 to 2 mL of anticoagulated blood in a large tube.
2. Fill the tube with saline and centrifuge the tube.
3. Aspirate or decant the supernatant saline.
4. Repeat washing (steps 2 and 3) until the supernatant saline is clear.
5. Pipette 10 mL of saline into a clean test tube.
6. Add 0.2 mL of the packed cell button to the 10 mL of diluent.
7. Rinse the pipette containing the red cells in the diluent until it is clear of cells.
8. Cover or stopper the tube until time of use. Immediately before use, invert the tube several times until the cells are in suspension.

Preparation of an accurate 5% red blood cell suspension is as follows:

1. Place 1 to 2 mL of anticoagulated blood in a large tube.
2. Fill the tube with saline and centrifuge the tube.
3. Aspirate or decant the supernatant saline.
4. Repeat washing (steps 2 and 3) until the supernatant saline is clear.
5. Pipette 10 mL of saline into a clean test tube.
6. Add 0.5 mL of the packed cell button to the 10 mL of diluent.
7. Rinse the pipette containing the red cells in the diluent until it is clear of cells.
8. Cover or stopper the tube until use. Immediately before use, invert the tube several times until the cells are in suspension.

An alternate procedure is as follows:

1. Using a disposable pipette, transfer approximately 0.2 mL (2 drops) of the patient's packed red cells to a 10 × 75 mm test tube.

2. Fill the tube with normal saline. Cover and mix by inversion.
3. Centrifuge the tube at 3400 rpm for 30 seconds.
4. Decant the saline.
5. Visually prepare a 3% or 5% suspension of red cells in saline by:
   A. Adding approximately 1 mL of saline to the washed red cells to prepare a 3% suspension.
   B. Adding approximately 0.5 mL of saline to the washed red cells prepare a 5% suspension.
6. The volume of saline (step 5) added to the packed red cells can be adjusted to prepare other percent concentrations, e.g., 2% or 4%.

Procedure Notes

The supernatant fluid should be clear after the final washing. If any evidence of hemolysis exists, additional washing should be performed.

REFERENCE

Turgeon, M.L., and Bender, J.: Routine Analysis. Corning, NY, Corning College Press, 1982.

TITLE: TREATMENT OF AN INCOMPLETELY CLOTTED SPECIMEN

Principle

Blood from patients who have received anticoagulant therapy may have a prolonged clotting time. Blood from those who have received heparin may not clot at all, and blood from patients with excessive fibrinolytic activity may reliquify. Serum separated from an incompletely clotted blood specimen will continue to produce fibrin, especially after 37° C incubation. The resulting strands of protein entrap erythrocytes as clotting progresses and make it difficult to evaluate agglutination.

Procedure

To accelerate clotting, one of the following techniques can be used:

1. Thrombin solution (50 units/mL) can be added to whole blood at the rate of one drop per mL of blood. Dried thrombin can also be added by placing a small amount on the tip of an applicator stick.
2. Small glass beads can be added to separated serum and gently agitated at 37° C for several minutes. After centrifugation, the supernatant serum can be used.

To neutralize heparin, one or more drops of a 1% saline solution of protamine sulfate (10 mg/mL) can be added to whole blood. Protamine sulfate should be used sparingly because it can promote rouleaux formation or, if added in great excess, can inhibit clotting.

To inhibit fibrinolytic activity, 0.1 mL of a solution containing 5 g epsilon-amino caproic acid in 20 mL saline can be added to 4 mL of freshly drawn whole blood.

TITLE: TYPE AND SCREEN PROTOCOL

Principle

On the basis of past experience, the amount of blood generally used in a specific surgical procedure can be established in advance. The amount of blood needed varies depending on the technique used by the surgeon and other factors such as the initial condition of the patient due to age or the existence of chronic disease. If the surgeon's order for blood varies from the established protocol of a blood bank (see Chapter 6, Pretransfusion Testing), the physician should be contacted to verify that the type and screen guideline is being overruled.

General guidelines to blood utilization (Table 13-8) can prevent unnecessary crossmatching of blood for procedures in which blood is rarely used. For surgical proce-

Table 13-8. Surgical Blood Order Schedule

Type of Surgery	Maximum Standard Crossmatch Order (Units)	Type of Surgery	Maximum Standard Crossmatch Order (Units)
Dental Surgery		Meniscectomy	0
Full mouth extraction	0	Minor hand or foot surgery	0
Extraction, impacted molars	0	Open reduction	T&S
		Osteotomy	1 PC
General Surgery		Removal of hip pin	T&S
Abdominal–perineal resection	4 PC	Shoulder reconstruction	T&S
Amputation	T&S	Spinal fusion	2 PC
Anal fistula excision	T&S	Synovectomy	0
Breast biopsy	T&S	Total hip replacement	4 PC
Cholecystectomy	T&S	Total knee replacement	T&S
Colon resection	2 PC		
Colostomy or closure	T&S	*Plastic Surgery*	
Esophageal resection	4 PC	Augmentation mammoplasty	T&S
Excision of anal fissure or fistula/		Facelift	0
sphincterotomy	0	Reduction mammoplasty	T&S
Excision of skin lesions	0	Rhinoplasty	0
Exploratory laparotomy	T&S	Skin flap	T&S
Gastrectomy	4 PC	Skin graft, minor	T&S
Gastroscopy	0	Skin graft, major (severe burns)	T&S
Hemicolectomy	2 PC		
Hemorrhoidectomy	0	*Pulmonary and Vascular Surgery*	
Hernia repair, hiatal	2 PC	Abdominal aortic aneurysm	4 WB and 2 PC
Hernia repair, inguinal or femoral	0	resection	
Hernia repair, ventral	T&S	Aortofemoral bypass graft	4 WB and 2 PC
Lymph node biopsy	0		
Mastectomy, modified radical	2 PC	Aortoiliac bypass graft	4 WB and 2 PC
Mastectomy, simple	T&S		
Parathyroidectomy	T&S	Bronchoscopy	0
Sigmoidectomy	2 PC	Endarterectomy:	
Splenectomy	T&S	Femoral or carotid	2 PC
Thyroid lobectomy	T&S	Femoral bypass graft	2 PC
Vagotomy and antrectomy	T&S	Femoral-popliteal bypass graft	2 PC
Vein stripping	T&S	Thoracotomy	4 PC
Ear, Nose, and Throat		*Gynecologic and Obstetric Surgery*	
Caldwell-LUC	T&S	Cesarean section	T&S
Excision of submandibular gland	0	Dilatation, curettage, and conization	0
Myringotomy	0	Hysterectomy, radical and pelvic	4 PC
Insertion of ear tubes	0	lymphadenectomy	
Laryngectomy	1 PC	Hysterectomy, simple (including	T&S
Mastoidectomy	0	TAH/BSO)	
Neck dissection (radical)	4 PC	Hysterectomy and antero-posterior	1 PC
Parotidectomy	0	repair	
Septoplasty	0	Laparoscopic tubal ligation	T&S
Tonsillectomy and adenoidectomy	T&S	Marshall-Marchetti procedure	0
Transantral ethmoidectomy	T&S	Ovarian wedge resection, ovarian	T&S
Tympanoplasty	0	cystectomy	
		Stamey procedure	T&S
Orthopedic Surgery		Tuboplasty	T&S
Amputation, toe	0	Uterine suspension, fulguration of	T&S
Arthroscopy	0	endometrial implants	
Arthrotomy—removal of loose body	0	Vaginal plastic procedures	T&S
Carpal tunnel repair	0		
Excision, Morton's neuroma	0	*Neurosurgery*	
Fracture, closed reduction	0	Carpal tunnel release	T&S
Fracture, open reduction, internal		Craniotomy for aneurysm	T&S
fixation	2 PC	Craniotomy for tumor	T&S
Hip nailing/hip screw	3 PC	Craniotomy for traumatic hematoma	T&S
Leg amputation	T&S	(acute)	

Table 13-8. (Continued)

Type of Surgery	Maximum Standard Crossmatch Order (Units)
Craniotomy for chronic subdural hematoma	T&S
Craniotomy for AVM	T&S
Craniotomy for rhizotomy	T&S
Craniotomy for EC-IC	T&S
Depressive laminectomy (cervical, thoracic, or lumbar)	T&S
Laminectomy for disc removal (lumbar)	T&S
Laminectomy for rhizotomy	2 WB + 2 PC
Bilateral T$_{2-3}$ sympathectomy	0
Laminectomy for spinal tumor	2 WB + 2 PC
Shunts (VP and VA) (if an alloantibody is detected 2 WB should be available)	T&S
Laminectomy for chordotomy	2 WB + 2 PC
Percutaneous chordotomy	T&S
Craniotomy for excision of abscess	2 WB
Burr hole for tapping of cyst or abscess	T&S
Carotid endarterectomy	T&S
Opthalmologic Surgery	
Cataract removal	0
Recession, eye	0
Entropion or extropion repair	0
Urologic Surgery	
Cystectomy, radical	4 WB
Cystectomy, segmental	T&S
Cystoscopy	0
Cystourethropexy	0
Fulguration of bleeding bladder tumor	1 PC
Hydrocelectomy	0
Ileal conduit-colon conduit	1 PC
Needle biopsy, prostate	0
Nephrectomy, radical	4 WB
Nephrectomy, simple	T&S
Nephrostomy	T&S
Orchiectomy	T&S
Orchiopexy	T&S
Penile prosthesis	T&S
Perineal prostatectomy	2 PC
Prostate biopsy	0
Pyelolithotomy	T&S
Suprapubic prostatectomy	2 PC
Transurethral resection of bladder tumor	T&S
Transurethral resection of prostate	T&S
Ureteral dilatation	0
Ureteral reimplantation	T&S
Ureterolithotomy	T&S

Key: T&S = Type and Screen
WB = Whole Blood
PC = Packed Red Blood Cells

dures rarely requiring transfusion, the type and screen procedure has been established as a safe and cost-effective measure that promotes more effective use of the blood supply. If unusual complications produce a need for hemotherapy on a patient who has had a type and screen only, the patient can receive ABO group and Rh type specific blood with safety even without a crossmatch.

Specimen

A blood specimen from a patient who has been typed and screened for alloantibodies should be held for 48 hours. This specimen can be used for crossmatching, if needed.

Procedure

1. Perform ABO grouping and Rh typing.
2. Perform an indirect antiglobulin test for alloantibodies.
   A. If this test is negative, verify that 2 units of the patient's ABO and Rh type are available for crossmatching in case of an emergency.
   B. If this test is positive, identify the alloantibody.
   C. Prescreen blood for the absence of the corresponding antigen to the patient's alloantibody and crossmatch 2 units of appropriate blood to ensure compatibility.
3. If uncrossmatched blood is issued for a patient who has had a type and screen *only,* the physician does not need to sign a special release form intended for the issuing of blood in an emergency with no previous type and screen.

REFERENCES

Boral, L.I., and Henry, J.B.: The type and screen: A safe alternative and supplement in selected surgical procedures. Transfusion, *17*:163-168, 1977.
Schmidt, P.J., Samia, C.T., Gregory, K.R., Leparc, G.F.: Rationale reduction in pretransfusion testing. Lab. Med. *17*(8): 467-479, 1986.

Special Blood Banking Procedures

At the conclusion of this chapter, the reader will be able to:
- Discuss the general principles of specialized procedures in blood banking.
- Describe the proper type of specimen needed for each procedure.
- Prepare the necessary reagents for each procedure.
- Describe the quality control steps needed for each procedure.
- Perform the stated procedure.
- Calculate any quantitative results needed for reporting the results of a procedure.
- State the normal results for each procedure.
- Describe the sources of error and clinical applications of each procedure.

Chapter Outline

ABH Secretor Status

Absorption of Cold Autoagglutinins

Absorption of Warm Autoagglutinins

Alloantibody Identification

Alloantibody Titration

Compatibility Testing (Crossmatching): Prewarmed Technique

Donath-Landsteiner Screening Test

D^u Rosette Test

Elution Techniques

Hemoglobin F Determination by Acid Elution

Immunoglobulin D (Rh_o) Protocol

Penicillin or Cephalosporin Antibody Screening

Transfusion Reaction Protocol

TITLE: ABH SECRETOR STATUS

Principle

Certain blood group substances, namely A, B, H, and Le^a, occur in soluble form in secretions such as saliva in a large proportion of individuals, referred to as *secretors*.

These water-soluble substances are readily detected in small quantities because they neutralize or inhibit the capacity of their corresponding antibodies to agglutinate erythrocytes possessing the corresponding antigen. These reactions, termed *hemagglutination inhibition*, provide a means of assaying the relative strength or potency of the water-soluble blood group substances. Identifying the presence of ABH or Le^a substance can be important in blood type problem-solving.

Specimen

The collection and processing of the patient specimen are as follows:

1. Have the patient chew a piece of paraffin wax (gum or anything else that contains sugar or protein cannot be used) to stimulate salivation.
2. Collect about 2 to 3 mL of saliva in a test tube.
3. Place the stoppered tube of saliva in a boiling waterbath for 10 minutes. Heating the specimen inactivates enzymes that might destroy blood group substances.
4. Centrifuge at 3400 rpm for 10 minutes.
5. Transfer the clear or slightly opalescent supernatant to a clean tube. Dis-

card any opaque or semi-solid material.

6. The supernatant fluid should be refrigerated until the time of testing. If testing will not be done on the day of collection and processing, it should be frozen. Frozen samples retain their activity for several years. *Do not refreeze an aliquot once it has been defrosted.*

Reagents, Supplies, and Equipment

Commercial lectin anti-H
2 to 5% washed erythrocytes, group O
10 × 75 mm or 12 × 75 mm disposable test tubes
Disposable pipettes, 4⅝" plastic or Pasteur
Normal saline (0.9%)
Centrifuge
High intensity lamp / optical magnifying lens
Microscope (optional)

Quality Control

Saliva from patients who are known ABH secretors, for example of Se and sese, can be used as positive and negative controls, respectively. Aliquots of saliva or processed supernatant from suitable individuals can be frozen for later use.

A reagent control can be simultaneously assayed by:

1. Adding 1 drop of the highest diluted antiserum with 2+ agglutination to a test tube.
2. Adding 1 drop of a 2 to 5% saline cell suspension of the appropriate blood group, e.g., group O.
3. Incubating 30 to 60 minutes (in parallel with testing).
4. Centrifuging for 15 seconds at 3400 rpm.
5. Reading for agglutination. The agglutination should be 2+.

Procedure

PRELIMINARY ANTISERA DILUTION

1. Prepare serial dilutions, e.g., 1:2, 1:4, of lectin anti-H.
2. Label a clean 12 × 75 test tube for each dilution and add 1 drop of the dilution to the appropriately labelled tube.
3. Add 1 drop of the 2 to 5% saline suspension of group O red blood cells to each of the tubes.
4. Centrifuge for 15 seconds at 3400 rpm and observe macroscopically for agglutination.
5. Select the highest dilution of antiserum that produces 2+ macroscopic agglutination as the *working antiserum (antibody dilution).* Record results.
6. Prepare a sufficient quantity of this dilution to complete the test procedure.

DETECTION OF SECRETION

1. Label four 12 × 75 mm test tubes: Patient, Reagent Control, Se, and sese.
2. Add 1 drop of the patient's supernatant saliva to the Patient tube. Add 1 drop of saline to the Reagent Control tube, and 1 drop of known Se and sese controls to their respective tubes.
3. Add 1 drop of working antibody dilution to all tubes.
4. Incubate all of the tubes at room temperature for 10 minutes.
5. Add 1 drop of the 2 to 5% red blood cell saline suspension of group O cells to each tube.
6. Incubate all the tubes at room temperature for 30 to 60 minutes.
7. Centrifuge for 15 seconds at 3400 rpm.
8. Observe for macroscopic agglutination and record results.

Reporting Results

The reagent control should demonstrate 2+ agglutination. The Se control should demonstrate no agglutination and the sese control should be negative (agglutination). A *nonsecretor* shows agglutination of red blood cells by antiserum-saliva mixture. A *secretor* shows no agglutination of red blood cells by antiserum-saliva mixture.

Procedure Notes

The absence of agglutination in saliva is a *positive* test for the presence of ABH soluble antigens and indicates that an individual is a secretor. The diluted reagent antiserum has been neutralized by soluble blood group antigens in the saliva. Hence, no antibodies in the antiserum are free to react with the antigens on the reagent red cells introduced into the test.

To detect or measure salivary A or B substance in addition to H substance, the same procedure can be used with diluted anti-A and anti-B reagents. The appropriate dilutions of anti-A or anti-B are obtained by preparing serial dilutions with A or B cells, respectively.

The quantity of H as well as A and B substance varies depending on the ABO type of an individual (Table 14-1). The screening procedure just described can be adapted for semiquantitative estimations of blood group activity by testing serial saline dilutions of processed saliva. Processed saliva should be diluted before incubation with diluted antiserum. The higher the dilution needed to remove inhibitory activity, the more salivary blood group substance is present.

Excessive levels of soluble ABH substances can be observed in rare cases, such as ovarian cysts, carcinoma of the stomach or pancreas, or intestinal obstruction. The level of ABH substance in a person's serum may be so high that it inhibits the anti-A or anti-B reagent sera. This interference with ABO blood grouping is due to neutralization of the reagent anti-A or anti-B by the excess specific soluble substances, which leaves no unbound antibody to react with the person's erythrocytes.

PROCEDURE FOR DETECTION OF LEWIS SECRETIONS

Controls: Use saliva from a person whose red cells are Le^a positive and from one who is Lewis-negative.

1. Prepare working Le^a antiserum in the same manner as lectin anti-H.
2. Label four 12 × 75 mm test tubes: patient, reagent control, Lewis-positive, and Lewis-negative.
3. Add 1 drop of processed saliva to the appropriate tubes and a drop of saline to the reagent tube.
4. Add 1 drop of working diluted antiserum to all of the tubes.
5. Incubate for 10 minutes at room temperature.
6. Add 1 drop of 2 to 5% saline suspension of washed Le^a red blood cells to each tube.
7. Incubate for 30 to 60 minutes at room temperature.
8. Centrifuge at 3400 rpm for 15 seconds.
9. Observe macroscopically for agglutination.
10. Record results.

Interpretation: A nonsecretor of Lewis substance demonstrates agglutination; a secretor has no agglutination of the Le^a positive indicator cells. The reagent control should exhibit 2+ agglutination.

A Lewis-positive person who is a secretor of ABH can be assumed to have Le^b as well as Le^a in the saliva. A Le(a+) person who is sese and does not secrete ABH substance will have only Le^a in saliva.

Limitations

Detection of soluble blood group substances in saliva should be used in conjunction with blood group testing for erythrocyte antigens.

Table 14-1. ABH Substances in Saliva

	ABO Type	ABH Substances in Saliva		
		A	B	H
Secreters	A	Much	None	Some
	B	None	Much	Some
	O	None	None	Much
	AB	Much	Much	Some
Nonsecretors	A, B, O, and AB	None	None	None

REFERENCES

Henry, J.B. (Ed.): Clinical Diagnosis and Management by Laboratory Methods, 17th ed. Philadelphia, W.B. Saunders Co., p. 988.

Zonijewski, C.M.: Immunohematology, 2nd ed. NY, Appleton-Century-Crofts, 1972, p. 263.

TITLE: ABSORPTION OF COLD AUTOAGGLUTININS

Principle

Cold-reacting autoantibodies can interfere with the identification of alloantibodies in a patient's serum. Absorption of the patient's serum with autologous red blood cells can remove autoantibody from the serum, permitting detection of underlying alloantibodies.

Specimen

No special preparation of the patient is required before specimen collection. The patient must be positively identified when the specimen is collected. The specimen must be labelled at the bedside and the label must include the patient's full name, the date when the specimen is collected, and the patient's hospital identification number. The time of collection and the phlebotomist's initials should be written on the required form.

Blood should be drawn by an aseptic technique and the specimen should be tested as soon as possible. The required specimens are 5 to 7 mL of clotted blood (red top evacuated tube) and 7 mL of EDTA blood (lavender top evacuated tube). Processing of the specimen is described in the following procedure.

Reagents, Supplies, and Equipment

10 × 75 mm or 12 × 75 mm disposable test tubes
13 × 100 mm or 16 × 100 mm test tubes

Disposable pipettes, $4\frac{5}{8}''$ plastic or Pasteur
Normal saline (0.9%) warmed to 37° C
Centrifuge
37° C waterbath or heat block
Ice bath
Test tube rack

Quality Control

An autologous control (a mixture of 1 drop of patient's absorbed serum + one drop of patient's red blood cells) should be tested at room temperature and with AHG sera. If this control is negative, most of the cold-reacting autoantibody has been removed and further testing should not be compromised.

Procedure

1. After properly obtaining the specimens, the red top or nonanticoagulated tube may be allowed to clot in the refrigerator. This step is usually *not sufficient* to remove all of the autoagglutinin, but it does begin the process of removing autoantibodies from the serum. If the patient's blood is already clotted or time is limited, this step may be deleted.
2. Wash the patient's own (autologous) red blood cells from the anticoagulated (lavender top or EDTA) specimen tube with warm 37° C saline at least four times. Care should be taken to remove all the saline after each wash.
3. After the last wash, centrifuge the cells for 5 minutes at 3400 rpm.
4. Remove any remaining saline. This step is very important because residual saline may dilute out an alloantibody in the serum that is being autoabsorbed.
5. Obtain the patient's clotted blood from the refrigerator and centrifuge.
6. Remove all available serum from this clotted specimen. If any red blood cells are unintentionally removed with the serum, centrifuge the serum and transfer it to a clean test tube.

7. Transfer enough serum to perform all necessary postabsorption testing, e.g., compatibility tests, antibody screening, etc., in a large test tube, e.g., 13 × 100 or 16 × 100.

8. Add an equal volume of the well-washed, tightly-packed autologous red blood cells prepared in steps 2 through 4.

9. Mix the serum and red cells thoroughly and place in a slush ice bath in a 4° C refrigerator for 15 to 30 minutes. Note: A longer incubation of this aliquot of red cells does not remove additional antibody because all the antigen sites are covered within the first 15 to 20 minutes.

10. Remove the tube from the ice bath and centrifuge for 3 minutes at 3400 rpm. Note: A refrigerated centrifuge or an ice-packed test tube holder is preferred.

11. After centrifugation, *immediately* place the tube in the refrigerator without disturbing the red blood cells. This step increases the amount of antibody removed with each absorption.

12. After 5 minutes, carefully transfer the serum to a clean test tube. The serum must be cell-free. Repeat step 10 if necessary.

13. At this point, the serum has been autoabsorbed *once.*

14. To perform subsequent autoabsorption, add the previously autoabsorbed serum to a fresh aliquot of well-washed, tightly packed autologous red blood cells and repeat steps 8 through 12.

15. After the serum has been removed from the last aliquot of autologous red blood cells, it should be warmed up to room temperature before being used for testing.

Reporting Results

The use of autoabsorbed serum should be noted on any tests performed with this processed serum.

Procedure Notes

In most cases, at least 2 autoabsorptions are necessary to remove even low-titered cold autoagglutinins. It is preferable to perform several absorptions with fresh aliquots of autologous red blood cells rather than to extend the cold incubation phase. For example, four 15-minute absorptions on four fresh aliquots of autologous RBCs are preferable to one hour-long incubation.

Exercise care when autoabsorbing the serum of a recently transfused patient because an alloantibody may be absorbed from the serum. The prewarmed compatibility test may be substituted.

Limitations

Cold-reacting antibodies, specific as well as nonspecific, will be removed by this procedure if the erythrocytes have expressed the corresponding antigen.

REFERENCE

Widmann, F.K. (Ed): AABB Technical Manual, 9th Ed. Arlington, VA, American Association of Blood Banks, p. 466.

TITLE: ABSORPTION OF WARM AUTOAGGLUTININS

Principle

Absorption of a patient's serum with autologous red blood cells can remove autoantibodies from the serum and permits detection of specific alloantibodies. Because circulating autologous red blood cells are already coated with autoantibody, they are pretreated with a proteolytic enzyme. This technique uncovers antigen sites, which are then capable of binding free autoantibody from the serum during incubation and producing an absorbed serum. In some cases, warm-reactive autoagglutinins can mask underlying clinically significant alloantibodies.

Specimen

No special preparation of the patient is required before specimen collection. The patient must be positively identified when the specimen is collected. The specimen must be labelled at the bedside and the label must include the patient's full name, the date when the specimen is collected, and the patient's hospital identification number. The time of collection and the phlebotomist's initials should be written on the required form.

Blood should be drawn by an aseptic technique and the specimen should be tested as soon as possible. The required specimens are 5 to 7 mL of clotted blood (red top evacuated tube) and 7 mL of EDTA blood (lavender top evacuated tube). Processing of the specimen is described in the following procedure.

Reagents, Supplies, and Equipment

6% bovine albumin
1% ficin (available commercially or prepared as follows)

PHOSPHATE BUFFER

Acidic Stock Solution. Dissolve 22.16 g of $NaH_2PO_4 \cdot H_2O$ in 1 L of distilled H_2O. This 0.16M solution of the monobasic phosphate salt (monohydrate) has a pH of 5.0.

Alkaline Stock Solution. Dissolve 17.2 g of Na_2HPO_4 in 1 L of distilled H_2O. This 0.126M solution of the dibasic phosphate salt (anhydrous) has a pH of 9.0.

Working Buffer Solution (pH 7.3). Mix 16 mL of acidic stock solution and 84 mL of alkaline stock solution. Check the pH of the working solution before using it.

Phosphate-Buffered Saline. The ratio of one volume of working buffer solution (pH 7.3) to nine volumes of normal (0.9%) saline to prepare the phosphate-buffered saline. To prepare a total of 100 mL, 10 mL of working buffer solution is added to 90 mL of normal saline.

1% FICIN SOLUTION

Caution: Ficin is harmful if it is inhaled or gets in the eyes. Wear gloves, a mask, and an apron, and work under a hood.

Place 1 g of powdered ficin in a 100 mL volumetric flask. Dissolve in phosphate-buffered saline, pH 7.3, to 100 mL. Agitate vigorously by inversion or on a rotator for 15 minutes, or with a magnetic stirrer for 30 to 90 minutes. The powder will not dissolve completely. Collect clear fluid by filtration or centrifugation. Dispense small aliquots of the solution into clear test tubes and stopper. Store aliquots at $-20°$ C. *Do not refreeze thawed solution.*

10 × 75 mm disposable test tubes
13 × 100 mm or 16 × 100 mm test tubes
Test tube rack
Disposable pipettes, $4\frac{5}{8}''$ plastic or Pasteur
Normal saline (0.9%)
Centrifuge
37° C waterbath or heat block

Quality Control

The patient's red blood cells can function as a negative control. If all of the autoantibody can be eluted from the patient's red blood cells (a nonreactive DAT following step 5 of the procedure), these cells can be used to check the efficacy of the absorption process. When the red blood cells no longer demonstrate autoantibody absorption from the serum (a negative DAT), the serum is ready for alloantibody testing.

Procedure

1. Wash 2 mL of patient red blood cells from an EDTA anticoagulated specimen four times in saline. Discard the supernatant fluid from the final centrifugation.
2. Add an equal volume of 6% albumin to the packed red blood cells and mix thoroughly.
3. Incubate the red blood cells-albumin mixture at 56° C for 3 to 5 minutes.

Gently agitate the mixture during incubation.

4. Centrifuge at 3400 rpm for 2 minutes.
5. Transfer the supernatant fluid to a clean test tube. Note: this supernatant fluid may be used as an eluate for testing, if a limited quantity of autologous red cells are available.
6. Wash the red cells three times with normal saline. Discard the final supernatant.
7. Add 1 mL of 1% ficin to the packed red cells. Mix thoroughly.
8. Incubate at 37° C for 15 minutes.
9. Wash the ficin-RBC mixture three times in saline.
10. Centrifuge the final wash for at least 5 minutes at 3400 rpm. Remove as much of the supernatant as possible.
11. Divide the red cells into two equal aliquots.
12. Centrifuge the nonanticoagulated red top specimen. To one aliquot of the washed red cells (step 11), add 2 mL of the patient's serum, mix, and incubate at 37° C for 30 minutes.
13. Centrifuge at 3400 rpm for 2 minutes and transfer the serum to the second aliquot of red cells.
14. Mix and incubate this mixture at 37° C for 30 minutes.
15. Centrifuge at 3400 rpm for 2 minutes. Immediately transfer the absorbed serum to a clean test tube. The serum must be cell-free. Recentrifuge the specimen if any red cells are inadvertently transferred with the serum.
16. At least two autoabsorptions are needed to remove enough autoantibodies to test for alloantibody reactivity.

If the patient's red cells can be shown to be nonreactive with DAT following step 5, these cells can be used to check the efficacy of the absorption process. When the red cells no longer demonstrate autoantibody absorption from the serum with the DAT procedure, the serum is now ready for alloantibody testing using group O reagent screening cells.

Reporting Results

If no reactivity with group O reagent red cells is observed (see the procedure for this test in Chapter 13, Routine Procedures), it is unlikely that alloantibody is present.

Procedure Notes

If there is reactivity against both the patient's treated red cells and the group O reagent red cells, further absorption of the serum is necessary.

If the absorbed serum reacts with one or both of the group O reagent screening red cells but not with the autologous red cells, the serum contains one or more alloantibodies. Further antibody identification (see Alloantibody Identification, this chapter) should be performed using the absorbed serum.

Limitations

Autoabsorption should not be performed on cells from a recently transfused patient because the circulating allogeneic RBCs may adsorb the alloantibodies that are being sought for identification.

REFERENCES

Hendry, E.B.: Osmolarity of human serum of chemical solution of biologic importance, Clin. Chem. 7:156-164, 1961.
Morel, P.A., Bergren, M.O., and Frank, B.A.: A simple method for the detection of alloantibody in the presence of autoantibody, Transfusion, 18:388, 1978.
Widmann, F.K. (Ed.): AABB Technical Manual, 9th Ed. Arlington, VA, American Association of Blood Banks, 1985.

TITLE: ALLOANTIBODY IDENTIFICATION

Principle

The antibody panel test is a qualitative test for the identification of alloantibodies in patient or donor serum. Serum from patients, for example a surgical or obstetric patient, or from a blood donor, which has exhibited reactivity with group O reagent screening red blood cells is further tested against a panel of 8, 10, or more red blood cells that represent a variety of blood group antigens.

Identification and initial detection of an antibody depend on the method, medium, and temperature of reactivity as well as the titer of the antibody. Hemolysis or agglutination of reagent red blood cells in the presence of serum at any stage of the test demonstrates the presence of an antibody (a positive test) with specificity to a corresponding antigen on the reagent red blood cells. The absence of hemolysis and / or agglutination indicates that the serum being tested does not contain detectable antibodies directed at antigens present on the reagent red cells being used.

Specimen

No special preparation of the patient is required before specimen collection. The patient must be positively identified when the specimen is collected. The specimen must be labelled at the bedside and the label must include the patient's full name, the date when the specimen is collected, and the patient's hospital identification number. The time of collection and the phlebotomist's initials should be written on the required form.

Blood should be drawn by an aseptic technique and the specimen should be tested as soon as possible. The required specimens are 5 to 7 mL of clotted blood (red top evacuated tube) and 7 mL of EDTA blood (lavender top evacuated tube). The presence of hemolysis in the specimen makes the specimen unsuitable for testing.

Antibodies that depend on the binding of complement for their detection may not be detected if aged serum or plasma from an anticoagulated sample is used for antibody detection testing. Samples for antibody screening may be used up to 48 hours after collection. The specimen must be stored at 1 to 6° C and kept for 7 days.

Reagents, Supplies, and Equipment

10 × 75 mm disposable test tubes
Disposable pipettes, 4⅝″ plastic or Pasteur
Normal saline (0.9%)
Bovine albumin* (Optional)
Antiglobulin reagent antiserum*
Coombs control or check cells (IgG-sensitized cells)*
Group O reagent panel cells*
Centrifuge
37° C waterbath or heat block
Test tube rack
High intensity lamp / optical magnifying lens
Microscope (optional)
*Should be refrigerated when not in use

Quality Control

The test reagents should be monitored daily or at the time of use, as described in Chapter 1 and according to the Daily Reagent Quality Assurance procedure in Chapter 13.

An autocontrol, a mixture of the patient's erythrocytes and serum, must be tested simultaneously with each antibody panel. This control must be negative for the test results to be valid.

All negative antiglobulin reactions must be tested with Coombs control check cells. A positive test result at this point confirms that active antiglobulin was added to the test system and was present when the original antiglobulin test was interpreted as negative. If a positive result is *not* obtained with the control cells, the test is invalid and must be repeated.

Procedure

1. Label a tube for each of the reagent panel cells, for example, 1-8 or 1-10, and an autocontrol (AUTO).
2. Using a disposable pipette, add 2 drops of the patient's serum to each tube.
3. Add 2 drops of bovine albumin to each tube (optional).

4. Add 1 drop of reagent red blood cells to each, except the autocontrol.
5. Add 1 drop of the patient's 2 to 5% red blood cell suspension to the tube labeled AUTO.
6. Mix all tubes and centrifuge for 15 seconds at 3400 rpm.
7. Gently resuspend the cells in all tubes and examine macroscopically for agglutination or hemolysis. Record the results as immediate spin (IS) reactions. Positive reactions should be graded from 1 to 4+ at each stage of observation (see Grading Agglutination Reactions, Chapter 13). Complete hemolysis precludes further testing and must be interpreted as a positive result. If partial hemolysis is observed, record and proceed. All positive and negative tests should be continued through all phases of testing.
8. Incubate all tubes for 30 minutes at 37° C.
9. Centrifuge all the tubes for 15 seconds at 3400 rpm.
10. Gently resuspend the cells in all tubes and examine macroscopically for agglutination or hemolysis. Record results as 37° C reactions.
11. Wash each tube 3 times. Decant completely after the last wash.
12. Add 2 drops of antiglobulin (AHG) reagent to each tube.
13. Mix and centrifuge for 15 seconds at 3400 rpm.
14. Gently resuspend the cells and examine macroscopically with the aid of magnification (microscopic examination is optional). Record results as antiglobulin (AHG) reactions.
15. To each tube that exhibits no agglutination, add 1 drop of Coombs check cells. Mix well and centrifuge for 15 seconds at 3400 rpm. Resuspend the cells and examine macroscopically for agglutination. Record these results as control cells (CC).

Reporting Results

Agglutination or hemolysis of any screening cell suspension in the immediate-spin, 37° C, or antiglobulin (AHG) phase indicates a positive reaction. The absence of hemolysis or agglutination constitutes a negative test and indicates the absence of detectable antibodies to specific antigens present on the reagent erythrocyte.

If a pattern of positive and negative reactions is observed with different test cells, antibody identification is simplified by eliminating antibodies specific for antigens present on any nonreactive cells. Comparisons of the pattern of positive and negative reactions with the known antigen makeup of the reagent red blood cells enable the specificity of the antibodies or antibodies to be determined (see Chapter 6, Pretransfusion Testing).

Procedure Notes

If the autocontrol is positive, absorption and/or elution tests need to be performed to separate the autoantibody from any underlying alloantibody. In the case of a recently transfused patient, a positive autocontrol may indicate the presence of an alloantibody directed at an antigen present on surviving donor cells. In such cases, a mixed-field agglutination reaction may be observed.

The reagent panel cells can be modified with enhancement media such as albumin, enzymes, polybrene, or LISS. If albumin is used as an enhancer, the reactivity of low-titered antibodies may be increased by washing the reagent erythrocytes once with normal saline, decanting the saline completely, and using the "dry button" of cells for the test. If a low ionic strength test procedure is used, the cell suspensions should be prepared according to the manufacturer's directions.

Limitations

See Antibody Screening (Indirect Antiglobulin or Indirect Coombs' Test with Autocontrol) in Chapter 13.

REFERENCES

Gamma Biologicals, Inc., Houston, Texas: Reagent Red Blood Cells, package insert, January, 1986.

Huestis, D., et al. Practical Blood Transfusion, 3rd Ed. Boston, Little, Brown and Co., 1982, pp. 106-107.

Issitt, P.: Applied Blood Group Serology, 2nd Ed. Oxnard, CA, Spectra Biologics, 1975, pp. 273-274.

Mollison, P.L. Blood Transfusion in Clinical Medicine, 6th Ed. Oxford, Blackwell Scientific Publications, 1979, p. 556.

TITLE: ALLOANTIBODY TITRATION

Principle

Titration is a semiquantative method of measuring the concentration of antibody in serum. Serial dilutions, for example, 1:2 or 1:4, of serum containing an antibody are tested with a constant volume of red blood cells. The test result is expressed as the reciprocal of the highest dilution that exhibits agglutination. Observation of agglutination is usually macroscopic; however, it may be microscopic with antibodies such as high-titer, low-avidity antibodies.

Titration is clinically most useful as a comparison of one specimen with another. Although it may be used for other purposes, for instance, to identify "least incompatible" donor units when crossmatching difficulties exist, the antibody titration procedure is most frequently used to detect changing antibody concentrations in obstetrical patients. When a significant increase in antibody concentration does occur, intrauterine transfusions can be performed between 28 and 32 weeks gestation. After 32 weeks, labor is usually induced.

Specimen

No special preparation of the patient is required before specimen collection. The patient must be positively identified when the specimen is collected. The specimen must be labelled at the bedside and the label must include the patient's full name, the date when the specimen is collected, and the patient's hospital identification number. The time of collection and the phlebotomist's initials should be written on the required form.

Blood should be drawn by an aseptic technique and the specimen should be tested as soon as possible. The required specimens are 5 to 7 mL of clotted blood (red top evacuated tube) and 7 mL of EDTA blood (lavender top evacuated tube). The presence of hemolysis in a specimen makes it unsuitable for testing.

Antibodies that depend on the binding of complement for their detection may not be detected if aged serum or plasma from an anticoagulated sample is used for antibody detection or titration. The serum from this specimen should be *frozen* for future comparative study.

Note: The previously titrated serum should be defrosted in a 37° C waterbath for simultaneous testing with the fresh specimen.

Reagents, Supplies, and Equipment

10 × 75 mm disposable test tubes
Graduated serologic pipettes or disposable pipette tips and aspirator
Normal saline (0.9%)
Bovine albumin* (Optional)
Antiglobulin reagent antisera*
Coombs control or check cells (IgG-sensitized cells)*
Reagent screening red blood cells I*
Reagent screening red blood cells II*
Patient's cumulative record (if previously tested)
Centrifuge
37° C waterbath or heat block
Test tube rack
High intensity lamp/optical magnifying lens
Microscope (optional)
  *Should be refrigerated when not in use

Quality Control

An autocontrol, a mixture of patient's erythrocytes and serum, must be tested simultaneously with each antibody screening test.

The test reagents should be monitored daily or at the time of use as described in

Chapter 1 and according to the Daily Re-agent Quality Assurance procedure in Chapter 13.

All negative antiglobulin reactions must be tested with Coombs Control/Check Cells. A positive test result at this point will confirm that active antiglobulin was added to the test system and was present when the original antiglobulin test was interpreted as negative. If a positive result is *not* obtained with the control cells, the test is invalid and must be repeated.

Procedure

PRELIMINARY

1. Compare information on specimen with request form: full name, full hospital number, and date. If this information is *not identical,* obtain a new specimen.
2. Prepare a 2 to 4% suspension of patient's red cells (see Preparation of Red Cell Suspensions in Chapter 13).
3. Centrifuge the clotted specimen for 5 minutes at 2500 rpm.
4. Determine if the patient has been previously tested by checking past records in a cumulative patient file.
5. Perform an antibody screening and panel cell procedure. This step is important even if the patient has had an antibody identified previously. It is important to establish the identity of the antibody or antibodies as well as the optimum phase of reactivity.
6. Prepare separate serial dilutions of both the fresh serum and the previous specimen (if available). The dilution should begin with 1:2 and extend to at least 1:132 according to the previous titer. The diluent may be either saline or albumin depending upon the optimum medium of reactivity observed in the screening procedure. If albumin is used as the diluent, the reagent red blood cells must also be suspended in albumin.

ANTIBODY TITRATION

1. Label two sets of 10 × 75 mm test tubes, one set for the present serum

and the other for the past serum. Each dilution must be represented by a separate tube.
2. Using a disposable pipette, add 2 drops of the diluted serum to each of the respective tubes.
3. Add 1 drop of reagent red cells to each of the tubes. The reagent red cell suspension should be chosen from the most reactive red cells from the screening or panel cells used in the preliminary testing.
4. Mix all tubes and centrifuge for 15 seconds at 3400 rpm.
5. Gently resuspend the cells in all tubes and examine macroscopically for agglutination or hemolysis. Record the results as immediate-spin (IS) reactions. Positive reactions should be graded from 1 to 4+ at each stage of observation (see Grading Agglutination Reactions in Chapter 13). Complete hemolysis precludes further testing and must be interpreted as a positive result. If partial hemolysis is observed, record and proceed. All positive and negative tests should be continued through all phases of testing.
6. Incubate all tubes for 30 minutes at 37° C.
7. Centrifuge all tubes for 15 seconds at 3400 rpm.
8. Gently resuspend the cells in all tubes and examine macroscopically for agglutination or hemolysis. Record results as 37° C reactions.
9. Wash each tube three times. Decant completely after the last wash.
10. Add 2 drops of antiglobulin (AHG) reagent to each tube.
11. Mix each tube and centrifuge for 15 seconds at 3400 rpm.
12. Gently resuspend the cells and examine macroscopically with the aid of magnification (microscopic examination is optional). Record results as antigloblin (AHG) reactions.
13. To each tube that exhibits no agglutination add 1 drop of Coombs check cells. Mix well and centrifuge for 15 seconds at 3400 rpm. Resuspend the cells and examine macroscopically for agglutination. Record these results as control cells (CC).

Grading the strength of agglutination is critical to the accuracy of the procedure. It is not uncommon to find that the end point (titer) may be the same for two successive specimens, but the strength of the reactions from the dilutions is not the same. Therefore, to determine antibody strength, both the *avidity* (the strength of the reaction at each dilution) and the titer should be considered. This is done by giving numeric values to each degree of agglutination and totaling the results of all tubes. Although the numeric score may vary from one blood bank to another, uniformity should be demonstrated within a blood bank. An example of a grading system is presented in Table

Table 14-2. Representative Grading System

Qualitative Notation	Score
4+	12
3+	10
2+	8
1+	5
W+	2
0	0

14-2. Complete or partial hemolysis cannot be easily quantitated; however, it usually denotes a highly positive reaction.

An example of an antibody titration follows.

Both of these sera have titers of 64, yet the difference in scores indicates that there has been an increase in antibody strength:

1st specimen

Dilution	1	2	4	8	16	32	64	128	Total Score
strength of reaction	4+	3+	3+	2+	2+	1+	1+	0	
score	12	10	10	8	8	5	5	0	58

2nd specimen

Dilution	1	2	4	8	16	32	64	128	Total Score
strength of reaction	4+	4+	4+	4+	3+	2+	1+	0	
score	12	12	12	12	10	8	5	0	71

Reporting Results

The previous and present antibody titers should be reported. If an antibody is increasing in strength but not titer, it should be noted. Only a titer change of two tubes (fourfold) or more is clinically significant.

Procedure Notes

If the autocontrol demonstrates a positive reaction, the serum contains an autoantibody. The presence of an autoantibody can conceal an underlying alloantibody in the serum. Autoabsorption (see sections on absorption of cold and warm agglutinins, this chapter) may be required to test the serum for the presence of alloantibodies.

The optimum mode and medium of reactivity as well as the most reactive red blood cells should be determined in preliminary evaluation of the antibody. Once determined, these should be used consistently. It is also important to establish the identity of the antibody at each testing and to detect the presence of any additional antibodies.

A variety of factors can affect an antibody titration:

1. The same cell suspension must be used for both sera. Any variation in the strength of suspension or antigen will introduce a variable into the comparison.

2. Meticulous pipetting technique is needed. Mouth pipetting is prohibited. A semi-automatic pipetter is recommended and a clean pipette tip should be used for each dilution.
3. The prozone phenomenon can produce weaker reactions in the initial tubes than in higher dilution. It is important to evaluate the dilution series, starting with the most dilute and ending with the most concentrated specimen.

Some additional applications of antibody titration include:

1. Selection of blood for patients with autoimmune hemolytic anemia
2. Study of the characteristics of one antibody or a mixture of antibodies in a single serum
3. Determination of the reactivity of the antigenic determinants on various red blood cells
4. Testing of antibodies for reagent use

Limitations

The detection of antibodies in serum can be compromised if the serum dilutions are incorrectly prepared or the ratio of diluted serum to cells in the test is incorrect.

Other limitations are comparable to the limitations encountered in the antibody screening and panel cell identification procedures.

REFERENCES

Gamma Biologicals, Inc., Houston, Texas: Reagent Red Blood Cells, package insert, January, 1986.
Huestis, D., et al.: Practical Blood Transfusion, 3rd Ed. Boston, Little, Brown and Co., 1982, pp. 106-107.
Issitt, P. Applied Blood Group Serology, 2nd Ed. Oxnard, CA, Spectra Biologics, 1975, pp. 273-274.
Mollison, P.L.: Blood Transfusion in Clinical Medicine, 6th Ed. Oxford, Blackwell Scientific Publications, 1979, p. 556.
Widmann, F.K. (Ed.): AABB Technical Manual, 9th Ed. Arlington, VA, American Association of Blood Banks, 1985, pp. 238-240.

TITLE: COMPATIBILITY TESTING (CROSSMATCHING): PREWARMED TECHNIQUE

Principle

Pretransfusion compatibility testing combines a potential recipient's blood specimen with a blood specimen from an intended donor. This procedure is based on the principle that warming the constituent ingredients to 37° C before mixing bypasses the phase in which the cold-reacting antibodies react by either direct agglutination or binding of complement that demonstrates reactivity in the AHG phase. By avoiding the in vitro interference produced by such antibodies, the prewarming technique ensures that agglutination is not present due to clinically significant antibody-antigen reactions that could have in vivo consequences; that is, antibodies that are reactive at 37° C.

Specimen

No special preparation of the patient is required before specimen collection. The patient must be positively identified when the specimen is collected. The specimen must be labelled at the bedside and the label must include the patient's full name, the date when the specimen is collected, and the patient's hospital identification number. The time of collection and the phlebotomist's initials should be written on the required form.

Blood should be drawn by an aseptic technique and the specimen should be tested as soon as possible. Approximately 5 to 7 mL of blood should be collected in a red top (no anticoagulant) or lavender top (EDTA) evacuated tube.

It is preferable to place the specimens immediately in a container of warm water en route to the blood bank. If the specimen is rapidly centrifuged, special techniques are not usually needed to keep the specimen at 37° C before testing. All specimens must be retained under refrigeration for 7 days after transfusion of a unit of blood.

Reagents, Supplies, and Equipment

Commercial antiglobulin (AHG) reagent (broad-spectrum or IgG)
  Note: The AHG should be brought to room temperature for this procedure.
10 × 75 mm disposable test tubes
Disposable pipettes, 4 5/8″ plastic or Pasteur
Scissors
Test tube rack
Normal (0.9%) saline
  Note: Warm saline to 37° C by placing in a 37° C waterbath for at least 30 minutes before beginning the test. Use prewarmed saline throughout the procedure.
37° C waterbath or heat block
High intensity lamp/optical magnifying lens
Centrifuge

Quality Control

Reagent erythrocytes should be tested daily with known antisera (see Daily Reagent Quality Assurance testing procedure in Chapter 13). All negative AHG reactions must be tested with IgG-sensitized erythrocytes and produce a positive reaction. If the AHG control cells do not agglutinate, the compatibility test is invalid.

Procedure

Preliminary

1. Compare the information on the patient's specimen with the information on the test requisition: name, identification number, date. If this information is not identical, obtain a new specimen.
2. Centrifuge the clotted specimen for 5 minutes at 2000 rpm.
3. Check past blood bank records to determine if the patient has even been screened for antibodies or previously transfused.

4. Perform an ABO grouping (forward and reverse), Rh typing, and antibody screen on the recipient's specimen. Record all test results in the blood bank log as well as on the crossmatch requisition.
5. Check data on previous records. If the ABO and Rh are not identical, obtain a new specimen for repeat testing.
6. Procure the whole blood or packed cells to be crossmatched from the blood bank refrigerator. Check all identification on the units, e.g., group and Rh, expiration date, and the physical characteristics of the units, including absence of hemolysis or abnormal color.
7. Detach a segment from the unit of blood. Cut the ends of the segment and drain the contents into a 10 × 75 mm test tube. Label the tube with the donor unit identification number. Recheck number.
8. Wash the donor specimen 3 times with normal saline. Decant the last wash completely and prepare a 3 to 5% suspension of the erythrocytes.
9. Enter the donor number and expiration date on the test requisition. If the donor unit has not been retyped on entering the blood bank inventory, an ABO typing and Rh typing should be performed.

Compatibility Procedure

The following is an example of a typical crossmatch configuration including both phases.

1. Label two 10 × 75 mm test tubes. One tube should be labelled Suspension; the other XM for control.
2. To the Suspension tube add 2 or 3 drops of donor cell suspension.
   To the XM tube add 2 drops of patient serum.
3. Prewarm both tubes at 37° C for 15 minutes.
4. Without removing the tubes from the incubator, add 1 drop of prewarmed cell suspension to the tube labelled XM containing the patient's serum.

5. Mix the XM tube thoroughly.
6. Discard the Suspension tube.
7. Incubate the tube labelled XM at 37° C for 30 minutes.
8. Following the 30-minute incubation, wash the contents of the tube labelled XM three times using the prewarmed saline.
9. Decant completely after the final wash.
10. Add 2 drops of AHG to the tube labelled XM and mix thoroughly. Note: the AHG should be at room temperature.
11. Centrifuge the tube at 3400 rpm for 15 seconds.
12. Gently resuspend the cell button, read macroscopically (see Grading Agglutination Reactions in Chapter 13) and examine for agglutination. Record the results.
13. Add 1 drop of Coombs control check cells to the tube if no agglutination is present. Centrifuge the tube at 3400 rpm for 15 seconds. Gently resuspend the cell button and read macroscopically. Record results.
14. If the Coombs control check cells do *not* agglutinate, the test is not valid and must be repeated.

Reporting Results

A compatible crossmatch is indicated by the absence of agglutination and/or hemolysis. The absence of agglutination indicates that the patient has no demonstrable antibodies at 37° C with a specificity for any of antigens on the donor erythrocytes.

Procedure Notes

Albumin should *not* be used in this technique because it has a tendency to enhance the reactivity of cold agglutinins.

If incompatibility is demonstrated by agglutination or hemolysis at any stage of the crossmatch, the donor unit should not be used for transfusion. Exceptions might include "least compatible" units in patients with autoantibodies.

The crossmatch should be reported as using *prewarmed technique.* The use of a warming coil is generally recommended for the administration of a unit crossmatched by the prewarming technique.

Limitations

In addition to the general limitations of the routine compatibility procedure, such as failure to prevent immunization of the patient or guaranteeing normal survival of transfused erythrocytes, the prewarming technique does not detect IgM antibodies such as anti-A or anti-B. Cold-reacting alloantibodies such as anti-M may be missed.

REFERENCE

Widmann, F. K. (Ed.): AABB Technical Manual. Arlington, VA, American Association of Blood Banks, 1985, p. 212.

TITLE: DONATH-LANDSTEINER SCREENING TEST

Principle

The Donath-Landsteiner antibody test is used to demonstrate the presence of this extremely potent hemolysin. This antibody requires cold incubation to exhibit hemolysis in the patient's serum. A positive test is diagnostic of paroxysmal cold hemoglobinuria (PCH), the rarest form of auto-immune hemolytic anemia.

Specimen

Fresh venous blood should be used. Care must be taken to avoid hemolyzing the specimen during venipuncture.

Reagents, Supplies, and Equipment

1. 16 × 100 mm test tubes
2. Crushed ice water bath (4° C)
3. 37° C water bath or heat block

Quality Control

A normal patient control specimen is run concurrently with the patient's test specimen.

Procedure

1. Place two test tubes in a 37° C waterbath or heat block. Warm a 10 cc syringe by holding it in the palm of the hand for a few minutes.
2. Draw 10 mL of blood and transfer 5 mL to each test tube. Label one tube "Control" and immediately place at 37° C. Label the other tube "Test" and place in an ice water bath at 4° C. Incubate both tubes for 1 hour. At the end of 1 hour, move the "Test" sample to the 37° C waterbath for an additional 30 minutes.
3. At the end of 90 minutes, carefully remove the tubes and examine for hemolysis.

Reporting Results

If the serum in both tubes is free of hemolysis, the test is negative. If a pink or red color is present in the serum of the "Test" and the "Control" is free of hemolysis, the test is positive. Normal blood will exhibit no hemolysis in either tube.

Procedure Notes

A positive test is diagnostic of paroxysmal cold hemoglobinuria (PCH). This disease is caused by a cold autoantibody with several unique characteristics. It is a complement-dependent, 7S IgG cold antibody; hemolysis occurs only after warming, even though complement activation may initially occur in the cold. The causative antibody, the Donath-Landsteiner antibody, is extremely lytic and is one of the most potent hemolysins known.

REFERENCES

Bauer, J. D.: Clinical Laboratory Methods (9th Ed.), St. Louis, C.V. Mosby Company, 1982, pp. 426-27.
Seiverd, C. E.: Hematology for Medical Technologists. Philadelphia, Lea & Febiger, 1972, p. 553.

TITLE: Dᵘ ROSETTE TEST

Principle

This screening procedure detects fetal D positive cells in the circulation of a D negative postpartum woman. The test uses D positive red blood cells as the indicators to demonstrate antibody coating. These indicator cells combine with the anti-D present on the coated red cells to form easily visible rosettes of several cells clustered around each antibody-coated D positive red blood cell in the maternal specimen. The number of rosettes is roughly proportional to the number of D positive red blood cells present in the mixture. Because this procedure is considered only a screening test, specimens producing a positive result should be tested with a quantitative method, such as Kleihauer-Betke acid elution, to quantitate the number of fetal cells present.

Specimen

No special preparation of the patient is required before specimen collection. She must be positively identified when the specimen is collected. The specimen must be labelled at the bedside and the label must include the patient's full name, the date when the specimen is collected, and the patient's hospital identification number. The time of collection and the phlebotomist's initials should be written on the required form.

Blood should be drawn by an aseptic technique and the specimen should be tested as soon as possible. Approximately 5 to 7 mL of blood should be collected in a red top (no anticoagulant) evacuated tube or lavender top (EDTA) evacuated tube. All specimens must be retained under refrigeration for 7 days.

Reagents, Supplies and Equipment

Indicator red blood cells:	0.2 to 0.5% saline suspension of type O, R_2R_2 red blood cells (cDE/cDE). Either enzyme-treated or untreated red blood cells in an enhancing medium can be used.

Commercial anti-D antisera
Commercial antihuman globulin (AHG) reagent (broad-spectrum or IgG)
10 × 75 mm or 12 × 75 mm disposable test tubes
Disposable pipettes, $4\frac{5}{8}''$ plastic or Pasteur
Test tube rack
Normal (0.9%) saline
37° C waterbath or heat block
High intensity lamp/optical magnifying lens
Centrifuge or cell washer

Quality Control

Negative control: A 3 to 4% saline suspension of washed D (Rh₀) D-negative cells
Positive control: A 3 to 4% saline suspension of a mixture of D positive and D negative red blood cells. This mixture of 0.5% D positive cells can be prepared as follows:

1. Add 1 drop of a 3% saline suspension of washed D positive red blood cells to 15 drops of a 3% saline suspension of washed D negative red blood cells. Mix well.
2. Add 1 drop of the mixture prepared in step 1 to 9 drops of the 3% suspension of D negative cells. Mix well.

Procedure

1. Prepare a 3 to 4% saline suspension of washed red blood cells from the patient's postpartum blood sample.
2. Label three 10 × 75 mm or 12 × 75 mm tubes: test, positive, and negative control.
3. Add 1 drop of anti-D antisera (or follow manufacturer's instructions) to each test tube.
4. Add 1 drop of maternal red blood cells, negative control cells, or positive control red blood cells to the respectively labeled tubes.
5. Incubate at 37° C for 15 to 30 minutes.
6. Wash the cell suspensions at least four times. Decant the saline completely after the last wash.
7. To the dry cell buttons, add 1 drop of indicator red blood cells to each tube and mix thoroughly to resuspend.
8. Centrifuge the tubes for 15 seconds at 3400 rpm.
9. Resuspend the cell button and examine the cell suspension microscopically at 100 × magnification.
10. Examine at least 10 fields and count the number of cell rosettes in each field.

Reporting Results

The absence of rosettes is a negative result. However, if enzyme-treated indicator red blood cells were used, a maximum of 1 rosette per 3 fields is considered a negative result. If the indicator red blood cells were treated with another type of enhancement media, a maximum of 6 rosettes per 5 fields constitutes a negative result.

If the number of rosettes exceeds the allowable maximums previously stated, the test is considered positive. In these cases, a quantitative test for the amount of fetal blood in the maternal circulation should be conducted.

Procedure Notes

The presence of rosettes or agglutination in the negative control tube indicates inadequate washing after incubation. If washing is inadequate, enough residual anti-D antiserum is present to agglutinate the D positive indicator red blood cells.

Limitations

Blood from a D^u positive mother produces strongly positive results. It is important to establish that the mother is D and D^u negative before performing the rosetting test. A massive fetal-maternal bleed may produce a rosetting pattern that is difficult to distinguish from D^u blood.

REFERENCE

Sebring, E.S., and Polesky, H.F.: Detection of fetal maternal hemorrhage in Rh immune globulin candidates. Transfusion, *22*:468-471, 1982.

TITLE: ELUTION TECHNIQUES

Principle

Several methods are used to elute antibody that is attached to red blood cells, including

1. Heat elution
2. Ether elution
3. Cold alcohol precipitation
4. Acid elution
5. Freeze-thaw elution
6. Xylene elution

The preparation of an antibody-containing eluate will be successful only if the processed red cells are adequately coated with antibody. Before an elution is actually performed, free (unbound) antibody is removed from the suspension by washing the cells thoroughly with saline. One of the elution methods is then used to free the antibody bound to the red blood cells. An eluate can be tested with reagent red blood cells to test for specificity in the same manner as for serum.

Elution is clinically useful in any situation in which antibody is attached to red blood cells, for example hemolytic disease of the newborn (HDN). Even in cases of very weakly positive (or even negative) direct antiglobulin tests, cell-bound antibody may be present, for example HDN due to ABO incompatibility.

Eluates are not stable. If not tested on the day of preparation, the eluate should be frozen and stored at $-20°$ C. Most eluates contain hemoglobin but cellular debris, if present, should be completely removed by centrifugation.

Specimen

An anticoagulated specimen of whole blood in EDTA from an adult, or a cord specimen from a newborn should be tested while it is still fresh. If a delay in testing is necessary, the specimen must be stored at 2 to 8° C for no longer than 7 days. Note: The yield of antibody evaluated from stored cells may be less than from fresh cells.

Reagents, Supplies, and Equipment

10 × 75 mm disposable test tubes
Disposable pipettes
Normal saline (0.9%)
Antiglobulin sera
Coombs' control check cells
6% Albumin prepared by adding 4 mL of normal saline to 1.5 mL of 22% bovine albumin
7 mL test tubes
Large centrifuge
56° C waterbath
Test tube rack

Quality Control

A small volume of thoroughly washed patient red blood cells is tested with AHG to ensure that the cells are coated. Add 2 drops of antiglobulin serum to 2 drops of the final saline wash. Mix well and let stand at room temperature for 5 minutes. Add 1 drop of Coombs' control cells. Mix and centrifuge at 3400 rpm for 15 seconds. Agglutination indicates that the cells have been washed free of any free antibody. No agglutination indicates that additional washing is necessary.

Procedures

ETHER ELUATE

Caution: Ether is highly volatile and explosive. Be careful to avoid sparks or flame.

1. Wash approximately 1 mL of packed red cells six times with saline.
2. To the washed, packed cell volume, add ½ volume of saline.
3. Add a volume of reagent grade diethyl ether, equal to the total volume of saline plus packed red cells.
4. Close with stopper and mix by inversion for about 1 minute, removing stopper occasionally to release volatile ether.
5. Centrifuge for 1 minute at 3600 rpm.
6. There will be three distinct layers: upper, containing clear ether; middle, containing denatured red cell stroma; and bottom, containing hemoglobin-stained eluate. Remove the ether layer by aspiration with suction. Carefully insert pipette tip through the stroma layer and remove the eluate (bottom layer) to another tube.
7. Incubate in unstoppered tube at 37° C for 30 to 45 minutes, in an open waterbath to drive off any residual ether.
8. Centrifuge for 1 minute at 3600 rpm to separate any remaining particles.

LUI EASY FREEZE ELUTION TECHNIQUE

1. To six or eight drops of washed, packed red cells add 1 or 2 drops 0.9% NaCl, mix and stopper.
2. Coat sides of tube by rotation. Place the slanted tube at −6 to −30° C for 10 minutes.
3. Thaw rapidly (under running tap water).
4. Centrifuge the hemolyzed cells.
5. Test clear hemolysate against group A, B, and O cells by routine technique.

LANDSTEINER AND MILLER HEAT ELUTION TECHNIQUE

1. Wash antibody-coated red cells 4 times with normal saline.
2. To one volume of packed red cells add one-half the volume of normal saline.
3. Agitate this suspension *continuously* in a waterbath kept at 56° C for 10 minutes.
4. Centrifuge for 3 minutes at 3000 rpm. Preheated centrifuge cups are recommended.
5. Remove the supernatant, containing the eluted antibody, as quickly as possible. Test the eluate by appropriate techniques.

PREPARATION OF ELUATE

1. Break up the clotted specimen of cord blood with applicator sticks or obtain 1 or 2 mL of free cells from an EDTA specimen. Wash the cells by hand at least three times with large quantities of saline. If less than 1 mL of free cells is used, there will be insufficient eluate for testing.
2. Pack the cell mass and remove all of the last wash completely.
3. To one volume of packed cord cells, add one volume of 6% bovine albumin and resuspend.
4. Constantly agitate the cell-albumin mixture in a 56° C waterbath for 7 minutes.
5. Preheat centrifuge holders by placing them in the 56° C water bath.
6. Immediately centrifuge the cell-albumin mixture at 2000 rpm for 5 minutes.
7. Immediately remove the supernatant (eluate) and use it for testing. Do not remove any cells with the eluate because they will reabsorb the antibody. This eluate is used in the same manner as serum.
   Note: If antibodies other than anti-A or anti-B are suspected, identify the antibody using a reagent red blood cell panel with the eluate (see Alloantibody Identification, this chapter).

Testing Procedure

1. Label 4 10 × 75 mm test tubes: A, B, I, and II
2. Add 2 drops of eluate to each tube.
3. To each of the labelled tubes add one drop of 3% suspension of adult A_1 cells, B cells, and I, II.
4. Mix the cells thoroughly and incubate at 37° C for 30 minutes.
5. Wash the contents of each tube three times with normal saline. Decant completely after the last wash.
6. Add 2 drops of antiglobulin serum to each tube.
7. Mix all tubes and centrifuge at 3400 rpm for 15 seconds.
8. Gently resuspend the cells and examine each tube macroscopically and microscopically for agglutination. Record the results.
9. To each tube showing no agglutination, add 1 drop of Coombs' control check cells.
10. Mix the tubes and centrifuge for 15 seconds at 3400 rpm.
11. Gently resuspend the cells and examine each tube macroscopically for agglutination. If any of the tubes show no agglutination, the entire procedure is invalid and must be repeated.

Reporting Results

Agglutination occuring when the eluate is tested against RBCs of appropriate phenotypes, indicates that an antibody has been recovered from the original cells, if the controls are satisfactory.

The absence of agglutination or of protein indicates that no antibody has been recovered from the cells.

Procedure Notes

When cells are used to absorb antibody from serum, the lag periods between the adsorption, washing of the cells, and elution should be as short as possible. If the cells are allowed to remain in the serum after incubation, some of the adsorbed antibody may elute back into the original serum.

The strength of the AHG on a sample of the cells is an indication of the amount of antibody adsorbed onto them. This will help to determine the amount of fluid to be added to the cell mass for elution. If the AHG reaction is 3+ or 4+, the antibody can be eluted into a volume of fluid $1\frac{1}{2}$ × the volume of the cells, the reaction of the eluate will still be strong enough for definitive testing. If the AHG reaction is 2+, an equal volume of fluid and cell mass is used. If the AHG reaction is less than 2+, a smaller volume of fluid than the cell mass is indicated, thereby concentrating the antibody.

The Lui Freeze and Landsteiner-Miller Heat Elution techniques are the most simple techniques available for eluting antibodies. Both are very effective for eluting ABO antibodies.

Example

Results of eluate from group A cord cells:

Test Cells	Antiglobulin Test Results
A^1	3+
B	1+
O	Neg.
O	Neg.

Note: A weak reaction of the eluate with B cells indicates cross-reactivity of the antibody.

Clinical Applications

Once an antibody has attached to red blood cells, either in vivo or in vitro, it can be recovered from these cells by a process called elution. The recovered antibody, in whatever fluid has been used, is called an eluate. Antibody elution is a valuable serologic tool and can be applied to:

1. Identification of antibodies from sera containing mixtures of antibodies.
2. Confirmation of antibody specificity.
3. Confirmation of the presence of weak antigens of red cell samples.

4. Identification of antibodies causing hemolytic disease of the newborn.
5. Identification of antibodies that have caused transfusion reactions.
6. Investigation of antibodies of patients with acquired hemolytic anemia.

Limitations

Although heat elution is an easy and rapid procedure, it does not demonstrate good recovery of antibodies. Preparation of an eluate with ether is dangerous.

If washing is not adequate, the eluate will actually be a combination of free and eluated antibody. As many as a dozen or more washes may be necessary to remove free antibodies.

REFERENCES

Feng, C.S., Kirkley, K. C., Eicher, C. A. and DeJongh, D. S.: The Lui elution technique. Transfusion, 25:433-434, 1985.
Issitt, P. H.: Applied Blood Group Serology, 2nd Ed. Oxnard, CA, Spectra Biologicals, 1975, p.28.
South, S. F., Rea, A. E., and Tregellas, W. M.: An evaluation of 11 red cell elution procedures. Transfusion, 26(2):167-170, 1986.
Stec, N., Shirey, R. S., Smith, B., Kickler, T. S., and Ness, P. M.: The efficacy of performing red cell elution studies in the pretransfusion testing of patients with positive direct antiglobulin tests. Transfusion, 26(3):225-226, 1986.
Widmann, F. K. (Ed.): AABB Technical Manual, 9th Ed. Arlington, VA, American Association of Blood Banks, 1985, p. 429.

TITLE: HEMOGLOBIN F DETERMINATION BY ACID ELUTION (KLEIHAUER-BETKE METHOD MODIFIED BY SHEPARD, WEATHERALL, AND CONLEY)

Principle

After blood smears are fixed with ethyl alcohol, a citric acid-phosphate buffer solution removes (elutes) hemoglobin other than hemoglobin F from erythrocytes. The hemoglobin F (fetal hemoglobin)-containing erythrocytes are visibly identifiable upon microscopic examination when appropriately stained. Shortly after birth, the amount of hemoglobin F in humans decreases to low levels. Increased amounts of hemoglobin F are found in various hemoglobinopathies such as hereditary persistence of fetal hemoglobin, sickle cell anemia, and thalassemias.

Specimen

Capillary blood or EDTA anticoagulated blood should be used. Smears made from fresh blood give the best results. Whole blood drawn into EDTA anticoagulant can be stored under refrigeration for no longer than 2 weeks. However, as soon as the blood smears are made, the test must be performed.

Reagents, Supplies, and Equipment

1. Ethyl alcohol, 80% (v / v)
2. Citric acid-phosphate buffer
   A. Stock Solutions
      (1) 0.2 M dibasic sodium phosphate (Na_2HPO_4). Weigh 2.84 g of dibasic sodium phosphate and transfer to 100 mL volumetric flask. Dilute to the 100 mL calibration mark with distilled water. Transfer to a dark brown bottle. Label the container with the reagent name and date. Refrigerate this stock solution.
      (2) 0.1 M citric acid. Weigh 2.1 g of citric acid. Transfer to a 100 mL volumetric flask and dilute to the 100 mL calibration mark with distilled water. Transfer to a dark brown bottle. Label the container with the reagent name and date. Refrigerate this stock solution.
   B. Working Solution
      Before use, prepare the citric acid-phosphate buffer by mixing 13.3 mL of 0.2M dibasic sodium phosphate and 36.7 mL of 0.1M citric acid. A pH of 3.2 to 3.3 is critical; check with pH meter.

3. An aqueous solution of 0.1% erythrosin B. Weigh 0.2 g of erythrosin B and transfer to a 200 mL volumetric flask. Add approximately 170 mL of distilled water. Add two to three drops of glacial acetic acid. Dilute to the 200 mL calibration mark with distilled water. Mix and filter through #42 Whatman filter paper. Transfer to a labelled brown bottle. Store at room temperature and filter before use.

4. Mayer's hematoxylin. To prepare this solution, add 1 gram of hematoxylin (color index #75290) to an Erlenmeyer flask containing 500 mL of distilled water. Heat just to boiling on a hot plate and add another 500 mL of distilled water. Mix. Add 0.2 grams of sodium iodate. Mix. Add 50 grams of aluminum potassium sulfate (12 H_2O). Mix. Transfer to a large stoppered bottle and shake for 1 minute. Filter. Transfer to a brown bottle, label with reagent name and date. This solution should be stored at room temperature and keeps indefinitely.

5. 6 staining containers with covers and a timer.

6. Microscope, immersion oil, lens paper.

Quality Control

Control tests using normal adult blood as well as blood from a neonate should be performed simultaneously with a patient specimen. The adult blood sample should have only a rare cell containing hemoglobin F, while the newborn infant sample should have a high percentage of acid resistant cells per microscopic field.

Procedure

1. Make four thin blood smears from each specimen: patient, normal control, and neonatal control. Label.

2. Allow these smears to air-dry for 10 to 60 minutes.

3. Prepare the working citric acid-phosphate buffer solution. Transfer to a staining jar and cover. Incubate at 37° C for 30 minutes.

4. The solutions needed for steps 5 to 9 should be prepared and filtered (if needed) and dispensed into labelled containers before proceeding with the next step.

5. Place the dry slides into 80% ethyl alcohol for about 5 minutes. At the end of this time, gently rinse or dip the smears in distilled water and allow to air-dry.

6. After the smears are completely dry, place the slides in the prewarmed citric acid-phosphate buffer solution for 5 minutes. At the end of 1 minute, dip the slides up and down. Repeat again at 3 minutes.

7. After 5 minutes, remove the slides from the citric acid-phosphate buffer solution and rinse with distilled water. Air-dry.

8. After the smears are completely dry, stain in Mayer's hematoxylin for 3 minutes. Rinse with distilled water.

9. Place the slides in Erythrosin B for 4 minutes. Rinse with distilled water and allow to air-dry.

10. Examine with (100×) oil immersion objective for hemoglobin F. Cells containing hemoglobin F stain a dark red-orange color depending upon the concentration of hemoglobin F. Normal adult erythrocytes appear as ghost cells. The neonatal blood sample should have many dense-appearing erythrocytes per field.

Calculations

The percentage of hemoglobin F-containing cells can be determined by counting the number of dense-staining cells and the number of ghost cells per field. Using the high dry (43-44×) objective, count 500 ghost cells and record the number of dense hemoglobin F-containing cells seen during the count.

Reporting Results

An adult specimen should have approximately the same number of dense hemoglobin F-containing cells as the normal adult blood. These cells should appear rarely. The results are expressed in percentage. Normal adults have less than 1% hemoglobin F-containing cells. Infant values are higher, with newborn infants having 70 to 90% hemoglobin F-containing cells.

Procedure Notes

False positive results may be obtained if anticoagulated blood is allowed to stand overnight or if a patient has a very high percentage of reticulocytes. Reticulocytes may resist elution and give the appearance of cells containing hemoglobin F. To cross-check high concentrations of hemoglobin F, a reticulocyte count can be performed.

In hemoglobinopathies such as sickle cell disease, the amount of hemoglobin F varies, producing inconsistent staining results. Cells containing small amounts of hemoglobin F stain lightly.

Clinical Applications

Increased amounts of hemoglobin F are found in various hemoglobinopathies such as hereditary persistence of fetal hemoglobin, sickle cell anemia, and thalassemias. Refer to the Clinical Applications section of Hemoglobin F Determination by Alkaline Denaturation, this chapter, for additional special examples of disorders in which hemoglobin F is increased.

Limitations

This procedure is a semiquantitative method. Hemoglobin electrophoresis can provide quantitative measurements of specific types of hemoglobin.

REFERENCE

Shepard, M.K., et al.: Semiquantitative estimation of the distribution of fetal hemoglobin in red cell populations. Bull. John Hopkins Hosp. *110*:293, 1962.

TITLE: IMMUNOGLOBULIN D (Rh$_o$) PROTOCOL

Principle

Refer to Chapter 10, Hemolytic Disease of the Newborn.

Specimen

MATERNAL SPECIMEN

No special preparation of the mother is required before specimen collection. She must be positively identified when the specimen is collected. The specimen must be labelled at the bedside and must include the patient's full name, the date the specimen is collected, and the patient's hospital identification number. The time of collection and the phlebotomist's initials should be written on the required form.

Blood should be drawn by an aseptic technique and the specimen should be tested as soon as possible. Approximately 5 to 7 mL of blood should be collected in a red top (no anticoagulant) or lavender top evacuated tube. All specimens must be retained under refrigeration for seven days.

INFANT SPECIMEN

Either a cord blood specimen collected in an EDTA or anticoagulated tube or a capillary blood specimen collected by the heel-stick method can be used.

LABORATORY CRITERIA

The laboratory criteria for Rh IgG administration are as follows:

1. The mother is D and D^u negative.
2. The mother's screening test for alloantibodies is negative for anti-D.
3. The infant is D or D^u positive. In obstetric cases where the Rh cannot be determined, it must be assumed that this criterion has been met.
4. The direct antiglobulin test on cord cells or infant's cells, if available, is

negative. If a positive DAT test result is obtained, an elution technique should be employed to establish that anti-D is not the coating antibody.

Procedure Notes

Using an assay such as the Kleihauer-Betke test (in this chapter), the number of vials of Rh IgG can be determined. Calculation of the number of vials needed is presented in Chapter 10, Hemolytic Disease of the Newborn.

The criteria for the administration of antenatal Rh$_o$ Immune Globulin omits the infant requirements because the Rh status of the fetus is unknown. A complete discussion of antenatal prophylaxis can be found in Chapter 10.

REFERENCES

Bowman, J. M. (Ed).: Rh$_o$ (D) Immune Globulin. Berkeley, CA, Cutter Biological, 1984.
Cheng, M. S., and Lukomskyj, L.: Postpartum D^u-positive women and Rh immune globulin. Lab. Med., 17(12):748-749, 1986.

TITLE: PENICILLIN OR CEPHALOSPORIN ANTIBODY SCREENING

Principle

Drug-coated red blood cells demonstrate agglutination if the serum or eluate from a patient's red cells contains an antibody to the drug. This procedure is helpful in identifying penicillin or cephalosporins as the cause of a positive direct antiglobulin test.

Specimen

No special preparation of the patient is required before specimen collection. The patient must be positively identified when the specimen is collected. The specimen must be labelled at the bedside and must include the patient's full name, the date

when the specimen is collected, and the patient's hospital identification number. The time of collection and the phlebotomist's initials should be written on the required form.

Blood should be drawn by an aseptic technique and the specimen tested as soon as possible. Approximately 5 to 7 mL of blood should be collected in a red top (no anticoagulant) evacuated tube.

Reagents, Supplies, and Equipment

Drug-sensitized red cells, as follows:

Penicillin-treated red cells

1. Prepare 1 mL of packed, well-washed, fresh red cells.
2. Add 15 mL of penicillin solution prepared by dissolving 0.6 g of penicillin in 15 mL of TMA-buffer (pH 10.0). Swirl occasionally.
3. Incubate at room temperature for 1 hour.
4. Wash cells 4 to 8 times in saline.
5. Resuspend in saline to a 3 to 4% suspension.

or

Cephalothin-treated red cells

1. Prepare 1 mL of packed, well-washed, fresh red cells.
2. Add 10 mL of Keflin solution prepared by dissolving 0.4 g of sodium cephalothin in 10 mL of TMA-buffer (pH 10.0). Swirl occasionally.
3. Incubate at 37° C for 1 hour.
4. Wash cells 4 to 8 times in saline.
5. Resuspend in saline to a 3 or 4% suspension.

2 to 4% suspension of group O washed red cells
Antihuman globulin antisera
10 × 75 mm or 12 × 75 mm disposable test tubes
Disposable pipettes, 4⅝" plastic or Pasteur
Test tube rack
Normal (0.9%) saline

37° C waterbath or heat block
High intensity lamp / optical magnifying
  lens
Centrifuge or cell washer

Quality Control

Patient control and reagent control must
be included in the test procedure.

Procedure

1. Label four test tubes and add the following:

Patient Test	Patient Control
2 drops patient serum	2 drops patient serum
1 drop drug-coated red cells	1 drop washed group O red cells

Control Test	Control Control
2 drops positive control serum	2 drops of positive control serum
1 drop drug-coated red cells	1 drop washed group O red cells

2. Incubate all of the tubes at 37° C for
   30 minutes.
3. Centrifuge, read and record results.
4. Wash all tubes 3 to 4 times with saline.
5. Add 2 drops of antiglobulin serum.
6. Mix, centrifuge for 10 to 15 seconds,
   read and record results.
7. Add 1 drop of Coombs' control red
   cells to each tube.
8. Mix, centrifuge for 10 to 15 seconds,
   read and record results. All tubes
   should be agglutinated after this step.

Reporting Results

If the patient test is agglutinated in step
6, the patient has an antibody to the drug.
For the patient results to be valid, the following reactions must also be observed:
Patient Control—No agglutination

Control Test—Agglutination
Control Control—No agglutination

Procedure Notes

If the patient control exhibits agglutination, the patient may have an alloantibody.
The identity of the antibody must be determined. After identification, red cells that
lack the corresponding antigen should be
coated with the drug and the procedure
should be repeated.

If the control test demonstrates no agglutination, the cells are not adequately coated
with drug.

If the control control exhibits agglutination, the control serum is contaminated. The
procedure should be repeated with a new
control specimen.

Alternate Procedure

Prepare titrations of the patient's serum
or an eluate using serial doubling dilution
in saline of the patient serum or an eluate
of the patient's red blood cells. Follow the
previous procedure.

Reporting Results

If the eluate demonstrates agglutination
with the drug-coated red cells but fails to
agglutinate uncoated red cells, the positive
direct antiglobulin test has been caused by
antibodies directed against the drug.

Procedure Notes

Many normal sera have antibodies to
penicillin or cephalothin-coated red cells
that react at room temperature to a low
titer. Individuals who have an antibody to
the drug that is causing positive direct
antiglobulin tests show reactivity to higher
titers when tested with the indirect antiglobulin test. It is important to test the patient's serum to rule out a red cell
alloantibody directed against the normal
test cells.

REFERENCES

Levine, B. B., and Redmond, A.: Immunochemical mechanisms of penicillin-induced Coombs positivity and hemolytic anemia in man. Int. Arch. Allergy Appl. Immunol., 31:594, 1976.

Petz, L. D., and Garratty, G.: Acquired Hemolytic Anemias. In Clinical Practice of Blood Transfusion, New York, Churchill-Livingstone, 1981.

Ries, C. A., Rosenbaum, T. J., Garratty, G., Petz, L. D. and Fudenberg, H. H.: Penicillin-induced immune hemolytic anemia. JAMA, 233:432, 1975.

TITLE: TRANSFUSION REACTION PROTOCOL

Principle

A sample standard protocol is established for the routine workup of transfusion reactions other than hives and urticaria. Refer to Chapter 11 for a complete discussion of transfusion reactions.

Specimen

Approximately 5 to 7 mL. of blood should be collected in a plain (no anticoagulant) evacuated tube and an additional specimen should be collected in an EDTA evacuated tube. Blood samples should be collected as soon as possible after notification of an adverse transfusion reaction. The blood samples must be examined as soon as possible. Hemolysis due to conditions such as traumatic venipuncture produces an inappropriate specimen.

Reagents, Supplies, and Equipment

1. Antisera
   A. Direct blood grouping antisera: anti-A, anti-B, anti-A,B
   B. Rh typing antisera: anti-D, Rh control reagent
   C. Antiglobulin reagent polyspecific
2. Reagent red blood cells
   A. A$_1$ and B reagent red blood cells
   B. Coombs' control red blood cells
3. 10 × 75 mm disposable test tubes
4. Normal saline (0.9%).
5. Disposable pipettes, 4⅝″
6. Centrifuge
7. Cell washer (optional)
8. Magnifier
9. Transfusion Reaction Request Form

Quality Control

Quality control steps should be implemented for each of the specific procedures. Refer to each specific procedure.

Procedure

1. Symptoms: Hives, urticaria
   Response:
   A. The nurse in charge should notify the patient's physician for orders of treatment and should watch for more serious symptoms.
   B. Transfusion need not be stopped unless symptoms worsen.
   C. No lab workup is necessary unless the patient's physician requests it.
2. Symptoms: Chills, fever, pain (back, chest, local site of infusion), shortness of breath, hypotension, tachycardia, palpitations, hemorrhagic diathesis.
   Response on the floor:
   A. The nurse should stop the transfusion immediately and notify the patient's physician and the blood bank.
   B. A physician or nurse should evaluate the patient clinically for signs and symptoms of a severe reaction.
   C. A clerical check of the patient's identification and the blood unit identification must be conducted at the patient's bedside.
   D. The blood bag should be returned to the blood bank.
   Response in the laboratory:

IMMEDIATE STEPS

1. Check the identification of the patient and the transfused unit of blood or component. Notify the medical director of the blood bank if any clerical or

identification error exists. Check to see if any other patients are at risk.

2. Immediately obtain a post-transfusion blood specimen. Label appropriately as the *post-transfusion specimen.* Obtain the discontinued bag of blood, administration set, and any attached IV solutions. Request the collection of a urine sample from the patient as soon as possible. Intact red cells indicate hemorrhage into the urinary tract, not hemolysis. Test the urine specimen for the presence of free hemoglobin. If the urine specimen is not collected for several days, test for hemosiderin.

3. Examine the patient's post-transfusion specimens by:
   A. Visually examining the patient's post-transfusion specimen for hemolysis. A pink color indicates that intravascular hemolysis has recently taken place. A sample obtain 4 to 10 hours after transfusion will have a yellow or brown color from increased bilirubin and other hemoglobin breakdown products.
   B. Performing a direct antiglobulin test (DAT). If transfused incompatible cells (antibody or complement-coated) are not immediately destroyed, the direct AHG test will be positive with a mixed-field appearance.

If any of the above tests are positive or doubtful, perform the following laboratory procedures:

1. Perform ABO grouping and Rh typing of the pretransfusion, post-transfusion and blood from the bag or a segment attached to the unit.
2. Repeat the crossmatch with the pretransfusion and post-transfusion specimen.
3. Perform a direct antiglobulin test (DAT) on the pretransfusion specimen.
4. Repeat alloantibody screening tests on the pretransfusion and donor units as well as the post-transfusion specimen. If either the pretransfusion or donor unit has a previously unreported antibody, check for clerical errors in the pretransfusion testing. Perform a mi-

nor crossmatch using the patient's pretransfusion specimen if the donor unit has a previously unsuspected antibody.

5. If any of the alloantibody screening tests are positive, identify the antibody. Test the patient or donor erythrocytes for the corresponding antibody depending which serum contains the antibody.

ADDITIONAL TESTS

If routine testing fails to provide information and immune hemolysis is suspected, the following tests may be helpful:

1. Antibody screening and compatibility tests with enhancement media or by increasing the ratio of serum to cells.
2. Perform DAT and alloantibody screening tests on several post-transfusion specimens collected from the patient at daily or frequent intervals.
3. Monitor the hemoglobin/hematocrit levels. In a nonbleeding patient, a unit of packed erythrocytes should produce an increase of 1 g/dL or packed cell volume (hematocrit) of 3%.
4. Genotype the erythrocytes of the patient's pretransfusion specimen and the donor cells. Examine the patient's postreaction specimen for the presence of cells bearing foreign antigens. If an antigen can be found that is present on the donor cells and absent on the patient's cells, its presence or absence in the post-transfusion sample indicates the degree to which the transfused cells have survived and remain in the circulation.
5. Test post-transfusion serum samples for the presence of unconjugated bilirubin.
6. Measure serum haptoglobin in pre- and post-transfusion patient specimens.

Reporting Results

If a discrepancy occurs between the ABO grouping or Rh typing of the pretransfusion, post-transfusion, or donor unit, an error in patient identification, specimen labelling, donor unit identification or other clerical error is responsible. Notify the patient's physician and the medical director of the blood bank. Crosscheck all past patient records as well as the labelling of the blood product itself. The phlebotomist responsible for obtaining the blood specimen should be questioned *immediately* if the pretransfusion specimen does not agree with the post-transfusion specimen. Any other patient specimens drawn at approximately the same time should be rechecked, if the possibility of having another patient at risk exists.

An incompatible crossmatch with the pretransfusion specimen indicates that an error existed in the patient or donor specimen during pretransfusion testing. If the crossmatch is incompatible *only* with the post-transfusion specimen, an anamnestic reaction is suspect.

If only the DAT on the post-transfusion test is positive, the patient's erythrocytes have been coated with antibody or complement. Procedures for investigation of a positive DAT should be followed to determine the cause.

If the post-transfusion specimen has an alloantibody not present in the pretransfusion specimen, the cause may be an anamnestic reaction or passive administration of antibody in a transfusion component recently infused.

The presence of an alloantibody does not necessarily indicate that it is the cause of the reaction; the corresponding antigen must also be present.

A rising bilirubin may be detectable as early as 1 hour postreaction. Peak levels occur at 4 to 6 hours and disappear within 24 hours if bilirubin excretion is normal.

Visible hemoglobinemia develops only after haptoglobin depletion. Compare pretransfusion and post-transfusion values. A decline in haptoglobin is most useful in chronic hemolysis. If studies are performed several days after a hemolytic episode, normal levels may be restored because haptoglobin is an acute phase reactant that may regenerate rapidly after depletion.

Other Tests

BACTEREMIA

Carefully take specimens from the bag for cultures at 4° C, 20 to 24° C, and 35 to 37° C. Examine a smear of the blood stained with Gram stain or acridine orange (a DNA stain).

Physical Damage

Examine the donor unit for physical damage (heat, cold storage / transport, or excessive heat from an in-line blood warmer) or chemical damage (drugs, hypotonic solutions). Discoloration (pink or red) of the donor unit can result from osmotic hemolysis caused by a hypotonic or dextrose solution entering the unit or present in the administration unit.

REFERENCES

(See Chapter 11, Transfusion Reactions, for a full discussion of this topic.)

Holland, P. V. Other Adverse Effects of Transfusion. In Clinical Practice of Blood Transfusion, Petz, L. W., and Swisher, S. N. (Ed.): NY, Churchill-Livingstone Inc., 1981, pp. 783-801.

Huestis, D. W., Bove, J. R., and Case, J.: Practical Blood Transfusion. Boston, Little, Brown and Co., 1988, pp. 265-268.

Widmann, F. K. (Ed.): Adverse Effects of Blood Transfusion, AABB Technical Manual, 9th Ed. Arlington, VA, American Association of Blood Banks, 1985, pp. 325-331.

15

New Directions in Serologic Testing

At the conclusion of this chapter, the reader will be able to:
- Name the dates and locations of the beginning of microtechniques.
- Cite the two types of micromethods.
- List the applications of micromethods.
- Describe the advantages of microplate hemagglutination techniques.
- Explain the physical characteristics of microplates.
- Describe the principle of solid-phase assay.
- Compare the original method of automation in blood banking to the second-generation instruments.

Chapter Outline

Serologic testing in immunohematology has usually been performed by slide or test tube techniques, but increased emphasis on cost containment has stimulated interest in microtechniques as an alternative to conventional methods. Capillary tubes and microplates have been used in some laboratories for a long time. Capillary tube techniques have been used in the Rh Laboratory in Winnipeg since 1944 and microplates were invented in 1950 in Hungary by Takatsky. Microtesting for typing lymphocytes was introduced 20 years ago. This method has been adopted internationally and is basically the only method used for typing lymphocytes today.

The term microtechnique is deceptive because the amount of reagent is not as small as the quantities used in HLA testing. Micromethods for red cell antigen and antibody testing are either hemagglutination or solid phase adherence assays. These methods are still evolving, but are considered more economical than traditional methods because most methods require microliter quantities of reagent antisera or cells per test. These methods are also considered simpler to perform. Although the capillary tube technique has not yet been automated, the microplate method is the basis for several automated instruments.

Applications for micromethods include:

1. ABO grouping (forward and reverse)
2. Rh typing and Rh control
3. Alloantibody detection
4. Alloantibody identification
5. Antibody titration
6. Crossmatching
7. Reagent quality control

MICROPLATE HEMAGGLUTINATION TECHNIQUES

In the 1960s, microplate technology was applied to blood banking. Subsequent modifications of the initial technique have succeeded in developing a reproducible and reliable test system without loss of reaction

468

sensitivity. Use of microplates allows the performance of a large number of tests on a single plate, which eliminates time-consuming steps such as labelling test tubes. Although microplate testing was initially restricted to large-scale testing, the development of smaller microplates now allows smaller blood banks to use this technique.

The microplate is a compact plate of rigid or flexible plastic with multiple wells. The wells may be U-shaped or V-shaped or have a flat-bottom configuration. The U-shaped well has been the most commonly used in immunohematology. The volume capacity of each well is approximately 0.2 mL, which prevents spilling during mixing.

Samples and reagents are dispensed with small-bore Pasteur pipettes, recommended because they deliver 0.025 mL, which prevents splashing. After the specimens and reagents are added to the wells, they are mixed by gentle agitation of the plates. The microplate is then centrifuged for immediate reading. Countertop or floor model centrifuges are suitable if they are equipped with special rotors that can accommodate microplate centrifuge carriers and are capable of speeds between 400 and 2000 rpm. Smaller plates can be centrifuged in serologic centrifuges with an appropriate adapter.

After centrifugation, the cell buttons are resuspended by either gently tapping the microplate or using a flat-topped mechanical shaker. A shaker provides a more consistent and standard resuspension of the cells than manual tapping. After the cells are resuspended, the wells are examined with an optical aid or over a well-lighted surface. A positive reaction will settle in a diffuse, uneven button; negative reactions are manifested by a smooth, compact button (Fig. 15-1). Detection of weakly positive reactions is enhanced by allowing the red cells to settle.

It may be necessary to incubate the plates before centrifugation, depending on the type of test being performed. If a test requires a 37° C incubation, the plates are placed in a dry heat incubator or allowed to float in a waterbath. The wells must be covered during incubation to reduce evaporation of the specimen and reagents. An AHG test can be performed by washing the red cells manually with a dispenser designed to deliver a measured amount of saline to each well and centrifuging the plate between washings. After the last wash, AHG antiserum is added and the plate is recentrifuged. To read AHG reactions, the plate is placed at a 60 to 75-degree angle to allow the red cells to stream. Positive reactions remain in an aggregated button or stream very slowly; negative reactions stream down the well in a smooth flow. A weakly positive reaction may be detected by gently resuspending the red cells and allowing them to resettle.

Although this technique is considered highly reliable, one problem with the microplates is that new microplates may have static charges. Static can cause adherence of cells and antisera to the sides of the microplate well and prevent the smooth settling of cells. This problem can, however, be avoided by pretreatment of the microplates.

SOLID-PHASE TECHNIQUES

Solid-phase adherence assays are a recent advancement in blood group serology to test erythrocytes for selected antigens, including weak antigen expression, subgroups A and B, and red cells classified by D^u by conventional methods. These assays also test serum for erythrocyte antibodies, detect platelet antibodies, and perform compatibility and hepatitis testing. The sensitivity of solid-phase assays has been shown to be equivalent to or better than conventional agglutination methods.

For the past 90 years, the hemagglutination endpoint has remained the most widely used method in immunohematology to detect the interaction of erythrocyte antibodies and antigens. The major disadvantage of hemagglutination methods is the lack of an objective endpoint. Weakly positive reactions may be difficult to distinguish from negative reactions; therefore, test interpretation is subjective and relies on the technical ability and expertise of the technologist performing the test. By comparison, solid-phase assays have been designed to achieve endpoints that are more easily dif-

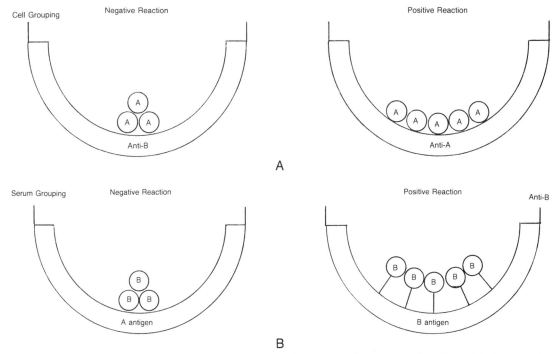

Figure 15-1. A, Solid-phase adherence assay results of A antigen grouping. B, Solid-phase adherence assay results of anti-B grouping.

ferentiated by manual or automated methods.

Solid-phase assays rely on adherence rather than hemagglutination for detection of antigen-antibody reactions. In 1976, it was demonstrated that monolayers of red cells could be immobilized on plastic tubes for the detection of antigen-antibody reactions. With this technique, either an antigen or an antibody is immobilized on a solid phase. Methods of immobilization are usually based on simple, passive adsorption of antibody or antigen onto the plastic surface. This phenomenon is believed to occur by hydrophobic bonding. Adsorption may be facilitated by pretreating the plates with chemicals such as glutaraldehyde before addition of antigen or antibody. Polystyrene microplates are the most commonly used, but polystyrene tubes and microplates or tubes made of polypropylene or polyvinyl plastics can also be used.

Erythrocyte antigen typing involves immobilization of specific antibodies such as anti-A or anti-D on the microplate wells. The red cells are enzyme-treated before testing to enhance antigen-antibody inter-

action. A dilute suspension of these treated red cells is prepared and added to the appropriate antibody-coated wells. Equipment used in solid-phase testing is the same as in microplate hemagglutination procedures. A centrifuge that can accommodate microplate centrifuge carriers and a 37° C dry heat incubator or waterbath are the minimum requirements. After addition of the appropriate reactants, the microplate is centrifuged and observed for a positive or negative reaction. A positive reaction is demonstrated by adherence of the red cells to the entire inner surface of the well; a negative reaction is exhibited by nonadherence. Nonadhering red cells pellet into a discrete, compact button in the bottom of the well when centrifuged (Figure 15-2).

Solid-phase assays for antibody detection are more involved than antigen detection. One method is used for detection of IgM antibodies such as anti-A or anti-B and another for detection of IgG antibodies such as anti-D. The assay for anti-A or anti-B requires the immobilization of a red cell monolayer of A_1 or B red cells, or purified antigens on an immunologically active sur-

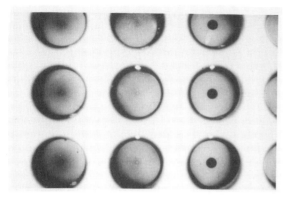

Figure 15-2. Buttons formed by nonagglutinated cells. Photograph courtesy of Olympus Corporation, Clinical Instruments Division, Lake Success, New York.

face of the microplate well. Test serum is added to the appropriate wells, incubated, and decanted. Enzyme-treated A_1, B, or A_1B indicator red cells are added to each well and the microplate is centrifuged. Positive reactions are indicated by adherence of the indicator cells to either anti-A or anti-B that has been previously bound to the immobilized red cell monolayer. The reaction can be visualized as a "sandwich" of two layers of antigen linked together by antibody. Negative reactions are demonstrated by no adherence.

The assay for the detection of IgG alloantibodies also uses the immobilization of a red cell monolayer of red cells with a known selection of erythrocyte antigens. Test serum and a low ionic enhancement medium are added to each well. The mixture is incubated at 37° C and then washed with saline to remove free serum. Antiglobulin antiserum facilitates the linking of the antibody-coated indicator cells to the antibody bound to the red cell monolayer. The presence or absence of adherence is interpreted as a positive or negative result, respectively.

In addition to the adherence of erythrocytes, other indicators may be used to determine the reaction results. The results can be decided using a spectrophotometer designed for microplate reading. Adhering erythrocytes can be hemolyzed with distilled water and the resulting hemolysis can be read as a positive result. A chromogenic substrate may also be added for test inter-

pretation. This type of substrate reacts with the hemoglobin peroxidase of the adhering erythrocytes to produce an interpretable color reaction.

The solid-phase antiglobulin test (SPAT) has been applied to crossmatching. This technique results in adherence of sensitized red cells to IgG-coated wells. Results can be read visually or automatically using a spectrophotometer designed for microplate readings. This application is considered to have more sensitivity than manual methods without loss of specificity.

AUTOMATED METHODS

A major achievement in the past several decades has been the introduction of automation into the blood bank. Automated systems have the capabilities of positive sample identification; automatic dispensing of specimens and antisera; and interpretation, recording, and storing of results. One of the problems associated with early automated systems was the inability to detect weak antibody-antigen interactions.

Original Approaches to Automation

THE CONTINUOUS-FLOW METHOD

In 1963, an adaptation of the continuous-flow method which was successfully implemented in clinical chemistry applications, was introduced to automate hemagglutination. Modifications of this basic technique have extended to applications such as special antigen typing, antibody screening, and antibody titration.

With the continuous-flow methodology, test specimens—erythrocytes, serum, or both—are aspirated, divided into aliquots, and routed through separate channels. Air bubbles are added to mechanically separate individual specimens and prevent liquid film formation on the mixing coils. The specimen mixes with appropriate reagents and agglutination occurs in a reaction coil. After mixing, a hypertonic salt solution is added to disperse clumps that are not bound by antibody. The mixture is sent through s settling coil to allow the resulting agglutinates to settle before passing over a T-fitting. As the mixture stream passes over the T-fitting, the agglutinates fall out of the sample stream.

Agglutination may be detected visually by examining deposits of agglutinates, which are removed at the T-fitting onto a strip of moving filter paper. If the stream is debubbled and infrared light-emitting diodes and sensors are positioned across the tubing, the optical density of the remaining liquid can be measured.

This type of instrumentation is limited to large blood processing centers because it is expensive and best suited for batch processing. A disadvantage of the system is that it is less effective than manual techniques in detecting all examples of clinically significant alloantibodies.

The Hemagglutination Method

Another system of automated hemagglutination is comparable to the manual tube method. Specimens and antisera are automatically dispensed into cuvettes. The mixtures are then incubated, centrifuged, and agitated. Agitation disperses all of the free erythrocytes into a homogeneous suspension and the clumps of agglutinated cells collect in the center of the cuvette. Agglutination is detected by comparing the optical density of the peripheral and central area of each cuvette.

A positive reaction is demonstrated by a reciprocal variation in the central and peripheral light intensities. The absence of variation in the optical density between the central and peripheral areas signifies a negative reaction. The instrument is interfaced to a computer, which interprets and prints the results.

This type of instrumentation is also limited to large blood processing centers because it is expensive and best suited for batch processing. A disadvantage of the system is that it is less effective than manual techniques in detecting all examples of clinically significant alloantibodies.

Second-Generation Instrumentation

Basic Considerations

Newer systems that use microplate technology have been developed for large- and small-scale applications. Automated microplate systems may be used for routine blood grouping and antibody detection. These systems are considered more economical in terms of equipment costs than older systems. A disadvantage of the automated microplate systems, in general, is difficulty in detecting weak antigen-antibody reactions. In such cases, visual observation of the microplate and on-line manual editing require technologist interpretation of questionable reactions. The basic principle of automated systems is similar to manual microplate hemagglutination. The systems have incorporated densitometers to read microplate hemagglutination and interfaced them with computers that interpret and print or store the serologic results.

Specimens are dispensed to microplate wells either manually or automatically. The plate is processed by incubation, centrifugation, and gentle agitation. Free erythrocytes are resuspended and agglutinated cells remain in the center of the well. The optical density of each well is then read; the actual number of readings per well varies with the type of densitometer used. The readings are transferred through an interface to a computer for processing. Depending on the number of readings conducted, hemagglutination may be determined by either histogram analysis or a comparison of peripheral and central optical densities.

Examples of Instrumentation

Two examples of second-generation instrumentation are the MicroBank™ Automated Blood Grouping System (Dynatech Laboratories, Inc., Chantilly, Virginia) and the Olympus PK 7100 (Olympus Corporation, Lake Success, New York).

The MicroBank system (Fig. 15-3) is designed to determine ABO grouping and Rh typing. A laser scanner identifies up to 8 bar code-labelled test tubes in the bar code-labelled microplate that is placed into a specially designed carrier (Fig. 15-4).

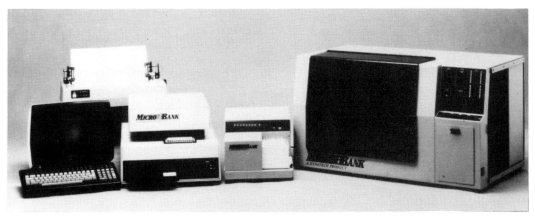

Figure 15-3. MicroBank system components. This system consists of the MicroBank™ reader (far right), which measures the optical density of red cell suspensions in U-bottom, 96-well microplates and processes the information by means of a resident computer and dedicated software. The reader microprocessor also accepts bar coded tube and microplate information from the laser scanner. The reader houses one floppy disk drive for storage and transfer. The video terminal (far left) allows the operator to control and monitor the reader, scanner, and microprocessor operation. The dot matrix printer (rear) produces a hardcopy printout of serologic tests results, quality control records, and administrative reports. The laser scanner (optional, second from right) reads bar-coded information from test tubes and microplates and transmits the information to the microprocessor for subsequent correlation of test sample numbers with blood group interpretations. The sample preparation device (optional, second from left) automatically prepares each test cell suspension and delivers the specimen and reagents to the appropriate microplate wells. Photograph courtesy of Dynatech Laboratories Inc., Chantilly, Virginia.

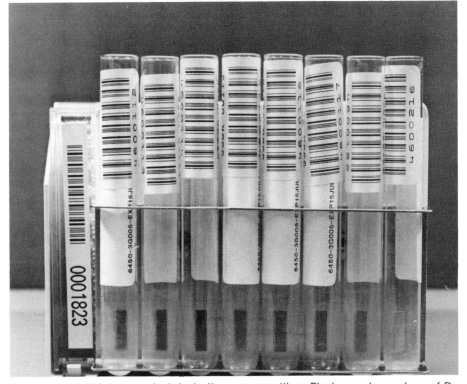

Figure 15-4. Bar-coded tubes and plate in the scan position. Photograph courtesy of Dynatech Laboratories, Inc., Chantilly, Virginia.

Specimens can be dispensed into the microplate by manual or semiautomated method and maintain the pre-established test sample/microwell configuration (Fig. 15-5). Specimens and reagents are mixed in the wells of rigid U-bottom microplates. After centifugation and resuspension of the test well mixtures, the microplate is placed on the reader platform. The microplate bar code is again scanned and multiple readings are made of each well (Fig. 15-6). The light absorbance of reactions is compared to preset threshold values for positive, negative, or questionable reactions. Specimens yielding negative results with anti-D require further manual testing before the Rh type can be determined. All results are stored on a floppy disk and/or transferred to a mainframe computer system.

The Olympus PK 7100 automated microplate-based, pretransfusion blood group system (Fig. 15-7) is a fully automated high-throughput instrument that performs forward and reverse ABO grouping and Rh typing. A bar code reader is standard for identification of patient specimens. Determination of ABO grouping is in saline without additives, but Rh typing includes treatment of the cells with bromelin using dual probes.

This system uses a unique terraced-well microplate (Fig. 15-8). The reaction wells have concentric rings cut into the walls, allowing agglutinated erythrocytes to settle evenly on the steps, or terraces, of the well. Nonagglutinated cells roll to the bottom of the well and form a tight concentric button, which will not dissociate or crumble due to automated handling.

Interpretation of reactions is made by comparing the optical densities at peripheral (P) and central (C) locations in each well, determining the P/C ratio, and comparing the results to the threshold levels of a known sample population. A built-in microcomputer records the results of each sample and controls the printout. Visual

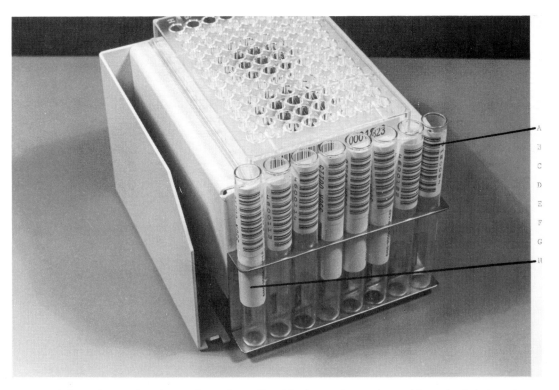

Figure 15-5. Test sample-microwell configuration. Photograph courtesy of Dynatech Laboratories, Inc., Chantilly, Virginia.

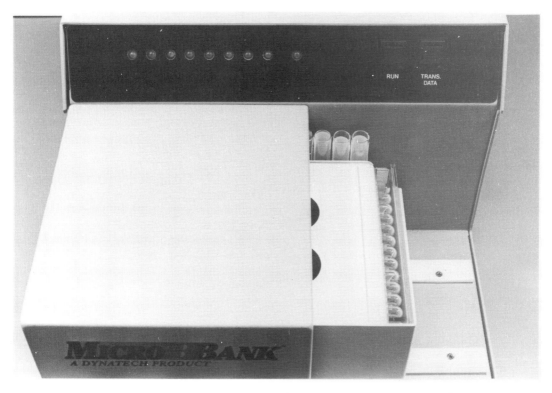

Figure 15-6. Laser scanner. Photograph courtesy of Dynatech Laboratories, Inc., Chantilly, Virginia.

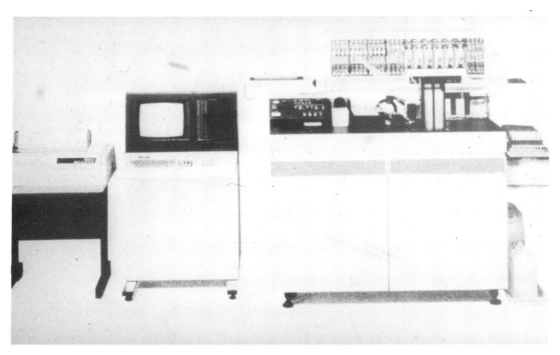

Figure 15-7. Olympus system. Photograph courtesy of Olympus Corporation, Clinical Instruments Division, Lake Success, New York.

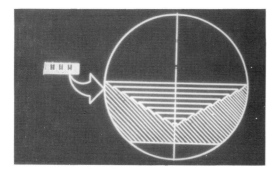

Figure 15-8. Olympus microwell construction. Photograph courtesy of Olympus Corporation, Clinical Instruments Division, Lake Success, New York.

evaluation can be performed as the microplate enters the viewing station located on the top surface of the analyzer.

CHAPTER SUMMARY

Microtechniques are becoming more popular because of an increased emphasis on cost containment. Micromethods for red cell antigen and antibody testing are hemagglutination or solid phase adherence assays. These methods are considered more economical than traditional methods. Applications of micromethods include ABO grouping, Rh typing and control, alloantibody detection and identification, antibody titration, crossmatching, and reagent quality control.

Microplate Hemagglutination Techniques

Use of microplates allows performance of a large number of tests on a single plate, which eliminates time-consuming steps such as labelling test tubes. The microplate is a compact plate of rigid or flexible plastic with multiple wells. The U-shaped well has been the most commonly used in immunohematology. Although this technique is considered highly reliable, one problem with the microplates is that new microplates may have static charges that can cause adherence of cells and antisera to the sides of the microplate well and prevent smooth settling of cells. This can lead to erroneous results.

Solid-Phase Techniques

Solid-phase assays rely on adherence rather than hemagglutination for detection of antigen-antibody reactions. With this technique, either an antigen or an antibody is immobilized on a solid phase. Erythrocyte antigen typing involves the immobilization of specific antibodies such as anti-A or anti-D on the microplate wells. Solid-phase assays for antibody detection are more involved than antigen detection. One method is used for the detection of IgM antibodies such as anti-A or anti-B and another for the detection of IgG antibodies such as anti-D. The solid-phase antiglobulin test (SPAT) has been applied to crossmatching. This technique results in adherence of sensitized red cells to IgG-coated wells. Results can be read visually or automatically using a spectrophotometer designed for microplate readings. This application is considered to have more sensitivity than manual methods without loss of specificity.

Automated Methods

Automated systems have the capabilities of positive sample identification; automatic dispensing of specimens and antisera; and interpretation, recording, and storage of results. The first blood bank automated hemagglutination instrument was a modification of the continuous-flow method which had been successfully implemented in clinical chemistry. This type of instrumentation is limited to large blood processing centers because it is expensive and best suited for batch processing. A disadvantage of the system is that it is less effective than manual techniques in detecting all examples of clinically significant alloantibodies.

Another system of automated hemagglutination is comparable to the manual tube method. The instrument is interfaced to a computer, which interprets and prints the results. This type of instrumentation is also limited to large blood processing centers because it is expensive and best suited for batch processing.

Newer systems that use microplate technology have been developed for large- and small-scale applications. Automated microplate systems may be used for routine blood grouping and antibody detection. These systems are considered more economical in terms of equipment costs than older systems. A disadvantage of the automated microplate systems, in general, is difficulty in detecting weak antigen-antibody reactions. In such cases, visual observation of the microplate and on-line manual editing require technologist interpretation of questionable reactions. The basic principle of these systems is similar to manual microplate hemagglutination. The systems have incorporated densitometers to read microplate hemagglutination and interfaced them with computers that interpret and print or store the serologic results. Two examples of second-generation instrumentation are the MicroBank™ Automated Blood Grouping System and the Olympus PK 7100.

REVIEW QUESTIONS

1. Capillary tube microtechniques have been used in blood bank testing since:
    A. 1908
    B. 1924
    C. 1944
    D. 1963
    E. 1980
2. Micromethods can be used for:
    A. ABO grouping
    B. Rh Typing
    C. Alloantibody detection and identification
    D. Crossmatching
    E. All of the above
3. The advantage or advantages of the microplate technique is (are):
    A. Eliminates time-consuming steps
    B. Uses less specimen and reagents
    C. Uses less personnel time
    D. Is reliable
    E. All of the above
4. Solid phase assays rely on ____ for detection of antigen-antibody reactions.
    A. Hemagglutination
    B. Adherence
    C. Differential solubility rates
    D. Differences in optical density
    E. Competitive inhibition
5. The first automated systems in blood banking were adaptations of ____ methodology.
    A. Microplate hemagglutination

B. Solid phase
C. Continuous-flow
D. Competitive inhibition
E. Fluorescent

6. Most second-generation instrumentation is based on:
    A. Microplate hemagglutination
    B. Solid phase
    C. Continuous flow
    D. Competitive inhibition
    E. Fluorescence

ANSWERS

1. C	4. B
2. E	5. C
3. E	6. A

BIBLIOGRAPHY

Crawford, M. C.: A review of micromethods for blood bank laboratories. Lab. Med., 18(3):149-152, 1987.

Douglas, R., Schneider, J. V., Wilkie, D., and Harden, P. A.: A solid phase antiglobulin test. Transfusion, 27(4):378-383, 1987.

Eisinger, R. W., Rolih, S. D., Moheng, M. C., and Eatz, R. A.: Transfusion, 24(5):417, 1984.

Friedman, L. I., Severns, M. L., Goodkofsky, I., and Holland, N.: The status of automation and data processing in the United States blood banking community. Transfusion, 26(6):514-518, 1986.

Gibbons, D. S., Kano, T., and Edelmann, M.: A terraced microplate system for automated ABO and Rh grouping. Am. Clin. Prod. Rev., 42-46, Nov. 1986.

Kohmann, T. F., Forey, J. E., Burch, J. W., and Au-Buchon, J. P.: Prelicensure evaluation of a microplate-based blood testing system. Transfusion, 26(6):550, 1986.

Kutt, S. M., Larison, P. J., and Lewis, C. A.: Evaluation of a microplate test system for blood banks. Am. Clin. Prod. Rev., 8-11, Jan., 1988.

Leong, S. W., and Terasaki, P. I.: Microtest for red cell typing. Transfusion, 25(2):149-151, 1985.

Moheng, M. C.: Blood Banking: State of the Art. In Pierce, S. R., and Wilson, J. K. (Eds.): Approaches to Serological Problems in the Hospital Transfusion Service. Arlington, VA, American Association of Blood Banks, 1985.

Peoples, J. C. A.: A retrospective survey of blood bank automation. Lab. Med., 16(12):763-765, 1985.

Rachel, J. M., Sinor, L. T., Beck, M. L., and Plapp, F. V.: A solid-phase antiglobulin test. Transfusion, 25(1):24-26, 1985.

Sinor, L. T., et al.: Solid-phase ABO grouping and Rh typing. Transfusion, 25(1):21-23, 1985.

Theuriere, M., Zelenski, K. R., Moore, V. K., and Logulo, A. C.: Automated detection of red cell antibodies in donor sera using an automated technology. Transfusion 25(3):257-260, 1985.

Tomchick, C., Piccirilli, R., and Schmidt, A. P.: Evaluation of an automated microplate blood grouping system. Transfusion, 24(5):441, 1984.

Fundamentals of Immunohematology Glossary

AABB. American Association of Blood Banks.

AB cis gene. A condition in which both the A and B genes seem to be inherited on a single chromosome.

abruptio placentae. The premature separation of a normally situated placenta.

acquired immunodeficiency syndrome (AIDS). An immune disorder affecting (T4) lymphocytes. This disorder is caused by the HTLV-III (human T cell leukemia virus) or LAV virus, also referred to as the human immunodeficiency virus (HIV).

acriflavin. The yellow dye used in some commercial anti-B reagents. This additive can produce false agglutination in some individuals but, this is rare.

acute. Term for a condition of sudden and short duration.

affinity. The bond between a single antigenic determinant and an individual combining site.

agammaglobulinemia. The absence of plasma gamma globulin due to either congenital or acquired states.

agglutination. The clumping of particles that have antigens on their surface, such as, erythrocytes, by antibody molecules that form bridges between the antigenic determinants.

agglutinin. The older term for an antibody.

agglutinogen. The older term for antigen.

alleles. Alternate forms of genes that code for traits of the same type; for example, the genes Fy^a and Fy^b are alleles.

allergic reaction. A reaction to soluble constituents in donor plasma.

alloantibodies. Immunoglobulins (antibodies) produced in response to exposure to foreign antigens of the same species.

allogenic. Denotes genetically different individuals of the same species.

amniocentesis. The process of removing fluid from the amniotic sac for study, for example, chromosome analysis or biochemical studies.

amorphic gene. A gene that produces no detectable gene product, i.e. antigen.

anamnestic antibody response. An antibody "memory" response. This secondary response occurs on subsequent exposure to a previously encountered and recognized foreign antigen. An anamnestic response is characterized by rapid production of IgG antibodies.

anaphylactic reaction. A severe allergic reaction that can develop in IgA-deficient patients who have developed anti-IgA antibodies.

anaphylactoid reaction. A severe reaction to soluble constituents in donor plasma which produces edema.

antenatal. Before birth.

antibodies. Specific glycoproteins (immunoglobulins) produced in response to an antigenic challenge. Antibodies can be found in blood plasma and body fluids such as tears, saliva, and breast milk.

antibody elution. See eluate.

antigen (antigenic, immunogenic). A foreign substance that can elicit an immune (antibody) response.

antigenicity. The ability of an antigen to stimulate the immune response. The antigenicity of a substance may be influenced by the number of antigen receptor sites.

antithetical antigens. Two antigens controlled by a pair of allelic genes such as Kell (K) and Cellano (k).

asymptomatic. Exhibiting no symptoms of a disease or disorder.

autocontrol. A test consisting of the patient's erythrocytes and serum.

autoimmune hemolytic anemia. A condition of destruction of erythrocytes by self-produced antibodies.

autologous donation. Donation of blood for one's self. Autologous donation may take the form of predeposit or autotransfusion, for example, intraoperative autotransfusion, hemodilution, or postoperative autotransfusion.

avidity. The strength with which a multivalent antibody binds to a multivalent antigen.

bilirubin. A breakdown product of erythrocyte catabolism.

blood substitutes. Artificial substances that mimic the effect of a natural blood constituent, such as erythrocytes.

Bombay phenotype. The failure of an individual to express inherited A or B genes because of the lack of at least one H gene and the subsequent lack of the resulting H precursor substance.

carrier state. The asymptomatic condition of harboring an infectious organism. This term may also refer to a heterozygous individual or the carrier of a recessive gene.

chimerism. A condition producing two cell populations in an individual.

chronic. Term for condition of long duration.

cis position. Refers to the situation in which a gene on one chromosome of a homologous pair affects the actions of a related gene on the same chromosome.

cold agglutinins. Antibodies that react at room or colder temperatures.

compatibility testing. A term frequently used synonomously with the term crossmatch. Compatibility testing includes ABO and Rh grouping, screening of serum for alloantibodies, and crossmatching.

complement. A complex of plasma proteins.

compound antigen. The term used to express the idea that certain combinations of antigens demonstrate a combined effect, for example, the ce or f antigen.

Coombs' test. The older term for the antiglobulin test.

critical incident. A problem or any deviation from the standard operating procedures of the blood bank.

Dane particle. The intact, double-shelled hepatitis B virus.

DAT. Direct antiglobulin test.

deglycerolized red blood cells. See frozen blood.

direct antiglobulin test (also called the direct antihuman globulin test.) A test performed to detect the coating of erythrocytes with antibodies.

disseminated intravascular coagulation (DIC). Secondary fibrinolysis in which excessive clotting and fibrinolytic activity occur.

dominant. The gene that is expressed if present.

dosage effect. A variation in strength of agglutination between homozygous and heterozygous erythrocytes. The presence of a homozygous genotype can express itself with more antigen than the heterozygous genotype and can produce a stronger degree of agglutination.

D^u. A phenotype of the Rh blood group system.

D^u rosette test. A procedure that uses D positive indicator erythrocytes to form identifiable rosettes around individual D positive fetal cells that may be in the maternal circulation.

ectopic pregnancy. The gestation of a fertilized egg outside the uterus, most commonly in a fallopian tube.

edema. Accumulation of fluid in the tissues that produces swelling.

EDTA. Tripotassium ethylenediamine tetraacetate. This is a type of anticoagulant that removes calcium (Ca^{++}) through the process of chelation.

eluate. The product of deliberate manipulation of a red cell suspension to break an antigen-antibody complex (elution), with subsequent release of the antibody into the surrounding medium.

endotoxemia. A condition of having bacterial cell wall heat-stable toxins in the circulation. These toxins are pyrogenic and increase capillary permeability.

Epstein-Barr virus (EBV). A human herpes DNA virus that is the causative agent of infectious mononucleosis.

erythrocytes. The scientific term for red blood cells.

erythropoiesis. The process of producing red blood cells.

etiology. A synonym for cause (of a disease or disorder).

exchange transfusion. The replacement of an infant's coated erythrocytes with donor blood until a one or two total blood volume transfer is accomplished.

extramedullary hematopoiesis. Production of erythrocytes outside the bone marrow which can produce enlargement of the liver and spleen.

extravascular hemolysis. The phagocytizing and catabolizing of erythrocytes by the reticuloendothelial system, for example, the spleen.

fab fragments. The two antigen-binding fragments that result from the digestion of an antibody by proteolytic enzymes, e.g., papain.

frozen blood. A term used to refer to red blood cells that are coated with a substance such as, glycerol, frozen to $-80°$ C, and deglycerolized when needed.

genotype. An individual's composite genetic inheritance of maternal and paternal genes. For example, A/O is one the genotypes that a group O person may have.

gestation. The period of development and growth of the unborn in viviparous animals, including humans, from fertilization of the ovum to birth.

glycosphingolipid. A sphingolipid containing the sugar glucose or galactose. Sphingolipids are phospholipids containing sphingosine. Examples are ceramide and cerebrosides.

goodness of fit. The complementary matching of antigenic determinants and the antigen-binding sites of corresponding antibodies that influences the strength of bonding between antigens and antibodies.

graft-versus-host disease. An intense and frequently fatal immunologic reaction of engrafted cells against the host caused by the infusion of immunocompetent lymphocytes into individuals with impaired immunity, such as organ transplantation patients.

granulocyte. A type of leukocytic white blood cell.

haplotype. The gene complex or genetic composition of an individual or population.

hapten. A very small molecule which can bind to a larger carrier molecule and behaves as an antigen.

haptoglobin. A plasma globulin which binds to hemoglobin alpha-beta dimers.

hematoma. A swollen are under the skin or membranes that results from blood collecting underneath. If this area is under the skin, a large bruised area results.

hematopoietic tissues. Blood-producing structures of the body, such as the liver, spleen, and bone marrow.

hemochromatosis. A condition of accumulation of iron in the tissues. This condition is likely to develop in chronically transfused patients.

hemolysis. The rupturing of a cell membrane, for example of an erythrocyte, with subsequent dumping of cytoplasmic contents.

hemolytic disease of the newborn (previously called *Erythroblastosis fetalis*). An immunologic incompatibility between mother and fetus that can produce severe or fatal consequences to the unborn or newborn infant due to destruction of erythrocytes and the accumulation of breakdown products.

hemopexin. A transport protein in the blood circulation.

hemosiderin. An insoluble storage form of iron.

heterozygous. The genetic state of having two dissimilar genes for the same trait.

high protein solution. A medium used in blood banking testing, for example, albumin.

high titer-low avidity (HTLA) antibodies. Antibodies with similar serologic characteristics which have a low antigen binding capacity and a high titration value.

histocompatibility (HLA) antigens. Cell surface protein antigens found on blood and body cells, such as leukocytes and platelets, that readily provoke an immune response if transferred into a genetically different (allogenic) individual of the same species.

HIV. See HTLV III.

homozygous. The genetic state of having two similar genes for the same trait, for example AA or cc.

HTLV III. Human T cell leukemia virus. A type of retrovirus that is also known as LAV or HIV.

hypochromic or hypochromia. A hematologic term used to describe erythrocytes that appear pale when examined microscopically.

hypogammaglobulinemia. A decreased gamma globulin fraction of plasma protein that can lead to errors in blood typing because of weak or missing antibodies.

hypothermia. A decrease in body temperature to below 30° C at the sino-atrial node of the heart that results in ventricular arrhythmias. The rapid infusion of large volumes of refrigerated blood can cause this condition.

hypovolemic shock syndrome. A physiologic condition, such as decreased blood pressure, resulting from the rapid loss of 15 to 20% or more of blood volume.

icterus. A synonym for jaundice or the yellow appearance of the skin and mucous membranes due to bilirubin (a product of red cell breakdown) accumulation.

immunocompetent. The term referring to lymphocytes that acquire thymus-dependent characteristics which allow them to function in an immune response.

immunodominant sugar. The carbohydrate residual that confers antigen specificity to a molecule.

immunogenic. See antigen.

immunoglobulins. A synonym for antibodies.

immunohematology. The study of blood-related antigens and antibodies as applied to situations such as blood transfusion and hemolytic disease of the newborn. Applications of immunohematology are related to blood transfusion therapy.

incompatibility. Agglutination of antigen-bearing erythrocytes and their corresponding antibodies.

intraperitoneal fetal transfusion (IPT). The administration of blood to an unborn infant through the abdominal cavity.

intrauterine. Within the uterus.

intravascular hemolysis. The lysing of erythrocytes within the vessels of the circulatory system.

intrinsic coagulation mechanism. The initial stage of blood coagulation that can be activated by antigen-antibody complexes.

in vitro. Outside the body, for example, in the test tube.

in vivo. In a living organism.

jaundice. See icterus.

kernicterus. The deposition of increased bilirubin, a red cell breakdown product in lipid-rich nervous tissue such as the brain, which can produce mental retardation or death in the newborn. This condition can occur when circulating plasma bilirubin levels reach 20 mg/dL in a full-term infant and at lower levels in a premature infant.

Kleihauer-Betke test. A procedure based on the differences in solubility between adult and fetal hemoglobin. The test is performed on a maternal blood specimen to detect fetal-maternal hemorrhage.

latent infection. Persistent infection characterized by periods of reactivation.

LISS. An antibody enhancement medium, low ionic strength salt solution.

low incidence antigens. Antigens that occur in very few individuals in a population.

massive transfusion. The administration of enough blood or components to constitute a complete volume replacement in 24 hours or less, for example, 8 to 10 or more units in an adult.

microspherocytosis. A hematologic term used to describe the microscopic appearance of smaller than normal, dense-appearing erythrocytes.

monoclonal antibodies. Purified immunoglobulins produced by cells that are cloned from a single fusion-type hybridoma cell.

murine hybridomas. A fusion product of malignant and normal cells which produces large quantities of monoclonal antibodies.

neocytes. Young red blood cells.

neonatologist. A physician specializing in the treatment of disorders of the newborn.

nonsecretor. The absence of water-soluble antigens in body fluids.

oncogenic. Associated with tumor formation.

paroxysmal cold hemoglobinuria (PCH). This form of destruction of erythrocytes is due to an IgG protein that reacts with the red blood cells in colder parts of the body and subsequently causes complement components to bind irreversibly to erythrocytes. It is commonly seen as an acute transient condition secondary to viral infection.

paroxysmal nocturnal hemoglobinura (PNH). A disorder in which the patient's erythrocytes act as a complement activator. The activation of complement results in excessive lysis of the patient's erythrocytes.

pathogenicity. The disease-producing potential of a microorganism.

phenotype. The detectable or expressed characteristics of genes.

phlebotomy. The process of withdrawing blood from the circulatory system. The usual site for the phlebotomy procedure is a vein.

phototherapy. The use of ultraviolet light to accelerate the breakdown of bilirubin that has abnormally accumulated in the skin.

plasma. The straw-colored fluid in circulating or anticoagulated blood.

polyagglutination. Agglutination of erythrocytes by most normal human sera. Examples of polyagglutination include T and Tn activation as well as Cad polyagglutinability.

postpartum. After birth.

post-transfusion viability. The length of survival of blood cells after infusion into the human body, believed to be related to the structural and metabolic status of the cell membrane.

prenatal. Before birth.

primary antibody response. An immunologic (IgM antibody) response following a foreign antigen challenge.

primiparous. Term for a woman who has had at least one pregnancy that resulted in a live infant.

properdin pathway. The former term for the alternate pathway of complement activation.

prophylaxis. Prevention.

prozone phenomenon. A possible cause of false-negative antigen-antibody reactions due to an excessive amount of antibody.

recessive. Term used for a gene which is not expressed unless it is in the homozygous form.

reticulocytosis. A condition in which the number of cells in the normal developmental stage preceding the mature erythrocyte stage is increased.

retrovirus. A type of virus that carries a single, positive-stranded RNA and uses a special enzyme, reverse transcriptase, to convert viral RNA into DNA.

Rh factor. A blood group antigen, named for the Rhesus monkey, originally identified because an antibody agglutinated the erythrocytes of all rhesus monkeys and 85% of humans. The antibody was later discovered to be the Landsteiner-Wiener antibody, which is dissimilar from the Rh antibody; the antigen was actually the Landsteiner-Wiener antigen.

Rh null. The term used for the phenotype in which no Rh antigens are expressed.

rouleaux. Pseudoagglutination or the false clumping of erythrocytes when the cells are suspended in their own serum. This phenomenon resembles agglutination and is due to the presence of an abnormal protein in the serum, plasma expanders such as dextran, or Wharton's jelly from cord blood samples.

secretions. Fluids such as tears, saliva, and semen that may contain water-soluble substances such as A, B, and/or H antigens.

secretor. The presence of water soluble antigens in body fluids.

sepsis. Microbial infection throughout the systemic circulation.

serum. The straw-colored fluid remaining when blood has clotted.

specificity. The complementary relationship between the binding sites of antibodies directed against determinants of a similar-type antigen.

spherocytes. Hematologic term to describe dense-appearing erythrocytes on microscopic examination.

steric hindrance. Mutual blocking of dissimilar antibodies with the same binding constant and directed against antigenic determinants located in close proximity to each other on a cell's surface.

storage lesion. The ATP-independent, irreversible loss of surface area of an erythrocyte stored in anticoagulant.

subclinical infection. An early or mild form of a disease without visible signs.

surface of shear. The outer edge of the ionic cloud surrounding a particle, for example erythrocytes, in an electrolyte solution.

surrogate tests. Tests that nonspecifically detect a condition or disorder. In hepatitis testing, the surrogate tests are the ALT and hepatitis B core antibody tests.

symptom. An indication of a disorder or disease, or a variation in normal body function.

therapeutic phlebotomy. The process of removing venous blood as a treatment for a condition or disorder such as polycythemia vera.

thrombocytopenia. A decrease in the normal number of circulating platelets.

titer. The concentration or strength of an antibody expressed as the highest dilution of the serum that produces agglutination, for example 1:4, 1:8.

transferase enzyme. A type of enzyme that catalyzes the transfer of a monosaccharide molecule from a donor substrate to the precursor substance. This type of biochemical activity is related to the development of A, B, and H antigens.

transplacental hemorrhage. The entrance of fetal blood cells into the maternal circulation.

transposition. The situation of having a gene on one chromosome of a homologous pair affect the actions of a related gene on the other homolog.

type and screen procedure. This technique consists of performing an ABO and Rh typing and an indirect antiglobulin test.

universal blood and body fluid precautions. Specific regulations that conform to current state and Federal requirements. These precautions assume that *all* blood and body fluid specimens have the potential for transmitting disease.

universal donor. A misnomer often used for group O Rh negative blood.

universal recipient. A general term used to refer to a group AB patient.

venous blood. The circulating blood in the veins.

WAIHA. Warm autoimmune hemolytic anemia. This form of autoimmune anemia is associated with antibodies reactive at warm temperatures.

zeta potential. The difference in electrostatic potential between the net charge at the cell membrane and the charge at the surface of shear.

Index

Page numbers in italics refer to figures. Page numbers followed by the letter "t" refer to tables.